# *Brahma Yoga*
# *Bhagavad Gītā*

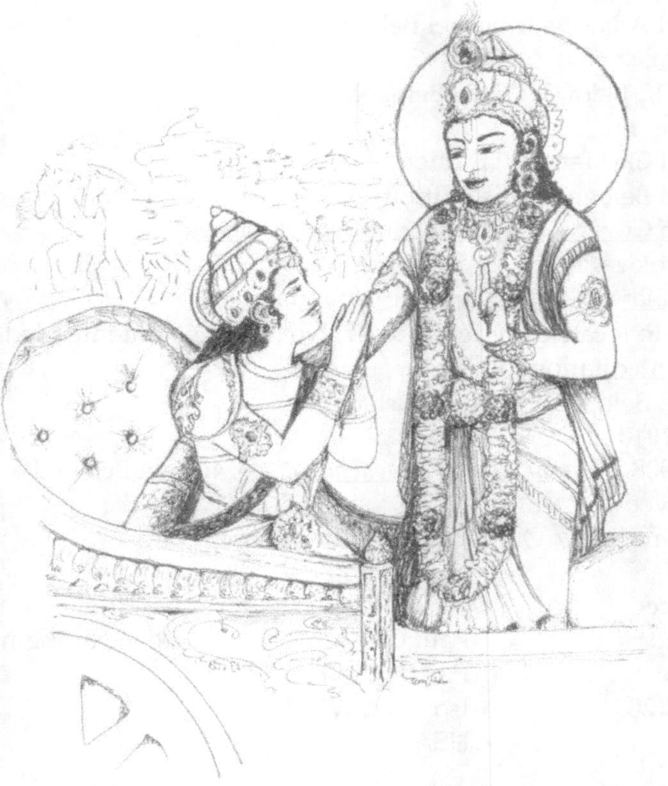

Michael Beloved/ Yogi Madhvācārya

Original Sanskrit text:

- Chapters 23 - 40 Bhishma Parva, *Mahābhārata*--granted and permitted by John Smith-University of Cambridge, Bhandarkar Oriental Research Institute.

Numbered, four-lined, formatted Sanskrit:

- Marcia & Michael Beloved (April 2008)

Devanagari script:

- Sanskrit 2003 Font

Transliteration:

- URW Palladio ITU font/ ITranslator

Word-for-Word typeset:

- Bernard Adjodha/Michael Beloved

Format assistants:

- Marcia K. Beloved/Dear Beloved

Cover Design:

- Sir Paul Castagna (1st.Edition)
- Michael Beloved (This Edition)

Universal Form Cover Art, Śrī Śrī Arjuna-Krishna Art:

- Terri Stokes-Pineda

Śrī Gopāl Krishna - Siddha Swami Nityānanda Photo:

- Unable to locate copyright holder. No infringement intended

Illustrations of meditation focus:

- Michael Beloved/Sir Paul Castagna

**2nd Edition --- 2010**



**Correspondence**
Michael Beloved
3703 Foster Ave
Brooklyn NY 11203
USA

Paul Castagna
P.O.Box 150
Iron Belt WI 54536
USA

**Email**
axisnexus@gmail.com

**ISBN**

**9780979391651**

**LCCN**

**2008906545**

# Brahma Yoga
# Bhagavad Gītā

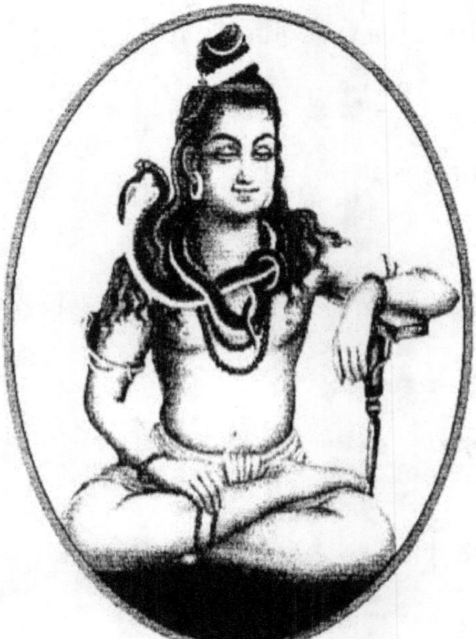

# Scheme of Pronunciation

## Consonants

| | | | | | |
|---|---|---|---|---|---|
| Gutturals: | क | ख | ग | घ | ङ |
| | ka | kha | ga | gha | ṅa |
| Palatals: | च | छ | ज | झ | ञ |
| | ca | cha | ja | jha | ña |
| Cerebrals: | ट | ठ | ड | ढ | ण |
| | ṭa | ṭha | ḍa | ḍha | ṇa |
| Dentals: | त | थ | द | ध | न |
| | ta | tha | da | dha | na |
| Labials: | प | फ | ब | भ | म |
| | pa | pha | ba | bha | ma |

**Semivowels:**

| | | | |
|---|---|---|---|
| य | र | ल | व |
| ya | ra | la | va |

**Numbers:**

० १ २ ३ ४ ५ ६ ७ ८ ९

0 1 2 3 4 5 6 7 8 9

**Sibilants:**

| | | |
|---|---|---|
| श | ष | स |
| śa | ṣa | sa |

**Aspirate:** ह ha

**Vowels:**

| | | | | | | | |
|---|---|---|---|---|---|---|---|
| अ | आ | इ | ई | उ | ऊ | ऋ | ॠ |
| a | ā | i | ī | u | ū | ṛ | ṝ |
| ए | औ | ओ | औ | ऌ | ॡ | < | : |
| e | ai | o | au | lṛ | lṝ | ṁ | ḥ |

**Apostrophe** ऽ

# Table of Contents

*Scheme of Pronunciation* .................................... 4

**How to use this book:** .................................... 8

**A note on the diacritical marks and pronounciation:** .................................... 8

*Introduction* .................................... 9

***CHAPTER 1*** .................................... *11*

***Śoka Samvigna Mānasah*** .................................... *11*

***Arjuna's Depression**** .................................... *11*

***CHAPTER 2*** .................................... *45*

***Buddhi Yoga*** .................................... *45*

***Intellectual Discipline through Yoga**** .................................... *45*

***CHAPTER 3*** .................................... *100*

***Karma Yogam*** .................................... *100*

***Regulating Work through Yoga Practice**** .................................... *100*

***CHAPTER 4*** .................................... *135*

***Bahuvidhā Yajñā*** .................................... *135*

***Disciplines of Accomplishment**** .................................... *135*

***CHAPTER 5*** .................................... *168*

***Brahma Yoga Yukta Ātmā*** .................................... *168*

***Linking the Spirit to the Spiritual Plane through Yoga**** .................................... *168*

***CHAPTER 6*** .................................... *189*

***Yogam Ātma Viśuddhaye*** .................................... *189*

***Purity of the Psyche Yoga **** .................................... *189*

***Special Notation:*** .................................... *224*

***CHAPTER 7*** .................................... *225*

*Vijñānam* ........ 225
*The Experience** ........ 225
*CHAPTER 8* ........ 245
*Paramam Puruṣam Divyam* ........ 245
*The Divine Supreme Person** ........ 245
*CHAPTER 9* ........ 264
*Bhaktyā* ........ 264
*The Devotional Attitude** ........ 264
*CHAPTER 10* ........ 286
*Tejah Amśa Sambhavam* ........ 286
*A Fraction of Krishna's Splendor** ........ 286
*CHAPTER 11* ........ 307
*Paramam Rūpam Aiśvaram* ........ 307
*The Supreme Form* ........ 307
*The Supernatural Glory** ........ 307
*CHAPTER 12* ........ 339
*Mad Yogam Āśritah* ........ 339
*Resorting to Krishna's Yoga Process ** ........ 339
*CHAPTER 13* ........ 354
*Anādimat Param Brahma* ........ 354
*The Beginningless Supreme Reality ** ........ 354
*CHAPTER 14* ........ 377
*Guṇāh Prakṛti Sambhavāh* ........ 377
*The Influences Produced of Material Nature ** ........ 377
*CHAPTER 15* ........ 397
*Dvau Imau Puruṣau* ........ 397
*Types of Spirits** ........ 397

*CHAPTER 16* ........ *409*

*Dvau Bhūta Sargau* ........ *409*

*Types of Created Beings** ........ *409*

*CHAPTER 17* ........ *431*

*Trividhā Bhavati Śraddhā* ........ *431*

*Three Types of Confidences** ........ *431*

*CHAPTER 18* ........ *450*

*Sarva Guhyatamam* ........ *450*

*The Most Secret of All Information** ........ *450*

*Concluding Remarks* ........ *491*

*Regarding the English Translation* ........ *491*

*Indexed Names of Arjuna* ........ *492*

*Indexed Names of Krishna* ........ *493*

*Names, Places and Things* ........ *496*

*Index To Verses: Selected Sanskrit Words* ........ *497*

*Index to Translation* ........ *505*

*LIST OF TEACHERS* ........ *537*

*About the Author* ........ *537*

*Publications* ........ *539*

English Series ........ 539

Meditation Series ........ 541

Explained Series ........ 542

Commentaries ........ 543

Specialty ........ 546

*Online Resources* ........ *547*

**How to use this book:**

*Make a casual reading of the entire text.*

*Make a second reading taking note of specific interests.*

*Make a third reading checking carefully for realisations and applications.*

*Finally, make an indepth study for integrating Bhagavad Gītā into your life.*

**A note on the diacritical marks and pronounciation:**

*Names like Krishna and Arjuna are accepted in common English usage. Their English spellings occur in the translation without diacritical marks.*

*There is a sanskrit lettering guide on page 4.*

***Here are some hints** on how to use the diacritical marks for near-exact pronunciation:*

*Letters with a **dot** below them, should be pronounced while the tongue touches and is released curling slightly at the top of palate.*

*The s sound for **ś** carries an h with it and is said as the **sh** sound in **she**.*

*The s sound for **ṣ** carries an h with it and is said as the **sh** sound in **shun**.*

*The h sound for **ḥ** carries an echoing sound of the vowel before it, such that **oḥ** is actually **oho** and **aḥ** is actually **aha**.*

*In many Sanskrit words the **y** sound is said as an **i** sound, especially when the y sound preceeds an a. For instance, prāṇāyāma should be praa-**nai**-aa-muh, rather than praa-naa-**yaa**-muh.*

*The **a** sound is more like **uh** in English, while the **ā** sound is like the a sound in **far**.*

*The **ṛ** sound is like the **ri** sound in **ridge**.*

*The **ph** sound is never reduced to an f sound as in English. The **p sound** is maintained.*

*Whenever **h** occurs after a consonant, its integrity is maintained as an air forced sound.*

*If the h sound occurs after a vowel and a consonant, one should let the consonant remain with the vowel which preceeds it and allow the h sound to carry with the vowel after it, such that Duryodhana is pronounced with the d consonant allied to the o before it and the h sound manages the a after it.Say Dur-**yod-ha**-na or Dur-**yod-han**. Do not say Dur-yo-**dha**-na. Separate the d and h sounds to make them distinct. In words where you have no choice and must combine the d and h sound, as in the word dharma. Make sure that the **h sound** is heard as an **air sound pushed out from the throat**. Dharma should never be mistaken for darma. But adharma should be **ad-har**-ma.*

*The **c** sound is **ch,** and the **ch** sound is **ch-h**.*

# Introduction

During a short stay in England, in September of 2004, I was requested by *Mahāsiddha* Swami *Nityānānda* to write this commentary on *Bhagavad Gītā*. To date I wrote two commentaries. The first, *Bhagavad Gītā Explained*, shed light on some distortions of commentators which became standardized in the process of time. The second, *Kriyā Yoga Bhagavad Gītā*, showed the *kriyā yoga* techniques which were revealed by *Śrī* Krishna to Arjuna. That second commentary was inspired by *Śrī Bābāji Mahāśaya* after he introduced me into the use of the critical energy. The first commentary was inspired by Lord Baladeva (*Śrī Balarāma*), for clarifying the distortions which entered into many spiritual lineages over time, and which since their entry became standard teachings.

This third commentary, which I hope will be my last, was inspired by one of my *brahma yoga* teachers to reveal some of the techniques of that process and to show that the basis for these lies in the *Bhagavad Gītā*.

*Brahma yoga* is built up on a foundation which is the stoppage of the automatic functions of the appropriation energy in the psyche. That energy is then diverted to or made to adhere itself to the naad subtle sound which is usually heard in the right subtle ear on the inside of the head of the subtle body. If the appropriation energy is not controlled, one cannot proceed in a systematic and sure way with *brahma yoga*.

A question arises as to what exactly is the nature and usage of the appropriation energy. And hopefully that will be answered in this commentary. Readers should assume that most of this work was dictated to me by *Mahāsiddha* Swami *Nityānānda*.

On October 14th, 2004, the day before I began this commentary, the *Mahāsiddha* was sitting with some of his disciples in the astral world. At the time some orthodox Hindus who successfully performed *agnihotra* fire sacrifices in this world in their last human forms, passed by in the sky. They were radiant with light energy and wore shining garments made of light. They were paired with spouses and were joyfully moving through the sky in celestial chariots. Looking down on the Siddha and his disciples, they pitied us. I was amazed but I felt sorry for the whole group who were heading for the Swarga heavenly world. At the time, Siddha Swami saw them. All of a sudden as if to call them, he waved and said:

"O fools! O fools! Why pity us? You are the ones who are lost, who are on the wrong path. What will you gain by going to the Swarga heavens? Why not come and join us in the venture to find the blue pearl? All other aims are futile."

Then he laughed, "Ha Ha Ha!" His laughter shook the sky and the chariots of those celestial people jerked erratically. However they continued on their journey, bewildered at the statement made by the almost-naked siddha.

***Regarding the exhaustive Indexes:***

*All entries* ***except*** *those for the Commentary give reference to verse numbers. The last Index which is to the Commentary is the only one which refers to page numbers.*

*Śrī Gopāl Krishna*

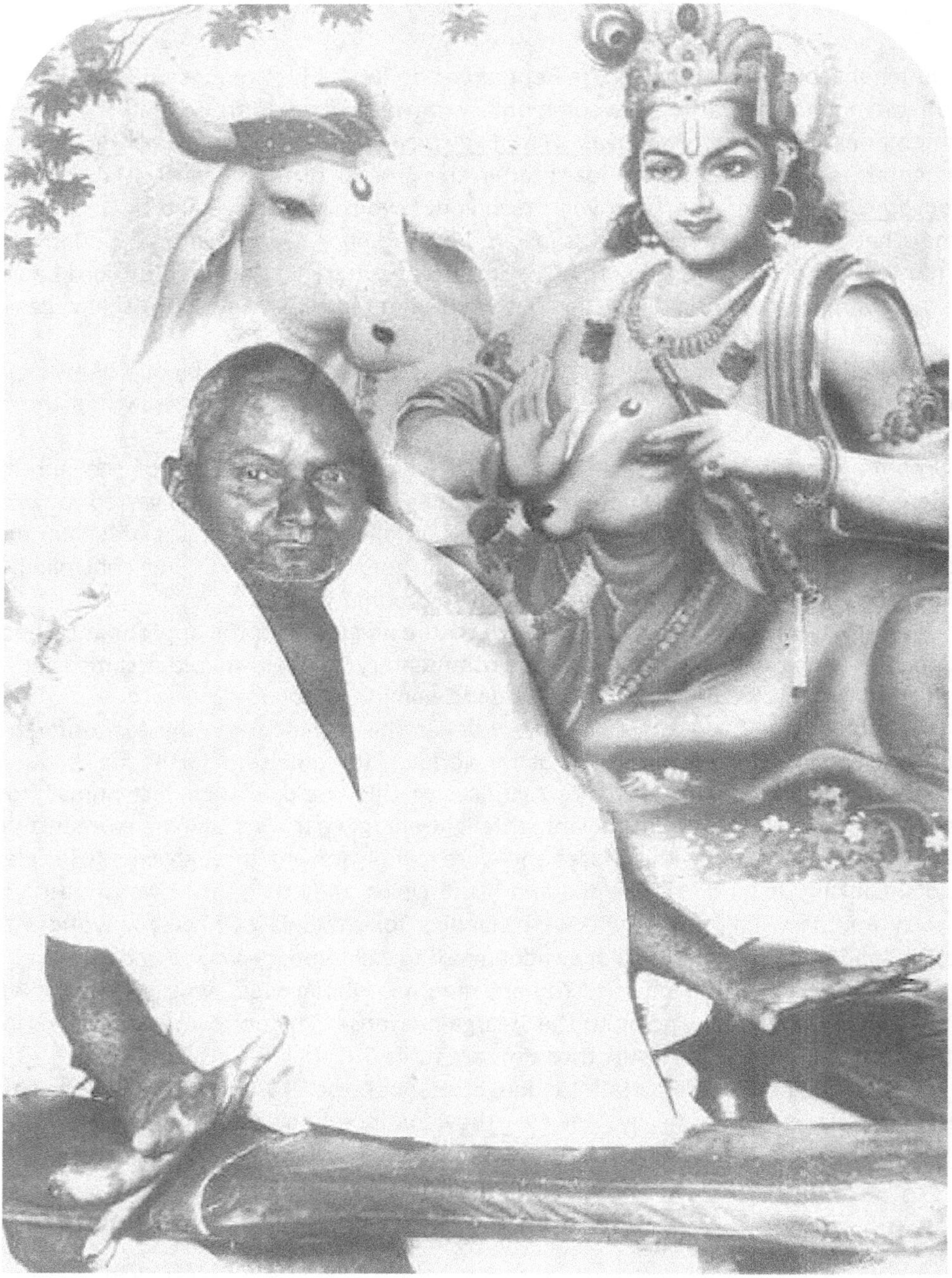

*Siddha Swami Nityānānda*

# CHAPTER 1

## Śoka Samvigna Mānasah

## Arjuna's Depression*

*evamuktvārjunaḥ saṁkhye rathopastha upāviśat*
*visṛjya saśaraṁ cāpaṁ śokasaṁvignamānasaḥ (1.46)*

***Having spoken, Arjuna, who was in the midst of the conflict, sat down on his chariot. Casting aside his arrow and bow, he was overwhelmed with sorrow. (1.46)***

***Siddha Swami assigned this chapter title on the basis of verse 46 of this chapter.**

धृतराष्ट्र उवाच
धर्मक्षेत्रे कुरुक्षेत्रे
समवेता युयुत्सवः ।
मामकाः पाण्डवाश्चैव
किमकुर्वत संजय ॥ १.१ ॥
dhṛtarāṣṭra uvāca
dharmakṣetre kurukṣetre
samavetā yuyutsavaḥ
māmakāḥ pāṇḍavāścaiva
kimakurvata saṁjaya (1.1)

*dhṛtarāṣṭra – Dhṛtarāṣṭra; uvāca — said; dharmakṣetre — at the place for settling political affairs; kurukṣetre — at Kurukṣetra, a small plain in Punjab, India; samavetā — meeting together; yuyutsavaḥ — being possessed with battle spirit; māmakāḥ — my sons; pāṇḍavāś — the sons of Pāndu; caiva — and indeed; kim — what; akurvata — did so; saṁjaya — Sanjaya*

**Dhṛtarāṣṭra said: O Sanjaya, being possessed with battle spirit and meeting together, what did my sons and the sons of Pāndu do at Kurukṣetra, the place for settling political affairs? (1.1)**

***Author's Commentary:***

Dhṛtarāṣṭra was physically blind. This is why he relied on Sanjaya to give him this news. For *brahma yoga*, a requirement is physical blindness but it must be voluntarily imposed. Thus *Dhṛtarāṣṭra*, who became blind because of the attitude of his mother during conception, was disqualified from the course of *brahma yoga*. All the senses and their attunement to this world must cease for success in *brahma yoga*. Thus if one can voluntarily become blind, physically insensitive, deaf, lose the sense of taste and lose the sense of smelling, one could, if properly directed by a *Mahāsiddha*, become a practicing *brahma* yogi over-night.

*Dhṛtarāṣṭra* did not qualify because he yearned for the physical vision. That yearning is itself a disqualification. It means that the self is allied with forces in the psyche which are habituated to appropriation, to seizing and stealing various aspects of reality. *Dhṛtarāṣṭra* was impelled by such forces to steal whatever information he could cull from Sanjaya. In *brahma yoga* one has to stop the psyche from executing such theft.

*Kurukṣetra*, the physical place in India, is like other places on this earth, where creatures meet to settle political affairs, either those of the family or of the state. And in all such cases, the appropriation or grand theft of the properties takes place. Possessed with a battle spirit and meeting together, we usually act out circumstances in order to lift off impressions which we enjoy mentally, using the faculty of imagination and the camera-recorder mechanism of memory. We usually perpetrate acts of grand larceny, bold theft. And that is the sum and substance of our mundane existence.

*Dhṛtarāṣṭra* was deprived of a full life because the body he received was blind. Thus he was even more eager to perpetrate the grand theft but he had to take help from Sanjaya who was a more able and fit camera man and recording expert. Whatever Sanjaya would steal, might be procured by *Dhṛtarāṣṭra* for a price. And Sanjaya's price was for *Dhṛtarāṣṭra* to bear with insults from time to time. *Dhṛtarāṣṭra* was forced to take selected merchandise which Sanjaya carefully presented to him, leaving out other details of other circumstances on the battlefield. But what could *Dhṛtarāṣṭra* do? After all, his physical body was blind and Sanjaya was placed before him by providence, as a secretary and eye piece.

संजय उवाच
दृष्ट्वा तु पाण्डवानीकं
व्यूढं दुर्योधनस्तदा ।
आचार्यमुपसंगम्य
राजा वचनमब्रवीत् ॥ १.२ ॥
saṁjaya uvāca
dṛṣṭvā tu pāṇḍavānīkaṁ
vyūḍhaṁ duryodhanastadā
ācāryamupasaṁgamya
rājā vacanamabravīt (1.2)

*saṁjaya uvāca — Sanjaya said; dṛṣṭvā — after observing; tu — indeed; pāṇḍavānīkaṁ — Pandava army; vyūḍhaṁ — which was set in battle formation; duryodhanas — Duryodhana, the eldest son of Dhṛtarāṣṭra, the crown prince of the Kurus; tadā — at that time; ācāryam — military teacher; upasaṁgamya — approaching; rājā — crown prince; vacanam — remark; abravīt — said*

**Sanjaya said: Indeed, after observing the Pandava army which was set in a battle formation, the Crown Prince Duryodhana, while approaching the Military Teacher, said this remark: (1.2)**

***Author's Commentary:***

This begins the report of Sanjaya, a discourse which King *Dhṛtarāṣṭra* relied on, and to which his nature responded in favorable, unfavorable and indifferent ways. Accurate conceptions formed and so did inaccurate ones. *Dhṛtarāṣṭra*'s nature responded on the basis of prejudices which were formed in many lives transmigrating in material forms. The Crown Prince Duryodhana was his son, and seeing the Pandavas army posing before them, the Prince decided to consult with his military teacher about the formations.

The problem with such episodes is this: One has to rely on one's own mind as well as on the minds of others. All these minds are prone to mistakes. Thus despite all precautions one is prone to error. Such are the probabilities. In *brahma yoga*, the whole idea of any material involvement is scrapped. It is because the mind is bound to make mistakes. That is the nature of it. There are always a group of good people, pious folk. And there will always be a group of bad fellows. Both groups are equipped with imperfect minds, which make miscalculations from time to time. Thus the only solution is to scrap such a mind. And that is one of the purposes of *brahma yoga*.

पश्यैतां पाण्डुपुत्राणाम्
आचार्य महतीं चमूम् ।
व्यूढां द्रुपदपुत्रेण
तव शिष्येण धीमता ॥ १.३ ॥
paśyaitāṁ pāṇḍuputrāṇām
ācārya mahatīṁ camūm
vyūḍhāṁ drupadaputreṇa
tava śiṣyeṇa dhīmatā (1.3)

*paśyaitāṁ — see this; pāṇḍuputrāṇām — of the sons of Pāndu; ācārya — sir; mahatīm — great; camūm — army; vyūḍhāṁ — which is set for combat; drupada putreṇa — by the son of Drupada; tava — your; śiṣyeṇa — by a student; dhīmatā — by perceptive*

**Sir, see this great army of the sons of Pāndu, which is set for combat by your perceptive student, the son of Drupada. (1.3)**

***Author's Commentary:***

In *kriyā yoga* which is the stage just below the last progression which is *brahma yoga*, one learns how to use the critical energy in the psyche for constructively criticizing the self. Instead of criticizing a teacher, one learns how to use the valuable critical force to locate and rectify faults in the psyche.

One learns both in *kriyā yoga* and in *brahma yoga* how not to hold resentments, since these do inflict self harm and hamper spiritual development. It is not worth it to hurt another person verbally, if it means that by doing so one would have hurt oneself to greater degree.

Thus, if indeed the military teacher of Prince Duryodhana had trained the son of *Drupada*, and had not foreseen that the student would fight against the teacher, then Duryodhana if he was versed in *kriyā yoga* or *brahma yoga*, would not have mentioned it. He would have overlooked it, or would have concluded silently, that it was a stroke of providence. A limited being is subordinate to providence, such that providence may not reveal the ulterior motives of every student. Providence has that power. All teachers should be accepting to that and should not be irritated when providence contravenes. Even if providence makes a fool out of someone, that person should not bear a grudge. The idea is: Providence knows best.

अत्र शूरा महेष्वासा
भीमार्जुनसमा युधि ।
युयुधानो विराटश्च
द्रुपदश्च महारथः ॥१.४॥
atra śūrā maheṣvāsā
bhīmārjunasamā yudhi
yuyudhāno virāṭaśca
drupadaśca mahārathaḥ (1.4)

*atra — here; śūrā — heroes; maheṣvāsā — great bow men; bhīmārjunasamā — equal to Bhīma and Arjuna; yudhi — in battle; yuyudhāno — Yuyudhāna; virāṭaś — Virāṭa; ca — and; drupadaś — Drupada; ca — and; mahārathaḥ — the great chariot fighter*

**Here are heroes, great bowmen, who are equal in battle to Bhīma and Arjuna. There is Yuyudhāna, Virāṭa, and Drupada, the great chariot fighter. (1.4)**

***Author's Commentary:***

Duryodhana was opposed on that war field by his cousins, the Pandavas. He was impressed with their army which is described as being great (*mahatīṁ*, verse 3). Even though they were dispossessed of the Kuru legacy of rulership, still these cousins of his, managed to acquire able allies and raise a formidable army.

Duryodhana, by impulsion within his mind and emotions, took note of the leading figures who opposed him on that war field. *Bhīma* and Arjuna are two of the five Pandavas. *Yuyudhāna*, *Virāṭa* and *Drupada* were their allies. In *brahma yoga*, the habit of taking note of nearly everything we encounter is greatly curtailed. This is because such note-taking is full of psychological hazards. Such note-taking is a source of on-going emotional stress.

धृष्टकेतुश्चेकितानः
काशिराजश्च वीर्यवान् ।
पुरुजित्कुन्तिभोजश्च
शैब्यश्च नरपुंगवः ॥१.५॥

*dhṛṣṭaketuś — Dhṛṣṭaketu; cekitānaḥ — Cekitāna; kāśirājaś — the king of Kāśi; ca — and; vīryavān — valiant man; purujit — Purujit; kuntibhojaś — Kuntibhoja; ca — and; śaibyaś — Śaibya; ca — and;*

dhṛṣṭaketuścekitānaḥ
kāśirājaśca vīryavān
purujitkuntibhojaśca
śaibyaśca narapuṁgavaḥ (1.5)

*narapuṅgavaḥ — bull among men*

**There is Dhṛṣṭaketu, Cekitāna, and the Kāśi ruler, that valiant man. There is Purujit and Kuntibhoja and Śaibya, the bull-bodied man. (1.5)**

***Author's Commentary:***

So long as one is carrying on the material existence, such details in the struggle for existence are important, for one must assess situations as one proceeds in any dimension. However, when the time comes to depart from the material existence in a meaningful way, one must take to *brahma yoga*, an area in which such painstaking observations have little or no meaning. Whatever was important in the country of his birth becomes very insignificant to one who leaves for a foreign country. He has to orient himself to a new territory or sociology, and so it is with higher yoga.

As far as their political attainments and martial skills were concerned, *Dhṛṣṭaketu, Cekitāna*, the *Kāśi* king, *Purujit, Kuntibhoja* and *Śaibya* were of value to the Pandavas. They were a threat to Duryodhana. In terms of *brahma yoga* those persons were very irrelevant, because they were focused into the material existence, in the old territories, which the *brahma yogi*s abandoned or were about to relinquish.

King *Dhṛtarāṣṭra* is tormented by what he heard from Sanjaya, the reporter of the battle details. This inner harassment administered to the self by the mental and emotional energies of the very same self, comes to an end when one masters the techniques of *brahma yoga*, which are mystic procedures described in this commentary.

युधामन्युश्च विक्रान्त
उत्तमौजाश्च वीर्यवान् ।
सौभद्रो द्रौपदेयाश्च
सर्व एव महारथाः ॥ १.६ ॥
yudhāmanyuśca vikrānta
uttamaujāśca vīryavān
saubhadro draupadeyāśca
sarva eva mahārathāḥ (1.6)

*yudhāmanyuś — Yudhāmanyu; ca — and; vikrānta — valiant; uttamaujāś — Uttamauja; ca — and; vīryavān — heroic; saubhadro — the son of Subhadra; drāupadeyāś — the sons of Draupadī; ca — and; sarve — all; eva — indeed; mahārathāḥ — champions of chariot warfare*

**There is the valiant Yudhāmanyu and the heroic Uttamauja. There are the son of Subhadra and the sons of Draupadī, who indeed, are all champions of chariot warfare. (1.6)**

***Author's Commentary:***

*Brahma yoga* means to turn away from the social advantages and disadvantages. Thus a *brahma yogi* would not be ranging over objects to determine their value for usage in political conquest. Duryodhana would have preferred that *Yudhāmanyu, Uttamauja* and the sons of *Subhadra* and *Draupadī*, be loyal to him in one unified government for the peaceful rulership of society by his view. And thus he strained himself psychologically when he made this assessment, seeing that these champions of chariot warfare joined his opponents, who were his cousins and who refused to subordinate themselves to him.

However to a *brahma yogi*, all this is irrelevant, for the conquest must occur within the nature of the yogi. It is a war on the psychological plane, if any, between his core self and his psychological machinery.

अस्माकं तु विशिष्टा ये
तान्निबोध द्विजोत्तम ।
नायका मम सैन्यस्य
संज्ञार्थं तान्ब्रवीमि ते ॥१.७॥
asmākaṁ tu viśiṣṭā ye
tānnibodha dvijottama
nāyakā mama sainyasya
saṁjñārthaṁ tānbravīmi te (1.7)

*asmākaṁ — our men; tu — but; viśiṣṭā — distinguished; ye — who; tān — them; nibodha — be informed; dvijottama — O best of the initiates; nāyakā — commanders; mama — of my; sainyasya — of the army; saṁjñārthaṁ — for the sake of giving information; tān — them; bravīmi — I mention; te — to you*

**But, O best of the initiates, be informed of our men who are distinguished. For the sake of giving information to you, I mention the leaders of my army. (1.7)**

***Author's Commentary:***

In his time, *Droṇa*, the military teacher of Duryodhana was in fact the best of the initiates, in both spiritual and material development. Despite his skill *Droṇa* was a poor man, made so by destiny. Hence *Droṇa*, that greatly learned person, had to take a job from Duryodhana as commander of the Prince's army. *Droṇa* had to compromise his values. He had to be humble to a haughty ruler like Duryodhana. He had to keep his mouth shut on occasion even when he knew for certain that Duryodhana was vicious and irresponsible.

Getting initiated into material and spiritual skills does not protect a person from making mistakes. The only protection we can have is perfect character, but such a trait eludes us repeatedly. In *kriyā yoga*, we work on creating for ourselves such perfect character. It is a spiritual skill.

The assessments made by Prince Duryodhana were done to calculate his chances of winning battle. His opponents, the Pandavas, had a sizeable army comprising of some skillful soldiers. What was Duryodhana to do? Since he was not conversant with *brahma yoga*, he could not divert his mind from the external world, and therefore his internal situation remained impulsive and uncontrolled.

भवान्भीष्मश्च कर्णश्च
कृपश्च समितिंजयः ।
अश्वत्थामा विकर्णश्च
सौमदत्तिस्तथैव च ॥१.८॥
bhavānbhīṣmaśca karṇaśca
kṛpaśca samitiṁjayaḥ
aśvatthāmā vikarṇaśca
saumadattistathaiva ca (1.8)

*bhavān — your qualified self; bhīṣmaś — Bhishma; ca — and; karṇaśca — Karṇa; kṛpaś — Krpa; ca — and; samitiṁjayaḥ — victorious in battle; aśvatthāmā — Aśvatthāmā; vikarṇaś — Vikarṇa; ca — and; saumadattis — the son of Somadatta; tathaiva — as well; ca — and*

**There is your qualified self, and Bhishma, Karṇa and Krpa who are victorious in battle. There is also Aśvatthāmā, Vikarṇa and the son of Somadatta. (1.8)**

***Author,s Commentary:***

In contrast to Duryodhana, a *brahma yogi* must also make assessments about the energies and mechanisms within his subtle nature, within his mind compartment and his emotional reach. Duryodhana listed his assistants such as the qualified teacher, *Droṇa*, the eldest of the generals, his great uncle Bhishma, the marksman, his friend, *Karṇa*, *Droṇa's* son, the skilled and capable *Aśvatthāmā*, and others like the notable *Vikarṇa* and the son of Somadatta. These people were well known in their own time. Their histories are enumerated in the *Mahābhārata* literature.

But for *brahma yogi*s who left aside or who are leaving aside the gross material existence, to go into the more substantial realms of the mind and emotions, which persons and what forces are allies and which are opponents?

Which person can a yogi rely on to be his military commander in the conquest of his own nature? And should he insult that person from time to time, when he discovers that such a teacher made a decision which compromises victory over the psyche? Which grandfather or great uncle would advise a *yogin* on how to proceed in political dominance within the psyche? Which friend like *Karṇa* can be relied on to help in the battle between the core self and the emotions? Are there non-personal forces involved in this battle, just as there are weapons, chariots and locations involved in a physical war? Should a truce be declared? Should the yogi adopt a non-violent stance in the hope of pressuring the unruly forces in his nature to give up their aggressive postures?

अन्ये च बहवः शूरा
मदर्थे त्यक्तजीविताः ।
नानाशस्त्रप्रहरणाः
सर्वे युद्धविशारदाः ॥१.९॥
anye ca bahavaḥ śūrā
madarthe tyaktajīvitāḥ
nānāśastrapraharaṇāḥ
sarve yuddhaviśāradāḥ (1.9)

*anye — other; ca — and; bahavaḥ — many; śūrā — heroes; madarthe — for my sake; tyakta jīvitāḥ — would give their lives; nānā śastra praharaṇāḥ — wielding various weapons; sarve — all; yuddha viśāradāḥ — being experts in warfare*

**And many other heroes wielding various weapons, being experts in warfare, would give their lives for my sake. (1.9)**

***Author's Commentary:***

There are certainly persons who would support a man, no matter what, no matter if he was right or wrong. But what part of his mind or emotions would support him when he was morally-inclined? Which part would give him great impetus of energy when he was immorally determined? Would a *yogin*'s mind give full support in the effort to eliminate vices? Would his emotions even tolerate it, if the *yogin* became determined to avoid social contacts? What weapons do the mind and emotions wield? And are these energies assisted by any other types of subtle energies? Is the mind just one singular unit or is it comprised of parts? What is the relationship between the mind and the emotions? Do the emotions work hand-in-hand in a joint enterprise to cajole and intimidate the core self? Would there be a sharp divide, a psychological conflict of sorts, if the core self decided that it no longer wanted to have a give and take relationship with the mind and emotions?

अपर्याप्तं तदस्माकं
बलं भीष्माभिरक्षितम् ।
पर्याप्तं त्विदमेतेषां
बलं भीमाभिरक्षितम् ॥१.१०॥

*aparyāptaṁ — inadequate; tad — this; asmākaṁ — of ours; balaṁ — military force; bhīṣmābhi rakṣitam — supervised by Bhishma; paryāptaṁ — sufficient; tvidam = tu — however + idam — this; eteṣām — of*

aparyāptaṁ tadasmākaṁ
balaṁ bhīṣmābhirakṣitam
paryāptaṁ tvidameteṣāṁ
balaṁ bhīmābhirakṣitam (1.10)

*these; balam — military power; bhīmābhirakṣitam — protected by Bhīma*

**Inadequate is this military force of ours which is supervised by Bhishma. Sufficient, however, is their military power which is protected by Bhīma. (1.10)**

***Author's Commentary:***

Duryodhana ascertained that the Pandavas, his opponents, had sufficient soldiers to combat him effectively. He could see that he would have to fight for victory. It would not be easy to dispose of the Pandavas, his rivals for political power. Their army which was protected by his cousin *Bhīma*, was adequate for a counter-offensive against him while his own force seemed to be inadequate for a crushing victory or an effective show of military intimidation. What could he do, now that a battle seemed inevitable and there would certainly be casualities? And what should a *yogin* do after he turns away from the material world and then finds that he must fight a battle within his nature, one that he might not easily win.

अयनेषु च सर्वेषु
यथाभागमवस्थिताः।
भीष्ममेवाभिरक्षन्तु
भवन्तः सर्व एव हि ॥१.११॥
ayaneṣu ca sarveṣu
yathābhāgamavasthitāḥ
bhīṣmamevābhirakṣantu
bhavantaḥ sarva eva hi (1.11)

*ayaneṣu — in maneuvers; ca — and; sarveṣu — in all; yathā bhāgam — as by assignment; avasthitāḥ — positioned; bhīṣmam — Bhishma; evābhirakṣantu — definitely protect; bhavantaḥ — your honorable master; sarve — all; eva – indeed; hi — certainly*

**And in all maneuvers, as positioned by assignment, all your honorable masters should definitely protect Bhishma. (1.11)**

***Author's Commentary:***

Bhishma, the great uncle of Duryodhana and of the Pandavas, was the representative of tradition, being the eldest of soldiers on the battlefield. Due to his social experience, he was worthy of the protection requested by Duryodhana. If his body died, the Kauravas would lose the one man who was a treasury of advice.

In the field of *brahma yoga*, a person as old as Bhishma has value in two ways. If he is experienced in the higher yoga, his opinions about practice and his experiences during practice are taken seriously. If he made contributions to the moral order of society, to *dharma*, he is appreciated for protecting and fostering humanity.

Duryodhana's interest in Bhishma was one of appreciation for the elder's contribution to the society as well as his military and political expertise.

***Siddha Swami's Commentary:***

As in all maneuvers within the mind and emotions, as the subtle organs are positioned in their particular places, all the senses should act in such a way as to protect the *buddhi* organ. Even the effeminate emotions should take steps to facilitate the *buddhi* organ and that organ in turn, should only function for the spiritual welfare of the soul.

तस्य संजनयन्हर्षं
कुरुवृद्धः पितामहः ।
सिंहनादं विनद्योच्चैः
शङ्खं दध्मौ प्रतापवान् ॥ १.१२ ॥
tasya saṁjanayanharṣaṁ
kuruvṛddhaḥ pitāmahaḥ
siṁhanādaṁ vinadyoccaiḥ
śaṅkhaṁ dadhmau pratāpavān (1.12)

*tasya — of him (Duryodhana); saṁjanayan — producing; harṣaṁ — happiness; kuruvṛddhaḥ — the eldest Kuru; pitāmahaḥ — the grandfather; siṁha nādaṁ — a lion—like roar; vinadyo ccaiḥ — sounding a loud; śaṅkhaṁ — conchshell; dadhmau — blew; pratāpavān — voluminously*

**The eldest Kuru, the grandfather, voluminously blew his conchshell, sounding a loud lion-like roar, thus producing great happiness for Duryodhana. (1.12)**

***Author's Commentary:***

Duryodhana acted like the lusty emotions, which when they are facilitated by providence, expand immensely within the psyche and produce a type of happiness. For this to happen, the intellect and the sense of identity, the initiative, must give their approval to some plan or idea of the emotions. When the lusty emotions get the intellect and the sense of identity to be in agreement, a joy is felt within the psyche.

ततः शङ्खाश्च भेर्यश्च
पणवानकगोमुखाः ।
सहसैवाभ्यहन्यन्त
स शब्दस्तुमुलोऽभवत् ॥ १.१३ ॥
tataḥ śaṅkhāśca bheryaśca
paṇavānakagomukhāḥ
sahasaivābhyahanyanta
sa śabdastumulo'bhavat (1.13)

*tataḥ — then; śaṅkhāś— conches; ca — and; bheryaś — kettledrums; ca — and; paṇavānaka gomukhāḥ — cymbals, drums and trumpets; sahasaivā—bhyahanyanta = sahasā — simultaneously + eva — indeed + abhyahanyanta — were sounded; sa — that; śabdas — sound; tumulo — tumultuous; 'bhavat (abhavat) — was*

**And then the conches and kettledrums, the cymbals, drums and trumpets, were simultaneously sounded. That sound was tumultuous. (1.13)**

***Author's Commentary:***

All the various emotions and mental energies usually join in with the lusty emotions to enjoy real or imagined occurence. The feelings within the psyche may grow to an overwhelming intoxicating or deluding extent, thus destroying the objectivity of the self, making it feel as if it were in unity with these feelings, which soon subside, leaving the self in a sober state again.

ततः श्वेतैर्हयैर्युक्ते
महतिस्यन्दने स्थितौ ।
माधवः पाण्डवश्चैव
दिव्यौ शङ्खौ प्रदध्मतुः ॥ १.१४ ॥
tataḥ śvetairhayairyukte
mahatisyandane sthitau
mādhavaḥ pāṇḍavaścaiva
divyau śaṅkhau pradadhmatuḥ (1.14)

*tataḥ — then; śvetair — with white; hayair — with horses; yukte — harnessed; mahati — in a magnificent; syandane — swift-moving chariot; sthitau — standing; mādhavaḥ — the descendant of Madhu; pāṇḍavaś caiva — and indeed the son of Pāndu; divyau — supernatural; śaṅkhau — two conches; pradadhmatuḥ — blew*

**Then, standing in a magnificent, swift-moving chariot with white horses harnessed, the descendant of Madhu and the son of Pāndu blew two supernatural conchshells. (1.14)**

***Author's Commentary:***

Duryodhana made calculations on the basis of gross existence, but his opponents, the Pandavas, who were directed by *Śrī* Krishna, the descendant of Madhu, figured in the supernatural level. Sanjaya, a capable mystic, reported to King *Dhṛtarāṣṭra*, that while Prince Duryodhana and his men were relying solely on material means of conquest, their opponents had an additional dependence on the supernatural energies. Thus when *Śrī* Krishna and Arjuna picked up and blew their conchshells, that was both a physical and supernatural conscious act of theirs.

Everyone on that battlefield had physical, supernatural and spiritual segments in their activities, but *Śrī* Krishna and Arjuna were aware of theirs, while most other soldiers were focused on material gains.

***Siddha Swami's Commentary:***

King Pandu, the father of Arjuna, failed to protect the Kuru kingdom. This was due to complications of destiny which were intertwined with Pandu's sexual affairs. However, Pandu's son was determined to level with providence and to be successful as a moral man, a respecter of *dharma* or righteousness. Similarly, a yogi who failed to reach perfection in his last life should in a new body, try to gain full success by sidestepping the complications of destiny which are thrown on his path and by foregoing sexual indulgence.

Just as Arjuna has *Śrī* Krishna on his side to advise him every step of the way through that providence on the war field, a yogi should have a guru present with him at all times so that he can get timely advice on how to deal with the willy nilly time factor which baffles human beings, even the philosophers. Such a guru may or may not be physically present, but he must be present on the supernatural level for communication with the capable mystic disciple.

Just as you, *Madhvācārya*, agreed to accept my dictates into your head and to write these down in this commentary on the *Bhagavad Gītā*, so the yogi should develop the ability to communicate with a mahāyogīn guru who can guide one through the maze of material existence. Otherwise there will be no full success either in *kriyā yoga* or in this *brahma yoga*, which is the advanced stage of *kriyā* practice.

पाञ्चजन्यं हृषीकेशो
देवदत्तं धनंजयः ।
पौण्ड्रं दध्मौ महाशङ्खं
भीमकर्मा वृकोदरः ॥१.१५॥

pāñcajanyaṁ hṛṣīkeśo
devadattaṁ dhanaṁjayaḥ
pauṇḍraṁ dadhmau mahāśaṅkha
bhīmakarmā vṛkodaraḥ (1.15)

*pāñcajanyaṁ — the conch named Pāñcajanya; hṛṣīkeśo — Krishna; devadattaṁ — a conch named Devadatta; dhanaṁjayaḥ — conqueror of wealthy countries; pauṇḍraṁ — conch named Paundra; dadhmau — blew; mahāśaṅkha — great conch; bhīma karmā — one whose actions are terrible; vṛkodaraḥ — wolf—bellied man*

**The conchshell named Pāñcajanya was blown by Hṛṣīkeśa, Krishna. The Devadatta conch was sounded by the conqueror of wealthy countries, Arjuna. Bhīma, the wolf-bellied man whose actions are terrible, blew the great conch named Paundra. (1.15)**

***Siddha Swami's Commentary:***

*Pāñcajanya* may be taken to mean something that produced *(janya)* the five senses *(pāñca).* Lord Krishna, the supreme *brahma yogi,* controlled the mind which produced the five senses. In that way there was no scope for chaos in the psychology of Lord Krishna. Chaos exists in the psyche of the limited being in this world but such a person has the possibility of order if he takes instruction from *Śrī* Krishna. Thus *Śrī* Krishna blew the conchshell and effectively handled the mind but the limited being is usually compelled by impulses to act in this world and he is effectively handled by the mind.

Arjuna's conchshell is named *Devadatta* which may indicate that it was given over *(datta)* for control by the supernatural rulers (the *devas*). Thus accordingly, the limited being in this world should follow Arjuna's example and give over his mind for control by the *devas* who may guide him in how to acheive order in the confused and disordered psyche. It is believed that an ordinary person cannot control his mind. He must take help from superior personalities. This instruction begins when the mother stops the child from eating dirt and other refuse. Later, the child is scolded by the mother when he hits her to show that he should get what he desires. And still later the child is taught moral values. These begin with the teaching of, "You should not steal. You should not speak an untruth."

Even though the mother is the first teacher, still she may not be a superior personality. But that is not the point since she is usually guided by superior persons in the forms of priests and the writers of scriptural text. Ultimately, moral instructions *(dharma)* come down to human beings from superior souls.

These restrictions are part of the first course in yoga which is called *yama* or restraints of the nature of the living being. This is followed by the 2nd stage of yoga which consists of approved behaviors called *niyama*. These encourage one to do things which facilitate an orderly spiritually-indicative psyche. These consist of instructions like: *This is yours. Take it. It was assigned for your use. What you just said is truthful, therefore you may be rewarded.*

Initially when one gives over one's mind to the supernatural rulers, one gets moral values. These are ways of lubricating the social order in the material world. These do not give an absolute grip over the psyche or the internal mechanism which one thinks is one's personality. To get control over the psyche, one has to give the mind over to *Śrī* Krishna for its control internally. The mind is a very private part of the self, even more private than the sexual organs, but the emotions are just as private as the analytical functions. Inside the mind, memory and the imagination or visualization organ are even more private. Any circumstance one remembers can be hidden from others. One may visualize something without revealing it to others. For the purpose of *brahma yoga* one should give the mind over to *Śrī* Krishna. This is what Krishna requested Arjuna to do but the details of how to submit are generally unknown to spiritual teachers. In the first place, *Śrī* Krishna may not agree to control a person's mind. He may send that person to another person, a capable yogi or another divine personality. Or *Śrī* Krishna may even instruct the person rather than control the person's mind directly.

In most cases the student yogi reaches a stage where his mystic perception becomes sensitive. Then a mahāyogī enters into his mind space and shows how to control the various parts of the psyche.*

*This writer attests to the fact that Siddha Swami Nityananda and specifically Yogiraj Yogeshwarananda did and do enter into his mind space to show how to control the organs of perception.

Arjuna was given over to the supernatural people and thus he could not possibly lose at the battle of *Kurukṣetra*. Correspondingly, a *yogin* who gives his mind for control by greater yogis, will be successful in the quest for control of the psyche.

*Bhīma*, Arjuna's elder brother, blew the great *(mahā)* shell named *Pauṇḍram*. That is a physical fact of history, but *pauṇḍram* indicates something specific, a particular tool. *Bhīma* carried a particular tool which on occasion would be used by the supernatural people. A yogi should get particular techniques if he is to escape from material existence. *Puṇḍah* means a sign or mark.

*Bhīma* had a reputation as a crude person. On occasion a yogi does vulgar things like passing stool or passing air. Eventually in *haṭha* yoga practice, one learns how to control and greatly reduce the various vulgarities like sexual indulgence and over-eating. If a yogi is specially marked *(puṇḍah)* by his teachers they will assist him in a way that causes success in higher yoga, otherwise he will remain as a mediocre student.

अनन्तविजयं राजा
कुन्तीपुत्रो युधिष्ठिरः ।
नकुलः सहदेवश्च
सुघोषमणिपुष्पकौ ॥१.१६॥
anantavijayaṁ rājā
kuntīputro yudhiṣṭhiraḥ
nakulaḥ sahadevaśca
sughoṣamaṇipuṣpakau (1.16)

*anantavijayaṁ — name of a conchshell; rājā — king; kuntī putro — son of Kuntī ; yudhiṣṭhiraḥ — Yudhishthira; nakulaḥ — Nakula; sahadevaś — Sahadeva; ca — and; sughoṣa maṇipuṣpakau — names of two conchshells: Sughosha and Manipushpaka*

**The King, Kuntī's son, Yudhishthira, blew the Anantavijayam. Nakula and Sahadeva blew the Sughosha and Manipushpaka respectively. (1.16)**

***Author's Commentary:***

Yudhishthira is the eldest Pandava. He is the king of their family dynasty. Though a Prince, he was not arrogant or self-conceited like his cousin Duryodhana. He was reluctant to oppose his conniving cousin but as urged by his mother Kunti and by his friend and God, *Śrī* Krishna, he took it as a duty to fight for a kingdom. He was reputed to be the son of Righteousness.

***Siddha Swami remarked:***

Any yogi who is expert at upholding righteous behavior with good judgment and discrimination, may be compared to Yudhishthira. Such a person is rare even among the millions of religious people and yogis. Such a person gets unlimited (*ananta*) victory (*vijayam*) even in the material world. And it is not that such people are exempt from frustrations. Generally they attain great prosperity without much endeavor and without being stigmatized with sinful reactions.

Due to righteous tendency, a person like Yudhishthira does not need to give over his mind to anyone for moral guidance. Such a person has an internal affinity for morality and even God does not need to advise him in moral issues. However morality is not a part of *brahma yoga*. Hence even such a morally-inclined yogi must take help from *Śrī* Krishna or from a great yogi on how to regulate the psyche in order to be transferred out of this material world.

Nakula is the fourth Pandava. His conchshell *Sughoṣa* may indicate the naad sound in the right ear of the yogi. This sound or *ghoṣa* becomes pleasant or nice to hear (*su*), as soon as the yogi settles down, when he stops pursuing objects in the outside gross and subtle world and becomes content to not ingest anything from this mundane existence. Sahadeva is the fifth and youngest Pandava. His conchshell, the *Maṇipuṣpaka*, may be taken as the visualization organ in the mind compartment. This organ is like a jewel *(mani)*. It is like a beautifully designed flying conveyance. This is held in awe and veneration by the evolving soul who is bewildered by its swiftness. Such a person, when he becomes a *yogin*, thinks that whatever is said by the *mahāyogī* is fantastic and incredible. When told of the subtle objects which comprise the mind, he admits to his teacher, "My mind and I are one and the same. I do not experience mental objectivity. My person and mind are one and the same."

काश्यश्च परमेष्वासः
शिखण्डी च महारथः ।
धृष्टद्युम्नो विराटश्च
सात्यकिश्चापराजितः ॥१.१७॥
kāśyaśca parameṣvāsaḥ
śikhaṇḍī ca mahārathaḥ
dhṛṣṭadyumno virāṭaśca
sātyakiścāparājitaḥ (1.17)

*kāśyaś — King of Kāśi; ca — and; parameṣvāsaḥ — superior bowman; śikhaṇḍī — Śikhandī; ca — and; mahā rathaḥ — great chariot fighter; dhṛṣṭadyumno — Dhṛṣṭadyumna; virāṭaś — Virāṭa; ca — and; sātyakiś cā 'parājitaḥ = sātyakiś — Satyaki + ca — and + aparājitas — unconquered one*

**The King of Kāśi, the superior bowman, and Śikhandī, the great chariot fighter, Dhṛṣṭadyumna and Virāṭa and Sātyaki, the unconquered one, (1.17)**

***Siddha Swami's Commentary:***

These allies of the Pandavas, as well as others, came to *Kurukṣetra* with their armed forces to show their objections to Duryodhana's unfair handling of the Kuru kingdom. Each of these generals, each of their soldiers, came with karmic packages which were intertwined in the past and present. Sometimes destiny is hazy. At other times it is clear. A person loses out today, but gains tomorrow. Thus in *brahma yoga* one is trained to carefully remove the strand of one's karmas from the yarn of destiny. At one stage the strand is dyed black, at another white. In part of one's life, one acts sensibly. In another, one acts silly. The solution is to remove oneself from this type of destiny, since here one cannot always have full discrimination and one is not always afforded a comprehensive view of any circumstance.

द्रुपदो द्रौपदेयाश्च
सर्वशः पृथिवीपते ।
सौभद्रश्च महाबाहुः
शङ्खान्दध्मुः पृथक्पृथक् ॥१.१८॥
drupado draupadeyāśca
sarvaśaḥ pṛthivīpate
saubhadraśca mahābāhuḥ
śaṅkhāndadhmuḥ pṛthakpṛthak (1.18)

*drupado — Drupada; draupadeyāś — sons of Draupadī; ca — and; sarvaśaḥ — all together, being grouped together; pṛthivī pate — O King of the province; saubhadraś — son of Subhadra; ca — and; mahābāhuḥ — strong-armed; śaṅkhān — conchshells; dadhmuḥ — blew; pṛthak pṛthak — one by one*

**...O king of the province, Drupada and the sons of Draupadī, being grouped together, and the strong-armed son of Subhadra, blew conchshells in series. (1.18)**

***Author's Commentary:***

As *pṛthivīpate*, the king of a province, *Dhṛtarāṣṭra* was being ridiculous. Full of conceit, impulsively ambitious, not scaling down his desires, he pretended to be a capable monarch, even though he could not even set eyes on those who stood before him. Destiny robbed him of the physical vision and still it gave him a chance to be king. What a joke destiny was to play on him! By its actions, destiny said to him, "I do not approve of your desire to rule a kingdom. If, however, you are determined in this regard, you may do so while using a blind body. Go ahead. Try your best. Pretend that you can be a king."

***Siddha Swami's Commentary:***

In this world, destiny is perverse. It is quite contrary. One person may be deemed wise in one lifetime and be considered foolish in another. The same man who we acclaim today as being far-sighted may be ridiculed as the greatest idiot tomorrow. He who is blessed with good luck today, may be struck with misfortune and be pitiable tomorrow. Such is this existence.

In India we believe that the Goddess of fortune is shifty. This means that whosoever she associates with today, will cry for her when she leaves his company and he becomes poverty-stricken tomorrow. We should also know that the Goddess of nature, *Durgā*, and the goddess of education, *Sarasvatī*, are shifty. They too support a fellow today and leave him to languish on the following day. None of these blessings are permanent in the material existence. I may be quite capable of taking care of an adult body but what would I do with an infant one which cannot clean its stool or direct its urine into a urinal?

My son, since you allow me to use your body to give this commentary on the *Bhagavad Gītā* of Lord Krishna, I bless you. Even for liberated entities like me, certain duties must be performed. Some of these tasks require a material body. Since I can use your body, it would not be necessary for me take on another material form to do this. I am therefore appreciative of your willingness to let me use your brain and publishing power to complete this. May you be successful in *kriyā* and *brahma yoga* practice.

स घोषो धार्तराष्ट्राणां
हृदयानि व्यदारयत् ।
नभश्च पृथिवीं चैव
तुमुलो व्यनुनादयन् ॥ १.१९ ॥
sa ghoṣo dhārtarāṣṭrāṇāṁ
hṛdayāni vyadārayat
nabhaśca pṛthivīṁ caiva
tumulo vyanunādayan (1.19)

*sa — the; ghoṣo (ghoṣaḥ) — noise; dhārtarāṣṭrāṇāṁ — the men of Dhṛtarāṣṭra; hṛdayāni — emotions; vyadārayat — disrupted; nabhaś — the sky; ca — and; pṛthivīṁ — the earth; caiva — and indeed; tumulo — vibrating sound; vyanunādayan — cause to resonate*

**The noise disrupted the emotions of the sons of Dhṛtarāṣṭra, and the vibrating sound caused the sky and earth to resonate. (1.19)**

***Author's Commentary:***

Since their intellects and sensing mechanisms were outwardly focused with intent to exploit the situations which would arise in this material world, the sons of *Dhṛtarāṣṭra* were emotionally unsettled when the Pandavas blew their conchshells in defiance to the plans of Prince Duryodhana. This is only relevant if we are focused into this dimension. Here one must consider if something is good or bad, moral or immoral, alive or dead, according to the whim of providence.

***Siddha Swami's Commentary:***

Since providence must balance various forces, it cannot be partial to any specific good or bad power at any given time. It can only seem to facilitate one or the other, from time to time. It is foolish to think that destiny will support what is good or moral at all times, for such an expense is not permitted in this world.

Since we cannot permanently adjust for all good at all times, we should realize the futility of any short-ranged or long-ranged attempt for such order. Thus we should strive for success in *brahma yoga* and leave this world to go its own way.

By causing the sky and earth to resonate, the sound of the conches of the Pandavas and their supported forces, gave a portent for victory. All the same, it spoke of their ultimate defeat. No one can be victorious forever, since no one is allowed to keep an unchanging material body. No one is allowed to rule over this world forever. Time itself, which indicated the victory of the Pandavas, would in turn, ruin that same dynasty.

अथ व्यवस्थितान्दृष्ट्वा
धार्तराष्ट्रान्कपिध्वजः ।
प्रवृत्ते शस्त्रसंपाते
धनुरुद्यम्य पाण्डवः ॥१.२०॥
atha vyavasthitāndṛṣṭvā
dhārtarāṣṭrānkapidhvajaḥ
pravṛtte śastrasaṁpāte
dhanurudyamya pāṇḍavaḥ (1.20)

*atha — then; vyavasthitān — in battle formation; dṛṣṭvā — after observing; dhārtarāṣṭrān — the sons of Dhṛtarāṣṭra; kapidhvajaḥ — the man with a monkey insignia; pravṛtte — in the challenge; śastrasaṁpāte — in the clash of weapons; dhanur — bow; udyamya — raising; pāṇḍavaḥ — son of Pāṇḍu*

**Then after observing the sons of Dhṛtarāṣṭra in battle formation, the man with a monkey insignia, that son of Pandu, raised his bow in the challenge of the clash of weapons. (1.20)**

***Siddha Swami's Commentary:***

*Dhṛtarāṣṭra* wanted to know how the battle evolved. He heard of it from the reporter Sanjaya. All of a sudden after the sounding of musical instruments, the man with a monkey insignia raised his bow in the challenge of the clash of weapons. What exactly motivated this one warrior to take precedence? There are many forces, some within and some outside one's psyche. Which of these sponsored that lone warrior to set himself apart from the others? Was he inspired only by forces within his own mind and emotions? Or was he motivated by conjoint powers springing from his own psyche and from that of others in his own and in the opponents' camp?

Why did Sanjaya not give that warrior's name outright? Why did he indicate who it was by naming the warrior's insignia? Obviously, Sanjaya wanted to guide the blind king through a maze of difficult emotions, by flashing certain sensitive symbols in the mind. The warrior was Arjuna. The insignia used was *Hanumān*, a man-monkey of repute, who exhibited remarkable intelligence, who was successful in assisting a certain Prince *Rāma* of *Rāmāyaṇa* fame.

By the time of the *Kurukṣetra* war, both *Hanumān* and Prince *Rāma* were accredited as being divine personages, in whom many people rested their hopes and faith. Thus Sanjaya disrupted the peace of *Dhṛtarāṣṭra*, by bringing it to his attention that Arjuna was reliant on *Hanumān*, a victor in the war of *Rāma* against Rāvaṇa, the abductor of *Rāma*'s wife, Sītā. Sanjaya did effectively sabotage King *Dhṛtarāṣṭra*'s confidence, for in the material world, regardless of whether one is right or wrong, or whether one is the offender or victim, some forces will in effect erode one's confidence.

हृषीकेशं तदा वाक्यम्
इदमाह महीपते ।
सेनयोरुभयोर्मध्ये
रथं स्थापय मेऽच्युत ॥ १.२१ ॥

hṛṣīkeśaṁ tadā vākyam
idamāha mahīpate
senayorubhayormadhye
rathaṁ sthāpaya me'cyuta (1.21)

*hṛṣīkeśaṁ — Hṛṣīkeśa, Krishna; tadā — then; vākyam — request; idam — this; āha — he spoke; mahīpate — O Lord of the earth; senayoḥ — of the two armies; ubhayoḥ — of the two; madhye — in the midst; rathaṁ — chariot; sthāpaya — cause to be parked; me — my; 'cyuta = acyuta — unaffected*

**Then he spoke this request to Hṛṣīkeśa, Krishna: O Lord of the earth, cause my chariot to be parked in the midst of the two armies, O unaffected one, (1.21)**

***Author's Commentary:***

Arjuna, as a warrior on Yudhishtira's side, addressed his charioteer as *mahīpate*, lord of the earth. But Sanjaya addressed *Dhṛtarāṣṭra* as lord of the earth (*pṛthivīpate*, verse 18). Both *pṛthivī* and *mahī* mean the earth. Who, therefore, is the real lord of the earth?

Arjuna addressed *Śrī* Krishna as the unaffected person (*'cyuta, acyuta* ), as if to say, "O Krishna I know that these circumstances are no bother to you. Still I request you to put me in a position so that I can be subjected to the full impact of this confrontation between members of the same family. It is difficult for me to understand how you can remain undisturbed in times like this. However, since I must do this, please drive the chariot forward and forgive me for requesting this of you."

***Siddha Swami's Commentary:***

One is compelled to act in this world by a sense of importance. This arrogance is temporary, because it is reliant on factors which are not the self. Thus one must learn from a *brahma yoga* teacher how to abandon such prominence, which fosters conceit. This world will go on with or without a particular limited being. Hence no limited being really has importance. This is to be realized factually by higher yoga meditation.

We know now that *Śrī* Krishna is the God in Person. Arjuna did not realize that at the time of making this request. When dealing with the God, our position should be one of subordination. Instead of requesting that *Śrī* Krishna take our chariot somewhere, we may instead ask *Śrī* Krishna if we can take His chariot anywhere. But if it is that *Śrī* Krishna asked us to be served by Him, then we have to be very careful to get advice on how we should request divine services. God should not be used by a limited being, even though the same limited person cannot exist without accepting services from God. It is a dilemma. All these perplexities motivate a *yogin* to strive for liberation from his ignorant and inept condition in this world.

यावदेतान्निरीक्षेऽहं
योद्धुकामानवस्थितान् ।
कैर्मया सह योद्धव्यम्
अस्मिन्रणसमुद्यमे ॥ १.२२ ॥

yāvadetānnirīkṣe'haṁ
yoddhukāmānavasthitān
kairmayā saha yoddhavyam
asminraṇasamudyame (1.22)

*yāvad — so that; etān — these; nirīkṣe — I can see; 'ham = aham — I; yoddhu kāmān — battle-hungry; avasthitān — armed warriors; kair — with whom; mayā — with myself; saha — with; yoddhavyam — should be fought; asmin — in this; raṇasamudyame — in the battle engagement*

**...so that I can see those battle-hungry, armed warriors, with whom I should fight in this battle engagement. (1.22)**

***Author's Commentary:***

Arjuna drew conclusions. He named the opponents as battle hungry warriors. To his mind, they were a vicious lot. If so, what would he achieve by ranging over them? What else but his own frustration? It is said that if looks could kill, many of us would be dead already. Arjuna's viewing of the soldiers would not stop their enthusiasm for war. But Arjuna would get the fulfillment of seeing their valor in war. What would he do with the energy of that fulfillment? Where in his nature would it go? Why did he have a need for it, even as *Śrī* Krishna remained cool-headed and unaffected (*'cyuta acyuta*)?

योत्स्यमानानवेक्षेऽहं
य एतेऽत्र समागताः ।
धार्तराष्ट्रस्य दुर्बुद्धेर्
युद्धे प्रियचिकीर्षवः ॥ १.२३ ॥
yotsyamānānavekṣe'haṁ
ya ete'tra samāgatāḥ
dhārtarāṣṭrasya durbuddher
yuddhe priyacikīrṣavaḥ (1.23)

*yotsyamānān — those who are about to fight; avekṣe — I wish to observe; 'ham = aham — I; ya — who; ete — these; 'tra = atra — here; samāgatāḥ — assembled together; dhārtarāṣṭrasya — of the son of Dhṛtarāṣṭra; durbuddher — of the evil-minded; yuddhe — in battle; priyacikīrṣavaḥ — desiring to please*

**I wish to observe these who are to fight, who assembled here desiring to please the evil-minded son of King Dhṛtarāṣṭra, in battle. (1.23)**

***Author's Commentary:***

This was an act of censorship. Arjuna wanted to purview everyone who dared to support Duryodhana. He thought, "Let me take a good look at these people. Where is their conscience?"

The material existence sponsors both good and evil. This cannot be stopped by anyone. What appears to be evil may sometimes bring about good and what appears to be beneficial may sometimes bring misfortune. This does not mean that human beings should not have conventions and standards of behavior. But it does mean that over all, the situation is a mix of good and evil always, and there is absolutely nothing anyone can do to permanently change these conditions.

Each opponent in a political or military contest has supporters who are helplessly attached. There are also supporters who owe favors to one party. Some supporters render favors to gain other favors. Thus Prince Duryodhana had his allies. And Arjuna's eldest brother, Prince Yudhishthira, had his too.

Some good people like *Droṇa* and Bhishma supported Duryodhana. Some not-so-good people supported Yudhishthira. Such is the way of circumstance. Yudhishthira had an edge, however, since his main supporter was Lord Krishna, the God of the world according to the *Bhagavad Gītā*. But if to win one has to have God on one's side, then how do we explain the victory of evil rulers? Did God support their temporary conquests?

**Siddha Swami *Nityānānda* said this**:

A student of *brahma yoga* should forego or give up the habit of surveying the world and the circumstances which are formed within the material existence. If he does this he will see success in higher yoga, otherwise he will stagnate and be a failure, mediocre at best. Whatever concerns this world, does concern this world, but it has nothing to do with the world in the *brahman* energy. Thus if one wants to be transferred there, one should leave aside the details of what occurs here.

This world will go on regardless. A particular limited being is not necessary. Thus as a *brahma yogi* one should practice detachment. One should not apply the energy of appropriation to this dimension. Instead one should turn one's attention to the naad transcendental sound in the right ear, and from that posture develop the supernatural vision to see into the spiritual dimensions.

Just as Arjuna lived, surveyed the world, was concerned with law order and then had to leave it aside because his body aged and circumstances pushed him out of political importance, so a *yogin* must push himself out of the world and leave its functioning to others. The world will not perish merely because a particular yogi's mind is absent from it.

In cases where it is one's divinely-ordained duty to act in the world, one should do so with detachment just as an employee acts with professional concern while doing a task for an employer. One should remember always that the concerns of the world are the concerns of the God of the world and that one's puny self is not necessary unless the God Himself deems one to be, and only for as long as that God assigns. It is foolish to be self-righteous and to feel that unless one acts, nothing will happen for the good of the world.

संजय उवाच
एवमुक्तो हृषीकेशो
गुडाकेशेन भारत ।
सेनयोरुभयोर्मध्ये
स्थापयित्वा रथोत्तमम् ॥ १.२४॥
saṁjaya uvāca
evamukto hṛṣīkeśo
guḍākeśena bhārata
senayorubhayormadhye
sthāpayitvā rathottamam (1.24)

*saṁjaya — Sanjaya; uvāca — said; evam — thus; ukto — being addressed; hṛṣīkeśo — Hrisikesa; guḍākeśena — by the thick—haired baron; bhārata — O descendant of Bharata; senayor — of the two armies; ubhayor — of the two; madhye — in the middle; sthāpayitvā — caused to be positioned; rathottamam — best of the chariots*

**Sanjaya said: O descendant of Bharata, thus being addressed by Arjuna, the thick-haired baron, Krishna, who is known as Hṛṣīkeśa, caused the best of the chariots to be positioned in the midst of the two armies. (1.24)**

***Author's Commentary:***

It is difficult to know exactly who is who in material existence, for we hear of the God, of *Śrī* Krishna, taking instructions willingly from Arjuna, a warrior and friend of the God.

Sanjaya addressed King *Dhṛtarāṣṭra* as a descendant of *Bharata* because *Dhṛtarāṣṭra* identified himself by the clan of his body. He did not perceive himself as a spirit who would take various bodies in various families here or there in the material creation. It was this stubborn tendency to identify oneself as one's developed body, which stymied *Dhṛtarāṣṭra* and kept him from making decisions which were in his spiritual and moral interest.

भीष्मद्रोणप्रमुखतः
सर्वेषां च महीक्षिताम् ।
उवाच पार्थ पश्यैतान्
समवेतान्कुरूनिति ॥ १.२५॥

*bhīṣma droṇa pramukhataḥ — in the presence of Bhisma, Droṇa; sarveṣām — of all these; ca — and; mahīkṣitām — rulers of the earth; uvāca — (Krishna) said; pārtha — O son of Pṛthā; paśyai 'etān — behold them;*

bhīṣmadroṇapramukhataḥ
sarveṣāṁ ca mahīkṣitām
uvāca pārtha paśyaitān
samavetānkurūniti (1.25)

*samavetān — are assembled together; kurūn — Kurus; iti — thus*

**In the presence of Bhishma, Droṇa and all those rulers of the earth, Krishna said: O son of Pṛthā, behold these Kurus who are assembled here together. (1.25)**

***Author's Commentary:***

In any situation one has to decide whether to act or not act, to respond or to ignore. On what basis should one decide to participate or not participate? How would one face the reaction if one acted indifferently, or if one participated fully? Agreeing with Arjuna's request, the God said, "Please look on, for this is what you wanted to see."

***Siddha Swami said:***

In each life one comes out into the material world with a set of senses for perceiving in the particular dimension of that birth. One ranges over objects and responds to various situations. Each of the worlds one may appear in, is already existing and progressing, in one's absence. Thus to assume that one is essential to any of those places is ridiculous.

Naturally then, as soon as one enters into a dimension one tries to participate. Usually one does not enter with a developed discrimination. One enters without memory of past lives and without an understanding of the history of the place. Thus inevitably one makes wrong, ill-timed decisions. Arjuna is rare, because God stood beside him. God supplemented Arjuna's ignorance. Others are not as fortunate.

Arjuna went forward, not as a living entity who was transmigrated here or there but as a descendant of the Kurus, and specifically as the son of *Pṛthā*, who was the wife of King Pandu, *Dhṛtarāṣṭra*'s brother. Since Arjuna lost sight of himself as a transmigrating personality and identified himself only as a descendant of the Kurus, Lord Krishna sarcastically called Arjuna, *Pārtha*, which meant the person who is a son of *Pṛthā*. Until Arjuna is able to lift his awareness from the identity as a descendant of the Kurus, he will suffer emotionally from the confrontation. And even after it was brought to Arjuna's attention that he was a transmigrating soul and only superficially, was he a Kuru, even then whenever Arjuna would lose sight of that, he would again suffer emotionally in any such plight of the Kurus.

तत्रापश्यत्स्थितान्पार्थः
पितृनथ पितामहान् ।
आचार्यान्मातुलान्भ्रातृन्
पुत्रान्पौत्रान्सखींस्तथा ।
श्वशुरान्सुहृदश्चैव
सेनयोरुभयोरपि ॥ १.२६ ॥
tatrāpaśyatsthitānpārthaḥ
pitṝnatha pitāmahān
ācāryānmātulānbhrātṝn
putrānpautrānsakhīṁstathā
śvaśurānsuhṛdaścaiva
senayorubhayorapi (1.26)

*tatra apaśyat — there he saw; sthitān — standing; pārthaḥ — the son of Pṛthā; pitṝn — fathers; atha — then; pitāmahān — grandfathers; ācāryān — revered teachers; mātulān — maternal uncles; bhrātṝn — brothers; putrān — sons; pautrān — grandsons; sakhīṁs — friends; tathā — as well as; śvaśurān — fathers-in-law; suhṛdaś = suhṛdaḥ — well-wishing men; caiva — and indeed; senayoḥ — in the two armies; ubhayoḥ — in the both; api — also*

**The son of Pṛthā saw men who were fathers, grandfathers, revered teachers, maternal uncles, brothers, sons, grandsons, as well as friends, fathers-in-law and well-wishing friends, standing there in both armies. (1.26)**

***Siddha Swami's Commentary:***

Arjuna's psychology at the time of this view was based on taking a body from Pandu and *Pṛthā*, without consideration for all of Arjuna's previous manifested existences in different families at different places, at different times. Naturally one forgets all past births because usually a limited being is unable to repossess the memories. Thus nearly everyone is fooled in each birth. This gives providence the upper hand over most limited beings.

In retrospect when we consider the whole of the *Bhagavad Gītā* discourse and the way the God explained this existence, Arjuna's spirit took that body as the son of Pandu and *Pṛthā*, for the purpose of helping the Supreme Spirit with His self-ordained duties in maintaining righteousness. The posture as the son of Pandu and *Pṛthā* was to be used by the Supreme Spirit for His own purposes and not to uphold all or part of the Kuru family. But Arjuna, naturally, was overwhelmed with the relationships within the Kuru family and society. Arjuna was out of touch with the divine mission of his birth.

If he could have steadied himself and tuned into the divine mission, he would not have perceived the relatives in their clan designations. He would have seen them as they were seen by the Universal Form of *Śrī* Krishna. Those are distinct visions. For all practical purposes Arjuna, who had a divine mission, shifted from the mission and indulged in a materialist life based only on the current social relations. Thus *Śrī* Krishna had the task of resituating Arjuna for divine usage.

तान्समीक्ष्य स कौन्तेयः
सर्वान्बन्धूनवस्थितान् ।
कृपया परयाविष्टो
विषीदन्निदमब्रवीत् ॥ १.२७ ॥
tānsamīkṣya sa kaunteyaḥ
sarvānbandhūnavasthitān
kṛpayā parayāviṣṭo
viṣīdannidamabravīt (1.27)

*tān — them; samīkṣya — observing; sa — he; kaunteyaḥ — son of Kuntī; sarvān — all; bandhūn — relatives; avasthitān — armored; kṛpayā — with compassion; parayāviṣṭaḥ — overwhelmed by deep; viṣīdann — feeling discouraged; idam — this; abravīt — he said*

**Observing all his relatives in the armored state, that son of Kuntī was overwhelmed by deep compassion. Feeling discouraged, he spoke this: (1.27)**

***Siddha Swami's Commentary:***

In material existence, any limited being is bound to be aware of family designation and local conditions for behavior. A special endeavor should be made to see life apart from the family situation. A higher intelligence and a more flexible outlook is required before a limited person can act in a detached but righteous manner. The utility of family life need not encumber the spiritual view of a limited spirit who transmigrates.

Arjuna, because his entire self was given over to the family designation, could not regard himself and his relatives as spirits apart from their bodies. Arjuna could not see that righteousness was a priority over family security. Thus he fell under the influence of family emotions without regard for any other reality.

The relationship between one spirit and another is rarely coincidental with the relationship between one body and another. Thus generally, the bodily relationship denies the spiritual one. *Śrī* Krishna, for example, the God Himself, was born as the son of a lady named *Devakī*. Thus physically and even emotionally *Devakī* was *Śrī* Krishna's producer. But spiritually that is not the fact, as explained elsewhere in the *Bhagavad Gītā*. There is kinship between spirits but that usually does not coincide with the family orders in this world. Thus one must learn how to minimize family relations and bring forward the spiritual connections.

*Śrī* Krishna was Arjuna's cousin. Arjuna was not required by social rules of seniority to do everything *Śrī* Krishna recommended. But from the spiritual relationship, *Śrī* Krishna is Arjuna's God, and as such Arjuna should comply with all of *Śrī* Krishna's requests. Thus to honor the spiritual life, Arjuna would be required to take advice from *Śrī* Krishna, who from the material view, was only a cousin.

*Śrī* Krishna was a relative to the Kurus, but from the social view, he had no right to interfere in their quarrel. He was an unwelcome involvement for Duryodhana. But from the spiritual family view, *Śrī* Krishna, as He portrayed himself as the supreme father, had every right to interfere, not only in the Kuru affairs but in everyone else's social concerns.

दृष्ट्वेमान्स्वजनान्कृष्ण
युयुत्सून्समवस्थितान् ।
सीदन्ति मम गात्राणि
मुखं च परिशुष्यति ॥ १.२८ ॥
dṛṣṭvemānsvajanānkṛṣṇa
yuyutsūnsamavasthitān
sīdanti mama gātrāṇi
mukhaṁ ca pariśuṣyati (1.28)

*dṛṣṭvemāṁ — having seen this; svajanān — my people; kṛṣṇa — Krishna; yuyutsūṁ — eager for combat; samavasthitān — standing near; sīdanti — collapse; mama — my; gātrāṇi — legs; mukhaṁ — mouth; ca — and; pariśuṣyati — dries up*

**Having seen this situation of my own people, standing near, eager for combat, my legs collapse and my mouth dries up. (1.28)**

***Siddha Swami's Commentary:***

This is a case of the social perspective overriding the spiritual relationship. Arjuna was much closer to *Śrī* Krishna than to any other person on the battlefield. But that is an estimate of spiritual connection. From the social connection of the gross body, Arjuna is closer to the Kurus. This contradiction of the spiritual and the social should be settled in favor of the spiritual.

Instead of standing close to *Śrī* Krishna emotionally, Arjuna stood close to the Kurus. He was overwhelmed with deep compassion towards them, fearing their injuries or death. It would only be the injury or death of their bodies, but Arjuna saw it differently as the injury or death of their personalities, which to him meant their bodies. He moved away from the spiritual connection with *Śrī* Krishna at the time of viewing the circumstance in that way. He got closer to the biological relatives, most of whom were prejudiced by the same consciousness.

Arjuna regarded the Kurus as his own people (*svajanān*), but spiritually this was not the truth. Arjuna's estimation was from his view of having taken a body as the son of King Pandu and Queen *Pṛthā*. Arjuna's emotions and vital energies also sensed the material connection between Arjuna's body and the forms of the relatives of his body. And thus, his legs collapsed. His mouth dried up. This indicates that the emotions and life force usually promote bodily connections, even at the expense of spiritual relationships.

वेपथुश्च शरीरे मे
रोमहर्षश्च जायते ।
गाण्डीवं स्रंसते हस्तात्
त्वक् चैव परिदह्यते ॥ १.२९ ॥
vepathuśca śarīre me
romaharṣaśca jāyate
gāṇḍīvaṁ sraṁsate hastāt
tvak caiva paridahyate (1.29)

*vepathuś — trembling; ca — and; śarīre — in the body; me — my; romaharṣaś — bristling of hair; ca — and; jāyate — takes place; gāṇḍīvaṁ — Gāṇḍīva bow; sraṁsate — falls; hastāt — from the hand; tvak — skin; caiva — and indeed; paridahyate — burns*

**A trembling is in my body and a bristling of my hairs takes place. The Gāṇḍīva bow falls from my hand. Indeed, my skin burns. (1.29)**

***Siddha Swami's Commentary:***

Some of Arjuna's emotions and vital energy, some of his psychology, gave way with fear and anxiety over the safety of the Kurus. Under that influence, Arjuna lost touch with the spiritual relationship. His life force and emotions refused to cooperate in the warfare. It did not want any of the Kurus to be harmed.

न च शक्नोम्यवस्थातुं
भ्रमतीव च मे मनः ।
निमित्तानि च पश्यामि
विपरीतानि केशव ॥ १.३० ॥
na ca śaknomyavasthātuṁ
bhramatīva ca me manaḥ
nimittāni ca paśyāmi
viparītāni keśava (1.30)

*na — not; ca — and; śaknomy — I can; avasthātuṁ — to remain standing; bhramatīva — as if it wanders; ca — and; me — my; manaḥ — the mind; nimittāni — indications; ca — and; paśyāmi — I perceive; viparītāni — bad; keśava — beautiful-haired one*

**I cannot remain standing. My mind feels as if it wavers. I perceive bad indications, O beautiful-haired one. (1.30)**

***Siddha Swami's Commentary:***

On each level of existence, there are *dharmas* which are rules for righteous lifestyle. If one breaks such rules, the consequence is discomfort and violence. Thus each *yogin* in any circumstance acts on one level or another, reacting in part and generating new impetuses in part. Any other warrior who entered into the emotional plane which Arjuna endured, would have felt the same way and would have come under the same weakening influences. It was not Arjuna but it was rather the particular emotional plane which he entered.

One must therefore learn about the various levels of energization in the psyche and avoid those which are deluding, avoid those which lack clarity. Judgments are made by the intellect on the basis of its contact with one level or the other. Therefore one should keep the intellect in touch with higher levels and not let it descend to lower emotional planes, where the dharmas or the rules of behavior there, dictate that one should not have insight but should be emotionally encumbered.

न च श्रेयोऽनुपश्यामि
हत्वा स्वजनमाहवे ।
न काङ्क्षे विजयं कृष्ण
न च राज्यं सुखानि च ॥ १.३१ ॥

*na — no; ca — and; śreyaḥ — benefit; 'nupaśyāmi = anupaśyāmi — I can imagine; hatvā — killing; svajanam — my folks; āhave — in battle; na — nor; kāṅkṣe — desired;*

na ca śreyo'nupaśyāmi
hatvā svajanamāhave
na kāṅkṣe vijayaṁ kṛṣṇa
na ca rājyaṁ sukhāni ca (1.31)

*vijayaṁ — victory; kṛṣṇa — O Krishna; na — nor; ca — and; rājyaṁ — political power; sukhāni — good feelings; ca — and*

**And I can imagine no benefit in killing off my kinfolk in battle. I do not desire victory, O Krishna, or political power, or good feelings. (1.31)**

***Siddha Swami's Commentary:***

On the emotional plane which Arjuna's mind entered, the ultimate value was kindness towards loved-ones and indulgence of loved ones. On that level one must act in such a way as not to discipline anyone, even if anyone offends another or acts unfairly and unjustly to another. On that plane there is no motivation for a victory over others, or for political control or good feelings, so long as there is continued effort to be kind to others at all costs, even if such others indulge in vices detrimental to their well-being.

किं नो राज्येन गोविन्द
किं भोगैर्जीवितेन वा ।
येषामर्थे काङ्क्षितं नो
राज्यं भोगाः सुखानि च ॥१.३२॥
kiṁ no rājyena govinda
kiṁ bhogairjīvitena vā
yeṣāmarthe kāṅkṣitaṁ no
rājyaṁ bhogāḥ sukhāni ca (1.32)

*kiṁ — what value would there be; no — to us; rājyena — with political control of a nation; govinda — Chief of the cowherds; kiṁ — what use would there be?; bhogair — with enjoyments; jīvitena — with life; vā — or; yeṣām — whose; arthe — in the interest; kāṅkṣitaṁ — was desired; no — of us; rājyaṁ — political control; bhogāḥ — enjoyable aspects; sukhāni — pleasures; ca — and*

**What value to us would there be with political control of a nation, O Chief of the cowherds? What use would there be with the enjoyable aspects or with life? Those in whose interest, the political control, the enjoyments and pleasures, were desired by us, (1.32)**

***Siddha Swami's Commentary:***

Arjuna succumbed so much to the emotional feelings, that he considered *Śrī* Krishna to be under the same power, even though *Śrī* Krishna was thoroughly resistant to that plane of consciousness. Speaking as if they were both sharing the same views, Arjuna appealed to *Śrī* Krishna to look at the situation from that perspective. Arjuna felt that the war would benefit the Kurus and therefore it made no sense to kill or discipline them with lethal weapons. After all, why kill those very same people whom one wishes to please?

त इमेऽवस्थिता युद्धे
प्राणांस्त्यक्त्वा धनानि च ।
आचार्याः पितरः पुत्रास्
तथैव च पितामहाः ॥१.३३॥
ta ime'vasthitā yuddhe
prāṇāṁstyaktvā dhanāni ca
ācāryāḥ pitaraḥ putrās
tathaiva ca pitāmahāḥ (1.33)

*ta — they; ime — these; 'vasthitā = avasthitā — are armored; yuddhe — in battle formation; prāṇāṁs — lives; tyaktvā — having left aside; dhanāni — financial assets; ca — and; ācāryāḥ — revered teachers; pitaraḥ — fathers; putrās — sons; tathaiva — also; ca — and; pitāmahāḥ — grandfathers*

**...(they) are armed in battle formation, having left aside their lives and financial assets. These are revered teachers, fathers, sons and also grandfathers, (1.33)**

***Siddha Swami's Commentary:***

From the emotional plane which Arjuna endured, it made no sense for his relatives to be on the war field, fighting over land and political control of a kingdom. It was better for them to enjoy the kingdom, even if perchance they were vice-ridden and wronged other people and Arjuna's siblings. Because this view did not take into account the desires of the Supreme Being, it was flawed. It was not up to Arjuna or to anyone on the battlefield, except for *Śrī* Krishna and the laws of nature, which dictate how a person would be penalized or rewarded for activities. Activities which are hostile to morality and which support and develop vices, do cause hardships for all concerned. Therefore the God requested that human beings adhere to rules of conduct which greatly decrease harsh reactions from material nature. Arjuna was not aware of these issues because he fell under the influence of emotions.

मातुलाः श्वशुराः पौत्राः
स्यालाः संबन्धिनस्तथा ।
एतान्न हन्तुमिच्छामि
घ्नतोऽपि मधुसूदन ॥ १.३४ ॥
mātulāḥ śvaśurāḥ pautrāḥ
syālāḥ saṁbandhinastathā
etānna hantumicchāmi
ghnato'pi madhusūdana (1.34)

*mātulāḥ — brothers of mothers; śvaśurāḥ — fathers of wives; pautrāḥ — grandsons; śyālāḥ — brothers-in-law; saṁbandhinas — relatives; tathā — also; etān — them; na — not; hantum — to kill; icchāmi — I desire; ghnato — those who are intent on killing; 'pi = api — even though; madhusūdana — slayer of Madhu.*

**...brothers of our mothers, fathers of our wives, grandsons, brothers-in-law, and also their relatives. O slayer of Madhu, I do not desire to slay them even though they are intent on killing, (1.34)**

***Siddha Swami's Commentary:***

In *brahma yoga*, one is trained how to see the family relationships as utilities of providence and not as realities unto themselves. One's social teacher, father, son, grandfather, uncle, in-laws, grandson, cousin, aunt and other relatives are there as utilities of providence. They are not to be seen as direct relations of oneself. They are placed in position by providence for its utility. Oneself is also in the same position as a utility of time. The bodies of clan members are at the disposal of providence and a *brahma yogin* should not attempt to exploit them for fulfilling desires or for extracting affections.

Arjuna did not desire to kill them but he desired their affectionate dealings. He wanted to be approved by them and to be accredited as being beneficial to them. However, a *brahma yogi* should not desire to kill them, or be honored by them, or to honor them, except as stipulated in his duty by providence. A *brahma yogi* should not want to discipline his relatives but he should also not want to offend providence by excusing them for sinful or immoral acts. All the same he should not be eager to discipline anyone on his own behalf, but should be willing to do so if he is assigned the task by providence. If it is his responsibility, he should discipline any family member who is his dependent, but only on behalf of providence, not for his own sake, and not with pride, thinking that he was instrumental in bringing them to morality.

अपि त्रैलोक्यराज्यस्य
हेतोः किं नु महीकृते ।
निहत्य धार्तराष्ट्रान्नः
का प्रीतिः स्याज्जनार्दन ॥ १.३५॥
api trailokyarājyasya
hetoḥ kiṁ nu mahīkṛte
nihatya dhārtarāṣṭrānnaḥ
kā prītiḥ syājjanārdana (1.35)

*api — even; trailokya — of the three sectors, of the universe; rājyasya — political control; hetoḥ — on account of; kiṁ — what; nu — then; mahīkṛte — for the sake of the earth; nihatya — killing; dhārtarāṣṭrān — the sons of Dhṛtarāṣṭra; naḥ — to us; kā — what; prītiḥ — joy; syāj — might it be; janārdana — O motivator of people*

**...even for political control of the three sectors of the universe, how then for the earth? O motivator of people, what joy should be had by killing the sons of Dhṛtarāṣṭra? (1.35)**

***Siddha Swami's Commentary:***

Arjuna's statement shows only one side of the argument which may be adapted by a *brahma yogin*. A brahmin should like Arjuna, be unwilling to kill relatives or even enemies, or to discipline or ridicule any of these for the sake of gaining control of a kingdom or even for many planets of real estate. All the same, the *brahma yogin* must also be willing to comply with duties imposed by providence in terms of doing just that, disciplining, even if there is no benefit from it or if there will be much reward offered by providence.

The *brahma yogin* must be sensitive and flexible to providence. A servant who refuses to do menial tasks or horrible activities is not a servant. Likewise a servant who refuses to do an honored, approved, pleasant or glorious task is also not a servant.

Arjuna went along with providence when there was a nice relationship with the Kauravas, but as soon as there was hostile dealings with them, Arjuna became unwilling and rejected providence. In *brahma yoga*, one develops a dislike for worldly association of the family, the friends and the general mass of people, but this does not mean a dislike for the unfavorable aspects only, but a dislike for the favorable ones as well. One sees clearly that in most cases, what is liked as a circumstance, what is convenient for the time being, usually turns into something contrary. With that vision one seeks to decrease both the favorable and unfavorable offerings of providence.

Arjuna asked the Lord of providence, *Śrī* Krishna, about the joy to be had by killing the sons of *Dhṛtarāṣṭra*. That is not an issue for a *brahma yogi*. The issue is this: What would the Supreme Being gain, if we were to follow an instruction for disciplining relatives either superficially by harsh words or physically by capital punishment? The answer to this is indicated when we consider that the Supreme Being, if indeed *Śrī* Krishna is that Supreme Person, does not have to explain His acts or His assignment of such acts to any limited being. As a *brahma yogin*, one should be satisfied with this but, regardless, Krishna explained Himself later on in the Gita. Providence can do as it likes, because it takes into account the complete past. It has within its scope the entire future. Therefore we should deliberately have faith in providence. Such faith should not be that providence will do us good but rather that providence does not have to do good for anyone. It satisfies itself and works out the equations of energy and circumstance for its own ease. Whether it damages one man or one woman is of little consequence.

पापमेवाश्रयेदस्मान्
हत्वैतानाततायिनः ।
तस्मान्नार्हा वयं हन्तुं
धार्तराष्ट्रान्स्वबान्धवान् ।
स्वजनं हि कथं हत्वा
सुखिनः स्याम माधव ॥ १.३६ ॥

pāpamevāśrayedasmān
hatvaitānātatāyinaḥ
tasmānnārhā vayaṁ hantuṁ
dhārtarāṣṭrānsvabāndhavān
svajanaṁ hi kathaṁ hatvā
sukhinaḥ syāma mādhava (1.36)

*pāpam — sin; evāśrayed = eva — even + āśrayed — should take hold; asmān — to us; hatvaitān = hatvā — having killed + etān — these; ātatāyinaḥ — offenders; tasmān — therefore; nārhā — unjustified; vayaṁ — we; hantuṁ — to kill; dhārtarāṣṭrān — sons of Dhṛtarāṣṭra; svabāndhavān — our relatives; svajanaṁ — our own people; hi — indeed; kathaṁ — how; hatvā — having killed; sukhinaḥ — happiness; syāma — should be; mādhava — descendant of Madhu*

**Having killed the offenders, sin will take hold of us. Therefore we are not justified to kill the sons of Dhṛtarāṣṭra, our relatives. Having killed our own people, how should we be happy, O descendent of Madhu? (1.36)**

***Siddha Swami's Commentary:***

Arjuna was correctly concluded that if one killed even an aggressor, there would be a sin or reaction for it. This material energy is reactive to all action. Nothing done here avoids a reaction. Still Arjuna was incorrect in thinking that in every case the reactions finds the actor. Sometimes the reaction cannot latch on to the actor and then it remains as an impersonal energy or it latches on to someone else, an innocent by-stander. If the reaction has sufficient force, it will go on to the actor or to someone else or it will move about as weather, disease or some other type of calamity.

For a *brahma yogi,* it is unreasonable to think that one may avoid unfavorable acts and only perform pleasant, approved ones. Material existence does not operate like that. To be practical, one should prefer favorable acts and one must also hold the courage to perform unfavorable acts when providence pressures one to do so. Providence needs servants to do both its good and bad acts, both its pleasant and unpleasant acts, both its acceptable and horrible tasks. Thus one must be willing to do either if one is so selected.

Providence has the upper hand and can inconvenience and force us in the future; we must find a way to perform unfavorable activities without getting the inevitable reaction. We must find a method of avoiding it, so that it may manifest without our presence. And if perchance we must be present for the reaction, then we must find a way of taking that with ease, without resentment to anyone or even to providence. The correct statement for a *brahma yogin* is: Having killed the offenders, a reactionary energy will be released in the environment and if we are not careful, if we did not act with detachment, that energy will take hold of us.

Arjuna explained that they were not justified to kill the sons of *Dhṛtarāṣṭra*, their relatives. This is correct, but it is incorrect to think that providence was not justified in appointing Arjuna and his brothers to the task. Providence has that power. It may do what it likes. Arjuna or his brothers were not justified in refusing to do the tasks assigned by providence. When completing an assignment of providence, one should neither be happy nor sad. That is not the objective. Happiness is pursued by childish entities. For *brahma yoga*, one has to develop further.

यद्यप्येते न पश्यन्ति
लोभोपहतचेतसः ।
कुलक्षयकृतं दोषं
मित्रद्रोहे च पातकम् ॥१.३७॥
yadyapyete na paśyanti
lobhopahatacetasaḥ
kulakṣayakṛtaṁ doṣaṁ
mitradrohe ca pātakam (1.37)

*yadyapyete = yadi — if + api — even + ete — these; na — not; paśyanti — see; lobhopahata cetasaḥ = lobha — greed + upahata — possessed by + cetasaḥ — thoughts; kulakṣayakṛtaṁ = kula — clan + ksaya — destruction + kṛtaṁ — caused; doṣaṁ — fault; mitradrohe = mitra — friend + drohe — harm; ca — and; pātakam — crime*

**Even if these persons, their minds being possessed by greed, do not see the fault caused by the destruction of the clan and the crime of hurting a friend, (1.37)**

***Siddha Swami's Commentary:***

The faults of the Kauravas or their supposed crimes against man and nature, was the concern of providence, not of other beings who were just as limited as the Kauravas themselves. Arjuna was being judgmental, but he was not hired by providence to levy opinions. Providence already made its move by setting the armies against each other on the battlefield. Providence intended to complete that. If Arjuna did not like the actions of providence, he might turn away from the battlefield and so refuse to participate in that drama. But would Arjuna's refusal to participate come with greater consequences for him? This is the question. Before refusing to do something menial or horrible, one should find out if one may be forced to do something even more menial or horrible in the future. For after all, providence does have the upper hand. It can force a future situation where one cannot resist it.

If a man plays God by being judgmental when he should not form an opinion, then what would happen when that same man is placed in a position where he cannot form any opinions at all, but is forced to act in horrible ways merely because he entered into a life form which is innately vicious?

कथं न ज्ञेयमस्माभिः
पापादस्मान्निवर्तितुम् ।
कुलक्षयकृतं दोषं
प्रपश्यद्भिर्जनार्दन ॥१.३८॥
kathaṁ na jñeyamasmābhiḥ
pāpādasmānnivartitum
kulakṣayakṛtaṁ doṣaṁ
prapaśyadbhirjanārdana (1.38)

*kathaṁ — how; na — not; jñeyam — to be understood; asmābhiḥ — by us; pāpād — from sin; asmān — from this; nivartitum — turn away; kulakṣaya = kula — clan + kṣaya — destruction; kṛtaṁ — caused; doṣaṁ — crime; prapaśyadbhiḥ — by due reason; janārdana — O motivator of human beings*

**...O motivator of human beings, why, by due reason, should we not understand that we should turn away from this sin, the crime caused by the destruction of the clan? (1.38)**

***Siddha Swami's Commentary:***

Arjuna felt that life should be discussed among human beings. Opinions should be formed and unnecessary risks should not be taken even for political control and financial gain. This is all well and good for human beings but there are other factors, namely, the Supreme Being and the force of providence. These two factors should also be figured into any discussion.

It may be proven that destruction of any clan, or of anything, is harmful and therefore is criminal. Still, that does not give us a practical way of functioning. Nature itself is the greatest of the criminals in that case, since nature is obsessed with destruction. Destruction is part and parcel of the subtle and gross material existence. Parts of our psyche are continually being subjected to destruction.

It is criminal to kill one's relatives but it is also criminal to allow one's relatives to perform criminal acts on the families of others and within one's family itself. The question is: "What is my duty in terms of disciplining my relatives?"

कुलक्षये प्रणश्यन्ति
कुलधर्माः सनातनाः ।
धर्मे नष्टे कुलं कृत्स्नम्
अधर्मोऽभिभवत्युत ॥ १.३९ ॥
kulakṣaye praṇaśyanti
kuladharmāḥ sanātanāḥ
dharme naṣṭe kulaṁ kṛtsnam
adharmo'bhibhavatyuta (1.39)

*kulakṣaye — in destruction of the family clan; praṇaśyanti — vanish; kuladharmāḥ — family traditions; sanātanāḥ — ancient; dharme — in the traditional values; naṣṭe — in the removal; kulaṁ — clan; kṛtsnam — whole; adharmo — lawlessness; 'bhibhavatyuta = abhibhavati — it overpowers + uta — even*

**In the destruction of the clan, the ancient family traditions vanish. In the removal of the traditional values, the entire clan is overpowered by lawlessness. (1.39)**

***Siddha Swami's Commentary:***

Arjuna assumed that protection of the family rested with himself and *Śrī* Krishna, as well as others. However, that does not take into account that if one protects one's clan today, one might be born into another clan tomorrow. If the purpose of this life is to protect the clan, it is reduced to the tendency of protection in each living entity. Since we may not return into the same family in the next life, the consistent aspect is our protection tendency. We impulsively apply that to whatever family we take birth in.

In the destruction of a clan, its traditions vanish, but other clans flourish proportionately and their traditions are established in turn. If, however, one clan loses its traditional values, then the members of the family become open to new values which might spur social degeneration or conversely, a social upgrade. In all such cases, the person who worked for the elevation of a particular clan, cannot guarantee that he would be born into that clan again. He might take birth in an opposing clan, in one which was suppressed or inconvenienced by the clan from his former birth. Then he would become a victim of the very same clan which he worked to establish.

If a *brahma yogi* is duty bound to the Supreme Being to assist the clan in which his body was born, he should do so with detachment. He should not make it a personal agenda for he cannot control the misuse of his contribution in the future. Since he must change bodies and since he must by nature, lose influence, someone in the clan might abuse his contribution in the future. Therefore he should not ignore the request of the Supreme Being and should not substitute personal ideas for those of the Supreme Being. It is the Supreme Being alone Who can and Who does monitor the various movements of providence. Thus He alone is able to make the proper adjustments. He alone is able to carry the liability in all circumstances.

अधर्माभिभवात्कृष्ण
प्रदुष्यन्ति कुलस्त्रियः ।
स्त्रीषु दुष्टासु वार्ष्णेय
जायते वर्णसंकरः ॥ १.४० ॥
adharmābhibhavātkṛṣṇa
praduṣyanti kulastriyaḥ
strīṣu duṣṭāsu vārṣṇeya
jāyate varṇasaṁkaraḥ (1.40)

*adharmābhibhavāt = adharma — lawlessness + abhibhavāt — from predominant; kṛṣṇa — O Krishna; praduṣyanti — are degraded; kulastriyaḥ — the women of the clan; strīṣu — in women; duṣṭāsu — degraded; vārṣṇeya — O clansman of the Vṛṣṇis; jāyate — there arises; varṇasaṁkaraḥ — sexual intermixture of the classes*

**Due to the predominance of lawlessness, the women of the clan are degraded. In such women, O clansman of the Vṛṣṇis, there arises the sexual intermixture of the classes. (1.40)**

***Siddha Swami's Commentary:***

This is certainly true, but this is not the concern of a limited being like Arjuna. This is the business of the Supreme Being, to protect or not to protect such women. It is good to want to correct every mistake and to wipe every tear from every crying face but it is not practical and no person can complete that. At all times there is danger, harm and trouble in the material world. It cannot be otherwise, due to the nature of the energy. This does not mean that we should stand by passively, but it does mean that we should not over-state our cause or pretend that we can permanently impact the conditions of this world.

Everywhere in nature we see the organization of classes of beings, and everywhere we also see the disorganization of it. Both occur at all times in one place or another. We also observe distortions in the classes, whereby a certain species of deer roam together in the forest but some are more capable of out-running their predators than others. This means that the classes of beings are haphazardly categorized. A group of human beings who form a clan, might feel that they are superior to another family clan. They might feel that such persons are below their level and that intermarriage should be prohibited. However history does not necessarily support such a claim. We find that some persons in a clan are below the standard of behavior advocated by the clan for itself. Thus the entire caste idea is flawed. This does not mean, however, that society should not be organized or that families should not protect themselves from cultural dilution. *Brahma yogi*s, however, should be level-headed and realize that the flaws in human nature are recurrent, and that human beings should endeavor to do their best, as guided by the Supreme Being. One should not exploit another class or set of human beings just to advance the family of one's birth. Such exploitation equates to the abuse of others, and it feeds a vicious, predatory attitude.

A human being from a high social order with a high standard of behavior, might in the next life, display vulgar and immoral behavior. Thus one's efforts at moral elevation may be thwarted, if not reversed entirely, by pressures of desire and circumstance. Unless one is commissioned by the Supreme Being, one should tend to one's purity and not be so concerned with others, since one cannot express the proper influence over any of them eternally.

संकरो नरकायैव
कुलघ्नानां कुलस्य च ।
पतन्ति पितरो ह्येषां
लुप्तपिण्डोदकक्रियाः ॥ १.४१ ॥

*saṁkaraḥ — sexual intermixture; narakāyaiva = narakāya — to hell + eva — indeed; kulaghnānāṁ = kula — clan + ghnānāṁ — destroyers; kulasya — of the clan; ca — and; patanti — are degraded; pitaro — the departed ancestors; hyeṣāṁ = hi — indeed +*

saṁkaro narakāyaiva
kulaghnānāṁ kulasya ca
patanti pitaro hyeṣāṁ
luptapiṇḍodakakriyāḥ (1.41)

*eṣām — of these; luptapiṇḍodakakriyāḥ = lupta — deprived of + piṇḍa — psychic cakes + udaka — psychic water + kriyāḥ — ceremonial rites*

**Indeed, the sexual intermixture causes the destroyers of the clan and the clan itself to go to hell. The departed ancestors of those clansmen, being deprived of the psychic cakes and water which are offered ceremonially, are degraded. (1.41)**

***Siddha Swami's Commentary:***

The departed ancestors *(pitaro, pitarah)* are those forbearers who left old bodies but did not acquire new ones. Every human being is potentially a departed ancestor. When one has a material body, one is addressed as a living human being. When one loses that body and has not acquired another, one is regarded as a departed ancestor or pitri. It is the duty of those who have living human forms to facilitate the entry of those without such bodies. This entails much responsibility since in the human form, a child's body does not reach maturity as quickly as it does in other life forms.

Responsibility is therefore the hedge that keeps the human species segregated from other life forms. If we do not help the departed ancestors, we imperil ourselves, for if we require bodies in the future, we will have to get such forms from the departed ancestors who became our children, grandchildren, and great grandchildren. If we circumvent the births of the ancestors, we, in effect, short-circuit our own chances for birth later on.

It does not matter if one is a *siddha* or an elevated being or a divine being; if one requires a human body, one will have to get that through sexual intercourse. It is irrelevant as to how the first man and woman came about, for regardless of that original procedure, it is now inoperative. What we must do now to generate human forms, is to perform an act of sexual intercourse. Hence that procedure is sacred and most valuable to anyone requiring a human form. The most important contribution one can make therefore as a human being is to give someone else a human body by sexual intercourse, but for responsibility sake, one should care for the off-spring until he or she reaches sexual maturity.

I am a *siddha*. I was known as *Bhagavān Nityānanda* to my disciples. But if I need a human body I will have to take one through sexual intercourse. Of course there are other dimensions where one can acquire a body without sexual intercourse. But If I require a body on earth, sexual intercourse is the means. Thus to me that is sacred. I do not take it lightly. No one should abuse sexual intercourse because it is our very lifeline to a body on the sacred earth. Arjuna was right to consider that careless sexual intercourse and permissive sexual life is ruinous to one and all.

If you take birth, you want it to occur in a decent family. You do not want to take it in a low class, vulgar family. You want to have a responsible father and mother. You do not prefer to be in an orphanage or to be eating food off the ground without the direction of a caring mother. And if you lose your body and have not become liberated, you will want to get back into the human world quickly so that you can again play some small or great part in history. Therefore everyone should think ahead and work for a bright future.

दोषैरेतैः कुलघ्नानां
वर्णसंकरकारकैः ।
उत्साद्यन्ते जातिधर्माः
कुलधर्माश्च शाश्वताः ॥ १.४२ ॥
doṣairetaiḥ kulaghnānāṁ
varṇasaṁkarakārakaiḥ
utsādyante jātidharmāḥ
kuladharmāśca śāśvatāḥ (1.42)

*doṣair — with sins; etaiḥ — by these; kulaghnānāṁ — of the family destroyers; varṇasaṁkarakārakaiḥ = varṇasaṁkara — sexual intermixture of classes + kārakaiḥ — by producing; utsādyante — disappeared; jātidharmāḥ — individual skills; kuladharmāś — family duties; ca — and; śāśvatāḥ — long-standing, traditional*

**By the sins of the family destroyers and by the sexual intermixture of the classes, individual skills and traditional family duties disappear. (1.42)**

***Siddha Swami's Commentary:***

Establishment of individual skills and relevant family duties help human beings to suppress animal urges. Thus when a culture of values and skills for saving time from animal pursuits is pursued, human beings rise up to advancement in religion and philosophy. This allows for curtailing animal tendencies which involve eating flesh and waging war on other clans.

Instead of a culture of living by killing, instead of barbarism, there develops a need to live by letting others survive as well, and this is civilization. In such an atmosphere, education becomes formalized and humanity begins to tame its animal tendencies.

This does not enable the human being to understand birth and death and what happens in between, but it does give some human beings more time to consider the realities which are unmanifested to physical eyes. From these considerations, they develop an inquest into the transcendental. Some human beings, however, do not take this opportunity to inquire into birth and death, but rather they try to increase the pursuits of science or pleasure. From science they derive sophisticated and more efficient ways of waging war and dominating others. From pleasure they gain more insight into how to expand vices. Thus the development of individual skills and family values (*jātidharmāh kuladharma*) leads in two separate directions, one for the development of transcendental insight and the other for the dominance of vices.

उत्सन्नकुलधर्माणां
मनुष्याणां जनार्दन ।
नरके ऽनियतं वासो
भवतीत्यनुशुश्रुम ॥ १.४३ ॥
utsannakuladharmāṇāṁ
manuṣyāṇāṁ janārdana
narake 'niyataṁ vāso
bhavatītyanuśuśruma (1.43)

*utsanna kula dharmāṇāṁ = utsanna — destroyed + kuladharmāṇāṁ — of family customs; manuṣyāṇām — of men; janārdana — O Kṛṣṇa; narake — in hell; 'niyataṁ = aniyatam — indefinitely; vāso — dwelling; bhavatītyanuśuśruma = bhavati — it is + iti — was developed + anuśuśruma — we heard repeatedly*

**O Krishna, those who destroy the family customs dwell in hell indefinitely. This was declared repeatedly. (1.43)**

***Siddha Swami's Commentary:***

Only those who destroy good family traditions and maintain bad ones go to hell. Arjuna's contention that he would go to hell if he opposed the corrupt Kauravas led by Duryodhana is incorrect. In protecting the family traditions, one is also required to prevent the family from corruption and unfair dominance, for that too is a cause for taking oneself and the family to hell. One must protect the family by not condoning its vices and by having in it a moral sense which results in political self-discipline.

A yogi should not be involved in politics but all the same, he has a responsibility to advise those receptive politicians who are. He should not be attached to family and should not encourage its promotion at the expense of others. If anything, his family mood should be directed to those who excel in dharmic, righteous lifestyle. The example is shown by Lord Krishna, the God, who supported King Yudhishthira, the man who symbolized righteousness. Since God backs righteousness, we yogis should do so vigorously, regardless of whether the proponent of fair means is a relative or not. And we should be against any relative who executes the unfair means.

The instruction from me is this: Resist and speak out against unfair means in your family. Support and praise fair means in any other family. If you can destroy corruption in your own family, do so. And if you can encourage fair means and righteous dealings in others, do so.

अहो बत महत्पापं
कर्तुं व्यवसिता वयम् ।
यद्राज्यसुखलोभेन
हन्तुं स्वजनमुद्यताः ॥ १.४४ ॥
aho bata mahatpāpaṁ
kartuṁ vyavasitā vayam
yadrājyasukhalobhena
hantuṁ svajanamudyatāḥ (1.44)

*aho — O!; bata — what a wonder!; mahat — great; pāpaṁ — sin; kartuṁ — to perform; vyavasitā — committed to; vayam — we; yad — which; rājyasukhalobhena = rājya — aristocratic + sukha — pleasure + lobhena — with greed; hantuṁ — to kill; svajanam — own folks; udyatāḥ — eager for*

**O! What a wonder! We are committed to perform a great sin, being eager to kill our kinfolk, through greed for aristocratic pleasures. (1.44)**

***Siddha Swami's Commentary:***

Somehow or the other Arjuna got under the emotionally perverse influence of the Kaurava people. Thus his line of reasoning was corrupted. *Śrī* Krishna was not there to obtain aristocratic pleasures, nor was the righteous Prince Yudhishthira, Arjuna's eldest brother. That reason was projected into the mind of Arjuna by the opponents in order to demotivate and demoralize him. It was effective because Arjuna began thinking in that way and was unable to take up the task which God assigned him.

A yogi should note that when one's attention shifts into a lower plane of consciousness, one views life in a completely different way. The same person who would make one decision on a certain level, would in turn make a completely opposite decision if his attention were shifted to another level. Hence a siddha yogi should study the way consciousness shifts from plane to plane and how it is influenced on the various levels.

Usually one mobilizes an army and attacks others for the sake of conquest to take their resources, to suppress them and to subjugate them. Still, there are other reasons for mobilizing an army. King Yudhishthira mobilized because he had a duty to represent righteousness and to suppress those who excelled at injustice.

Contrary to what Arjuna said, Prince Yudhishthira committed a great service, a pious act, in being eager to discipline or even to kill his own kinfolk, through the need to stop unfair politics and diplomatic corruptions.

यदि मामप्रतीकारम्
अशस्त्रं शस्त्रपाणयः ।
धार्तराष्ट्रा रणे हन्युस्
तन्मे क्षेमतरं भवेत् ॥ १.४५ ॥
yadi māmapratīkāram
aśastraṁ śastrapāṇayaḥ
dhārtarāṣṭrā raṇe hanyus
tanme kṣemataraṁ bhavet (1.45)

*yadi — if; mām — me; apratīkāram — unresisting; aśastraṁ — without weapons, unarmed; śastrapāṇayaḥ — those bearing weapons; dhārtarāṣṭrā — sons of Dhṛtarāṣtra; raṇe — in battle; hanyuḥ — they may kill; tan — this; me — to me; kṣemataraṁ — greater happiness; bhavet — would be*

**If the weapon-bearing sons of Dhṛtarāṣṭra should kill me in battle, while I was unresisting and unarmed, this to me would be greater pleasure. (1.45)**

***Siddha Swami's Commentary:***

This is the attitude of a martyr. Usually one adopts this attitude on the basis of inability to convince others to adopt one's views and in the hope of gaining the admiration of the public and those who doubted one's conviction. A *brahma yogi* avoids such a posture, because he realizes he has nothing to gain in this existence and that whatever is achieved here, will be wiped out by time. Nothing is permanent here. Everything is *asat* or temporarily manifested and then everything is changed by the sweep of time, without regard for one's objective. It is a sheer coincidence when time favors a man's plan, because the same time again reverses whatever it awarded the same man.

Many who are enslaved are freed in time and then are enslaved again. Those who are treated unfairly are compensated in time and then they are battered again. Thus whatever one may do for social equality or any such lofty human ideal, will be reversed by time. A *brahma yogi* may do good when allowed but he does not feel that it is permanent. He knows well that it is the play of time. He is merely an employed actor in the drama of time. It is not his mission to arouse feelings of pity or guilt in others about their activities. Everything is to be censored by the Supreme Being only. Others are merely assigned the task of levying the views of the Supreme; otherwise their reforming actions have little, if any, value.

Arjuna hoped to gain happiness by being killed while unarmed, in order to shame the Kauravas, instead of disciplining them outright. He preferred a non-violent, non-disciplinary approach. The Supreme Being, *Śrī* Krishna, did not agree to Arjuna's preference, because some persons do not feel guilty after committing horrible acts. Guilt is felt in those who have a conscience about the matter, but some do not have such a degree of judgment. Thus martyrdom does not affect their demeanor. Arjuna assumed that Duryodhana had guilt sensitivity but this was not the case, because Duryodhana was built with a different psychology. It would be left to Lord Krishna to effectively deal with Duryodhana. Persons like Duryodhana have yet to develop the sense of conscience of a person like Arjuna. Only the Supreme Being is masterful and perceptive enough to know what methods will cause a person like Duryodhana to develop the proper conscience.

एवमुक्त्वार्जुनः संख्ये
रथोपस्थ उपाविशत् ।
विसृज्य सशरं चापं
शोकसंविग्नमानसः ॥ १.४६ ॥

*evam — thus; uktvā — having spoken; arjunaḥ — Arjuna; saṁkhye — in the conflict; rathopastha = ratha — chariot + upastha — seat; upāviśat — sat down; visṛjya — casting aside; saśaraṁ — together*

evamuktvārjunaḥ saṁkhye
rathopastha upāviśat
visṛjya saśaraṁ cāpaṁ
śokasaṁvignamānasaḥ (1.46)

*with arrow; cāpaṁ — bow; śokasaṁvignamānasaḥ = śoka — sorrow + saṁvigna — overwhelmed + mānasaḥ — heart*

**Having spoken, Arjuna, who was in the midst of the conflict, sat down on his chariot. Casting aside his arrow and bow, he was overwhelmed with sorrow. (1.46)**

***Siddha Swami's Commentary:***

A limited being should not be caught in the middle of a conflict, unless he is authorized by providence to apply a solution. A person besieged in his own nature, ambivalent and emotionally-distressed, is of no use to providence when a decisive factor is required. Such a person should step aside from the occasion. The Supreme Being cannot be confused about any issue because He has the capacity to deal with any and all situations. Thus if someone is empowered by Him, that person should look to the God to get hints on what to do.

A limited being when left to his own devices, will more often than not, become confused. He will be emotionally distressed and agonized in many situations. A yogi should not take life upon his own shoulders but should realize that this life is governed by supernatural personalities. One should take hints from these people on the proper course of action.

# CHAPTER 2

## Buddhi Yoga

## Intellectual Discipline through Yoga*

*dūreṇa hyavaraṁ karma buddhiyogāddhanaṁjaya*
*buddhau śaraṇamanviccha kṛpaṇāḥ phalahetavaḥ (2.49)*

***Surely, cultural action is by far inferior to intellectual discipline through yoga. O victor of wealthy countries. (2.49)***

****Siddha Swami assigned this chapter title on the basis of verse 49 of this chapter.***

संजय उवाच
तं तथा कृपयाविष्टम्
अश्रुपूर्णाकुलेक्षणम् ।
विषीदन्तमिदं वाक्यम्
उवाच मधुसूदनः ॥२.१॥
saṁjaya uvāca
taṁ tathā kṛpayāviṣṭam
aśrupūrṇākulekṣaṇam
viṣīdantamidaṁ vākyam
uvāca madhusūdanaḥ (2.1)

*saṁjaya — Sanjaya; uvāca — said; taṁ — to him; tathā — in this way; kṛpayāviṣṭam — overcome with pity; aśrupūrṇākulekṣaṇam = aśru — tear + pūrṇa — filled + ākula — perplexed + īkṣaṇam — eyes; viṣīdantam — saddened with hopelessness; idaṁ — this; vākyam — response; uvāca — spoke; madhusūdanaḥ — killer of Madhu*

**Sanjaya said: To him who was overcome with pity, whose eyes were filled with tears, who was perplexed and saddened with hopelessness, the killer of Madhu spoke this response: (2.1)**

***Siddha Swami's Commentary:***

When overcome with pity, perplexed and saddened with hopelessness, one must either wait for the emotions to subside or act in the emotional state. If one waits, one may miss an opportunity. If one acts under impulse, one may regret the activity. If one is lucky, one may immediately seek out a wise personality in whom one has a great degree of faith.

Pity, perplexity, sadness and hopelessness are all banished in *brahma yoga*, because the yogi no longer takes shelter in the emotions of the psyche. This is in compliance with the instruction of *Śrī Patañjali*, that a yogi must by all means abandon the various operations of the *buddhi*. Pity is relational, being based on forgetting or ignoring the existence of the Supreme Being, and establishing relationships independent of His authority. Perplexity occurs when one feels that one should solve a problem but does not have the intellectual grasp of the factors which operate to produce the circumstance. Sadness comes about in the emotional nature when it is exposed to adversity. Hopelessness is felt when one is baffled by reality, whereby one feels that one cannot control a situation and that everything goes against one's favor. All of this is abandoned in the *brahma yoga* practice, by escaping from the levels where these occurences manifest. The occurences continue on their specific planes of existence, but since one abandons or becomes absent on such levels, one is unaffected and unaware of them. Other beings, however, continue to respond to those realities in their particular locale. They are affected in the normal way. A *brahma yogi* realizes that he is not needed in the world of pity, perplexity, sadness and hopelessness. Then he abandons those levels of psychology and allows others to flourish or perish there accordingly.

Sanjaya reported the hopelessness of Arjuna but *Dhṛtarāṣṭra* would soon be disappointed, because a very rare occurrence would take place, the speech of *Śrī* Krishna. Arjuna's hopelessness was favorable for *Dhṛtarāṣṭra*. If Arjuna gave in completely to dejection, then Yudhishthira could hardly win the war. Duryodhana would certainly achieve an easy victory, without having many casualties on the war field. King *Dhṛtarāṣṭra* hoped for this, but Sanjaya disturbed the King by reporting that *Śrī* Krishna would speak in response to Arjuna's emotional upset. It is a rare fortune to have *Śrī* Krishna or even a great *yogin* by one's side in times of perplexity. We must listen to *Śrī* Krishna, because He is the greatest of the *brahma* yogis. Thus whatever He said would be digested by all of us for upliftment.

श्रीभगवानुवाच
कुतस्त्वा कश्मलमिदं
विषमे समुपस्थितम् ।
अनार्यजुष्टमस्वर्ग्यम्
अकीर्तिकरमर्जुन ॥२.२॥
śrībhagavānuvāca
kutastvā kaśmalamidaṁ
viṣame samupasthitam
anāryajuṣṭamasvargyam
akīrtikaramarjuna (2.2)

*śrī bhagavān — the Blessed Lord; uvāca — said; kutastvā = kutas — how + tvā — to you; kaśmalam — sickly emotion; idaṁ — this; viṣame — at a crucial time; samupasthitam — come; anāryajuṣṭam — not suitable for a cultured man; asvargyam — not facilitating heaven in the hereafter; akīrtikaram — causing disgrace; arjuna — O Arjuna*

**The Blessed Lord said: How has this sickly emotion come to you at a crucial time? It is not suitable for a cultured man. It does not facilitate heaven in the hereafter. It causes disgrace, O Arjuna. (2.2)**

***Siddha Swami's Commentary:***

Who exactly is a cultured man by *Śrī* Krishna's definition? Who is the *ārya*? That person must be the *brahma yogi*, as we will see as we continue through the discourse. But if it were proven that to be cultured a person need not be as advanced as a *brahma yogin*, then at least that person should be expert in Vedic rites for promotion to the Swarga heavenly world hereafter *(svargyam).* By what operation did the sickly emotion take possession of Arjuna's psyche and compel him to abandon his caste duties?

क्लैब्यं मा स्म गमः पार्थ
नैतत्त्वय्युपपद्यते ।
क्षुद्रं हृदयदौर्बल्यं
त्यक्त्वोत्तिष्ठ परंतप ॥२.३॥
klaibyaṁ mā sma gamaḥ pārtha
naitattvayyupapadyate
kṣudraṁ hṛdayadaurbalyaṁ
tyaktvottiṣṭha paraṁtapa (2.3)

*klaibyaṁ — cowardly behavior; mā — not; sma — in fact; gamaḥ — should entertain; pārtha — O son of Patha; naitat — not this; tvayyupapadyate = tvayi — in your + upapadyate — is suitable; kṣudraṁ — degrading; hṛdayadaurbalyaṁ — emotional weakness; tyaktvottiṣṭha = tyaktva — give up + uttiṣṭha — stand up; paraṁtapa — scorcher of the enemy*

**O son of Pṛthā, you should not entertain cowardly behavior. This is not suitable for you. Give up this degrading emotional weakness. Stand, O scorcher of the enemy. (2.3)**

***Siddha Swami's Commentary***

It is possible to give up the degrading emotional weakness. One can do so suddenly and abruptly just as *Śrī* Krishna requested of Arjuna. As we see, Arjuna was unable to give it up that quickly, because Arjuna was not, at the time of his crisis, in the *brahma yoga* frame of mind. Unless one is established and recently practiced in the technique, one will succumb to the weakness and will have to wait until it wears off or has expended itself, before one can be freed from it. One will continually fall under its influences as soon as it draws sufficient energy and again overpowers the consciousness.

Arjuna was a scorcher of the enemy but he was yet to master the technique for scorching the emotional forces which carry the self in disillusionment and disempowerment. *Brahma yogis* get concerned with scorching the hostile influences within their nature. They use chivalry to master psychic influences. Arjuna focused on mastering persons who violated social laws. Thus he did not have the required proficiency in dealing with his emotional energies.

अर्जुन उवाच
कथं भीष्ममहं संख्ये
द्रोणं च मधुसूदन ।
इषुभिः प्रतियोत्स्यामि
पूजार्हावरिसूदन ॥२.४॥
arjuna uvāca
kathaṁ bhīṣmamahaṁ saṁkhye
droṇaṁ ca madhusūdana
iṣubhiḥ pratiyotsyāmi
pūjārhāvarisūdana (2.4)

*arjuna — Arjuna; uvāca — said; kathaṁ — how; bhīṣmam — Bhisma; ahaṁ — I; saṁkhye — in battle; droṇaṁ — Droṇa; ca — and; madhusūdana — O killer of Madhu; iṣubhiḥ — with arrows; pratiyotsyāmi — I will attack; pūjārhāv arisūdana = pūjārhāu — worthy of reverence + arisūdana — killer of the enemy, Krishna*

**Arjuna said: How will I attack in battle, Bhishma and Droṇa, who are worthy of reverence, O Krishna? (2.4)**

***Siddha Swami's Commentary:***

Arjuna discussed social reverence, social seniority, and not spiritual reverence which is due because a teacher mastered more advanced techniques and teaches the same. Social reverence, though important, is superficial to the soul. It addresses the status of one's body. Spiritual respect involves the relationship between one's soul and its subtle energies.

Both Bhisma and *Droṇa* were yogis of worth, who practiced *brahma yoga* and had some proficiency. However, their presence on the battlefield was for cultural reasons and not spiritual endeavors. In fact, both of them intended to use whatever mystic power they developed by yoga practice, for military proficiency. That is a misuse of yoga practice. *Śrī* Krishna chastised both of them for this.

When practicing yoga, one works for purity. That is a prime objective. If there is insufficient purity, one will fall back into the socio-cultural world and be forced to misuse whatever psychological expertise one developed through yoga. This will cause one to commit crimes against the Supreme.

There is certainly a social use for yoga, as we will hear from Lord Krishna about King Janak who was proficient in *karma yoga*. However, such social use of it is risky, unless one has the direct guidance of *Śrī* Krishna. Arjuna was lucky to have the Divine Lord as advisor.

So how can Arjuna attack revered seniors like Bhishma and *Droṇa*?: He can do so if he is instructed by the Supreme God, otherwise it would be risky for him to challenge any of them, even if they did something which appeared to him as wrong. Correcting others to establish righteousness is always risky if one is a limited being.

गुरूनहत्वा हि महानुभावान्
श्रेयो भोक्तुं भैक्ष्यमपीह लोके
हत्वार्थकामांस्तु गुरूनिहैव
भुञ्जीय भोगान्रुधिरप्रदिग्धान् ॥२.५॥
gurūnahatvā hi mahānubhāvān
śreyo bhoktuṁ bhaikṣyam
apīha loke
hatvārthakāmāṁstu gurūn ihaiva
bhuñjīya bhogān rudhira-
pradigdhān (2.5)

*gurūn — the revered teachers; ahatvā — not killing; hi — in fact; mahānubhāvān — great-natured; śreyo — better; bhoktuṁ — to eat; bhaikṣyamapīha = bhaikṣyam — begging + api — also + iha — here; loke — on earth; hatvārthakāmāṅs = hatvā — having killed + artha — on the basis of + kāmān — impulsive desires; tu — but; gurūn — revered teachers; ihaiva = iha — here + eva — indeed; bhuñjīya — I would enjoy; bhogān — luxuries; rudhirapradigdhān = rudhira — bloody + pradigdhān — stained*

**In fact, it is better to eat by begging in this world than by killing the revered teachers who are great-natured. But having slain the venerable teachers on the basis of impulsive desires, I would enjoy blood-stained luxuries here on earth. (2.5)**

***Siddha Swami's Commentary:***

Bhishma and *Droṇa* were fond of Arjuna. Both taught Arjuna many valuable lessons and shared with him skills in martial arts and political science. He was taught ideal social behavior by them. Remembering this, Arjuna can only respond to them with humility and appreciation. Because he took much from these persons in the social way, he felt that he could not enforce their reform. In the social world, one good turn deserves another. A person is therefore forced, by his own mood, not to correct a friend or a dear well wisher. In that way, one contributes to the downfall of a dear acquaintance or conscientious donor. One develops a predisposition of love, hate or indifference towards other living entities on the basis of social bodily interactions, irrespective of the spiritual relationship of the souls involved. These aspects are part of material creature existence and thus not part of the course of *brahma yoga*.

In this course, *Śrī* Krishna spoke of those who feel that this world is produced by lust only and that there is no God in control of the world to enable law and order. Arjuna is under the influence of a similar view that no one has a right to chastise another and that everyone should only see good in the other, always overlooking faults. This philosophy does not hold well with Lord Krishna.

If there is a God of this world, what are our duties to Him? Are we to form conclusions and act accordingly in each case? Should we act on His prompting? What part should any of us play in manifesting the desires of that God? Does that God have a right to use any of us to reform our fellows, elders, mothers and fathers? Are there consequences if we refuse to comply with that God? How can a person be sure that an action is God-ordained and not concocted by his own mind, leaving him with dire consequences?

न चैतद्विद्मः कतरन्नो गरीयो
यद्वा जयेम यदि वा नो जयेयुः ।
यानेव हत्वा न जिजीविषामस्
तेऽवस्थिताः प्रमुखे धार्तराष्ट्राः ॥२.६॥
na caitadvidmaḥ kataranno garīyo
yadvā jayema yadi vā no jayeyuḥ
yāneva hatvā na jijīviṣāmas
te'vasthitāḥ pramukhe
dhārtarāṣṭrāḥ (2.6)

*na — not; caitad — and this; vidmaḥ — we know; kataran — which of the alternatives; no = nah — for us; garīyo — is better; yad – which; vā — other; jayema — we should conquer; yadi — if; vā — or; no = naḥ — to us; jayeyuḥ — they should triumph over; yān — who; eva — indeed; hatvā — having killed; na — us; jijīviṣāmas — we desire to outlive; te — they; 'vasthitāḥ = avasthitāḥ — stand armed; pramukhe — before us; dhārtarāṣṭrāḥ — the sons of Dhṛtarāṣṭra*

**And this we do not know, which of the alternatives is better; whether we should conquer or if they should triumph over us. It concerns these sons of Dhṛtarāṣṭra who stand armed before us, and whom we would not desire to outlive, if they are killed. (2.6)**

***Siddha Swami's Commentary:***

The pros and cons, advantages or disadvantages of social life, and the participation or lack of it, hardly concerns a *brahma yogi*. He is not seeking results in this world. He is done with the idea that he can reap benefits or contrary results. By higher perception gained from *kriyā yoga*, he understands that the fulfilling or frustrating circumstances are there to be enjoyed or endured by the mento-emotional energies and its configurations, which are highlighted in female forms. The soul, stooge that it may be in this configuration, supplies energy which is magnetically drawn into the mindal space and emotional body. The soul does not directly connect to the mundane social circumstance. It cannot directly enjoy the material world. This is unknown except to those who mastered higher yoga.

One has nothing to gain in this material world, except to understand that one is always at a disadvantage in it and should strive to be liberated. Externally one cannot permanently conquer anyone, because all circumstances are washed out by the time factor and nearly every occurrence is upturned. One cannot be conquered in truth either, for even if one's body is killed by another, the person cannot enslave the spirit within the body. Once released from a body, a spirit usually goes into another dimension and, for the time being, escapes from the dimension of the dead body.

Since one may not be allowed to re-enter into a baby form in the same family in the next life, it is not a good idea to balance one's life on the scale of family relationship. One should strive to satisfy the Supreme Person since He is in a position to monitor future births. One should link up with spiritually perceptive teachers who are aware of transmigration and whose decisions are not based on having one body in a particular family.

कार्पण्यदोषोपहतस्वभावः
पृच्छामि त्वां धर्मसंमूढचेताः
यच्छ्रेयः स्यान्निश्चितं ब्रूहि तन्मे
शिष्यस्तेऽहं शाधि मां त्वां प्रपन्नम्
॥२.७॥

kārpaṇyadoṣopahata-
svabhāvaḥ
pṛcchāmi tvāṁ dharma-
saṁmūḍhacetāḥ
yacchreyaḥ syānniścitaṁ
brūhi tanme
śiṣyaste'haṁ śādhi māṁ
tvāṁ prapannam (2.7)

*kārpaṇyadoṣopahatasvabhāvaḥ = kārpaṇya — mercy-prone + doṣa — faulty weakness + upahata — overcome + svabhāvaḥ — my feelings (a person being afflicted with inappropriate mercy, a compulsive mercy-prone man); pṛcchāmi — I ask; tvāṁ — you; dharmasaṁmūḍhacetāḥ = dharma — sense of duty + sammūḍha — clouded by confusion + cetāḥ — mind (one whose sense of duty is clouded by confusion of mind); yacchreyaḥ = yac (yad) — which + chreyaḥ (śreyah) — is better; syān — it should be; niścitaṁ — for certain; brūhi — tell; tan — this; me — to me; śiṣyas — student; te — of yours; 'haṁ = aham — I; śādhi — instruct; mām — me; tvāṁ — you; prapannam — submission*

**As a mercy-prone man, overcome by these feelings of pity, with my sense of duty clouded by mental confusion, I ask You to tell me with certainty, what is preferable. I am a student of Yours. Instruct me, who submit to You. (2.7)**

***Siddha Swami's Commentary:***

Even though Arjuna was emotionally inclined, still he had the inclination to get advice from *Śrī* Krishna. He had confidence in *Śrī* Krishna. He wanted to lean on that confidence, since he reached an impasse after seeing the Kurus assembled in a violent mood.

Arjuna did not, however, just accept what *Śrī* Krishna told him initially. Instead Arjuna raised counter-questions. Finally *Śrī* Krishna instructed Arjuna to resolve the crisis within his nature by consultation with the Supreme Spirit who resides in the psyche of every living creature. This means that one who is very emotional will not accept what he is told by the Supreme Lord, nor by a valid agent of God. Such a person will raise doubts and related queries. If these are unresolved in a discourse with the God or agent of God, then that person will leave aside the divine advisory.

Ultimately one has to make up one's mind. Therefore it is important to advance to higher yoga, where one develops higher intuition and direct insight into higher realities. Since each spirit is a person, each must form opinions based on a certain amount of direct experience. Part of the divine life involves the cultivation of faith in the God as well as in His agents. That is not all. One must also develop higher sense perception to see into the workings of higher realities; otherwise one will always have doubts about the Supreme Being. On a lower level, certain laws of function play out, but on a higher level other methods operate. Therefore one must strive to reach the higher planes by developing the subtle body and then branching off to the causal. This will give one direct insight.

न हि प्रपश्यामि ममापनुद्याद्
यच्छोकमुच्छोषणमिन्द्रियाणाम् ।
अवाप्य भूमावसपत्नमृद्धं
राज्यं सुराणामपि चाधिपत्यम् ॥२.८॥

na hi prapaśyāmi mamāpanudyād
yacchokamucchoṣaṇam indriyāṇām
avāpya bhūmāvasapatnam ṛddhaṁ
rājyaṁ surāṇāmapi cādhipatyam (2.8)

*na — not; hi— in fact; prapaśyāmi — I see; mamāpanudyād = mama — of me + apanudyāt — should remove; yac (yad) — which; chokam (śokam) — sadness; ucchoṣaṇam — absorbs; indriyāṇām — sensual enthusiasm; avāpya — acquiring; bhūmāvasapatnam = bhūmau — on earth + asapatnam — unrivaled; ṛddham — prosperity; rājyaṁ — rulership; surāṇām — of the angelic kingdom; api — also; cādhipatyam = ca — and + adhipatyam — sovereignty*

**In fact, I do not see, what would remove the sadness that absorbs my enthusiasm, even unrivaled rulership and prosperity on earth or sovereignty over the angelic kingdom. (2.8)**

***Siddha Swami's Commentary:***

Each level of consciousness has particular moods and justifications for actions. Anyone on a certain plane, makes generally the same type of decision because the energy acts and reacts in one way. Arjuna mentioned all his perceived outcomes to the battle, namely, unrivaled rulership over the Kuru kingdom with prosperity on earth, or alternately, if he lost his body in battle or after ruling justly, sovereignty in the astral regions, the angelic worlds. None of this, however, is the objective of a *brahma yogi*. A *brahma yogi* in the same position as Arjuna, viewing the same battle, would not be looking for such outcomes. Arjuna perceived in this way because his senses remained under the influence of a lower emotional force, and those emotions sort through existence for those types of advantages.

Even though Arjuna tried to deny himself the benefits of winning the war or dying as a hero, still his nature held on to those benefits for the purpose of contrasting the sadness it endured. His nature itself relished the sadness and could not free itself from trauma. Thus Arjuna had no control over the fluids of emotion which flooded his psyche. Fighting a battle for the sake of establishing righteousness and removing a corrupt brazen government has nothing to do with a desire for rulership or a desire for heaven. It deals with duty for a just human society. That is how a *brahma yogi* would view this.

संजय उवाच
एवमुक्त्वा हृषीकेशं
गुडाकेशः परंतप ।
न योत्स्य इति गोविन्दम्
उक्त्वा तूष्णीं बभूव ह ॥२.९॥
saṁjaya uvāca
evamuktvā hṛṣīkeśaṁ
guḍākeśaḥ paraṁtapa
na yotsya iti govindam
uktvā tūṣṇīṁ babhūva ha (2.9)

*saṁjaya – Sanjaya; uvāca — said; evam — thus; uktvā — having appealed to; hṛṣīkeśaṁ — Kṛṣṇa; guḍākeśaḥ — Arjuna; paraṁtapa — scorcher of enemies; na – not; yotsya — I will fight; iti — thus; govindam — chief of the cowherds; uktvā — having spoken; tūṣṇīṁ — silently; babhūva — became; ha — indeed*

**Sanjaya said: O Dhṛtarāṣṭra, scorcher of enemies, after appealing to Krishna, Arjuna said to Govinda, the chief of cowherds, "I will not fight." Having said this, he became silent. (2.9)**

***Siddha Swami's Commentary:***

A person who is saturated with emotional energy will cooperate with the Supreme Lord, when the Lord contributes to the flow of that energy. If the Lord's instructions run contrary to the pleasurable aspirations of that energy, the person will be unable to cooperate.

Sanjaya rightfully addressed blind King *Dhṛtarāṣṭra*, as scorcher of the enemies, since the king and his sons were expert at intimidation. Arjuna was humbled by the experience of the war-ready Kauravas and thus he told *Śrī* Krishna that he would not fight. This was a victory for *Dhṛtarāṣṭra*, who was hopeful that somehow by emotional means there would be a truce prior to the battle of *Kurukṣetra*.

By practicing *brahma yoga*, one can move one's nature into a new state, whereby one cooperates with *Śrī* Krishna at all times, not just when Krishna facilitates one's emotions. But who is Krishna? Sanjaya addressed the Lord as Govinda, the chief of the cowherds. Actually *Śrī* Krishna's material status is not important. It is His spiritual power. The Kurus were in charge of that area of India, not *Śrī* Krishna. *Dhṛtarāṣṭra* was the king there. Still, because Krishna is God, His lowly status as a cowherd did not decrease His influence and power. Arjuna's refusal to fight dealt little with *Śrī* Krishna's enforcement of righteous living. Thus *Dhṛtarāṣṭra*'s hopes for victory were frustrated by the design of Krishna. If all the powerful rulers of the earth were to stand together against *Śrī* Krishna, they would lose, what to speak of the clan of King *Dhṛtarāṣṭra*. *Śrī* Krishna explained that it was His war, this war of the Kurus. Thus Arjuna's crippling emotions could not stop the victory of Prince Yudhishthira.

तमुवाच हृषीकेशः
प्रहसन्निव भारत ।
सेनयोरुभयोर्मध्ये
विषीदन्तमिदं वचः ॥२.१०॥
tamuvāca hṛṣīkeśaḥ
prahasanniva bhārata
senayorubhayormadhye
viṣīdantamidaṁ vacaḥ (2.10)

*tam — to him; uvāca — spoke; hṛṣīkeśaḥ — Kṛṣṇa; prahasan — smiling; iva — like; bhārata — O descendant of Bharata; senayoḥ — of the two armies; ubhayoḥ — of both; madhye — in the middle; viṣīdantam — dejected; idaṁ — this; vacaḥ — speech*

**Then, in the middle of both armies, Krishna, who was smiling, spoke this speech to the dejected Arjuna. (2.10)**

***Siddha Swami's Commentary:***

Since the king only regarded himself as a clansman and not as a servant of the God of the creation, Sanjaya sarcastically addressed him as descendant of *Bharata*. Such a title however is superficial, for in the past life, the blind king may have been in another family line, and in the future, he could be assigned to any planet or dimension or to different parents.

What was a disturbance to the emotions of Arjuna was no irritation to the feelings of *Śrī* Krishna. Krishna smiled and spoke to the dejected warrior. *Dhṛtarāṣṭra* may have wondered why *Śrī* Krishna smiled while Arjuna was shocked with dejection and grief.

श्रीभगवानुवाच
अशोच्यानन्वशोचस्त्वं
प्रज्ञावादांश्च भाषसे ।
गतासूनगतासूंश्च
नानुशोचन्ति पण्डिताः ॥२.११॥
śrībhagavānuvāca
aśocyānanvaśocastvaṁ
prajñāvādāṁśca bhāṣase
gatāsūnagatāsūṁśca
nānuśocanti paṇḍitāḥ (2.11)

*śrī-bhagavān — the Blessed Lord; uvāca — said; aśocyān — that which should be regretted; anvaśocas — mourned; tvaṁ — you; prajñāvādāṁś — intelligent statements; ca — and; bhāṣase — you express; gatāsūn — departed souls; agatāsūṁś — those not departed; ca — and; nānuśocanti = na — not + anuśocanti — mourn; paṇḍitāḥ — educated persons*

**The Blessed Lord said: You mourned for that which should not be regretted. And you expressed intelligent statements. Educated persons mourn neither for those who are embodied nor departed. (2.11)**

***Siddha Swami's Commentary:***

Even though Arjuna made statements which would have legal value in a court of law, still Arjuna's application of those rulings was perverse. This meant that Arjuna's emotions took support from the philosophy of great sages who transcended bodily social life. Arjuna had, in effect, misused the philosophy.

From the perspective of the Upanishads and the *Smṛti* law books, the material body should not be regretted even though social laws are, ultimately, for the protection of that very same form. It is the value of the form for cultivating spiritual realization, which gives the form its importance. Irreligious activities damage a person's ability to pursue spiritual life. Therefore the law books do not issue rulings to protect irreligion. In fact such books condemn and give methods for the suppression of vices.

न त्वेवाहं जातु नासं
न त्वं नेमे जनाधिपाः ।
न चैव न भविष्यामः
सर्वे वयमतः परम् ॥२.१२॥
na tvevāhaṁ jātu nāsaṁ
na tvaṁ neme janādhipāḥ
na caiva na bhaviṣyāmaḥ
sarve vayamataḥ param (2.12)

*na — no; tvevāhaṁ = tv (tu) — in fact + eva — alone + aham — I; jātu — ever; nāsaṁ = na — not + āsam — I did exist; na — nor; tvaṁ — you; neme = na — nor + ime — these; jana-adhipāḥ — rulers of the people; na — not; caiva — and indeed; na — nor; bhaviṣyāmaḥ — we will exist; sarve — all; vayam — we; ataḥ — from now; param — onwards*

**There was never a time when I did not exist, nor you, nor these rulers of the people. Nor will we cease to exist from now onwards. (2.12)**

***Siddha Swami's Commentary:***

This basic knowledge of the yogis and basic belief of the Vedic religion underscores the contrasting value of the temporary body, taken on by the same eternal spirit described in this verse. The singularity of a spirit, as well as his eternity is asserted here by the Supreme Lord. Arjuna put all value on the temporary bodies of family members. He felt that their bodies should not be harmed, even if their greed-possessed minds caused them not to see the fault caused by destruction of the family or the crime of hurting a friend in social dealings. Arjuna was against stringent disciplines.

A material body holds value but never the value of an eternal spirit. The Supreme Being would never levy a greater value for the temporary body. The body may be dispensed with for the sake of the spirit. And for that matter, the Supreme Spirit is more concerned with the effects of the body on a spirit, than with the body itself for its own sake. If a body causes a spirit to develop bad habits, then that body may not be worth its continuation. These decisions should be made by the Supreme Spirit, since the cultivation of bad habits are necessary in the course of this existence, for the purpose of the individual spirits developing first-hand knowledge about the experiences.

Arjuna was not sorting between the value of the spirits of his relatives and the value of their bodies. He was rating their spirits and bodies as one composite personality. Such a vision is incorrect. All such calculations are flawed indeed. Thus *Śrī* Krishna corrected that error of Arjuna.

*Śrī* Krishna does not give Arjuna or anyone else a license to kill bodies. *Śrī* Krishna stated that in social life, when calculating how to act, one should always remember that none of the personalities involved is its body, and that each personality is eternally existing.

By a law of spiritual nature, no one is allowed to kill another person. The resentments which are highlighted by the killing of bodies, occur to the equipment of the spirits and not to the spirits themselves, but, since the spirits are temporarily fused to their psychologies, they are affected by the status of their acquired bodies. For a sensible discussion about social life, there must be agreement that the spirits are eternal, though they appear to be affected by the temporary bodies.

देहिनोऽस्मिन्यथा देहे
कौमारं यौवनं जरा ।
तथा देहान्तरप्राप्तिर्
धीरस्तत्र न मुह्यति ॥२.१३॥

dehino'sminyathā dehe
kaumāraṁ yauvanaṁ jarā
tathā dehāntaraprāptir
dhīrastatra na muhyati (2.13)

*dehinaḥ — of the embodied soul; 'smin = asmin — in this; yathā — as; dehe — in the body; kaumāraṁ — in childhood; yauvanam — in youth; jarā — in old age; tathā — so in sequence; dehāntaraprāptir = deha — body + antara — another + prāptiḥ — acquirement; dhīraḥ — wise person; tatra — on this topic; na — not; muhyati — is confused*

**As the embodied soul endures childhood, youth and old age, so another body is acquired in sequence. The wise person is not confused on this topic. (2.13)**

***Siddha Swami's Commentary:***

We must agree with *Śrī* Krishna that bodies are acquired one after another by each spirit. Sometimes it takes a year to acquire another body. Sometimes it takes a few hours. Sometimes it takes thousands of years. Regardless, in all cases, bodies are acquired by the spirit in sequence. We must accept this either as a belief handed down to us by Lord Krishna or as a psychic fact which we experience personally. With this premise, we may proceed in the lessons of the *Bhagavad Gītā*. Wise persons, whose psyches are stabilized in mystic perception, are not confused on this topic. This is due to spiritual perception, derived from the lack of a strong focus into material existence.

मात्रास्पर्शास्तु कौन्तेय
शीतोष्णसुखदुःखदाः ।
आगमापायिनोऽनित्यास्
तांस्तितिक्षस्व भारत ॥२.१४॥
mātrāsparśāstu kaunteya
śītoṣṇasukhaduḥkhadāḥ
āgamāpāyino'nityās
tāṁstitikṣasva bhārata (2.14)

*mātrāsparśāḥ — mundane sensations; tu — but; kaunteya — O son of Kuntī; śītoṣṇasukhaduḥkhadāḥ = śīta — cold + usna — heat + sukha — pleasure + duḥkha — pain + dāḥ — causing; āgamāpāyino = āgama — coming + apāyinaḥ — going; 'nityās = anityāḥ — not manifested continually; tāṁs — them; titikṣasva — you should cope; bhārata — O man of the Bharata family*

**O son of Kuntī, mundane sensations which cause cold and heat, pleasure and pain, do come and go. Cope with them, O man of the Bharata family. (2.14)**

***Siddha Swami's Commentary:***

In this existence, no one can permanently remove heat and cold, pleasure and pain and other types of polarity. These features are the natural potential of this location. Thus, one should learn to tolerate these, at least until one can relocate to a place with a different type of nature. Right now, so long as we are located in a place like this, our response will depend on the type of body we received. If, for instance, one has a very furry skin, then a hot place will be disliked. Another one with a thin skin which freezes easily will prefer a heated location. Thus the selections we make in the material world are usually based on the type of body we inhabit. It should not be said therefore that a bodily preference is a spiritual one. It is not necessarily so.

In advanced yoga practice, we sometimes meet persons who use fiery bodies or radioactive forms on the sun planet, but if those persons were transferred into earthly bodies, they could not tolerate being so close to the sun. This shows clearly that it is the body which usually dictates our preferences.

*Śrī* Krishna advised Arjuna to become detached from weather conditions and sensations. Weather conditions are external to one's body, while sensations concern the inner workings of one's form. It may be said that sensations are weather conditions within one's psyche. *Śrī* Krishna wanted Arjuna to practice detachment both outside and inside his body.

Even though, normally, *Śrī* Krishna does not regard a person by family designation, in this case, because of Arjuna's mental condition, the Lord addressed Arjuna in the conventional way as a member of the *Bhārata* family. This means that even if we insist on identifying ourselves only as our present family clan, then even so, we should keep in mind that the clan-body is temporary, and the feelings within the body are limited and prejudiced. Thus we should not allow such feelings to be our sole reference.

यं हि न व्यथयन्त्येते
पुरुषं पुरुषर्षभ ।
समदुःखसुखं धीरं
सोऽमृतत्वाय कल्पते ॥२.१५॥
yaṁ hi na vyathayantyete
puruṣaṁ puruṣarṣabha
samaduḥkhasukhaṁ dhīraṁ
so'mṛtatvāya kalpate (2.15)

*yaṁ — whosoever; hi — indeed; na — not; vyathayantyete = vyathayanti — afflict + ete — these mundane sensations; puruṣaṁ — that person; puruṣarṣabha — O bull among men; samaduḥkhasukhaṁ — steady in miserable and enjoyable conditions; dhīraṁ — wise man; so — he; 'mṛta tvāya = amṛtatvāya — to immortality; kalpate — is fit*

**O bull among men, these mundane sensations do not afflict the wise man who is steady in miserable or enjoyable conditions. That person is fit for immortality. (2.15)**

***Siddha Swami's Commentary:***

Besides the sensations which tell us that certain external conditions are unfavorable and that certain moods are unpleasant, there is a state of mind which is unresponsive to the miserable or enjoyable conditions. A trained yogi learns to cling to that sober state, even while enduring miserable external conditions and conflicting moods. Gradually his mind becomes more and more distant from the plane of consciousness where the moods predominate.

Every spirit is immortal, but in this world, most spirits identify with the temporary body. Subsequently, most spirits feel threatened by the changing structures in material nature. They do not realize their immortality. By remaining anchored in the sober mood, one becomes fit to know of one's eternal nature. Thus one loses the fear of the changing psychology and physiology.

नासतो विद्यते भावो
नाभावो विद्यते सतः ।
उभयोरपि दृष्टोऽन्तस्
त्वनयोस्तत्त्वदर्शिभिः ॥२.१६॥
nāsato vidyate bhāvo
nābhāvo vidyate sataḥ
ubhayorapi dṛṣṭo'ntas
tvanayostattvadarśibhiḥ (2.16)

*nāsato = na — no + asatas — of the non-substantial things; vidyate — there is; bhāvo — enduring existence; nābhāvo = na — no + abhāvaḥ — lack of existence; vidyate — there is; sataḥ — substantial things; ubhayoḥ — of the two; api — also; dṛṣṭaḥ — perceived; 'ntas = antaḥ — certainty; tvanayos = tu — but + anayoḥ — of these two; tattvadarśibhiḥ = tattva — reality + darśibhiḥ — by mystic powers*

**Of the non-substantial things, there is no enduring existence. Of the substantial things, there is no lack of existence. These two truths were perceived with certainty by the mystic seers of reality. (2.16)**

***Siddha Swami's Commentary:***

Non-substantial things are impressionable upon an untrained, mystically-unresponsive mind. Even though they have no enduring existence, they make their impact upon the untrained mind. They leave impressions as memory and tendency. These must be dealt with in higher yoga or there will be no success for the aspiring spiritualist. Whatever is substantial is enduring forever, but that is too subtle to make an impact on a normal mind. Thus one has to develop the supernatural insight to perceive that. This is why in this world, almost everything is ordered by the convention of non-substantial things.

Arjuna, being a representative of convention, can hardly agree with *Śrī* Krishna's idea, because normal insight tells the spirit, that the non-substantial is real and solid, while the substantial appears as unreal and non-existent. One must therefore agree to be trained by

*Śrī* Krishna or alternately by a mystic seer, in order to see objects in the transcendence.

The *tattvadarśis* see tangible objects in the subjective world, but these things are blank to others. The seers' research is given in the Upanishads, and in the *Purāṇas* and their subsidiary literature. We should have confidence in this. Still it is left to us to develop the insight for ourselves. Assuming that each spirit has the capacity to develop transcendental perception, each would have to apply disciplines which aid in its cultivation.

अविनाशि तु तद्विद्धि
येन सर्वमिदं ततम् ।
विनाशमव्ययस्यास्य
न कश्चित्कर्तुमर्हति ॥२.१७॥
avināśi tu tadviddhi
yena sarvamidaṁ tatam
vināśamavyayasyāsya
na kaścitkartumarhati (2.17)

*avināśi — indestructible; tu — indeed; tad — that factor; viddhi — know; yena — by which; sarvam — all; idaṁ — this world; tatam — is pervaded; vināśam — destructible; avyayasyāsya — of the everlasting principle; na — no; kaścit — anyone; kartum — to accomplish; arhati — can*

**Know that indestructible factor by which all this world is pervaded. No one can accomplish the destruction of that everlasting principle. (2.17)**

***Siddha Swami's Commentary:***

Most of what *Śrī* Krishna explained may be taken at face value, at least until one is able to develop the subtle and super-subtle perception required to deny or confirm it. If the spirit is eternal, then obviously its destruction could not be effected. It would have to be the basis for the transmigrations from one body to another. Everything is built on a foundation, just as we put buildings on the earth on the basis of the earth's location in space. Thus the subtle body which we use in dreams, our psychology, would have to function on another principle which is called the spirit. The gross body functions on the basis of the subtle one which is a psychology made up of mental energy and emotions, but those subtle powers themselves function on the basis of the indestructible factor, the spirit *(avināśi)*.

At first a human being identifies itself as a material body. Later after careful observation and some training, the human being may transcend the gross body and regard itself as a mentality with emotions or as emotions with a mentality. Then, the human being may go further to transcend the emotions and mentality. That is the science of *brahma yoga*. In a dream one may not identify with one's gross body; one may only identify with one's emotions and mentality. In some dreams one becomes shorn of one's mentality and experiences oneself as horrific or blissful emotions only, while in other dreams one may experience the predominance of rational mental energy. This all proves that the identification of the self may be applied to subtle or gross energies. Thus the identifier is separate from the linked energies or emotions. This must be carefully checked in higher meditation practice.

अन्तवन्त इमे देहा
नित्यस्योक्ताः शरीरिणः ।
अनाशिनोऽप्रमेयस्य
तस्माद्युध्यस्व भारत ॥२.१८॥

*antavanta — terminal; ime — these; dehā — bodies; nityasyoktāḥ = nityasya — of the eternal + uktāḥ — it is declared; śarīriṇaḥ — of the embodied soul; anāśinaḥ — of the indestructible; 'prameyasya = aprameyasya — of the*

antavanta ime dehā
nityasyoktāḥ śarīriṇaḥ
anāśino'prameyasya
tasmādyudhyasva bhārata (2.18)

*immeasurable; tasmāt — therefore; yudhyasva — fight; bhārata — O descendant of Bharata*

**It is declared that the bodies of the eternal, indestructible, immeasurable embodied soul are terminal. Therefore fight, descendent of the Bharatas. (2.18)**

***Siddha Swami's Commentary:***

If the spirit has a body, then what sort of body is it? Each student yogi must work to discover this for himself. Some say that it has no body. Others testify that it has a spiritual body. Which of these views is correct? In this instant, I speak neither of the material nor subtle body used in dreams. I speak of the spirit itself. Is the spirit itself a body? What is it? Does it have a form? Some say it has a form. Others argue that it is formless. There are many people who haggle over the nature of the super-subtle and illusive spirit, but most of them did not take the time to observe the spirit.

*Deha* means the material body, the one which develops from an embryo to an adult. That body is terminal. On this we agree. But what of the spirit itself? Is the spirit itself a body? Does its influence have a limit? Is there any type of edge to it? Is it enclosed? Does it have a membrane or border?

*Śrī* Krishna advised Arjuna to fight since the body which Arjuna was concerned about was terminal anyway. Nothing Arjuna or anyone could do would stop the physical body from deteriorating. It could not exist forever. Therefore it should not be treated as something eternal. If misused, the subtle body would be affected by a demerit. If used properly, there would be a merit.

य एनं वेत्ति हन्तारं
यश्चैनं मन्यते हतम् ।
उभौ तौ न विजानीतो
नायं हन्ति न हन्यते ॥२.१९॥
ya enaṁ vetti hantāraṁ
yaścainaṁ manyate hatam
ubhau tau na vijānīto
nāyaṁ hanti na hanyate (2.19)

*ya — who; enaṁ — this embodied soul; vetti — concludes; hantāraṁ — the killer; yaścainaṁ = yas — who + ca — and + inam — this embodied soul; manyate — thinks; hatam — is killed; ubhau — both; tau — two viewers; na— not; vijānītaḥ— understood; nāyaṁ = na — not + ayam — this embodied soul; hanti — kill; na — nor; hanyate — can be killed*

**Both viewers do not understand, namely: He who concludes that the embodied soul is the killer and he who thinks that the embodied soul is killed. The embodied soul does not kill nor can he be killed. (2.19)**

***Siddha Swami's Commentary:***

The embodied souls could not, by killing another's gross body, kill that other person's soul. A suicidist, for instance, cannot kill his own spirit. He cannot get rid of his subtle body, which is much more enduring than any gross form he may kill. The suicidist can only kill his gross body, and even that cannot be done in all circumstances. Sometimes a prisoner becomes so disillusioned, that he desires to find a means for killing his body. Some take to starvation, some strangulation, some to fatal wounds. Some others who try to kill their own bodies fail at it, either by too feeble an attempt or through circumstances which prohibit death. Since even killing a gross body can be perplexing, what can be said of killing the subtle body which is used in dreams, or the causal form which most human beings cannot perceive, or the spirit itself which is so abstract that its existence is questioned or disbelieved.

Unless it can control physical means, a spirit cannot kill the gross body of another spirit. Even those who succeed in killing other gross bodies, need to be expedited by providence, for unless one is in the right place at the right time, one cannot kill the body of another entity. One has to be graced by being in the proper location, having opportunity and having the right means for killing any other gross life form. The human beings, for instance, are the superior life form on this earthly planet. Still, we see that a small insect might outsmart the human being. A farmer might try to kill an agricultural pest but the creature might survive anyway. This is all due to providence. By fate, even the superior human being cannot protect his gross form from death.

न जायते म्रियते वा कदा चिन्
नायं भूत्वा भविता वा न भूयः ।
अजो नित्यः शाश्वतोऽयं पुराणो
न हन्यते हन्यमाने शरीरे ॥२.२०
na jāyate mriyate vā kadā cin
nāyaṁ bhūtvā bhavitā vā na bhūyaḥ
ajo nityaḥ śāśvato'yaṁ purāṇo
na hanyate hanyamāne śarīre (2.20)

*na — not; jāyate — is born; mriyate — dies; vā — either; kadācin — at any time; nāyaṁ = na — nor + ayam — this embodied soul; bhūtvā — having been; bhavitā — will be; vā — or; na — not; bhūyaḥ — again; ajo — birthless; nityaḥ — perpetual; śāśvataḥ — eternal; 'yaṁ = ayam — this; purāṇaḥ — primeval; na — not; hanyate — is killed; hanyamāne — in the act of killing; śarīre — in the body*

**This embodied soul is not born, nor does it die at any time, nor having existed will it not be. Being birthless, eternal, perpetual and primeval, it is not slain in the act of killing the body. (2.20)**

***Siddha Swami's Commentary:***

The gross body, which at this time, is the point of reference, is opposed to the spirit, for while the spirit will endure beyond the life of the body, the body itself as a conglomeration of energies, will separate from the spirit. This may cause psychological distress in the subtle body which is used in dreams. The body develops in the mother's womb by the subtle influences of the spirit, but the same body will in time become unresponsive to the same spirit which caused its development. Thus ultimately the body is opposed to the spirit. At times the subtle material energies respond favorably to the spirit and seem to compliment it, but at other times these same energies are hostile to it. So in *brahma yoga*, one is required to develop detachment, even to the favorable responses of material nature, since in time, these same powers will effectively resist one's influences.

वेदाविनाशिनं नित्यं
य एनमजमव्ययम् ।
कथं स पुरुषः पार्थ
कं घातयति हन्ति कम् ॥२.२१॥
vedāvināśinaṁ nityaṁ
ya enamajamavyayam
kathaṁ sa puruṣaḥ pārtha
kaṁ ghātayati hanti kam (2.21)

*vedāvināśinaṁ = veda — knows + avināśinam — indestructible; nityaṁ — eternal; ya = yaḥ — who; enam — this; ajam — not born, birthless; avyayam — imperishable; kathaṁ — how; sa = saḥ — he; puruṣaḥ — person; pārtha — O son of Partha; kaṁ — whom; ghātayati — causes to kill; hanti — kills (directly); kam — whom*

**O son of Pṛthā, how can the person who knows this indestructible, eternal, birthless and imperishable principle, cause someone to be killed or even kill someone directly? (2.21)**

***Siddha Swami's Commentary:***

One must start to not regard the physical body as the person. If we think that the cultural identity of the person is the person, then still we may sort that into a physical body, a subtle one used in dreaming, and a transcendental principle which goes dormant in sleep. *Śrī* Krishna's focus is on the transcendental principle, which is the most elusive to gross sense perception. The physical body does house the subtle form and the elusive transcendental principle, but that body itself is different from the other two factors which make up the human personality. In that case, if the gross body were to die, then the subtle body and the transcendental principle would continue to exist.

One cannot kill the subtle body or the transcendental principle due to the subtlety of such forms. *Śrī* Krishna chided Arjuna over his lamentation for the possible deaths of the personalities of Bhishma and *Droṇa*. Only the gross bodies of those two men would be killed. Arjuna was incapable of eradicating their subtle forms and their transcendental selves. The subtle form may be hurt emotionally. In fact Arjuna was himself hurt in that way, when he casts aside weapons and sat on the chariot. But even though it may be hurt emotionally, the subtle form cannot be killed by a limited being. And certainly the elusive, transcendental principle which appears to be dormant in deep sleep, cannot be touched by physical objects or even by emotional assaults.

वासांसि जीर्णानि यथा विहाय
नवानि गृह्णाति नरोऽपराणि ।
तथा शरीराणि विहाय जीर्णा;न्य्
अन्यानि संयाति नवानि देही ॥ २.२२ ॥
vāsāṁsi jīrṇāni yathā vihāya
navāni gṛhṇāti naro'parāṇi
tathā śarīrāṇi vihāya jīrṇāny
anyāni saṁyāti navāni dehī (2.22)

*vāsāṁsi — clothing; jīrṇāni — worn out; yathā — as when; vihāya — discarded; navāni — new; gṛhṇāti — takes; naro = naraḥ — person; 'parāṇi = aparāṇi — others; tathā — so; śarīrāṇi — bodies; vihāya — abandoned; jirṇāny = worn-out; anyāni — others; saṁyāti — encounters; navāni — new; dehī — the embodied soul*

**As when discarding old clothing, a person takes new garments, so the embodied soul abandons old bodies taking new ones. (2.22)**

***Siddha Swami's Commentary:***

We should always remember that a body-prone spirit, will take one body after another in sequence, as a matter of course, so long as the material nature permits. The proneness to taking bodies causes the spirit to helplessly achieve one body after another, as a function of its unexplained attraction to material nature.

The assumption of bodies in sequence does not depend on determination. It happens by a causeless attraction between a spirit and subtle material nature. In fact, the very same emotional energy which crippled Arjuna and forced him to reconsider his involvement at *Kurukṣetra*, is the force which operates the continuous quest for material forms.

This force can be neutralized if a particular spirit develops a resistance to it, not otherwise. That resistance does not come naturally. It comes by repeated effort at higher detachment in yoga practice. *Śrī* Krishna is correct in showing Arjuna that no one should be anxious about the possibility of taking another body, since that is the most natural occurrence. Unless he develops a special resistance, it is impossible for a disembodied soul not to take another physical body.

नैनं छिन्दन्ति शस्त्राणि
नैनं दहति पावकः ।
न चैनं क्लेदयन्त्यापो
न शोषयति मारुतः ॥२.२३॥
nainaṁ chindanti śastrāṇi
nainaṁ dahati pāvakaḥ
na cainaṁ kledayantyāpo
na śoṣayati mārutaḥ (2.23)

*nainaṁ = na — not + enam — this; chindanti — pierce; śastrāṇi — weapons; nainaṁ = na — not + enam — this; dahati — burns; pāvakaḥ — fire; na — not; cainaṁ = ca — and + enam — this; kledayantyāpo = kledayanti — soak + āpo = āpaḥ — water; na — nor; śoṣayati — dry out; mārutaḥ — the wind*

**Weapons do not pierce, fire does not burn, and water does not wet, nor does the wind dry that embodied soul. (2.23)**

***Siddha Swami's Commentary:***

This brings to our attention, that despite our impulsion for these material bodies, still our essential spirits are distinct from the temporary forms, which are pierceable, burnable, wetable and dryable. Even the subtle bodies which we use in dreams are distinguished from the gross ones which are not as durable. For instance, a bullet may kill the gross form, but it cannot kill the subtle one. Water may cause the gross one to drown but water cannot drown the subtle one. Even though it is not always possible to remember these distinctions, still a *yogin* should make every effort to recall and to integrate this information into his consciousness by repeated experiences of mystic yoga.

There one may research and properly understand by direct experience the various capacities of the various bodies which may be adopted in the course of this varied existence. Repeated experiences in the subtle world, day after day in conscious dreams and in the visions of meditation, gives a *yogin* direct insight into the nature of the various forms.

अच्छेद्योऽयमदाह्योऽयम्
अक्लेद्योऽशोष्य एव च ।
नित्यः सर्वगतः स्थाणुर्
अचलोऽयं सनातनः ॥२.२४॥
acchedyo'yamadāhyo'yam
akledyo'śoṣya eva ca
nityaḥ sarvagataḥ sthāṇur
acalo'yaṁ sanātanaḥ (2.24)

*acchedyaḥ — not to be pierced; 'yam = ayam — this; adāhyo = adāhyaḥ — not to be burnt; 'yam = ayam — this; akledyo = akledyaḥ — not to be moistened; 'śoṣya = aśoṣya — not to be dried; eva — indeed; ca — and; nityaḥ — eternal; sarvagataḥ — penetrant of all things; sthāṇuḥ — a permanent principle; acalo = acalaḥ — unmoving; 'yaṁ = ayam — this; sanātanaḥ — primeval*

**This embodied soul cannot be pierced, cannot be burnt, cannot be moistened and cannot be dried. And indeed, this soul is eternal. It can penetrate all things. It is a permanent principle and is stable and primeval. (2.24)**

***Siddha Swami's Commentary:***

As a tiny particle can enter the smallest spaces in any other coarse material, so the spirit may enter into the dimensional inter-layers which composite anything. It is this penetrating nature of the spirit which makes it difficult to define and near impossible to perceive except through its assumption of grossness by indirect influences.

In modern science, no one doubts that radio waves may pass through concrete. And yet, no human being has stated beyond a doubt that he has seen such radio frequencies. Still we take it for granted and accept the existence of transmitted pictures and sound. Therefore we may understand that the spirit is beyond such sound waves and can penetrate into anything. All material stuffs have interspaces. Some we see like the spaces in a sponge. Some we cannot see like the spaces in dense metal like steel. In addition, there are dimensional spaces which we may realize by studying how our subtle body separates and is then reunified with the gross one. To understand the soul, we have to study these dimensional aspects in higher yoga practice, through subtle meditation.

अव्यक्तोऽयमचिन्त्योऽयम्
अविकार्योऽयमुच्यते ।
तस्मादेवं विदित्वैनं
नानुशोचितुमर्हसि ॥२.२५॥
avyakto'yamacintyo'yam
avikāryo'yamucyate
tasmādevaṁ viditvainaṁ
nānuśocitumarhasi (2.25)

*avyakto = avyaktaḥ — undisplayed; 'yam = ayam — this; acintyo = acintyah — unimaginable; 'yam = ayam — this; avikāryo = avikāryaḥ — unchanging; 'yam = ayam — this; ucyate — it is declared; tasmāt — therefore; evaṁ — thus; viditvainaṁ = viditva — knowing + enam — this; nānuśocitum = na — not + anuśocitum — to lament; arhasi — you should*

**This embodied soul is undisplayed, unimaginable, and unchanging. Therefore knowing this, you should not lament. (2.25)**

***Siddha Swami's Commentary:***

Just about everything we encounter in the gross and subtle material world changes, even the subtle body. For instance, my subtle body resembles the last gross body I used. Now if I take another gross body from parents in a different family, my subtle body would be altered to look like those parents. Thus, repeatedly, the subtle body shows major or minor alterations. If I take a body from animal parents, my subtle body would go through a major alteration. Conversely, the spirit does not change in that way. The spirit does, however, provide the energy as the central power source for the subtle and the various gross forms. One changes many gross bodies but his subtle body remains the same, even though it goes through numerous adjustments and alterations, according to the parentage and location of its manifestation.

As the Supreme Being, *Śrī* Krishna could very well describe the limited spirits, but those spirits themselves may not understand their nature. This is due to their subtlety and their inability to objectify themselves. When *Śrī* Krishna said that the spirits are undisplayed, He referred to their inability to become matter. They cannot de-energize themselves or be de-energized by anyone. Thus, unlike a radioactive material which might degrade after thousands of years and be manifested into a lower plane of existence as lead or some other heavy material, the spirit cannot be degraded to the state of gross matter. This implies that the spirits are a perpetual energy source. They cannot be down-sized or exhausted. Their energy cannot be spent out.

In *brahma yoga* when we study the nature of the subtle body which is used in dreams, we find that it can be exhausted but that it is recharged repeatedly after each exhaustion. This is also the case with the gross body to a limited extent. The spirit, however, cannot be exhausted. Something that cannot be exhausted does not change in a downward direction. It does not deteriorate. All these statements about the soul, made to us by *Śrī* Krishna or by some other divinity or by a great *yogin*, or by Lord Shiva Himself, or by me, known in my last body as *Nityānanda*, should be verified by careful, painstaking mystic practice in higher yoga. *Śrī Patañjali Mahāmuni* gave many methods of doing this. A *yogin* is duty bound to spend much time making careful observation of these truths during *samādhi* practice.

अथ चैनं नित्यजातं
नित्यं वा मन्यसे मृतम् ।
तथापि त्वं महाबाहो
नैनं शोचितुमर्हसि ॥२.२६॥
atha cainaṁ nityajātaṁ
nityaṁ vā manyase mṛtam
tathāpi tvaṁ mahābāho
nainaṁ śocitumarhasi (2.26)

*atha — furthermore; cainaṁ = ca — and + enam — this; nityajātaṁ = nitya — continually + jātam — being born; nityam — continually; vā — or; manyase — you think; mṛtam — dying; tathā 'pi = tathā — so + api — also; tvam — you; mahābāho — strong-armed man; nainaṁ = na — not + enam — this; śocitum arhasi = śocitum — to mourn + arhasi — you can*

**And furthermore if you think that this embodied soul is continually being born or continually dying, even so, O strong-armed man, you should not lament. (2.26)**

***Siddha Swami's Commentary:***

Some persons maintain that a person is born, lives in the world and then dies whereby the animal or human form disintegrates by the laws of nature. After this, they opine that the person is again reformulated as a human being or animal according to his or her previous personality and is then again born, lives in the world and then again dies, repeatedly. This view comes about after observing how vegetation is produced. A tree lives year after year by consuming dirt and by eating decayed vegetation, some of which decayed from its own body. Thus after observing this, some ancient seers concluded that the human or animal personality is reformulated again and again according to this recycling of decayed or disintegrated materials.

*Śrī* Krishna was aware of this view and so was Arjuna. Thus the Lord said that even in that belief one should not worry about the death of the body, since the person is supposed to be reformulated repeatedly by the laws of transposition. Another similar view is the modern declaration that nothing can be created or destroyed. This view holds that whatever energy is existent will always be in existence, no matter what. This view presupposed that this is a contained situation, such that no portion of the energy can escape to another place. As such one may cause a shift of energy from one status to another or from one level or form to another, but one cannot in any way increase or decrease the amount of energy contained. Thus, this principle holds that energy is eternal. In this view no God is required, since energy itself is non-perishable and cannot be initiated into existence or originated; its origination is said to be spontaneous and causeless. In all such opinions, however, there is really no good reason to lament.

जातस्य हि ध्रुवो मृत्युर्
ध्रुवं जन्म मृतस्य च ।
तस्मादपरिहार्येऽर्थे
न त्वं शोचितुमर्हसि ॥२.२७॥
jātasya hi dhruvo mṛtyur
dhruvaṁ janma mṛtasya ca
tasmādaparihārye'rthe
na tvaṁ śocitumarhasi (2.27)

*jātasya — of that which is born; hi — in fact; dhruvo = dhruvaḥ — certain; mṛtyur = mṛtyuḥ — death; dhruvaṁ — certain; janma — birth; mṛtasya — of that which is dead; ca — and; tasmādaparihārye = tasmāt — therefore + aparihārye — in what is unavoidable; 'rthe = arthe — in the assessment; na — not; tvaṁ — you; śocitum — to lament + arhasi — you should*

**In fact, of that which is born, death is certain; of that which is dead, birth is certain. Therefore in assessing what is unavoidable, you should not lament. (2.27)**

***Siddha Swami's Commentary:***

For the average human being, for animals and for vegetation, birth and death are an absolute necessity. This process is the general experience of the living creatures. This is what they have to look forward to. Even though in higher yoga and in the Vedic religion there is heated discussion about going to a place where eternal life is possible, still in general, most of the spirits have only repeated birth and death to look forward to.

It requires a quantum leap, a great endeavor, to change from a birth and death outlook to one of eternity or immortality. It does not come easily. It does not come merely by grace of God. One has to endeavor as well. One has to change the natural tendency which is to give in to the psychological energies which construct the subtle material world.

*Śrī* Krishna admonished Arjuna that since most of the body-prone spirits will take new bodies, live in these, depart from them and again take new bodies and repeat the process all over again, there is no point in lamenting their fate. It is best, therefore, for the upkeep of righteous society to face what is unavoidable. And that means to do one's duty, make one's contribution for morality in the human world. At least if one does not believe in anything besides human existence, one should support righteous lifestyle and morality. This is the point.

अव्यक्तादीनि भूतानि
व्यक्तमध्यानि भारत ।
अव्यक्तनिधनान्येव
तत्र का परिदेवना ॥२.२८॥
avyaktādīni bhūtāni
vyaktamadhyāni bhārata
avyaktanidhanānyeva
tatra kā paridevanā (2.28)

*avyaktādīni = avyakta — undetected + ādīni — beginnings of a manifestation; bhūtāni — living beings; vyakta madhyāni = vyakta — visible + madhyāni — interim states; bhārata — O descendant of Bharata; avyakta nidhanāny eva = avyakta — undetected + nidhanāni — ends of a manifestation + eva — again; tatra — there; kā — what; paridevanā — complaint*

**The living beings are undetected in the beginning of a manifestation, visible in the interim stages, and are again undetected at the end of a manifestation. What is the complaint? (2.28)**

***Siddha Swami's Commentary:***

Even though living beings are undetected in the beginning and after the end of a manifestation, that is not proof of the non-existence of the spirit. Also, one should not feel that unless we can detect the living entity by modern technology, no other type of evidence is acceptable. In fact, the subtlety of the living entity is such that only the living entity can achieve the final proof of its own existence.

*Brahma yoga* concerns this matter, in that one is trained how to detect what is super-subtle. This begins in elementary yoga by tracing and analyzing the subtle body used in dreams. It is individual research. It is not done collectively as is modern science.

I was known as a yogi named *Nityānānda*. Due to my elevated status, people used to call me *Bhagavān*, which means Lord or God. Actually, *Śrī* Krishna is *Bhagavān*, but as a formality and to recognize a great *yogin*, people in India sometimes addresses a great person as Lord or God. Now in my case, I am using the brain and senses of this student of mine, Yogi *Madhvācārya*. By his cooperation, I write this commentary on the *Śrīmad Bhagavad Gītā*.

Because *Madhvācārya* advanced in higher yoga, he can detect another spirit and even allow another spirit to use his faculties and clearly discern between his ideas and that of the other person who inhabits his psychology. Therefore for the accomplished yogis, the living beings are detected in the beginning of a manifestation, in the interim stages and also at the end of a manifestation. Even though I departed my last body and did not develop any other one to this date, still *Madhvācārya* detects my existence. He can hear my subtle speech and converse with me through subtle senses just as if I were present physically.

आश्चर्यवत्पश्यति कश्चिदेनम्
आश्चर्यवद्वदति तथैव चान्यः ।
आश्चर्यवच्चैनमन्यः शृणोति
श्रुत्वाप्येनं वेद न चैव कश्चित् ॥२.२९॥
āścaryavatpaśyati kaścidenam
āścaryavadvadati tathaiva cānyaḥ
āścaryavaccainamanyaḥ śṛṇoti
śrutvāpyenaṁ veda na caiva kaścit (2.29)

*āścaryavat — wonderful; paśyati — perceives; kaścidenam = kaścid — someone + enam — this; āścaryavad — fantastic; vadati — describes; tathai 'va = tathā — so + eva — indeed; cānyaḥ = ca — and + anyah — another person; āścaryavaccainam = āścaryavat — amazing + ca — and + enam — this; anyaḥ — another; śṛṇoti — hears; śrutvāpyenaṁ = srutva — having heard + api — also + enam — this; veda — knows; na — not; caiva = ca — and + eva — in fact; kaścit — anyone*

**Someone perceives this embodied soul as being wonderful. Another person describes it as amazing. Another hears of it as being fantastic. And even after hearing this, no one knows this embodied soul in fact. (2.29)**

***Siddha Swami's Commentary:***

All opinions about the glory of the spirit are justified, because it is the ultimate energy source. It is wonderful. It is amazing. It is fantastic. And it is difficult to fathom in fact. It is only the Supreme Being who might look down upon the ordinary spirit. As He stated in the *Gītā*, the Supreme Person is even more glorious than the spirit. To know all this is fantastic, but one can only know this consistently if one becomes dedicated to the mystic and spiritual research, through which one can perceive these truths directly.

Since the spirit is intangible in the material sense, most human beings shy away from research into the nature of it. They prefer to deal with what is visible and tangible to their material bodies. Only a few stalwart souls might persevere in the quest for the spiritual truths.

देही नित्यमवध्योऽयं
देहे सर्वस्य भारत ।
तस्मात्सर्वाणि भूतानि
न त्वं शोचितुमर्हसि ॥२.३०॥
dehī nityamavadhyo'yaṁ
dehe sarvasya bhārata
tasmātsarvāṇi bhūtāni
na tvaṁ śocitumarhasi (2.30)

*dehī — embodied soul; nityam — eternally; avadhyo = avadhyaḥ — non-killable; 'yaṁ = ayam — this; dehe — in the body; sarvasya — of all, in all cases; bhārata — O descendant of Bharata; tasmāt — therefore; sarvāṇi — all; bhūtāni — beings; na — no; tvaṁ — you; śocitumarhasi = śocitum — to mourn + arhasi — should*

**In the body, in all cases, this embodied soul is always non-killable, O descendant of Bharata. Therefore you should not mourn for any of these beings. (2.30)**

***Siddha Swami's Commentary:***

*Śrī* Krishna disapproved of Arjuna's lamentation for the supposed deaths of any Kurus.

As Krishna said initially, Arjuna had mourned for that which should not be regretted. Arjuna lamented the death of the personalities of Bhishma, *Droṇa* and others who were dear to him, but such death was not possible. Thus Arjuna focused his emotional energy on something imaginary.

One may truthfully mourn for death of a person's body but not for death of the person. The person will move away from the body, entering another dimension in the hereafter, and will again appear somewhere else to live in another body or to be liberated as the bare spirit itself. Thus if we must mourn, we should at least be clear on this issue. One may also mourn the person's departure from this dimension if one feels that one will not be able to communicate with that person as easily if the person has to permanently leave the physical body.

This *Yogi Madhvācārya*, for instance, would not have mourned my departure from the physical world, since he can communicate with me just as well even though I no longer use a physical body. He does not feel a loss just because I lost my old body. This is basic spiritual life.

स्वधर्ममपि चावेक्ष्य
न विकम्पितुमर्हसि ।
धर्म्याद्धि युद्धाच्छ्रेयोऽन्यत्
क्षत्रियस्य न विद्यते ॥२.३१॥
svadharmamapi cāvekṣya
na vikampitumarhasi
dharmyāddhi
yuddhācchreyo'nyat
kṣatriyasya na vidyate (2.31)

*svadharmam — your assigned duty; api — also; cāvekṣya = ca — and + avekṣya — looking, mentally considering; na — no; vikampitum — to consider alternatives; arhasi — you should; dharmyād = dharmyāt — from righteousness; dhi = hi — indeed; yuddhācchreyo = yuddhāt — from battle + chreyo = śreyas — better; 'nyat = anyat — other; kṣatriyasya — of the son of a king; na — no; vidyate — there is*

**And considering your assigned duty, you should not look for alternatives. In fact, for the son of a king, there is no other duty which is better than a righteous battle. (2.31)**

***Siddha Swami's Commentary:***

*Śrī* Krishna with precision veered Arjuna away from cowardice and from a pretentious religious stance. Arjuna used religious and humanitarian arguments to avoid duty, but *Śrī* Krishna would have none of it. Everyone in this world is born in a particular family, educated in a particular way, and prepared to take on certain duties for the continuation of family and country. This is the way of the world. In that matter, the only thing to do, is comply with one's righteous duties.

As far as righteousness is concerned, every limited being has a part to play, in keeping the self in a moral lifestyle and in supporting government policies which afford fair living for one and all. Thus Arjuna would imperil himself if he avoided duty. There is a God of the world. That God can impose penalties upon a limited being. Apart from God, nature is very reactive to both morality and immorality. Each limited being should protect itself from harsh treatment which might be administered by God or by nature. This is intelligence.

यदृच्छया चोपपन्नं
स्वर्गद्वारमपावृतम् ।
सुखिनः क्षत्रियाः पार्थ
लभन्ते युद्धमीदृशम् ॥२.३२॥

*yadṛcchayā — by a stroke of luck; copapannaṁ = ca — and + upapannam — made available; svargadvāram = svarga — heaven + dvāram — gate; apāvṛtam — is open; sukhinaḥ — thrilled, happy; kṣatriyāḥ*

yadṛcchayā copapannaṁ
svargadvāramapāvṛtam
sukhinaḥ kṣatriyāḥ pārtha
labhante yuddhamīdṛśam (2.32)

*— warriors; pārtha — O son of Pṛthā; labhante — get; yuddham — battle opportunity; īdṛśam — such*

**And by a stroke of luck, the gate of heaven is opened. Thrilled are the warriors who get such a battle opportunity, O son of Pṛthā. (2.32)**

***Siddha Swami's Commentary:***

Even though one may do one's duty and become eligible for life in a heavenly world, still that depends on providence. If providence does not provide an opportunity, the performance of duty may not yield heavenly life in the hereafter, even though usually one is offered another body in the same species and often in the same family where one contributed cultural work.

*Śrī* Krishna encouraged Arjuna in taking what was a rare opportunity for life in the heavenly world hereafter. Without much endeavor such a world beckoned Arjuna for an easy transfer in the hereafter, if Arjuna would only take the opportunity to represent righteousness on that battlefield. Arjuna, however, saw the opportunity and rejected it in favor of not fighting and allowing the unruly Kauravas to continue their corrupted government. He wanted to influence them by pacifist means or by martyrdom.

For the purpose of *brahma yoga*, neither heavenly life through heroism nor righteousness on earth, nor martyrdom for proving that one has a benevolent nature, is suitable. *Brahma yoga* concerns neither happy conditions of living in the hereafter nor exhibitions of benevolence in the material world. It concerns spiritual awakening, sorting the various subtle objects in the psyche, and ridding the self of lower energies. Thus for a *brahma yogi*, there would be objections to heaven as an objective but not for the same reasons which Arjuna gave in Chapters One and Two. A *brahma yogi* should not waste his energy aspiring for heaven hereafter, or for displaying kindness to others and proving that pacifism is a better form of discipline than chastisement or judicial violence.

A *brahma yogin* requires the opportunity to do battle with the unruly forces in his nature and with all sorts of negative influences which come from others in the gross and subtle worlds. There cause him to decrease mystic practice for sorting the energies in the psyche and establishing his spirit as the master of his psychology.

अथ चेत्त्वमिमं धर्म्यं
संग्रामं न करिष्यसि ।
ततः स्वधर्मं कीर्तिं च
हित्वा पापमवाप्स्यसि ॥२.३३॥
atha cettvamimaṁ dharmyaṁ
saṁgrāmaṁ na kariṣyasi
tataḥ svadharmaṁ kīrtiṁ ca
hitvā pāpamavāpsyasi (2.33)

*atha — now; cet — if; tvam — you; imaṁ — this; dharmyaṁ — appropriate duty; saṁgrāmaṁ — warfare; na — not; kariṣyasi — will conduct; tataḥ — then; svadharmaṁ — own duty; kīrtiṁca = kīrtiṁ — reputation + ca — and; hitvā — having neglected; pāpam — sin, fault; avāpsyasi — will acquire*

**Now if you do not conduct this righteous war, then, by neglecting your duty and reputation, you will acquire a fault. (2.33)**

***Siddha Swami's Commentary:***

This was true for Arjuna because he took birth in a ruling family and was trained to establish righteousness at all costs. If Arjuna did not conduct that righteous war (*dharmyam samgrāmam*), then certainly by neglecting the duty and the reputation he earned by behaving properly, and by also tolerating irreligious life, he would acquire a fault in his record of cultural activities. For Arjuna there was no way out. He had to comply with unpalatable duties.

Pacifism and all such admirable ways of dealing with unruly people were tried with the Kauravas but they did not respond favorably. Their collective conscience was insensitive to humane methods of conciliation. Thus judicial violence had to be used as a last resort.

Does a brahma yogi have to use judicial force on his own nature, to get it in order? In fact, that is exactly the process of *haṭha* yoga. It is a way of austerities to bring the psychology under control. In the struggle for power between the forces which sponsor vice in the nature and those which sponsor virtuous conduct, a yogi has to apply austere methods of *haṭha* yoga, especially the methods pioneered by *Śrī* Gorakshanatha *Mahāyogin*. Kundalini yoga is especially expedient in conquering the lower nature and effectively moving the yogi out of the survival field of material nature.

अकीर्तिं चापि भूतानि
कथयिष्यन्ति तेऽव्ययाम् ।
संभावितस्य चाकीर्तिर्
मरणादतिरिच्यते ॥२.३४॥

akīrtiṁ cāpi bhūtāni
kathayiṣyanti te'vyayām
saṁbhāvitasya cākīrtir
maraṇādatiricyate (2.34)

*akīrtiṁ — downfall; cāpi = ca — and + api — also; bhūtāni — the people; kathayiṣyanti — will speak; te — of you; 'vyayām = avyayām — continually; saṁbhāvitasya — for an honored man; cākīrtir = ca — and + akīrtiḥ — loss of reputation; maraṇād = maraṇāt — than the loss of body; atiricyate — is harder to bear*

**The people will speak of your downfall continually. And for an honored man, the loss of reputation is harder to bear than the loss of his body. (2.34)**

***Siddha Swami's Commentary:***

For an emotionally-sensitive person like Arjuna, the loss of reputation affects the subtle body, hurting it grievously. That is hard for such a person to bear. Arjuna, if subjected to adverse criticism by not living up to social expectations, would be unsettled until he could explain himself to certain people satisfactorily. If he could not do so, he might pine away in sorrow or he might even attempt suicide. Thus *Śrī* Krishna hinted that Arjuna should evaluate his nature and act in a way which was beneficial in the long run.

*Brahma yoga* is different since a *yogin* learns how to disregard feelings of pity and such emotions which are necessary for good image and status in society. A *brahma yogin*, having turned away from the benefits and disappointments of social life, does not care about the loss of reputation or the acclaim of integrity. He knows very well that none of it has value anywhere else but in the material world. This does not mean that he acts whimsically or that he opposes righteous lifestyle. In fact, he supports that fully but he does not put an absolute value on that. He supports that as a routine, knowing that ultimately it is not the spiritual development he strives for.

भयाद्रणादुपरतं
मंस्यन्ते त्वां महारथाः ।
येषां च त्वं बहुमतो
भूत्वा यास्यसि लाघवम् ॥२.३५॥

*bhayād = bhayāt — because of fear; raṇād = raṇāt — from the excitement of battle; uparataṁ — withdraw from; maṁsyante — they think; tvāṁ — you; mahārathāḥ — great warriors; yeṣāṁ — of whom; ca — and; tvaṁ*

bhayādraṇāduparataṁ
maṁsyante tvāṁ mahārathāḥ
yeṣāṁ ca tvaṁ bahumato
bhūtvā yāsyasi lāghavam (2.35)

*— you; bahumato = bahumataḥ — high opinion; bhūtvā — had; yāsyasi — you will come; lāghavam — insignificance*

**The great warriors will think that because of fear, you withdrew from battle. And to those who held a big opinion, you will appear to be insignificant. (2.35)**

***Siddha Swami's Commentary:***

This was appropriate for Arjuna, a trained, duty-bound prince in the Kuru dynasty, but it is not suitable for a *brahma yogin*. Once a *yogin* decides to turn away from the material world, it is irrelevant what others might think. Those great leaders of society who saw promise and ambition in a neophyte *yogin*, are usually disappointed if he advances and decides to make an all-out effort for spiritual perfection. They try to discourage him by stating that he lost the vision of life, lost ambition and motivation, took to a lazy man's view of life and adopted a useless course which would benefit neither him, family, community nor country.

All the while that *yogin* observes that, in fact, he is not missed by the material energy, since her plans to expand the material world, go on in full force, even in his absence, even without his participation. Seeing this he ignores the criticism of others. A more advanced *yogin* begins to understand that unless he invests more time and energy in the practice, he cannot achieve perfection merely by complying with assigned social values which are approved even by God. Such assignments do help the righteous condition of the world, but it does not add an iota of spiritual development to anyone.

It was appropriate for Arjuna to stick to his duties as *Śrī* Krishna recommended, because Arjuna was on that level of consciousness where righteous acts are the highest attainment perceived. If and when Arjuna would advance further, he would not be in the socially, duty-bound position any longer; he would not have to satisfy the need for such performance of duty. *Śrī* Krishna requests this duty of Arjuna, only because of Arjuna's level of advancement at the time of the battle of *Kurukṣetra*.

अवाच्यवादांश्च बहून्
वदिष्यन्ति तवाहिताः ।
निन्दन्तस्तव सामर्थ्यं
ततो दुःखतरं नु किम् ॥२.३६॥
avācyavādāṁśca bahūn
vadiṣyanti tavāhitāḥ
nindantastava sāmarthyaṁ
tato duḥkhataraṁ nu kim (2.36)

*avācyavādāṁśca = avācya — not to be said, slurred + vādān — words, saying + ca — and; bahūn — many; vadiṣyanti — will speak; tavāhitāḥ = tava — about you + ahitāḥ — enemies; nindantas — laughed at; tava — of you; sāmarthyaṁ — capability; tato = tataḥ — from that; duḥkhataraṁ — greater grief; nu — but; kim — what*

**The enemies will say many slurs about you, thus laughing at your capability. But, what would be a greater grief than this? (2.36)**

***Siddha Swami's Commentary:***

Slurs and ridicule do not affect a *brahma yogi*, or a practicing *yogin* under the care of an advanced soul. But Arjuna was to be affected as *Śrī* Krishna stated. Because of emotional sensitivity towards others in the social field, Arjuna would be affected. A *brahma yogin* is also sensitive but only to his *brahma yogin* teachers, not to others on lower levels of existence which dictate other standards of behavior.

The main accomplishment for a neophyte *yogin* is this: He must learn how to be absent from such scenes like the battle of *Kurukṣetra*. This does not mean a convenient disappearance as Arjuna planned, but rather, an absence beforehand where one is not involved in those political affairs. One realizes that these things are necessary for human society and one appreciates those who are involved in it and who are duty-bound to righteous lifestyle. All the same, one keeps at a distance from those affairs, in order to conserve time for spiritual development in higher yoga practice.

हतो वा प्राप्स्यसि स्वर्गं
जित्वा वा भोक्ष्यसे महीम् ।
तस्मादुत्तिष्ठ कौन्तेय
युद्धाय कृतनिश्चयः ॥२.३७॥
hato vā prāpsyasi svargaṁ
jitvā vā bhokṣyase mahīm
tasmāduttiṣṭha kaunteya
yuddhāya kṛtaniścayaḥ (2.37)

*hato = hataḥ — be killed; vā — either; prāpsyasi — you will achieve; svargaṁ — angelic world; jitvā — having conquered; vā — or; bhokṣyase — you will enjoy; mahīm — the nation; tasmād = tasmāt — therefore; uttiṣṭha — stand up; kaunteya — O son of Kuntī; yuddhāya — to battle; kṛtaniścayaḥ — be decisive*

**Either be killed and achieve the angelic world or having conquered, enjoy the nation. Therefore stand up and be decisive, O son of Kunti. (2.37)**

***Siddha Swami's Commentary:***

Unless one has reached a level where one is no longer interested in the Swarga angelic paradises, one cannot be a *brahma yogin*. Neophytes who practice are still susceptible to such attraction but they are learning how to transcend and overcome that. At the time of the battle, Arjuna was still attracted to such paradise worlds, where one's every whim for pleasurable life may be fulfilled. In the *Mahābhārata* history, Arjuna went to the Swarga world and lived there. He was attracted to that. Now in *brahma yoga*, such a world only has value to a neophyte for testing his advancement before the time of death. He makes several trips into that world using his subtle body in dreams and visions. There as directed by his teachers, he observes his weakness for the paradises in which lovely, buxom angelic women draw pleasures and subtle sexual fluids through his souped-up, near-spiritual subtle body. He comes back to the earth after such encounters and perfects the kundalini yoga process, so that his psychology gets a resistance to such attractions in the angelic world. One has to work for this repeatedly, day after day, by deep meditation through mastery of *pratyāhār*, *dhāranā*, *dhyāna* and *samādhi*, the four higher stages of yoga.

Arjuna's status was different. His objective was performance of duty-bound social life for righteousness. Thus *Śrī* Krishna showed him the viable alternatives, which were to be killed in battle and then achieve the angelic world as a result of fighting on behalf of righteous lifestyle, or to conquer those unruly politicians who used irreligious means in government and then to rule the nation justly. Running away to be a political absentee or a pretend yogi would cause Arjuna to be neglectful towards a duty which he owed God, his family and human society.

सुखदुःखे समे कृत्वा
लाभालाभौ जयाजयौ ।
ततो युद्धाय युज्यस्व
नैवं पापमवाप्स्यसि ॥२.३८॥

*sukhaduḥkhe = sukha — happiness + duḥkhe — in distress; same — in the same emotions; kṛtvā — having regard; lābhālābhau — gains or losses; jayājayau — victory or defeat; tato = tataḥ — them; yuddhāya — to*

sukhaduḥkhe same kṛtvā
lābhālābhau jayājayau
tato yuddhāya yujyasva
naivaṁ pāpamavāpsyasi (2.38)

*battle; yujyasva — apply yourself; naivaṁ = na — not + evam — thus; pāpam — sin,demerit; avāpsyasi — you will get*

**Having regarded happiness, distress, gains, losses, victory and defeat, as the same emotions, apply yourself to battle. Thus you will get no demerit. (2.38)**

***Siddha Swami's Commentary:***

Arjuna was to take the path of *karma yoga*, to perform righteous cultural activities under the supervision of *Śrī* Krishna with the detachment gained from preliminary yoga practice. A person may take the path of *karma* without yoga and do so under the supervision of *Śrī* Krishna. That person, having not mastered even the preliminary steps in yoga, would be attached to whatever he does, but while acting in *Śrī* Krishna's influence he would, by the force of that association only and not on his own strength, express detachment even to his own emotional nature. That is described in Chapter Twelve specifically as an alternative way to have a relationship with *Śrī* Krishna.

That devotee must be able to regard happiness, distress, gains, losses, victory and defeat, as variations of the emotional energy in his nature. Thus being resistant to moods, he would perform duty dispassionately, even when disciplining others harshly. As *Śrī* Krishna guaranteed and explained, there would be no fault for that devotee.

*Brahma yogi*s should take note of this. Some *brahma yogi*s will have to perform *karma yoga* from time to time. If they do, they must tune into the views of *Śrī* Krishna and act accordingly so as not to create any sin in the material world. Of course, others who define sin differently might not agree with *Śrī* Krishna but we are not concerned with limited beings and their view points.

एषा तेऽभिहिता सांख्ये
बुद्धिर्योगे त्विमां श्रृणु ।
बुद्ध्या युक्तो यया पार्थ
कर्मबन्धं प्रहास्यसि ॥२.३९॥
eṣā te'bhihitā sāṁkhye
buddhiryoge tvimāṁ śṛṇu
buddhyā yukto yayā pārtha
karmabandhaṁ prahāsyasi (2.39)

*eṣā — this; te — to you; bhihitā = abhihitā — stated; sāṁkhye — in sāṁkhya philosophy; buddhir = buddhiḥ — insight; yoge — in yoga discipline; tvimām = tu — but + imāṁ — this; śṛṇu — hear; buddhyā — with the insight; yukto = yuktaḥ — yoked; yayā — by which; pārtha — O son of Pṛthā; karmabandhaṁ — complication of action; prahāsyasi — you will avoid*

**As explained in the Sāṁkhya philosophy, this vision is the insight, but hear of its application in yoga practice. Yoked with this insight, O son of Pṛthā, you will avoid the complication of action. (2.39)**

***Siddha Swami's Commentary:***

*Śrī* Krishna reminded Arjuna that such a vision of life, which is attained even by neophyte yogis, was itemized in the Samkhya philosophy. This vision is the basic insight. For neophytes, it was a theoretical foundation for their detachment while acting. Advanced yogis develop an actual insight which was applied in higher yoga practice.

Having developed it through yoga, one be may become an expert at avoiding the complications of action, something essential for attaining liberation from the material world. Continued action in this world automatically implies continued implication in further action. If one has that insight, one may avoid future implications and become free from certain actions, resulting in saved time that can be used to advance yoga practice.

नेहाभिक्रमनाशोऽस्ति
प्रत्यवायो न विद्यते ।
स्वल्पमप्यस्य धर्मस्य
त्रायते महतो भयात् ॥ २.४० ॥
nehābhikramanāśo'sti
pratyavāyo na vidyate
svalpamapyasya dharmasya
trāyate mahato bhayāt (2.40)

*nehābhikramanāśo = na — not + iha — in this insight + abhikrama — endeavor + nāśo (nāśaḥ) — loss; asti — it is; pratyavāyo = pratyavāyaḥ — reversal; na — not; vidyate — there is; svalpam — a little; apy = api — even; asya — of this; dharmasya — of righteous practice; trāyate — protects; mahato = mahataḥ — from the great; bhayāt — from danger*

**In this insight, no endeavor is lost nor is there any reversal. Even a little of this righteous practice protects from the great danger. (2.40)**

***Siddha Swami's Commentary:***

This insight, when applied while acting, causes the yogi to multiply his chances for release from social duties. It increases the time he may allot to practice. While before he could not find time or was not allowed to practice for long, he gains an exemption from some social duties. He practices for longer periods. Whatever cultural work he must perform is done more efficiently, because he is not distracted by moods of happiness, distress, gains, losses, victory or defeat (2.38).

Thus for such a *yogin*, there is no loss even in cultural participation. His insight into the conversion of emotions in varied moods, saves much time and causes him to cut through the social involvements. This is an insight into the fact that the basic emotional energy converts back and forth into varied moods which stymie the individual by entertaining or deluding him into feelings of happiness or distress, gains or losses, victory or defeat. This definition is derived from verse 38:

*sukhaduḥkhe same kṛtvā lābhālābhau jayājayau*
*tato yuddhāya yujyasva naivaṁ pāpamavāpsyasi (2.38)*

***Having regarded happiness, distress, gains, losses, victory and defeat, as the same emotions, apply yourself to battle. Thus you will get no demerit.*** *(2.38)*

*Śrī* Krishna guaranteed or at least brought to our attention, that a little insight into the conversion process of our emotions (into various types of moods), protects us from what He termed as the great danger *(mahato bhayāt)*. The key is to be free from the influence of one's emotions and its manifested or manifesting moods. If one resists that, one will fall under the influence of *Śrī* Krishna's Universal Form, which is described in Chapter 11. When someone gains the divine influence for righteous lifestyle, there is no loss or reversal, because that is the supreme power. It is an all-pervasive force, but to gain its influence one must be detached from emotions and from pleasant or unpleasant moods. This is a technique in elementary yoga.

As implied, the great danger is to act under the influence of one's emotions, since then one has no protection from the Supreme Person. Being restricted from the divine influence, one is automatically placed in great danger, because one is, after all, a limited being with limited insight into the perplexities of circumstance.

व्यवसायात्मिका बुद्धिर्
एकेह कुरुनन्दन ।
बहुशाखा ह्यनन्ताश्च
बुद्धयोऽव्यवसायिनाम् ॥२.४१॥
vyavasāyātmikā buddhir
ekeha kurunandana
bahuśākhā hyanantāśca
buddhayo'vyavasāyinām (2.41)

*vyavasāyātmikā — intentional determination; buddhir = buddhih — technical insight; ekeha = eka — one view + iha — in this instance; kurunandana — O dear man of the Kuru family; bahuśākhā — many offshoots; hyanantāś = hi — in fact + anantāḥ — endless; ca — and; buddhayo = buddhayaḥ — views; 'vyavasāyinām = avyavasāyinām — of the person with many hopes*

**When a person's intentional determination is guided by technical insight, he experiences one view, O dear man of the Kuru family. But the views of a person with many hopes are diverse and endless. (2.41)**

***Siddha Swami's Commentary:***

If a person is guided by his own emotions, then as those feelings are converted into various moods, he will adopt various psychological postures, some which are contrary to one another, and many which oppose the supreme will. Subsequently, he will be hurt emotionally. This will happen regularly. On the other hand, as *Śrī* Krishna explained, a person's intentional determination, when guided by the technical insight which is free from emotional moods, remains consistent. This is because his insight into the whimsical nature of his emotions, causes him to internally abandon the fluid and electrical workings of his psychology and to embrace the steady input from the Supreme Being.

Since a limited being has a jumpy mind and mixed-up emotions and prejudices, and since his nature is not properly ordered or sorted out, it is best that he abandon his own emotions and adopt the views of the Supreme Being as expressed in the *Gītā.* Until one is able to change his psychology, to alter it permanently, one should link up with and rely on the Supreme Being. Arjuna's pitiful condition, just before the battle of *Kurukṣetra*, dissipated as soon as he linked up with the mind of *Śrī* Krishna. In *brahma yoga*, the student learns how to transform his own mind into that higher state. Thus he becomes permanently altered into the divine way.

यामिमां पुष्पितां वाचं
प्रवदन्त्यविपश्चितः ।
वेदवादरताः पार्थ
नान्यदस्तीति वादिनः ॥२.४२॥
yāmimāṁ puṣpitāṁ vācaṁ
pravadantyavipaścitaḥ
vedavādaratāḥ pārtha
nānyadastīti vādinaḥ (2.42)

*yām — which; imām — this; puṣpitāṁ — poetic; vācaṁ — quotation; pravadantyavipaścitaḥ = pravadanti — they proclaim + avipaścitaḥ — ignorant reciters; vedavādaratāḥ — enjoying Vedic Sanskrit poetry; pārtha — O son of Pṛthā; nānyad = na — not + anyat — anything; astīti = asti — it is + iti — thus; vādinaḥ — saying*

**This is poetic quotation which the ignorant reciters proclaim, O son of Pṛthā. Enjoying the Vedic verses, they say there is no other written authority. (2.42)**

***Siddha Swami's Commentary:***

Some exponents of the Vedic way of life have no technical insight as described by *Śrī* Krishna. Thus they use the Vedic version in a perverse way, intending for it to support the human moody condition. Such reciters of the *Veda* pervert the text but they are appreciated by persons who are unable to work for the mood-free insight. Thus the Vedic system has two parts, one being superficial or poetic *(puṣpitām)* and the other being substantial or consistent with the views of the Supreme Being. *Veda* actually means the views of the Supreme Being; otherwise, it is pseudo *Veda*, which forms into a farcical religion.

Philosophical texts like the *Bhagavad Gītā* shed light on the actual meaning of *Veda*, but some speakers either ignore the *Gītā* or explain it superficially. These persons, perverse as they are, make claims about the authority of the *Veda* while striking down the deep explanations in the *Bhagavad Gītā*.

Somehow, even an intelligent person like Arjuna, fell into believing the superficial explanations of the *Veda*, and because he was unable to decipher his moods as whimsical operations of his emotions, he became convinced that the righteous war to be fought by his brother was irreligious, and so he wanted to abandon duty.

कामात्मानः स्वर्गपरा
जन्मकर्मफलप्रदाम् ।
क्रियाविशेषबहुलां
भोगैश्वर्यगतिं प्रति ॥२.४३॥
kāmātmānaḥ svargaparā
janmakarmaphalapradām
kriyāviśeṣabahulāṁ
bhogaiśvaryagatiṁ prati (2.43)

*kāmātmānaḥ — people of a sensuous nature; svargaparā — people intent on going to the swarga (angelic) world; janmakarmaphalapradām = janma — rebirth + karma — cultural act + phala – pay-off + pradām — offering; kriyāviśeṣabahulāṁ = kriyā — ceremonial rites + viśeṣa — specific + bahulām — various; bhogaiśvaryagatiṁ = bhoga — enjoyment + aiśvarya — political power + gatiṁ — aim; prati — toward*

**Those reciters, being people of a sensuous nature, being intent on going to the Svarga angelic world, offering such rebirth as payoff for cultural activities, make themselves busy in various specific ceremonial rites, and focus on enjoyment and political power. (2.43)**

***Siddha Swami's Commentary:***

It is one thing to understand the motives of the general public's attraction to pseudo religions, which offer them heaven in the hereafter or hell if they disobey, and it is a quite a different matter to see through the motives of the religious leaders who prey on a gullible and childish congregation.

The priests who advocate heaven hereafter are themselves persons of a sensuous nature. They themselves lack the insight which allows a yogi to see that his emotions are whimsically converted into happy, distressful, exciting, depressing, enthusing and gloomy moods. Being intent on going to the Swarga angelic world, they desire to greet their followers there in the future and to verify that what they advocated was true, thereby showing that they are agents of the rulers of heaven. They boldly offer rebirth in wealthy, educated families as a pay-off for the cultural activities which they so highly recommend. Making themselves busy in ceremonial rites, they excite a gullible public which consists of many adults with childish minds, who have no idea that they will be frustrated, and who are content to enjoy hearing of heaven and the possibility of future birth in aristocratic families here on earth.

As *Śrī* Krishna so vividly described, these priests pursue enjoyment of life and the acquirement of political power. With such motivation, they cannot be trusted but they do acquire large followings because most people are content with shallow promises and reduction of necessary austerities.

A *brahma yogi*, however, since he left aside this world and its concerns, does not envy or compete with such popular priests. Rather he leaves them to their devices and hardly seeks to alert the public to their dishonesty.

भोगैश्वर्यप्रसक्तानां
तयापहृतचेतसाम् ।
व्यवसायात्मिका बुद्धिः
समाधौ न विधीयते ॥२.४४॥
bhogaiśvaryaprasaktānāṁ
tayāpahṛtacetasām
vyavasāyātmikā buddhiḥ
samādhau na vidhīyate (2.44)

*bhogaiśvaryaprasaktānāṁ = bhoga — pleasure + aiśvarya — power + prasaktānāṁ — of the attached, of the prone; tayāpahṛtacetasām = tayā — by this + apahṛta — captivated + cetasām — idea; vyavasāyātmikā = vyavasāya — focused determination + ātmikā — self; buddhiḥ — intellect; samādhau — in meditation; na — not; vidhīyate — is experienced*

**Being absorbed by this way of life, pleasure-prone and power-seeking people, are captivated by this idea. Thus in meditation, the self-focused intellect is not experienced by them. (2.44)**

***Siddha Swami's Commentary:***

Generally a human being is absorbed in ideas about pleasure and control. These two features of lower consciousness dominate the psyche of the individual. The objective is pleasure, but that must be secured. Therefore the individual strives to gain control, so that he is not exploited, but can instead exploit either by benevolent or ruthless means. For a student of *brahma yoga*, this type of normal human life must be given up. The *brahma yogi* is taught to focus the intellect on the self *(ātmikā).* This is the reverse to normal living where the self focuses through the intellect into the senses, which are dedicated to objects in the gross and subtle world, for extracting the pleasures.

In this verse *Śrī* Krishna gave the basic *brahma yoga kriyā* of causing the intellect *(buddhih)* to focus on the *ātma*, the spirit. *Śrī* Krishna stated plainly that for those who are after pleasure and power, the experience of the intellect being turned towards the spiritual self does not occur in their consciousness. A neophyte yogi struggles with his psychology to turn it around, to reverse its organization, so that he can honor this basic requirement for higher yoga. This concerns focusing the intellect upon the *ātma* itself. This is an introversion.

The following drawings illustrate this reversal of the attention energy:

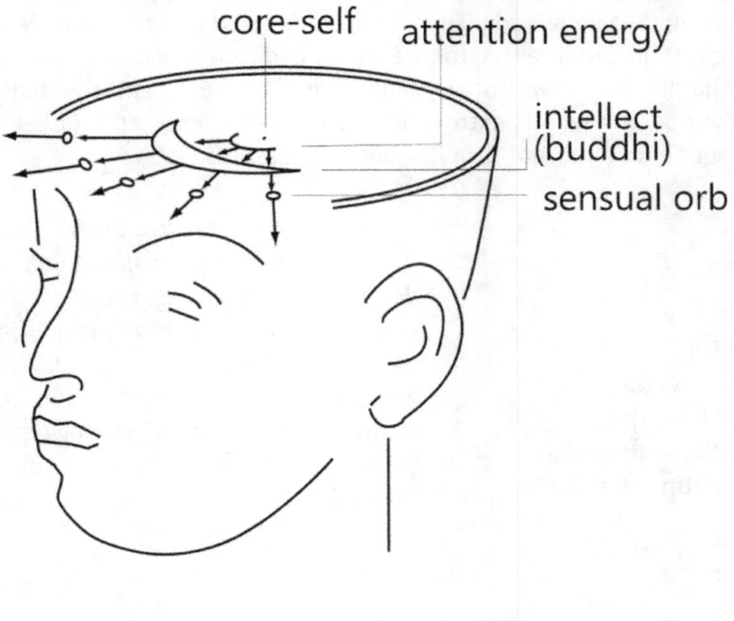

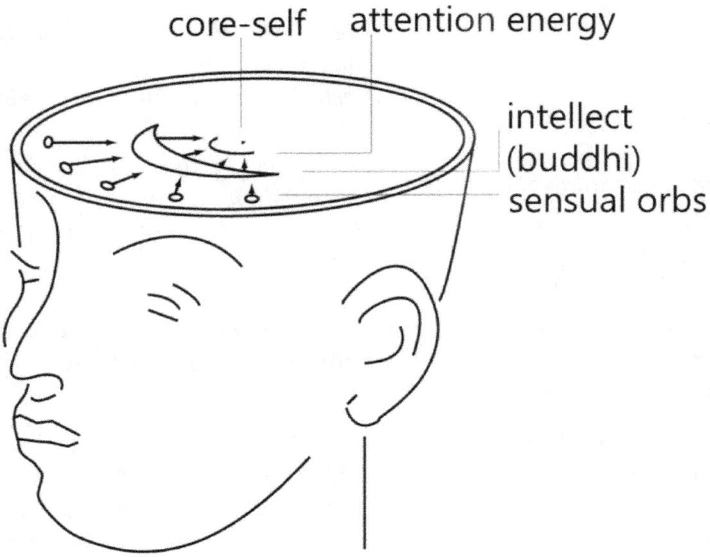


In the psyche, the pleasure-seeking need is expressed by the emotional energy. The power-seeking one is run by the intellect. Both of these work in cooperation. *Śrī Patañjali* gave an order that all yogis must curb the *vṛttis* which are the operations of the organs of subtle perception. Meditation becomes possible when the organs of subtle perception are curbed from their whimsical moves which are motivated by the emotional energy. A *yogin* must first master kundalini yoga, wherein he curbs the life force. Otherwise, *brahma yoga* will be a failure.

This is explained as follows: The intellect will not focus on the self merely by desire nor by will power. In fact, it is unable to focus like that so long as it is goaded or pushed by an unruly and impure life force. One must purify the life force by *prāṇāyāma*, by flushing out impure subtle air in the subtle body. Then it becomes possible. When the life air is dedicated to the spirit self, then the intellect too becomes dedicated, because the intellect is more attached to the life air than to anything else. The self-focused intellect cannot be experienced by a person who is extroverted, because his intellect is driven outwards into the gross and subtle material world, in its hunt for pleasures.

त्रैगुण्यविषया वेदा
निस्त्रैगुण्यो भवार्जुन ।
निर्द्वंद्वो नित्यसत्त्वस्थो
निर्योगक्षेम आत्मवान् ॥ २.४५ ॥
traiguṇyaviṣayā vedā
nistraiguṇyo bhavārjuna
nirdvaṁdvo nityasattvastho
niryogakṣema ātmavān (2.45)

*traiguṇya — three mood; viṣayā — phases; vedā — Vedas; nistraiguṇyo = nistraiguṇyaḥ — without the three moody phases; bhavārjuna = bhava — be + arjuna — Arjuna; nirdvandvo = nirdvandvaḥ — without fluctuation; nityasattvastho = nityasattvasthaḥ = nitya — always + sattva — reality + sthaḥ — fixed; niryogakṣema — without grasping and possessiveness; ātmavān — soul-situated*

**Three moody phases are offered by the Vedas. Be without the three moods, O Arjuna. Be without the moody fluctuations. Be always anchored to reality. Be free from grasping and possessiveness. (2.45)**

***Siddha Swami's Commentary:***

As I explained in detail to this writer, the yogi *Madhvācārya, brahma yoga* is based on the foundation of non-appropriation. In this technique, Lord Krishna established this fact by using the term *niryogakṣema*. This means non-appropriation of whatever is presented to the self by the pleasure-seeking, power-hungry senses. Of course, the senses do not relate directly to the spirit itself; they work through the intellect. In turn, the intellect works through the attention energy of the self. Without mastering *niryogakṣema*, non-appropriation, one cannot be a *brahma yogin* and one cannot effectively practice *samādhi* (*samādhau*, verse 44).

*Yogakṣema* means the acquisition and keeping of property. When the prefix *nir* is put before that word, the meaning is *not to acquire* and *not to keep property*. In yoga we discuss the more subtle phenomena. One should stop taking sensual pictures of any subtle or gross object encountered in the material world. Since the senses and the intellect are an automatic device for such picture taking, how is this done? One has to strive to be spirit self-centered *(ātmavan)*, rather than intellect-centered, to see the internal pictures visualized by the intellect from moment to moment. These pictures were appropriated by the senses initially and then displayed by the intellect and stored for later use by the memory. One has to forego all this to practice *brahma yoga*.

Since *Śrī* Krishna explained this to Arjuna early in the discourse, we have to assume that Arjuna was a very advanced *yogin*, but somehow he was unable to apply himself at *Kurukṣetra*. Somehow he lost touch with advanced practice. An ordinary person cannot even imagine that *Śrī* Krishna described *brahma yoga* techniques this early in the *Gītā*. Thus Arjuna was a great *yogin* at the time of the discourse, having taken lessons on higher yoga before.

As indicated in this verse, if one could stop the intellect from appropriating or taking things in this world, then one may be soul-situated *(ātmavan)*. The intellect is not a gross organ like the hand or the mouth. Thus whatever it possesses must be subtle. It may take possession of a photograph, or a sound from somewhere, or an odor, taste or feeling gained by contact with something. All these methods of appropriation must cease for establishing the foundation of *brahma yoga*.

यावानर्थ उदपाने
सर्वतः संप्लुतोदके ।
तावान्सर्वेषु वेदेषु
ब्राह्मणस्य विजानतः ॥२.४६॥
yāvānartha udapāne
sarvataḥ saṁplutodake
tāvānsarveṣu vedeṣu
brāhmaṇasya vijānataḥ (2.46)

*yāvān — as much; artha — importance; udapāne — in a well; sarvataḥ — in all directions; saṁplutodake = saṁpluta — flowing + udake — in water; tāvān — so much; sarveṣu — in the entire; vedeṣu — in the Vedas; brāhmaṇasya — of a brahmin; vijānataḥ — perceptive*

**For as much importance as there is in a well when suitable water flows in all directions, so much worth is in the entire Vedas for a perceptive brahmin. (2.46)**

***Siddha Swami's Commentary:***

Once the yogi begins to revert his intellect back to his core self, the external world does not attract him with such a force any longer. If one has no easy source of potable water, then wells become very important, and one may travel long distances just to reach them. If however, one has potable water in every direction, the wells lose their significance.

So long as one does not develop an intellect habituated to consulting the spirit self, one will be forced to do whatever is necessary to procure pleasures. A perceptive brahmin does not live like this, because he has found inner stability. His intellect serves to reinforce his spiritual self, rather than to be parasitic towards it.

All readers of the *Gītā* should take note of *Śrī* Krishna's definitions. Here He defined a perceptive brahmin as being a person who has a self-focusing intellect. This person must not be solely reliant on the *Vedas* but should be experienced in causing the intellect to turn away from the sensual energies to face the spirit self within the psyche.

कर्मण्येवाधिकारस्ते
मा फलेषु कदाचन ।
मा कर्मफलहेतुर्भूर्
मा ते सङ्गोऽस्त्वकर्मणि ॥२.४७॥
karmaṇyevādhikāraste
mā phaleṣu kadācana
mā karmaphalaheturbhūr
mā te saṅgo'stvakarmaṇi (2.47)

*karmaṇyevādhikāraste = karmaṇi — in performance + eva — alone + adhikāraḥ — command, privilege + te — your; mā — not; phaleṣu — in the aftermath of consequences; kadācana — at any time; mā — not; karmaphalahetur = karmaphala — a result + hetur (hetuh) — motivation; bhūr = bhūḥ — be; mā — not; te — your; saṅgo = sangah — attachment; 'stv = astu — should be; akarmaṇi — non-action, idleness*

**The command is yours while performing, but not at any time in the aftermath of consequences. Do not be motivated by a result, nor harbor an attachment to idleness. (2.47)**

***Siddha Swami's Commentary:***

This is a procedure for *karma yoga*, which consists of activities performed under the supervision of the Universal Form of *Śrī* Krishna and with a sense of detachment. In a sense a *karma* yogi has an easy-go-lucky, do-not-care attitude. He is not concerned with the outcome of what he does. His focus is on completion of duties.

Because he is employed by someone else, by *Śrī* Krishna specifically, the *karma* yogi does not have to be concerned with the outcome of what he does. At the same time, respecting the authority of the Supreme Being, he performs those duties industriously. He does not neglect the duties or maintain a sour attitude if they are unpalatable and cause him a bad reputation.

Someone who is employed to collect income taxes, should not regard the money or commodities collected as his own. Thus it does not disturb his mind if he has a large sum to collect on a specific day. In the same way, the *karma* yogi performs duties with detachment. Not all persons performing *karma yoga*, do so consciously. Many persons do so without knowing that they are serving the Universal Form of *Śrī* Krishna. However, whosoever willingly or accidentally, consciously or unconsciously, does comply with His way of running the world, that person attains merit in being favored by *Śrī* Krishna for the contribution to righteous lifestyle.

योगस्थः कुरु कर्माणि
सङ्गं त्यक्त्वा धनंजय ।
सिद्ध्यसिद्ध्योः समो भूत्वा
समत्वं योग उच्यते ॥२.४८॥
yogasthaḥ kuru karmāṇi
saṅgaṁ tyaktvā dhanaṁjaya
siddhyasiddhyoḥ samo bhūtvā
samatvaṁ yoga ucyate (2.48)

*yogasthaḥ — in yoga attitude; kuru — do perform; karmāṇi — actions; saṅgaṁ — attachment to crippling emotions; tyaktvā — having abandoned; dhanaṁjaya — conqueror of wealthy countries; siddhyasiddhyoḥ — to success or failure; samo = samaḥ — attitude of indifference; bhūtvā — be; samatvaṁ — indifference; yoga — yogic practice; ucyate — it is said*

**So perform actions in the yoga mood. Attachment to crippling emotions should be abandoned, O conqueror of wealthy countries. Be indifferent to success or failure. It is said that indifference denotes yoga. (2.48)**

***Siddha Swami's Commentary:***

Those who are ruled by emotions, will have some difficulty complying with this instruction for the *karma* yogis. It involves abandoning their natural obsession with emotions. Such persons believe in emotions more than anything else. Here *Śrī* Krishna instructs that they abandon or disregard crippling emotions.

Success is what motivates most people, but *Śrī* Krishna advised that one should be indifferent to that and not be disheartened by failure. If one acts for the Universal Form, for the Supreme Being, the venture might fail, even though the supreme will is behind it. In this world, the interaction of the supreme will and the puny wills spur action and reaction. In some circumstances, when the puny will encounters the supreme, the ultimate power fails to overcome the combined or individualized puny determinations. Thus if one acts for the supreme, one's action might still be thwarted by a lesser force. This does not mean that the puny will is just as powerful as the supreme, but it does mean that in this world, the supreme will is attenuated in contests with the puny determinations of the limited spirits.

It is sufficient to just represent the supreme will. One should not try to be the God but rather one should be an agent for the God and only for those duties assigned. One should be unconcerned in matters besides that.

Consequences are on-going. This means that whatever appears to be the outcome of an action, may very well not be related to that action at all. There is a backlog of reactions coming from previous actions. Some of these are coming from actions performed many millions of years ago. Hence at any given moment, in any circumstance, it is easy to confuse a fresh action with a reaction which might be coming from the long lost past. Only the Supreme Being has the supreme mind to analyze this. Therefore a *karma* yogi should never assume that he can understand the relationship between new actions and manifesting reactions, since those reactions may not relate to the new actions at all. This is why a *karma* yogi has to take *Śrī* Krishna's advice and not try to command consequences. He should not desire that consequences correspond to his actions.

In the case of a convicted man who is ordered to serve a prison sentence, it is hard to know whether the sentence is a consequence of his recent criminal action or if it is a reaction from an impious act from many lives before. How do we know that providence did not use his recent crime as an opportunity to deal with him for an impiety committed many, many lives before? Thus one should not jump to hasty conclusions, because one is normally unaware of the movements of providence. Ignorant persons who believe in the immediacy of the action-reaction cycle, profess that whatever a man does will definitely affect his future but there is no certainty about when the effects will come. It may be immediate or it may be delayed, all depending on providence.

दूरेण ह्यवरं कर्म
बुद्धियोगाद्धनंजय।
बुद्धौ शरणमन्विच्छ
कृपणाः फलहेतवः ॥२.४९॥
dūreṇa hyavaraṁ karma
buddhiyogāddhanaṁjaya
buddhau śaraṇamanviccha
kṛpaṇāḥ phalahetavaḥ (2.49)

*dūreṇa — by far; hyavaraṁ = hi — surely + avaraṁ — inferior + karma — cultural action; buddhiyogād = buddhiyogāt — intellectual discipline through yoga; dhanaṁjaya — victor of wealthy countries; buddhau — mystic insight; śaraṇam — location of confidence; anviccha — put; kṛpaṇāḥ — low and pathetic; phalahetavaḥ — people motivated for a result*

**Surely, cultural action is by far inferior to intellectual discipline through yoga, O victor of wealthy countries. One should take shelter in mystic insight, for how pathetic are those who are motivated by the promise of results. (2.49)**

***Siddha Swami's Commentary:***

*Karma yoga* without yoga is *karma* only. It is cultural activity only without the monitor of detachment gained though elementary yoga practice. As *Śrī* Krishna explained, the indifference to crippling emotions which is gained through yoga practice, is the very same indication that yoga is at work in the life of the *karma* yogi. Without that, one's cultural activities will be motivated by the various changing moods which emerge from the emotions in the psyche.

Cultural action alone is what motivates most human beings. They do so without the application of yoga maturity. Thus their actions are inferior because they do not have mystic insight. They hardly recognize a Supreme Controller, and as such their calculations are based on the family or species of their birth only. Intellectual discipline through yoga is *buddhi yoga*, and that entails forcing one's intellect to be subservient to one's *ātma* or spirit, as contrasted to the natural way of the intellect taking power from the spirit to foster pleasure and power in the gross world. It is natural to be motivated by the promise of results. This promise occurs in the mind, based on memory of previous enjoyments and hope for future ones, but this is haphazard and risky. Thus one is advised to come under the influence of the Supreme Lord and the great souls who adhere to Him. In that way, one can be trained to endeavor for more lasting benefits which involve the culture of the spirit and not just the status of the present body.

बुद्धियुक्तो जहातीह
उभे सुकृतदुष्कृते ।
तस्माद्योगाय युज्यस्व
योगः कर्मसु कौशलम् ॥२.५०॥
buddhiyukto jahātīha
ubhe sukṛtaduṣkṛte
tasmādyogāya yujyasva
yogaḥ karmasu kauśalam (2.50)

*buddhiyukto = buddhiyuktaḥ — a person disciplined by the reality-piercing insight; jahātīha = jahāti — he discards + iha — here; ubhe — both; sukṛtaduṣkṛte — pleasant and unpleasant work; tasmād = tasmāt — therefore; yogāya — to yoga; yujyasva — take yourself to; yogaḥ — yogic mood; karmasu — in performance; kauśalam — skill*

**A person who is disciplined by the reality-piercing insight discards in each life both pleasant and unpleasant work. Therefore take to the yogic mood. Yoga gives skill in performance. (2.50)**

***Siddha Swami's Commentary:***

We must note that this insight is gained when one sees clearly that one's emotions are usually converted into happy, distressful, exciting, depressing, enthusing and gloomy moods. Once this observation is made and the yogi keeps his emotions from being converted into moods, he develops the insight described by *Śrī* Krishna (2.38). Thus as *Śrī* Krishna stated in this verse, the *karma* yogi discards in life, both the pleasant and unpleasant work. For him work is work since his emotions do not react to the various circumstances. The prejudices and predispositions within his nature are no longer vented into his mind, and thus he becomes freed from the notions. Then he can take to the yogic mood. Subsequently, yoga gives him skill in performance, since he is no longer a pawn of his converted emotional energy in the form of moods.

कर्मजं बुद्धियुक्ता हि
फलं त्यक्त्वा मनीषिणः।
जन्मबन्धविनिर्मुक्ताः
पदं गच्छन्त्यनामयम् ॥२.५१॥
karmajaṁ buddhiyuktā hi
phalaṁ tyaktvā manīṣiṇaḥ
janmabandhavinirmuktāḥ
padaṁ gacchantyanāmayam (2.51)

*karmajaṁ — produced by actions; buddhiyuktā — disciplined mystic seers; hi — indeed; phalaṁ — result; tyaktvā — having abandoned; manīṣiṇaḥ — wise people; janmabandhavinirmuktāḥ = janma — rebirth + bandha — bondage + vinirmuktāḥ — freed from; padaṁ — place; gacchanty = gacchanti — go; anāmayam — misery-free*

**Having abandoned the results which are produced by actions, and being freed from the bondage of rebirth, those wise people, the disciplined mystic seers, go to the misery-free place. (2.51)**

***Siddha Swami's Commentary:***

Once the yogi gets free from moods, he gains ability to stop his emotions from being converted. These emotions remain stabilized and do not easily convert into various moods. When the moods no longer arise, the *yogin* no longer seeks, anticipates, or expects certain favorable results. Thus the petty gratifications no longer arise in his feelings and he abandons the results which are produced from actions.

Further practice causes one to transcend one's birth circumstance and to aim for full cooperation with the supreme will which calculates on a large scale, not just in relation to one life, but in relation to what should take place as a result of several lives. Thus the yogi becomes free from the bondage of rebirth, due to his cooperation with the Universal Form of *Śrī* Krishna.

One's nature, having been changed by this process of acting free from moods, develops compatibility with the spiritual places, the dimensions in which life is trouble-free.

यदा ते मोहकलिलं
बुद्धिर्व्यतितरिष्यति ।
तदा गन्तासि निर्वेदं
श्रोतव्यस्य श्रुतस्य च ॥२.५२॥

*yadā — when; te — you; mohakalilaṁ — delusion-saturated mind; buddhir (buddhiḥ) — discrimination; vyatitariṣyati — departs; tadā — then; gantāsi — you will become;*

yadā te mohakalilaṁ
buddhirvyatitariṣyati
tadā gantāsi nirvedaṁ
śrotavyasya śrutasya ca (2.52)

*nirvedaṁ — disgusted; śrotavyasya — with what is to be heard; śrutasya — what was heard; ca — and*

**When from your delusion-saturated mind, your discrimination departs, you will become disgusted with what is to be heard and what was heard. (2.52)**

Siddha Swami asked me to write what *Śrī Bābāji* instructed, since this is a *kriyā yoga* technique.

***Śrī Bābāji Mahāśaya's Commentary:***

Even though the yogi feels that his senses are going outwards, still he withdraws his intellect and lets it focus on the self. The sensual energy remains resistant and prejudiced towards the self. The sensual energies are parasitic on the self, only taking energy from it through the intellect and taking power from the kundalini shakti energy and from the diet eaten by the *yogin*. Thus the senses feel no necessity to cooperate with the self. They follow their own impulsions, which come from the emotional nature of the psyche. Still, the *yogin* must fight internally and command his intellect to give up its alliance with the senses. Some yogis use *japa*, the murmuring or loud repeating of Sanskrit phrases to keep the intellect occupied so that it does not chase after the senses. By nature the intellect chases after the senses and is indulged in related ideas by the memory. Thus the yogi must endeavor internally to cause the intellect to be introverted to the self.

Techniques are used in meditation, whereby a yogi pulls in the powers of his intellect even though he feels that his sensual energies resist him and keep going outwards regardless. The delusion-saturated mind *(moha kalilam)* consists of emotional energy which was converted into sensual energy. This might overpower the intellect, which in turn intimidates the core-self. Thus the self has to learn how to ignore the strength of the sensual energy and pull the intellect inwards towards the self, backwards into the head of the subtle body. So long as the intellect is focused outwards, it is hardly likely that it will be able to resist the strong sensual force. The technique is to pull the intellect backwards, away from the frontal lobe.

Please see these diagrams:

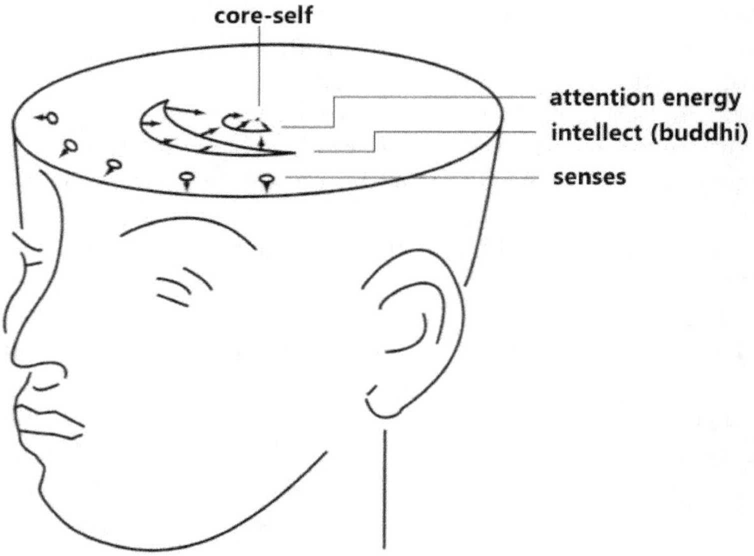

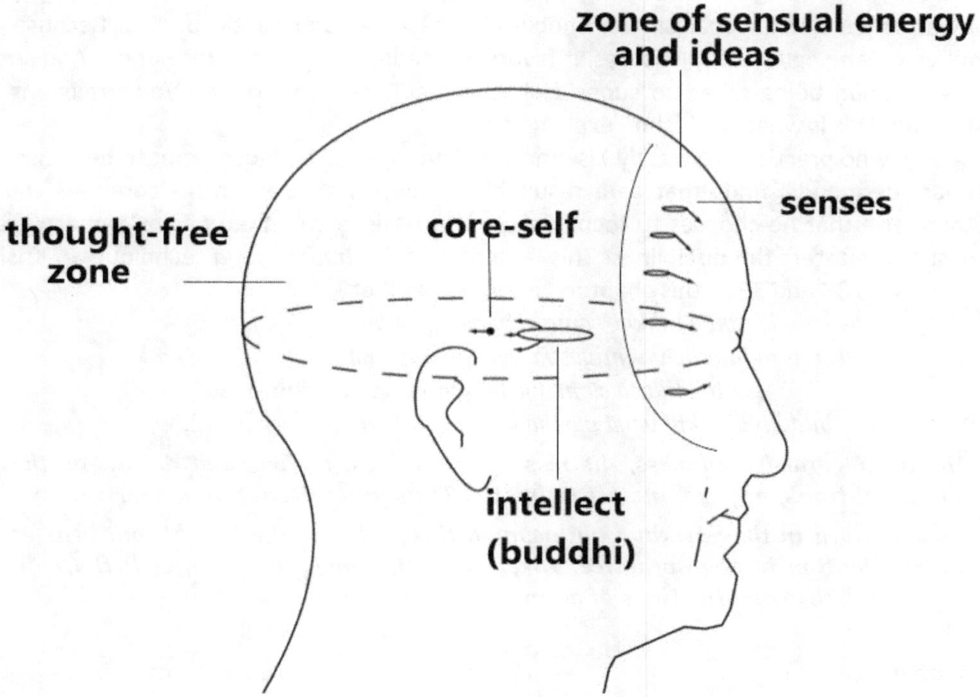


*Śrī* Krishna explained the outcome of this technique, whereby after mastering that, the yogi becomes disgusted with what is to be heard and was heard. He realizes that his progression hinges on individual effort to control the subtle parts of the psyche. He loses interest in superficial religions, because these usually focus on the external behavior of the body and hardly do they curb the organs in the subtle form.

श्रुतिविप्रतिपन्ना ते
यदा स्थास्यति निश्चला ।
समाधावचला बुद्धिस्
तदा योगमवाप्स्यसि ॥२.५३॥
śrutivipratipannā te
yadā sthāsyati niścalā
samādhāvacalā buddhis
tadā yogamavāpsyasi (2.53)

*śrutivipratipannā = śruti — scriptural information + vipratipannā — false, misleading; te — you; yadā — when; sthāsyati — will remain; niścalā — unmoving, steady; samādhāvacalābuddhis = samādhau — in deep meditation + acalā — without moving, stable + buddhis (buddhiḥ) — intelligence; tadā — then; yogam — yoga discipline; avāpsyasi — will master*

**When, rejecting misleading scriptural information, your intelligence remains steady without moody variation, being situated in deep meditation, you will master the yoga disciplines. (2.53)**

***Siddha Swami's Commentary:***

Initially a human being is attracted to misleading scriptural information *(śrutivipratipannā)*. This is because of a spirit's being under the influence of its psychology. The psychology itself is faulty. It consists of a sense of identity with attentive powers, an intellect with analyzing and visualizing capabilities, subtle senses with emotional energy, and a power-conversion mechanism for mobilizing the gross and subtle bodies. Because the primitive psychology seeks pleasures, it favors misleading scriptural information. And so the average human being takes up superficial religions. Even some of the Vedic religions are misleading. This is what *Śrī* Krishna explained here.

A yogi who practiced to steady his emotional energy and to cause it not to be converted into various moods, finds that as a result his intellect stabilizes on his core self and on anything else that he chooses to focus on. On this basis, a yogi then begins higher yoga in earnest and masters the disciplines. This is all part of the *buddhi yoga* technique *Śrī* Krishna gave in verses 38 and 39 of this chapter. Let us review that *kriyā*:

*sukhaduḥkhe same kṛtvā lābhālābhau jayājayau*
*tato yuddhāya yujyasva naivaṁ pāpamavāpsyasi (2.38)*
*eṣā te'bhihitā sāṁkhye buddhiryoge tvimāṁ śṛṇu*
*buddhyā yukto yayā pārtha karmabandhaṁ prahāsyasi (2.39)*

***Having regarded happiness, distress, gains, losses, victory and defeat, as the same emotions, apply yourself to battle. Thus you will get no demerit.***

***As explained in the Sāṁkhya philosophy, this vision is the insight, but hear of its application in yoga practice. Yoked with this insight, O son of Pṛthā, you will avoid the complications of action.* (2.38-39)**

अर्जुन उवाच
स्थितप्रज्ञस्य का भाषा
समाधिस्थस्य केशव ।
स्थितधीः किं प्रभाषेत
किमासीत व्रजेत किम् ॥ २.५४ ॥
arjuna uvāca
sthitaprajñasya kā bhāṣā
samādhisthasya keśava
sthitadhīḥ kiṁ prabhāṣeta
kimāsīta vrajeta kim (2.54)

*arjuna — Arjuna; uvāca — said; sthitaprajñasya — of the person who is situated in clear penetrating insight; kā — what; bhāṣā — description; samādhisthasya — one who is anchored in deep meditation; keśava — Keśava, Kṛṣṇa; sthitadhīḥ — one who is steady in objectives; kiṁ — whom; prabhāṣeta — should speak; kim — how; āsīta — should sit; vrajeta — move; kim — how*

**Arjuna said: In regards to the person who is situated in clear, penetrating insight, would you please describe him? Speak of the person who is anchored in deep meditation, O Keśava Krishna. As for the man who is steady in objectives, how would he speak? How would he sit? How would he act? (2.54)**

***Siddha Swami's Commentary:***

Arjuna asked a very important question. This is a worry for those who do not have mystic insight. How can a common person who evaluates external behavior, know if another person has penetrating insight? What are the external signs which denote a person who is advanced in *buddhi yoga*?

Arjuna categorized this *buddhi yoga* skill as *samādhi* practice, but this is only one type of such practice. In fact, this is a preliminary stage of *samādhi*, which consists of steadying *(sthita)* the intellect *(dhīh)* on the spirit *(ātma)*. When one does this consistently, then the spiritual research, the sorting out of the psychology, begins in earnest.

श्रीभगवानुवाच
प्रजहाति यदा कामान्
सर्वान्पार्थ मनोगतान् ।
आत्मन्येवात्मना तुष्टः
स्थितप्रज्ञस्तदोच्यते ॥२.५५॥
śrībhagavānuvāca
prajahāti yadā kāmān
sarvānpārtha manogatān
ātmanyevātmanā tuṣṭaḥ
sthitaprajñastadocyate (2.55)

*śrī bhagavān — the Blessed Lord; uvāca — said; prajahāti — abandons; yadā — when; kāmān — cravings; sarvān — all; pārtha — O son of Pṛthā; manogatān — escapes from mental dominance; ātmanyevātmanā = ātmani — in the spirit + eva — only + ātmanā — by the spirit; tuṣṭaḥ — being self-content; sthitaprajñastadocyate = sthitaprajñaḥ — one whose insight is steady + tadā — then + ucyate — is identified*

**The Blessed Lord said: When someone abandons all cravings, O son of Pṛthā, and escapes from mental dominance, being self-content, then that person is identified as one with steady insight. (2.55)**

Siddha Swami directed me to get a commentary from *Śrī Bābāji Mahāśaya*.

***Śrī Bābāji Mahāśaya's Commentary:***

To escape from mental dominance *(manogatān)*, one needs to perfect the *kriyā yoga* technique of separating the intellect from the sensual energies and memory (*mohakalikam buddhih vyatitarişyati*, 2.52). When this is done sufficiently, day after day in meditation practice, the intellect becomes resistant to the sensual energies, so much so that the intellect no longer follows the promptings of the senses without first consulting with the spiritual core-self. Gradually with time in practice, the *yogin* finds that his attention turns away from the intellect and begins to pay attention to the core self and to the naad subtle sound in the left ear. In addition, kundalini yoga has to be performed for the purification of the energy conversion mechanism which is in the spine. When the old energies are pushed out of the subtle spine, fresh, pranic subtle power enters. This causes a new type of sensual energy to be generated. This new energy is more interested in introspection and is resistant to the external reality.

In the advanced stage which is described in this verse, the yogi finds that his intellect loses its attractive power. Only his attention and sense of identity is felt as being turned inwards upon the core self. He is then said to be a *manogatān*, a person who has escaped from mental dominance.

Here is a diagram:

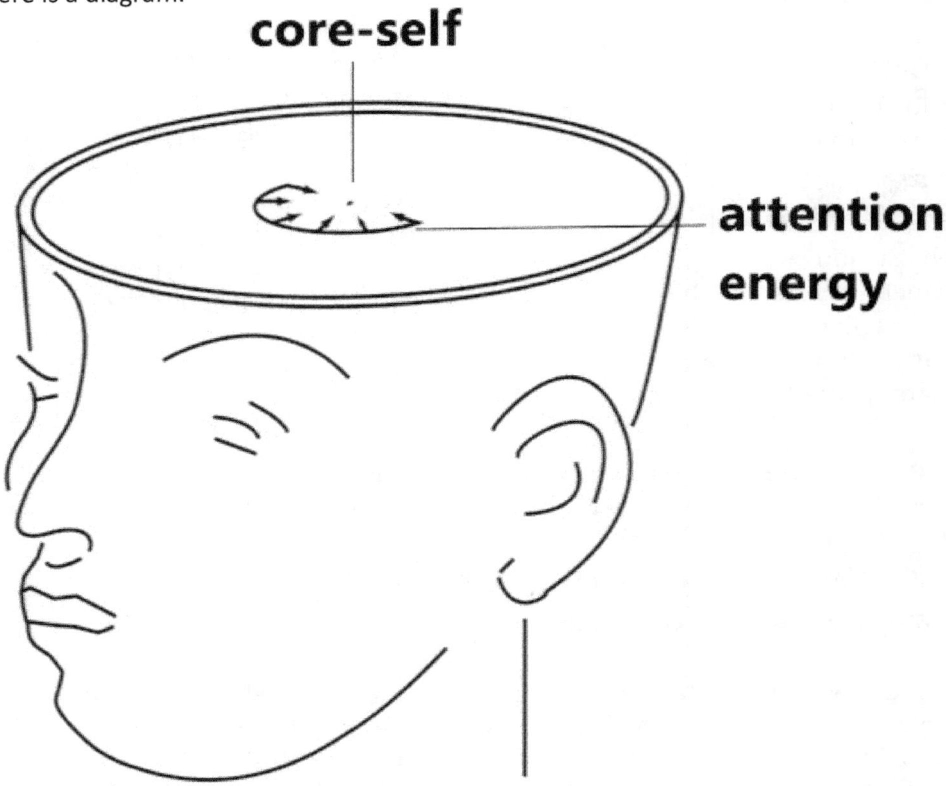


दुःखेष्वनुद्विग्नमनाः
सुखेषु विगतस्पृहः ।
वीतरागभयक्रोधः
स्थितधीर्मुनिरुच्यते ॥२.५६ ॥
duḥkheṣvanudvignamanāḥ
sukheṣu vigataspṛhaḥ
vītarāgabhayakrodhaḥ
sthitadhīrmunirucyate (2.56)

*duḥkheṣvanudvignamanāḥ = duḥkheṣv (duḥkheṣu) — in miserable conditions + anudvigna – free from worries + manāḥ — mind; sukheṣu — in good conditions; vigataspṛhaḥ — free from excitement; vītarāgabhayakrodhaḥ = vīta — steps aside + rāga — passion + bhaya — fear + krodhaḥ — anger; sthitadhīr = sthitadhīḥ — steady in meditation; munir = muniḥ — wise man; ucyate — is said to be*

**Furthermore, someone who in miserable conditions remains free from worries, and who in good conditions remains free from excitement, who steps aside from passion, fear and anger, and who is steady in meditation is considered to be a wise man. (2.56)**

***Siddha Swami's Commentary:***

Some external modes of behavior of the masterful *buddhi* yogi are given in this verse. These indications must be demonstrated consistently in the behavior of the said yogi. He must be able to ignore miserable conditions. He must overlook good conditions and be free of excitement in such circumstances. He must consistently be proven to have set aside passion, fear and anger. On the internal plane, to be verified by another mystic, his intellect must be steady in its focus on the core self, turning away consistently from the calls of the senses and from the pictures or sounds of the memory.

यः सर्वत्रानभिस्नेहस्
तत्तत्प्राप्य शुभाशुभम् ।
नाभिनन्दति न द्वेष्टि
तस्य प्रज्ञा प्रतिष्ठिता ॥२.५७॥
yaḥ sarvatrānabhisnehas
tattatprāpya śubhāśubham
nābhinandati na dveṣṭi
tasya prajñā pratiṣṭhitā (2.57)

*yaḥ — who; sarvatrā — in all circumstances; anabhisnehaḥ — without crippling affections; tattat = tad tad — this or that; prāpya — meeting; śubhāśubham — enjoyable and disturbing factors; nābhinandati = na — not + abhinandati — excited; na — nor; dveṣṭi — distressed; tasya — his; prajñā — reality-piercing consciousness; pratiṣṭhitā — is established*

**A person who, in all circumstances, is without crippling affections, who, when meeting enjoyable or disturbing factors, does not get excited or distressed, his reality-piercing consciousness is established. (2.57)**

***Siddha Swami's Commentary:***

More indications of the masterful *buddhi* yogi are given in this verse. Because his emotions usually remain unconverted into moods (verse 2.38), he usually remains poised to act but without crippling affections. When meeting enjoyable or disturbing factors, he does not get excited or distressed. He is said to be a reality-piercing ascetic *(prajñā pratiṣṭhitā)*. This is because his intellect is freed from sensual dominance and from addiction to being shown references by the memory mechanism. Thus he abandons prejudices and is free to act on behalf of the Supreme God.

यदा संहरते चायं
कूर्मोऽङ्गानीव सर्वशः ।
इन्द्रियाणीन्द्रियार्थेभ्यस्
तस्य प्रज्ञा प्रतिष्ठिता ॥२.५८॥
yadā saṁharate cāyaṁ
kūrmo'ṅgānīva sarvaśaḥ
indriyāṇīndriyārthebhyas
tasya prajñā pratiṣṭhitā (2.58)

*yadā — when; saṁharate — pulls; cāyaṁ = ca — and + ayam — this; kūrmo = kūrmaḥ — tortoise; 'ṅgānīva = aṅgānīva = aṅgāni — limbs + iva — like, compared to; sarvaśaḥ — fully; indriyāṇīndriyārthebhyas = indriyani — senses + indriyarthebhyaḥ — attractive things; tasya — his; prajñā — reality-piercing vision; pratiṣṭhitā — is established*

**When such a person pulls fully out of moods, he or she may be compared to the tortoise with its limbs retracted. The senses are withdrawn from the attractive things in the case of a person whose reality-piercing vision is established. (2.58)**

***Śrī Bābāji Mahāśaya's Commentary:***

This is an advanced stage of the same *buddhi yoga*, whereby the intellect is separated from the sensual energies and refocused on the core self. After much practice, the senses and their energies become attracted to the core self but they send their energies to it, through the intellect organ, the *buddhi*. During this state, the emotions are unable to convert their excess charges into moods. Thus *Śrī* Krishna compared such an accomplished *buddhi* yogi to a tortoise with its limbs retracted, not being interested in the external world, not procuring or showing interest in anything external to the psyche. It is due to a strong inner interest in the core self that the yogi develops this introverted state.

**Śrī *Bābāji Mahāśaya*** asked me to submit this diagram:

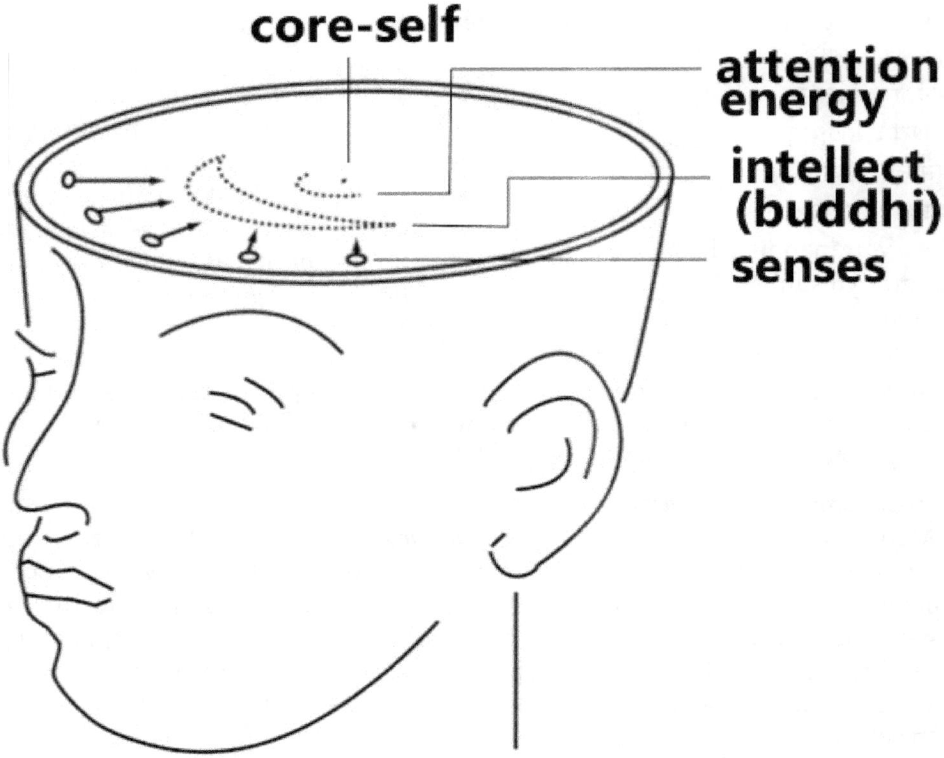


विषया विनिवर्तन्ते
निराहारस्य देहिनः।
रसवर्जं रसोऽप्यस्य
परं दृष्ट्वा निवर्तते॥ २.५९॥
viṣayā vinivartante
nirāhārasya dehinaḥ
rasavarjaṁ raso'pyasya
paraṁ dṛṣṭvā nivartate (2.59)

*viṣayā = viṣayāḥ — temptations; vinivartante — turn away; nirāhārasya — from (without) indulgence; dehinaḥ — of the embodied soul; rasavarjaṁ = rasa – memory or mental flavor of past indulgences + varjaṁ — except for, besides; raso = rasah — memories (mental flavors); 'pyasya = apyasya = apy (api) — even + asya — of him; paraṁ — higher stage; dṛṣṭvā — having experienced; nivartate — leaves*

**The temptations themselves turn away from the disciplinary attitude of an ascetic, but the memory of previous indulgences remain with him. When he experiences higher stages, those memories leave him. (2.59)**

***Siddha Swami's Commentary:***

This happens in a very advanced stage of *buddhi yoga*, when the ascetic has completely curbed his *buddhi* organ and when it has developed automatic resistance to the sensual energies, no longer trusting them, and no longer maintaining a romantic relationship with them. To such an ascetic, it seems that all of a sudden, even the temptations turn away from him. Objects which before used to call him, used to approach him enticingly, seem as if they are avoiding him with an ashamed attitude. People who formerly used to try to indulge him, now want to protect him from vices. Those who objected to his disciplines, now want to support him and to do whatever is possible for success.

However, despite that relief in social relationships and in the proposals of inanimate nature, the memory of previous indulgences haunt him.

***Śrī Bābāji Mahāśaya's Commentary:***

Initially in the practice of buddhi yoga, the ascetic does not know the irritation of memory. He feels that it is only the senses and their attractive objects (*indriyāṇīndriyārthebhyas,* 2.58) which pose a problem for him. Thus his introspection consists of pulling the buddhi intellect organ away from the senses. When he gets a foothold in mastering that, he gains sufficient courage to pull the sensual energies into the buddhi organ. This takes a tremendous amount of mental, muscular power. But if he persists day after day, after a time he gains success. Then he discovers that the memory is also a nuisance. This is a completely separate part of the mind mechanism. He has to study the memory at that stage. He must note its location and its operations. Then he may subdue it.

*Śrī Patañjali Mahārṣi* listed memory as one of the *vṛttis* or operative modes of the mento-emotional energy. Take note of it. Those who neglect to master the memory, cannot reach the advanced stages of *buddhi yoga,* the details of which are given by *Śrī* Krishna in this Chapter Two. One has to experience higher stages *(param dṛṣṭvā)* before the memory ceases its provocations. Unless one has experiences of higher dimensions in the brahma world, one cannot be free from the memory, because it is the nature of the core self to hunt for some type of experience. If it can no longer seek out experiences in the external world and feast on the mood changes of the emotions, then it takes experiences from the memory unless it finds another world for satisfactions.

***Śrī Bābāji Mahāśaya*** presented this diagram:

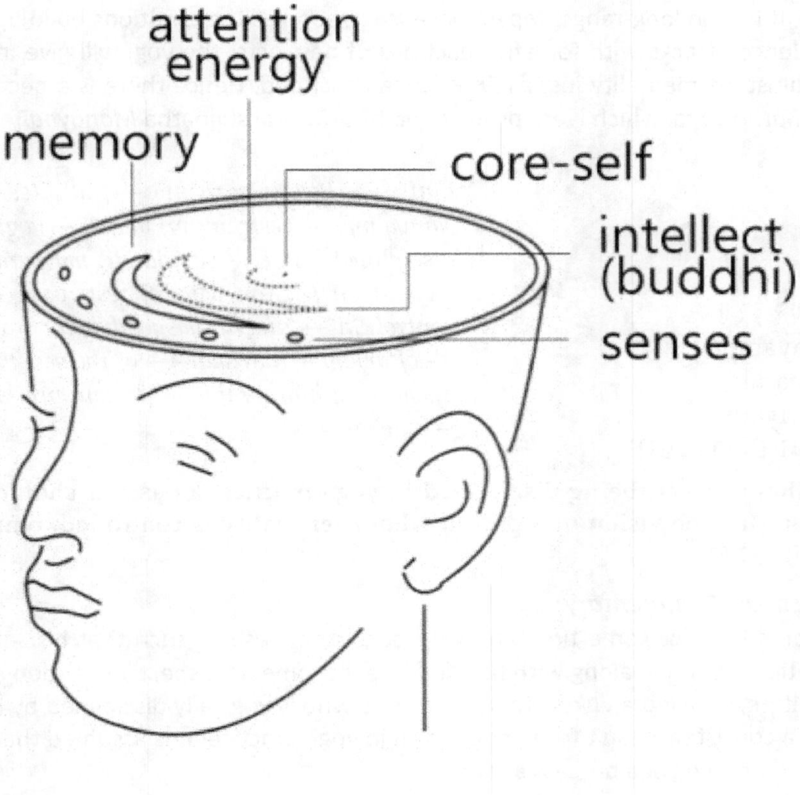

यततो ह्यपि कौन्तेय
पुरुषस्य विपश्चितः।
इन्द्रियाणि प्रमाथीनि
हरन्ति प्रसभं मनः ॥२.६०॥
yatato hyapi kaunteya
puruṣasya vipaścitaḥ
indriyāṇi pramāthīni
haranti prasabhaṁ manaḥ (2.60)

*yatato = yatataḥ — concerning an aspiring seeker; hyapi = hi — indeed + api — also; kaunteya — son of Kuntī; puruṣasya — of the person; vipaścitaḥ — of the discerning educated; indriyāṇi — the senses; pramāthīni — tormenting; haranti — seize, adjust; prasabhaṁ — impulsively, by impulse; manaḥ — mentally*

**Concerning an aspiring seeker, O son of Kuntī, concerning a discerned educated person, the senses do torment him. By impulses, the senses do adjust his mentality. (2.60)**

***Śrī Bābāji Mahāśaya's Commentary:***

This describes an intellectual who begins to observe how his mentality interacts with emotional moods to affect his determination and bring him to accept certain proposals of the senses which leak into the intellect and spur attachment. When pursuing spiritual life without following the eight part yoga system, one does so haphazardly and tries to regulate one's behavior by will power. This does not work because the will power may be charmed by the emotions. It may be neutralized by the memory images. It may be harnessed by the desires for pleasure. Aspiring celibates are quite familiar with this, since their desire for continence is often disrupted by emotions which overpower their determination and make them forcibly subscribe to schemes involving sexual indulgence. This may happen in the gross or subtle body. It can be observed by any honest celibate.

This technique for intellectual adjustment by will power and determination only works some of the time. It has no long-range impact because as soon as the emotions build up and as soon as providence attacks with forceful reactions of past acts, the yogi will give in and the senses will adjust his mentality just as *Śrī* Krishna described. Hence there is a necessity for austerities of *haṭha* yoga, which were propagated by *Śrī* Gorakshanatha *Mahāyogī*.

तानि सर्वाणि संयम्य
युक्त आसीत मत्परः।
वशे हि यस्येन्द्रियाणि
तस्य प्रज्ञा प्रतिष्ठिता ॥२.६१॥
tāni sarvāṇi saṁyamya
yukta āsīta matparaḥ
vaśe hi yasyendriyāṇi
tasya prajñā pratiṣṭhitā (2.61)

*tāni — these; sarvāṇi — all (senses); saṁyamya — restraining; yukta — yogically disciplined; āsīta — should sit; matparaḥ — focused on Me, on My interest; vaśe — in control; hi — indeed; yasyendriyāṇi = yasya — of whom + indriyāṇi — of the sensuality; tasya — of him; prajñā — vision; pratiṣṭhitā — anchored*

**Restraining all these senses, being disciplined in yoga practice, an ascetic should sit, being focused on Me. The vision of a person whose sensuality is controlled, remains anchored in reality. (2.61)**

***Śrī Bābāji Mahāśaya's Commentary:***

A yogi who practiced for some time and with consistent results, such that his senses, intellect and emotional energy, along with his life force, become introspective as soon as he sits down to meditate, is called a *yukta*. This means one who is yogically disciplined by habit and who accrued a consistent result from meditation in yoga practice. It is assumed that this person mastered the *haṭha* yoga process already.

First one must be a *vipaścitah*, a discerning educated person, who observed that the senses do adjust one's mentality. Then one has to reach a stage of knowing that mere will power cannot man-handle the sensual energies. In fact, one has to admit that it is more to the reverse. In more cases, the sensuality defeats the will power and enslaves it. Thus one has to move from the stage of being an intellectual to that of being a neophyte yogi. Such a yogi takes up *buddhi yoga* and when that is completed, he does kundalini yoga, which advances into *kriyā yoga* and then is finalized with *brahma yoga*.

What is now known as *bhakti yoga*, which is *bhakti* without the eightfold yoga practice, is not part of this system, except for the intellectual decisions made for detachment and observations of how forces in the psyche work. As such, those modern *bhakti* yogis are only intellectuals with impure emotions directed to *Śrī* Krishna, or to some other divinity.

The real *bhakti yoga*, which is *bhakti* and yoga practice combined, is part of *kriyā yoga* and *brahma yoga*. This text 61 of Chapter Two is the first *kriyā* for *bhakti yoga* given by *Śrī* Krishna in the *Gītā*. This is because before one can reach *Śrī* Krishna, one has to be very advanced in *buddhi yoga* and *kriyā yoga*, so advanced that one would have mastered the technique of causing the intellect to desist from the senses and to focus on the spirit self, the core self. One must also be so versed in this, that one's sensual energies would, of their own accord, follow the lead of the intellect to focus backwards onto the spirit self. Then when this is steadied, one would begin to submit to *Śrī* Krishna or alternately to one of the divinities who are parallel to Him or to a great *yogin* who is further along in the practice of these disciplines.

The spiritual existence of *Śrī* Krishna is not available to the polluted psyche of anyone. Therefore to focus on Him spiritually in the polluted state, is not possible. One must first gain the required purity by austerities in higher yoga, and then one must wait in *samādhi* for revelation about *Śrī* Krishna's spiritual condition and spiritual location. Only then, one can sit being focused on *Śrī* Krishna or on any of His parallel divinities. Unless one causes his core self and its attention to remain focused in the self for long periods of time in *samādhi*, one cannot reach *Śrī* Krishna and one cannot be a *bhakti* yogi in fact. This focus on Krishna *(matparah)* occurs through the reformed and transformed *buddhi* organ, which was reformed from external focus, liberated from dependence on the senses and freed from the hypnosis of the memory. When the *buddhi* organ is freed in that way, it develops into a spiritual tool of perception, whereby one can see into the chit akasha, the sky of consciousness, where *Śrī* Krishna resides in spiritual form. That is an entirely different dimension and one cannot see into it by any other means. The next diagram depicts this:

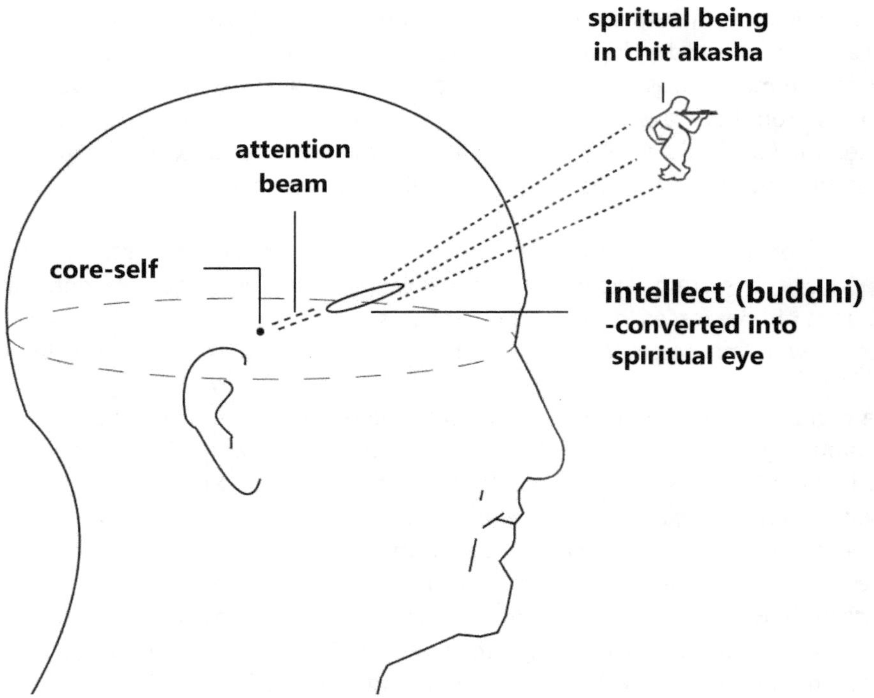


ध्यायतो विषयान्पुंसः
सङ्गस्तेषूपजायते ।
सङ्गात्संजायते कामः
कामात्क्रोधोऽभिजायते ॥ २.६२ ॥
dhyāyato viṣayānpuṁsaḥ
saṅgasteṣūpajāyate
saṅgātsaṁjāyate kāmaḥ
kāmātkrodho'bhijāyate (2.62)

*dhyāyato = dhyāyataḥ — considering; viṣayān — sensual objects; puṁsaḥ — a person; saṅgas — attachment; teṣupajāyate = teṣu — in them + upajāyate — is born, is created; saṅgāt — from attachment; saṁjāyate — is born; kāmaḥ — craving; kāmāt – from craving; krodho = krodhah — anger; 'bhijāyate = abhijāyate — is derived*

**The act of considering sensual objects, creates in a person, an attachment to them. From attachment comes craving. From this craving, anger is derived. (2.62)**

***Śrī Bābāji Mahāśaya's Commentary:***

These details are to be studied intellectually by the novice yogi and by those on the spiritual path who do not do yoga. This is an observational technique. The destruction of this detrimental process of sensual ingestion is not completed until one reaches the stage of non-appropriation in *brahma yoga*, but initially one makes many efforts to curtail this automatic process by partially curbing the sensual intake of data from this subtle and gross material world.

The appropriation or taking of sensual imprints of the subtle and gross objects is labeled in this verse as *dhyāyato viṣayān*. This is actually a form of theft of the imprints or images of the object. Once the item is imprinted in the senses, they relay the information to the intellect and memory. The memory takes the imprint as it is and files it in reference to other stored data. The intellect uses the information to form biases and make decisions about the value of items encountered by the senses. In *brahma yoga*, in higher yoga, a yogi is given an instruction not to appropriate, or ingest ideas and images which the senses steal from objects. However, neophyte yogis cannot do this. They endeavor to curb what the senses bring in but they cannot stop the senses altogether. They are unable to reject everything the senses steal and offer to the intellect and memory. This is due to a natural psychological weakness towards the power of the senses in its alliance with the memory and intellect.

Initially one cannot understand the details of a consideration. Therefore one has to regard it as one single occurrence. This is an intellectual observation. By such consideration one develops an attachment automatically. Even an aversion or repulsion from an object is an attachment. From such attachment, a craving develops in the emotional energy. If that craving is frustrated, it converts into a mood of anger or resentment. The craving may be positive or negative, meaning a desire to associate further with the object or a desire to be away from it. If one dislikes the object and comes near to it, one is frustrated. If one likes the object and is removed from it, one is frustrated as well. This occurs because one is confused about identity and one cannot sort between one's emotions, one's life energy, one's intellect and the moods which form from biases.

In *brahma yoga*, the act of considering is broken down into its constituent parts. These begin with the ranging of the senses into the subtle or gross material world. It proceeds to the absorption of images, recorded sounds, odors, taste or feelings. These impressions are then analyzed by the intellect and appropriated or held for storage by the memory. The practiced yogi greatly reduces the amount of sensual objects encountered by going into isolation. Then whatever imprints the senses take in from the subtle or gross material world, he intercepts and rejects before the memory and intellect are allowed to handle these. Initially there is a struggle for the yogi. Sometimes he stops the intellect and memory in their act of taking the stolen imprints from the senses but at other times, he is able to stop the senses from delivering their stolen imprints to either the intellect or the memory. When the yogi can stop the appropriation of the senses, he makes advancement in quieting the intellect and memory, for they are no longer encouraged and goaded by the imprints which strengthen them from the external world. Then there is hope for that yogi to enter into *samādhi* practice.

क्रोधाद्भवति संमोहः
संमोहात्स्मृतिविभ्रमः ।
स्मृतिभ्रंशाद्बुद्धिनाशो
बुद्धिनाशात्प्रणश्यति ॥२.६३॥
krodhādbhavati saṁmohaḥ
saṁmohātsmṛtivibhramaḥ
smṛtibhraṁśādbuddhināśo
buddhināśātpraṇaśyati (2.63)

*krodhād = krodhāt — from anger; bhavati — becomes (comes); saṁmohaḥ — delusion; saṁmohāt — from delusion; smṛti — conscience + vibhramaḥ — vanish; smṛtibhraṁśād = smṛtibhraṁśāt = smṛti — memory, judgment + bhraṁśāt — from fading away; buddhināśo = buddhināśaḥ = buddhi — discerning power + nāśaḥ — lose, affected; buddhināśāt = buddhi — discernment + nāśāt — from loss, from being affected; praṇaśyati — is ruined*

**From anger, comes delusion. From this delusion, the conscience vanishes. When he loses judgment, his discerning power fades away. Once the discernment is affected, he is ruined. (2.63)**

***Śrī Bābāji Mahāśaya's Commentary:***

Once a person is overcome by the conjoint influences of the senses, intellect and memory, his emotions side with the intellect in forming a bias. Thus his religious values may fade away. His power of discernment then serves the needs of the senses, instead of censoring their activity and condemning their theft of images, sounds, tastes, flavors and feelings. Such a person is, of course, ruined, as *Śrī* Krishna declared.

रागद्वेषवियुक्तैस्तु
विषयानिन्द्रियैश्चरन् ।
आत्मवश्यैर्विधेयात्मा
प्रसादमधिगच्छति ॥२.६४॥
rāgadveṣaviyuktaistu
viṣayānindriyaiścaran
ātmavaśyairvidheyātmā
prasādamadhigacchati (2.64)

*rāgadveṣaviyuktais = rāga — cravings + dveṣa — disliking + viyuktaiḥ — discontinued; tu — if, however; viṣayān — attractive objects; indriyaiścaran = indriyaiḥ — by the senses + caran — interacting; ātmavaśyair = ātmavaśyaiḥ — disciplined person; vidheyātmā — a well-behaved person; prasādam — grace of providence; adhigacchati — gets*

**If, on the other hand, cravings and dislikings are continued and the attractive objects and senses continue interaction, a disciplined person who is usually well-behaved, gets the grace of providence. (2.64)**

### *Śrī Bābāji Mahāśaya's Commentary:*

When a neophyte yogi first tries to discipline the senses, he discovers, to his dismay, that he cannot do so, because the senses are unsubmissive to him. The senses take cues from the intellect and the memory and from the external subtle and gross material world. They do not adhere to the desires of the core self, even though they are reliant on the attentive energy of the self. If he persists in the practice, the neophyte yogi discovers that the intellect will comply with his request more frequently than the senses and the memory. Thus he has no alternative but to curb the intellect first and to leave the senses and memory to their own devices until he can develop his psychological strength.

The craving and disliking of the intellect may be monitored successfully with due consideration in silent meditation and by taking help from more advanced yogins. In the meantime, the senses will continue to interact willy nilly with their objects and the memory will play havoc in assisting the senses and in trying to intimidate the intellect and the spirit self. But if the *yogin* keeps up his practice, if he maintains the disciplines of yoga which he learned, then he will get the grace of providence, provided he behaves himself socially by heeding moral laws and upholding a righteous lifestyle.

### *Siddha Swami's Commentary:*

The grace of providence, *prasādam*, is an absolute necessity for the neophyte yogi. Without it, he can advance no further. This is the helping energy from the divine beings and from greater, more advanced yogins. With this contribution, the neophyte yogi gets set in the higher yoga practice of *samādhi*. Normally a living being cannot get the best of his sensual energy and his memory which goad him to act in a prejudicial way. This is because the subtle body or psyche, which is awarded to a living being, is more than he can effectively control. Thus he must take help from superior beings. In India, there is a feeling that unless one gets the grace of a *Sat* guru, a person of reality, one cannot attain spiritual perfection. This belief is correct; it is because one has a complicated psyche which one cannot control alone. One must take assistance from the elevated beings.

प्रसादे सर्वदुःखानां
हानिरस्योपजायते ।
प्रसन्नचेतसो ह्याशु
बुद्धिः पर्यवतिष्ठते ॥२.६५॥
prasāde sarvaduḥkhānāṁ
hānirasyopajāyate
prasannacetaso hyāśu
buddhiḥ paryavatiṣṭhate (2.65)

*prasāde — the grace of providence producing spiritual peace of mind; sarvaduḥkhānāṁ = sarva — all + duḥkhāṇām — of the emotional distresses; hānir = hāniḥ — cessation, end; asyopajāyate = asya — of him + upajāyate — is produced; prasannacetaso = prasannacetasaḥ = prasanna – peaceful + cetasaḥ— of mind; hyāśu = hy (hi) — indeed + āśu — at once; buddhiḥ — intelligence; paryavatiṣṭhate — becomes stable*

**By the grace of providence, all the emotional distresses cease for him. Being of a pacified mind, his intelligence at once, becomes stable. (2.65)**

***Siddha Swami's Commentary:***

Those distresses cease for him because of sustained practice and eventual mastership of the *buddhi yoga* technique mentioned in verses 38 and 39 of this chapter. The sustained practice is caused by the divine grace, by the grace of providence, *prasādam*. Due to that he gets the strength to transcend, to actually ignore the moods. Eventually his emotions stop being transformed.

*Cetaso* means the combined energy which is emotional power, sensual energy and life force. This is usually experienced as consciousness in the mind. It is not one homogeneous energy. It is tripartite. Due to lack of clarity, a limited being does not understand these divisions or mixtures which make up what is termed consciousness. Thus one is misled into thinking that the cultural personality is an indivisible whole.

When the emotional energies no longer convert into various moods, one gets a more stable condition of consciousness, and one's intellect becomes steady, no longer being pulled haphazardly by the emotions, sensual energies and life force survival energy. This is the culmination of *buddhi yoga*, which was taught to Arjuna by *Bhagavān* Krishna in this chapter.

नास्ति बुद्धिरयुक्तस्य
न चायुक्तस्य भावना ।
न चाभावयतः शान्तिर्
अशान्तस्य कुतः सुखम् ॥२.६६॥
nāsti buddhirayuktasya
na cāyuktasya bhāvanā
na cābhāvayataḥ śāntir
aśāntasya kutaḥ sukham (2.66)

*nāsti = na— no + asti — is; buddhir = buddhiḥ — proper discernment; ayuktasya — of the uncontrolled person; na — not; cāyuktasya = ca — and + ayuktasya — of the uncontrolled person; bhāvanā — concentration; na — not; cābhāvayataḥ = ca — and + abhāvayataḥ — a person lacking concentration; śāntir = śāntiḥ — peace; aśāntasya — lacking emotional stability; kutaḥ — how is it to be achieved; sukham — happiness*

**In comparison, never is there proper discernment in an uncontrolled person. He is not capable of concentration. One who lacks concentration cannot get inner peace. For one who lacks emotional stability, how will happiness be achieved? (2.66)**

***Siddha Swami's Commentary:***

There are different types of concentration. This type is the yogic achievement. Everyone experiences concentration. Even animals, like tigers, concentrate on the animals they hope to kill for a meal. This is not yogic concentration. *Śrī* Krishna described a concentration which results from mood detachment and elimination and from which one's intellect becomes freed from its usual slavery to the emotional, sensual and involuntary survival energies. An uncontrolled person, lacking yoga expertise, cannot get that sort of psychological control. Plus, the happiness felt by that person differes from the happiness experienced by one whose nature no longer converts into various moods for excitement and depression.

Everyone achieves some type of happiness, even if it is not deliberate. Sometimes we see a baby smiling in a crib for no apparent reason. Sometimes persons who are insane exhibit great happiness. Hence the happiness and inner peace described here are gained when one abandons the mood swings of the emotions, when those emotions stabilize so that they do not convert into happiness, distress, feelings of gains and losses, victory and defeat, as stated in verse 38 of this chapter.

इन्द्रियाणां हि चरतां
यन्मनोऽनुविधीयते ।
तदस्य हरति प्रज्ञां
वायुर्नावमिवाम्भसि ॥२.६७॥
indriyāṇāṁ hi caratāṁ
yanmano'nuvidhīyate
tadasya harati prajñāṁ
vāyurnāvamivāmbhasi (2.67)

*indriyāṇām — of the senses; hi — indeed; caratāṁ — wandering; yan = yad — when; mano = manaḥ — the mind; 'nuvidhīyate = anuvidhīyate — is prompted; tadasya = tad — that + asya — of it; harati — it utilizes; prajñāṁ — of the discernment; vāyur = vāyuḥ — the wind; nāvam — a ship; ivāmbhasi = iva — like + ambhasi — in the water*

**When the mind is prompted by the wandering senses, it utilizes the discernment, just as in water, the wind handles a ship. (2.67)**

***Siddha Swami's Commentary:***

This is an observation made while trying to master *buddhi yoga*. One hears of this from the teacher; then in meditation, one sees this occurring. Here the word *mano (manah)* means the rim of the mind, the outer subtle membrane of it, where the senses burst out. The senses lie on the surface of the mind, just as hairs lie on and come out of the skin or just as a pimple erupts from the skin and oozes outwards. When the edge of the mind is alerted by any one or any combination of the senses, the sensual energies in the mind chamber direct themselves to the intellect which is deep in the mind. Receiving such information, the intellect feels forced to act. The memory is also alerted and it presents the intellect with impressions which might relate to the incoming information. The intellect then considers both the impressions from memory and the new information which was presented to it. From this a conclusion is derived. From that conclusion some action or some lack of action is decided. The spirit looks on as a neutral observer but it is usually influenced to endorse the plan of the intellect. With that endorsement, the intellect commands the psyche to operate to bring about a certain circumstance.

The intellect is identified here by the technical term *prajñām*. This is because by itself the spirit would not form any opinions about the material energy. But when it is connected to an intellect, it becomes subjected to the conclusions formed by that analyzing organ. The technique of *buddhi yoga* is to free the intellect from the dominance of the senses and the memory. The individual spirit must gain control of the intellect in such a way, that the senses are no longer free to influence it. That is the purpose of *buddhi yoga*.

As the wind will handle a ship in water, the senses will dominate the intellect. One has to stop this natural process. Thus one must learn *Śrī* Krishna's method of *buddhi yoga*.

तस्माद्यस्य महाबाहो
निगृहीतानि सर्वशः ।
इन्द्रियाणीन्द्रियार्थेभ्यस्
तस्य प्रज्ञा प्रतिष्ठिता ॥२.६८॥
tasmādyasya mahābāho
nigṛhītāni sarvaśaḥ
indriyāṇīndriyārthebhyas
tasya prajñā pratiṣṭhitā (2.68)

*tasmād — therefore; yasya — of the person who; mahābāho — O powerful Arjuna; nigṛhītāni — retracts; sarvaśaḥ — in every interaction; indriyāṇīndriyārthebhyas = indriyāṇi — sensual feelings + indriyārthebhyaḥ — of the attractive objects; tasya — his; prajñā — discernment; pratiṣṭhitā — remains constant*

**Thus, O Arjuna, concerning the person who, in every interaction retracts the sensual feelings from the attractive objects; his discernment remains constant. (2.68)**

***Siddha Swami's Commentary:***

One who practices this *buddhi yoga* must do much meditational observation of how the psyche operates. He must also observe the workings of the mind when not in meditation, when the senses are acting out their pursuits for attractive objects. This allows for the development of objectivity.

The retraction of the sensual feelings, just as they are going out through the senses or through the mind to reach the attractive objects, is a mystic act, mastered by steady meditation in *buddhi yoga* practice. So long as the senses are allowed to interact either externally with objects or internally with the memory or novel imagination of objects, the intellect may have to interact with the impressions it receives. It will, of necessity, have to analyze and then exhibit prejudices. Thus, for a constant discernment free from sensual dominance, the senses must be stopped from their procurement of impressions either from external real objects, from memories stored, or from mental creations manufactured in the imagination organ. A *buddhi* yogi must therefore practice day after day, during meditation and during external activity, to pull back or restrain the senses from their attractive objects.

या निशा सर्वभूतानां
तस्यां जागर्ति संयमी ।
यस्यां जाग्रति भूतानि
सा निशा पश्यतो मुनेः ॥२.६९॥
yā niśā sarvabhūtānāṁ
tasyāṁ jāgarti saṁyamī
yasyāṁ jāgrati bhūtāni
sā niśā paśyato muneḥ (2.69)

*yā — which; niśā — void; sarvabhūtānāṁ — all ordinary people; tasyāṁ — in this; jāgarti — is perceptive; saṁyamī — the sense-controlling person; yasyāṁ — in what; jāgrati — is exciting; bhūtāni — the masses of people; sā — that; niśā — is void; paśyato = paśyataḥ — of the perceptive; muneḥ — of the sage*

**The sense-controlling person is perceptive of that which is void to the ordinary people. What is exciting to the masses of people is void to the perceptive sage. (2.69)**

***Siddha Swami's Commentary:***

The *samyamī* yogi sees life in a different way, outside of convention. What has much value to others, may have no value at all to him. What interests him, appears worthless to others. *Śrī* Krishna titled such a person as a *muni*, a sagely philosopher. The opinions of such a *samyamī* yogi are based on his experiences of the various moods assumed by the emotions, such that the pleasures and pains of an ordinary person, are considered by him to be mere conversions of the one emotional energy as it is magnetized by the senses and their perceptions which influence the intellect. Due to stability in consciousness, others regard him as a person without feeling, without variety in moods. Understanding that the play of subtle forces motivates the psyche to act in prejudiced way, he avoids many circumstances which might trigger his attention, and so others regard him as being anti-social.

आपूर्यमाणमचलप्रतिष्ठं
समुद्रमापः प्रविशन्ति यद्वत् ।
तद्वत्कामा यं प्रविशन्ति सर्वे
स शान्तिमाप्नोति न कामकामी ॥ २.७० ॥
āpūryamāṇamacalapratiṣṭhaṁ
samudramāpaḥ praviśanti yadvat
tadvatkāmā yaṁ praviśanti sarve
sa śāntimāpnoti na kāmakāmī (2.70)

*āpūryamāṇam — becoming filled; acala – not moving about + pratiṣṭham — remaining stationary; samudram — the ocean; āpaḥ — the waters; praviśanti — they enter; yadvat — in which; tadvat — similarly; kāmā = kāmāḥ — cravings; yaṁ — whom; praviśanti — enter, arise; sarve — all; sa — he; śāntim — true satisfaction; āpnoti — gets; na — not; kāmakāmī — one who craves for every desire*

**Becoming filled, not flowing about, remaining stationary, the ocean absorbs the waters that enter it. Similarly, a person who remains calm when cravings arise gets true satisfaction, but not the person who craves for every desire. (2.70)**

***Siddha Swami's Commentary:***

This proves that the *samyamī yogin* might feel cravings from time to time, but he does not react to these by impulsion. He can see how the forces move within the psyche and he may resist them. Thus he discovers another type of satisfaction, besides the fulfillment of urges. That is the satisfaction of not having the emotions be converted into moods of excitement or depression, and knowing that one has, in fact, controlled the inner energies, particularly the sensual forces and the intellect which they once controlled.

The *kāmakāmī* is the ordinary person in this world. He does not understand the components of the psyche. He thinks that his psychology is one cohesive whole. He does not know that it has parts which work in tandem or in contrast. He feels that it is worth it to pursue nearly every desire which arises in the nature. He does not know how to trace the source of desires, regarding if they entered through the senses, or were stimulated by the images in the memory, or were created afresh by the imagination organ.

विहाय कामान्यः सर्वान्
पुमांश्चरति निःस्पृहः ।
निर्ममो निरहंकारः
स शान्तिमधिगच्छति ॥ २.७१ ॥
vihāya kāmānyaḥ sarvān
pumāṁścarati niḥspṛhaḥ
nirmamo nirahaṁkāraḥ
sa śāntimadhigacchati (2.71)

*vihāya — rejects; kāmān — cravings; yaḥ — who; sarvān — all; pumāṁścarati = pumān — person + carati — acts; niḥspṛhaḥ — free of lusty motivation; nirmamo = nirmamaḥ — indifferent to possessions; nirahaṁkāraḥ — free from impulsive assertion; sa — he; śāntim — contentment; adhigacchati — attains*

**The person who rejects all cravings, whose acts are free of lusty motivation, who is indifferent to possessions, who is free of impulsive assertion, attains contentment. (2.71)**

***Siddha Swami's Commentary***

This person has mastered the *buddhi yoga* techniques described by *Śrī* Krishna in this chapter. This procedure is standard. No one can invent another technique for freeing the intellect from sensual dominance. This is the method as given by *Śrī* Krishna.

The lusty motivations come up in the sensual energies when these are mixed with the emotions. This produces a craving for enjoyments yielded by the involvements with particular sense objects. Repeated involvement leads to either addiction or disgust. A person who becomes disgusted may not be able to give up the addiction however. The lusty energies are spear-headed by sexual intercourse. That is the leading way of expressing lust.

The senses usually try to procure attractive objects which are required by the psyche for some sort of nourishment or well-being. Frequently, however, the psyche procures more of these nourishing items than required. Thus complications arise due to competing claims by other living beings. This leads to violence. Animals in the same species cooperate together but they also fight for items of nourishment. This is conducted by an uncontrolled sense of possession. In *buddhi yoga*, one brings this sense under control.

*Nirahankārah* is very important since that is the skill of reducing the sense of identity to nil. This power is closer to the core self than the intellect. If controlled, all the other subtle mechanisms like senses, emotional energy, memory, intellect and vital energy would be automatically curbed, for all of these can only relate to the core self through its sense of identity. A yogi cannot discard it, nor can he discard any of the other psychological instruments, but he can curb it from abuse. That is the purpose of *buddhi yoga*.

एषा ब्राह्मी स्थितिः पार्थ
नैनां प्राप्य विमुह्यति ।
स्थित्वास्यामन्तकालेऽपि
ब्रह्मनिर्वाणमृच्छति ॥२.७२॥
eṣā brāhmī sthitiḥ pārtha
naināṁ prāpya vimuhyati
sthitvāsyāmantakāle'pi
brahmanirvāṇamṛcchati (2.72)

*eṣā — this; brāhmī — divine; sthitiḥ — state; pārtha — son of Pṛthā; naināṁ = na — not + enām — this; prāpya — does have; vimuhyati — is stupified; sthitvā — is fixed; 'syām = asyām — in this; antakāle — at the time of death; 'pi = api — also; brahma — divinity + nirvāṇam — full stoppage of mundane sensuality; ṛcchati — attains*

**This divine state is required, O son of Pṛthā. If a man does not have this, he is stupefied. At the time of death, the full stoppage of mundane sensuality and the attainment of divinity is attained by one who is fixed in this divine state. (2.72)**

***Siddha Swami's Commentary:***

Any person who does not master *buddhi yoga*, as *Śrī* Krishna elaborately described in this chapter, is certainly stupefied (*vimuhhyati*). This is because such a spirit is forced against its will to cooperate with the senses. This occurs indirectly through the intellect. Such a person must act impulsively. He or she has no choice in the matter.

*Śrī* Krishna guaranteed *nirvāṇam* or the full stoppage of the mundane sensuality and the attainment of the divine state to any person who mastered the *buddhi yoga* as He explained to Arjuna. Nowadays this *buddhi yoga* is called *kriyā yoga* and some call it *rāja* yoga.

Because the masterful *buddhi* yogi has isolated himself from the intellect, he is able to ward off the sensuality which causes a person to automatically enter into another physical womb after leaving the body. Thus, this *samyamī* yogi can attain the divine state.

# CHAPTER 3

## Karma Yogam

## Regulating Work through Yoga Practice*

*yastvindriyāṇi manasā niyamyārabhate'rjuna*
*karmendriyaiḥ karmayogam asaktaḥ sa viśiṣyate (3.7)*

***However, whosoever endeavors to control the senses by the mind, O Arjuna, and who restricts the limbs through regulating his work by yoga practice, without attachment, is superior. (3.7)***

****Siddha Swami assigned this chapter title on the basis of verse 46 of this chapter.***

अर्जुन उवाच
ज्यायसी चेत्कर्मणस्ते
मता बुद्धिर्जनार्दन ।
तत्किं कर्मणि घोरे मां
नियोजयसि केशव ॥ ३.१ ॥
arjuna uvāca
jyāyasī cetkarmaṇaste
matā buddhirjanārdana
tatkiṁ karmaṇi ghore māṁ
niyojayasi keśava (3.1)

*arjuna – Arjuna; uvāca — contested; jyāyasī — is better; cet = ced — if; karmaṇaḥ — than physical action; te — your; matā — idea; buddhirjanārdana = buddhiḥ — mental action + janārdana — motivator of men; tatkiṁ = tat (tad) — them + kiṁ — why; karmaṇi — in action; ghore — in horrible; māṁ — me; niyojayasi — you urge; keśava — handsome-haired one*

**Arjuna contested: O motivator of men, if it is Your idea that the mental approach is better than the physically-active one, then why do You urge me to commit horrible action, O handsome-haired One? (3.1)**

***Siddha Swami's Commentary:***

In Chapter Two, the previous chapter, *Śrī* Krishna condemned *karma* or cultural activity as being by far inferior to intellectual discipline through yoga. Here is that verse:

*dūreṇa hyavaraṁ karma buddhiyogāddhanaṁjaya*
*buddhau śaraṇamanviccha kṛpaṇāḥ phalahetavaḥ (2.49)*

***Surely, cultural action is by far inferior to intellectual discipline through yoga. O victor of wealthy countries. One should take shelter in mystic insight for how pathetic are those who are motivated by the promise of results. (2.49)***

Since *Śrī* Krishna promoted intellectual discipline through yoga, Arjuna wanted to know why *Śrī* Krishna urged action. But Arjuna forgot that *Śrī* Krishna also advocated *karma yoga*, which is cultural acts performed with the detachment gained from yoga practice (*yogah karmasu kauśalam* Bg. 2.50).

Arjuna being unable to grasp the line of action *Śrī* Krishna advocated, which was detached performance of duty, no matter what, spoke again about horrible action *(karmaṇi ghore)*. Arjuna thought that *Śrī* Krishna was contradicting Himself by recommending a mental method and then again advocating a physical way of action. Thus Arjuna failed to comprehend what *Śrī* Krishna spoke in Chapter Two. *Śrī* Krishna was not speaking of a mental approach, but rather a physical one with yogic detachment, using the developed *buddhi yoga* insight, which allows the actor to be free from moods because his emotions no longer convert into varying attitudes which cripple his ability to take instructions from somebody like Lord Krishna.

व्यामिश्रेणैव वाक्येन
बुद्धिं मोहयसीव मे ।
तदेकं वद निश्चित्य
येन श्रेयोऽहमाप्नुयाम् ॥ ३.२ ॥
vyāmiśreṇaiva vākyena
buddhiṁ mohayasīva me
tadekaṁ vada niścitya
yena śreyo'hamāpnuyām (3.2)

*vyāmiśreṇaiva = vyāmiśreṇa — with this two-way + iva — like this; vākyena — with a proposal; buddhiṁ — intelligence; mohayasīva = mohayasi — you baffle + iva — like this; me — of me; tad — this; ekaṁ — one; vada — tell; niścitya — surely; yena — by which; śreyo = śreyaḥ — the best; 'ham = aham — I; āpnuyām — I should get*

**You baffle my intelligence with this two-way proposal. Mention one priority, by which I would surely get the best result. (3.2)**

***Siddha Swami's Commentary:***

Arjuna requested *Śrī* Krishna to give a simply instruction, either for physical action or for mental considerations without physical motivation. This meant that Arjuna assumed the posture of an ordinary human being who cannot deal with complexities. Arjuna wanted to act for the best result. Again, even though *Śrī* Krishna tried to veer Arjuna away from a result-expectant course, still Arjuna stood his ground and requested something that would give the best result. This type of mentality is removed from the nature by the practice of *buddhi yoga*, *kriyā yoga*, and finally *brahma yoga*.

श्रीभगवानुवाच
लोकेऽस्मिन्द्विविधा निष्ठा
पुरा प्रोक्ता मयानघ ।
ज्ञानयोगेन सांख्यानां
कर्मयोगेन योगिनाम् ॥३.३॥
śrībhagavānuvāca
loke'smindvividhā niṣṭhā
purā proktā mayānagha
jñānayogena sāṁkhyānāṁ
karmayogena yogināṁ (3.3)

*śrī bhagavān — the Blessed Lord; uvāca — said; loke — in this physical world; 'smin = asmin — in this; dvividhā — of the two-fold; niṣṭhā — standard; purā — previously; proktā — was taught; mayā — by me; 'nagha = anagha — O blameless one, good man; jñānayogena — mind regulation by yoga practice; sāṁkhyānāṁ — of the Sāṁkhya philosophical yogis; karmayogena — action regulation by yoga practice; yoginām — of the non-philosophical yogis*

**The Blessed Lord said: In the physical world, a two-fold standard was previously taught by Me. O Arjuna, my good man. This was mind regulation by the yoga practice of the Sāṁkhya philosophical yogis and the action regulation by the yoga practice of the non-philosophical yogis. (3.3)**

***Siddha Swami's Commentary:***

We may assume here that *Śrī* Krishna is the Supreme God, the same person extolled by *Śrī Patañjali* as the instructor of the ancient teachers. By that, in ancient times, *Śrī* Krishna gave a two-fold process: one for those who were intellectually-inclined and one for others who were prone to practical means. Both types were trained in yoga but the intellectuals were trained in the Samkhya philosophy for a life beyond this physical world, while the others, the practical people, were trained in the rules for righteous lifestyle on earth.

Even though *jñāna yoga, or mind regulation by yoga practice,* is the higher of the two courses, still *karma yoga* has importance, since through it, human society became favorable and facilitative to those who practiced *jñāna yoga*.

न कर्मणामनारम्भान्
नैष्कर्म्यं पुरुषोऽश्नुते ।
न च संन्यसनादेव
सिद्धिं समधिगच्छति ॥३.४॥
na karmaṇāmanārambhān
naiṣkarmyaṁ puruṣo'śnute
na ca saṁnyasanādeva
siddhiṁ samadhigacchati (3.4)

*na — not; karmaṇām — concerning cultural activity; anārambhān — not being involved; naiṣkarmyaṁ — freedom from cultural activity; puruṣo = puruṣaḥ — a person; 'śnute = aśnute — attains; na — not; ca — and; saṁnyasanādeva = saṁnyasanād (saṁnyasanāt) — from renunciation + eva — alone; siddhiṁ — spiritual perfection; samadhigacchati — achieves*

**A man does not attain freedom from cultural activity merely by not being involved in social affairs. And not by renunciation alone, does he achieve spiritual perfection. (3.4)**

***Siddha Swami's Commentary:***

Generally each ascetic must follow a balanced life of action and renunciation. He must act when it is his duty and be renounced when he is not to participate. It is therefore a technique of knowing when to perform and when to restrain. Early on, the neophyte yogis have more cultural activities to perform, but as they advance they have more austerities to practice. This means less involvement in society in the later stages. Some advanced yogis, however, become involved in teaching to large numbers of students and they may give lectures on general religion to the public.

It is true what *Śrī* Krishna said, that a man does not attain freedom from cultural activity merely by not being involved in social affairs. It takes more than that, as *Śrī* Krishna will elaborate. On the other hand, as He described, it is not by renunciation alone that a person achieves spiritual perfection. It is very complicated, this business of spiritual life.

*Śrī* Krishna informed Arjuna and every other human being that there might be repercussions if one does not engage in cultural activity. If one merely renounces the world, one may fail to gain spiritual perfection.

न हि कश्चित्क्षणमपि
जातु तिष्ठत्यकर्मकृत् ।
कार्यते ह्यवशः कर्म
सर्वः प्रकृतिजैर्गुणैः ॥३.५॥
na hi kaścitkṣaṇamapi
jātu tiṣṭhatyakarmakṛt
kāryate hyavaśaḥ karma
sarvaḥ prakṛtijairguṇaiḥ (3.5)

*na — no; hi — indeed; kaścit — anyone; kṣaṇamapi = kṣaṇam — a moment + api — also; jātu — ever; tiṣṭhatyakarmakṛt = tiṣṭhati — exists + akarmakṛt — not acting; kāryate — caused to act; hyavaśaḥ = hi — indeed + avaśaḥ — against their wishes; karma — vibration; sarvaḥ — everyone; prakṛtijair = prakṛtijaiḥ — produced by material nature; guṇaiḥ — variations of mundane energy*

**No one, even momentarily, ever exists without vibration. By the variations of mundane energy in material nature, everyone, even against their wishes, is forced to perform. (3.5)**

***Siddha Swami's Commentary:***

Some type of action is always necessary in these material creations and in the spiritual creation as well, since the energies are always interacting and moving, no matter how slightly. Thus even if one decides not to act, that decision itself is an action. That decision itself is caused by moving energy. Material nature *(prakṛtijaih guṇaih)* will itself dictate certain actions, which its instruments will be forced to carry out, regardless of the will of an individual spirit. Thus a body, even of a great sage, might be forced to perform, even against his wish.

In *brahma yoga* and in *kriyā yoga* as well, we observe the workings of the subtle material energy, to see which of the operations occur independently, irrespective of our will. Thus we are able to gage the actual extent of our power and realize this information given by *Śrī* Krishna.

A warrior in a social circumstance like Arjuna, must either fight or run away from battle, and in either case he will be held accountable for the reactions of his decision. Running away may bring worse consequences than fighting the battle, or it may be the opposite. Thus in social situations, one must weigh the options properly.

कर्मेन्द्रियाणि संयम्य
य आस्ते मनसा स्मरन् ।
इन्द्रियार्थान्विमूढात्मा
मिथ्याचारः स उच्यते ॥३.६॥
karmendriyāṇi saṁyamya
ya āste manasā smaran
indriyārthānvimūḍhātmā
mithyācāraḥ sa ucyate (3.6)

*karmendriyāṇi — bodily limbs; saṁyamya — restraining; ya = yaḥ — who; āste — sits; manasā — by the mind; smaran — remembering; indriyārthān — attractive objects; vimūḍhātmā = vimūḍha — deluded + ātmā — self; mithyācāraḥ — deceiver; sa — he; ucyate — it is declared*

**A person who, while restraining his bodily limbs, sits with the mind remembering attractive objects, is a deceiver. So it is declared. (3.6)**

***Siddha Swami's Commentary:***

*Samyamya* is a term used for meditation. It is not meant to describe the state of a material body. Many creatures may sit still or stand in one place physically but their minds may be very active. Take the example of a crane. Sometimes a crane stands still for fifteen or twenty minutes on a river bank but the crane's mind remains ever active, waiting for a careless fish. Snakes sometimes remain still on the forest floor or on the branch of a tree for hours, only to catch their prey. Thus physical inactivity is not the criterion used to just judge *samyamya*.

*Śrī Patañjali Mahārṣi* explained *samyamya* as the three higher states of yoga in a progression one to another, from effortful focus on higher concentration forces or persons to effortless focus of the same, and then to continuous or spontaneous effortless focus, one progressing into the other as the yogi practices. A neophyte may begin by focusing within the mind chamber on the naad sound. When his attention settles down on that sound, abandoning all else including sense images and memory flashes, he will find that the focus becomes effortless and then it becomes continuous and spontaneous. If he continues that spontaneous contact with naad sound, then light appears before him. This is an example of *samyamya*.

*Śrī* Krishna did not think that Arjuna would, in his emotionally-disturbed condition, attain samyamya for internal organization and elevation of the instruments in his psyche. Thus the Lord chided Arjuna, indicating that Arjuna, even if he tried for yoga, would be a pretend ascetic.

A person who has problems or social entanglements cannot meditate successfully, even if he can make his body sit still for hours. His mind will not remain quiet at all. It will hash over the difficulties. The memory within it will flash related incidences, and the person will not be able to stop the film and sound show occurring on the mental screen. This happens because of the lack of power brought on by a preoccupation with social relationships. This lack of power was described by *Śrī* Krishna in Chapter Two and it is a law of our psychological nature.

*nāsti buddhirayuktasya na cāyuktasya bhāvanā*
*na cābhāvayataḥ śāntiraśāntasya kutaḥ sukham (2.66)*

***In comparison, never is there proper discernment in an uncontrolled person. He is not capable of concentration. One who lacks concentration cannot get inner peace. For one who lacks emotional stability, how will happiness be achieved? (2.66)***

*bhogaiśvaryaprasaktānāṁ tayāpahṛtacetasām*
*vyavasāyātmikā buddhiḥsamādhau na vidhīyate (2.44)*

***Being absorbed by this way of life, pleasure-prone and power seeking people, are captivated by this idea. Thus in meditation, the self-focused intellect is not experienced by them. (2.44)***

One who faces a situation of unpalatable duties, should find an advisor, just as Arjuna found Lord Krishna. It is not always in one's interest to side-step social obligations. Thus one should be advised by a superior personality. One cannot cheat in life merely by escaping from unpalatable tasks. One will not be allowed to escape drastic consequences by merely thinking or feeling that a certain obligation is not to one's liking or that it is vicious or mean. One also cannot meditate properly with problems pressing one's mind within its intellect and memory. One must first come to terms with the intellectual contents of mind and with the active memory. Meditation does not occur in the mind of a person who has pressing duties which should be performed.

यस्त्विन्द्रियाणि मनसा
नियम्यारभतेऽर्जुन ।
कर्मेन्द्रियैः कर्मयोगम्
असक्तः स विशिष्यते ॥३.७॥
yastvindriyāṇi manasā
niyamyārabhate'rjuna
karmendriyaiḥ karmayogam
asaktaḥ sa viśiṣyate (3.7)

*yas (yaḥ) — whosoever; tvindriyāṇi = tv (tu) — however + indriyāṇi — the senses; manasā — by the mind; niyamyārabhate = niyamya — controlling + ārabhate — endeavors; 'rjuna — Arjuna; karmendriyaiḥ — by the limbs; karmayogam — regulating his work by yoga practice; asaktaḥ — without attachment; sa = saḥ — he; viśiṣyate — is superior*

**However, whosoever endeavors to control the senses by the mind, O Arjuna, and who restricts the limbs through regulating his work by yoga practice, without attachment, is superior. (3.7)**

***Siddha Swami's Commentary:***

The first step for a worldly involved person is given in this verse. He must continue cultural life *(karma)* but he must begin the practice of yoga. Once he gets some expertise in yoga, he should apply that skill as he works, to become more efficient and to detach himself from the results of obligations. This is the scientific method propounded by *Śrī* Krishna. This means that a socially involved person should not abandon his obligations in order to meditate but should fulfill the obligations and begin lessons in the eight-part process of yoga. When he develops sufficient expertise in that, he should apply psychological pressure on himself to become detached from moods. When he attains that, he achieves steadiness when viewing the circumstances of life and that will give him a power of detachment from the results of action. The endeavor to control the senses by the mind *(indriyaṇi manasā niyamya ārabhate)* is part of *buddhi yoga*. When this *buddhi yoga* is somewhat mastered, the skill of it feeds into one's cultural life and permits one to perform *karma yoga* or the regulation of cultural activities by yoga skill. Such a person is superior, of course, to one who runs away from duties, claiming that he renounced what is unpalatable, when in fact, his mood changed and disempowered him to face the circumstance before him.

This verse seven of Chapter Three explains the process of *karma yoga* for the first time. Please note that for *karma yoga*, one must first master some of *buddhi yoga*. One cannot be a *karma* yogi if one does not have mastership in *buddhi yoga*.

नियतं कुरु कर्म त्वं
कर्म ज्यायो ह्यकर्मणः ।
शरीरयात्रापि च ते
न प्रसिध्येदकर्मणः ॥ ३.८ ॥
niyataṁ kuru karma tvaṁ
karma jyāyo hyakarmaṇaḥ
śarīrayātrāpi ca te
na prasidhyedakarmaṇaḥ (3.8)

*niyataṁ — moral; kuru — do; karma — cultural duty; tvaṁ — you; karma — performance; jyāyo = jyāyaḥ — better; hy akarmaṇaḥ = hi — indeed + akarmaṇaḥ — than non-action; śarīrayātrāpi = śarīra — body + yātrā — maintenance + api — even; ca — and; te — your; na — not; prasidhyet — could be achieved; akarmaṇaḥ — without activity*

**Moral action should be done by you. Performance is better than non-performance. Even the maintenance of your body could not be achieved without activity. (3.8)**

***Siddha Swami's Commentary:***

*Śrī* Krishna explained that it is better to act morally, than not to act at all. This means that in any given circumstance, one is duty-bound to act in support of righteous lifestyle. If one avoids a righteous act, one's subtle body will incur a blemish for indirectly supporting the irreligious way of life. Hence, it is important for an advanced *yogin* to be in isolation. If he remains in society, he will have to support all sorts of righteous activities and that will dissipate his energies and cause a reduction in practice. If he is unable to gain isolation, then he must engage in acts which are exemplary in the moral sense.

*Śrī* Krishna correctly pointed out that even the maintenance of Arjuna's body, or anyone else's, occurred only with activity. Even a yogi practicing *samādhi* must protect the body. He has to perform physical purification of the intestines. He has to do postures. He must carefully protect the body from being eaten by wild animals or from becoming diseased or infected through carelessness.

यज्ञार्थात्कर्मणोऽन्यत्र
लोकोऽयं कर्मबन्धनः ।
तदर्थं कर्म कौन्तेय
मुक्तसङ्गः समाचर ॥ ३.९ ॥
yajñārthātkarmaṇo'nyatra
loko'yaṁ karmabandhanaḥ
tadarthaṁ karma kaunteya
muktasaṅgaḥ samācara (3.9)

*yajñārthāt = yajña – religious fulfillment and ceremony + ārthāt — for the sake of; karmaṇo = karmaṇaḥ —from action; 'nyatra = anyatra — besides; loko = lokaḥ — world; 'yaṁ = ayam — this; karmabandhanaḥ — something bound by action; tadartham = tad — this + arthaṁ — purpose, value; karma — cultural activity; kaunteya — son of Kuntī; muktasaṅgaḥ — freedom from attachment; samācara — act promptly*

**Besides action for religious fulfillment and ceremony, this world, is action-bound. Act for the sake of religious fulfillment and ceremony, O son of Kuntī. Be free from attachment. Act promptly. (3.9)**

***Siddha Swami's Commentary:***

This is the action-prone world, the physical world. It signifies, encourages and operates on the basis of gross activity. *Śrī* Krishna labeled it as *karmabandhanah*, something that is bound by action. Thus, all who have material bodies must act, if for no other reason than the fact that the bodies themselves are ever-changing. The materials themselves are in an acting course of integration or disintegration, either forming or being dismantled. This is the fatigue of this world, where a spirit is forced to endorse these movements for formation or disintegration, not by its will but rather, by the nature of the material energy.

Arjuna had to act, either to fight at *Kurukṣetra* or to leave the battle scene. *Śrī* Krishna alerted us that Arjuna should act for the sake of religious fulfillment and ceremony, *yajñārthāt*. The point is this: Since one must act, one should prefer religious actions which support a righteous lifestyle. One should not rely on the prejudiced senses which always select what is palatable and pleasing.

For the proper selection, one must be free from attachment, *muktasaṅgah*. This attitude towards life comes about by mastership of *buddhi yoga*, where one's nature stops trying to convert one's unprejudiced feelings into happy, distressful, exhilarating, depressing and dispirited emotions.

सहयज्ञाः प्रजाः सृष्ट्वा
पुरोवाच प्रजापतिः ।
अनेन प्रसविष्यध्वम्
एष वोऽस्त्विष्टकामधुक् ॥३.१०॥
sahayajñāḥ prajāḥ sṛṣṭvā
purovāca prajāpatiḥ
anena prasaviṣyadhvam
eṣa vo'stviṣṭakāmadhuk (3.10)

*sahayajñāḥ — along with religious fulfillment and ceremony; prajāḥ — first human beings; sṛṣṭvā — having created; purovāca = pura — long ago + uvāca — said; prajāpatiḥ — procreator Brahmā; anena — by this; prasaviṣyadhvam — may you produce; eṣaḥ — this; vo = vaḥ — your; 'stviṣṭakāmadhuk = astviṣṭakāmadhuk = astu — may it be + iṣṭakāmadhuk — for granting desires*

**Long ago, having created the first human beings, along with religious fulfillment and ceremonies, the Procreator Brahmā said: By this worship procedure, you may be productive. May it cause the fulfillment of your desires. (3.10)**

***Siddha Swami's Commentary:***

*Śrī* Krishna as the Primeval Being, explained that initially, the conception for the existence of human beings happened simultaneously with the idea for religious fulfillment and ceremony *(sahayajñāh)*. The *prajāpatih* is the person who later become known as *Brahmā*, but here he is addressed as the Father of human beings. He conceived of the human race and of a worship procedure for their practice.

Therefore, there must have been other forces in the creation initially. Those other powers also influenced the human beings. Thus they deviated from the desire of the *Prajāpatih Brahmā*. Through good sense, however, some of the created persons adhered to *Brahmā*'s desires and they were blessed proportionately.

देवान्भावयतानेन
ते देवा भावयन्तु वः ।
परस्परं भावयन्तः
श्रेयः परमवाप्स्यथ ॥३.११॥
devānbhāvayatānena
te devā bhāvayantu vaḥ
parasparaṁ bhāvayantaḥ
śreyaḥ paramavāpsyatha (3.11)

*devān — supernatural rulers; bhāvayatānena = bhāvayatā — may you cause to flourish + anena — by this procedure; te — they; devā — the supernatural rulers; bhāvayantu — may they bless you; vaḥ — you; parasparaṁ — each other; bhāvayantaḥ — favorably regarding one another; śreyaḥ — well-being; param — highest; avāpsyatha — you will achieve*

**By this procedure, you may cause the supernatural rulers to flourish. They, in turn, may bless you. In favorably regarding each other, the highest well-being will be achieved. (3.11)**

***Siddha Swami's Commentary:***

The same *Prajāpatih* or Primal Father, *Brahmā*, did create or produce some supernatural beings, who were almost on par with him. They did not need physical bodies. They were naturally satisfied with the subtle existence. They became known as *devas* or beings of light. They had no need for physical forms, unlike the other entities whom *Brahmā* could only manifest as physical beings, human beings, animals and vegetation. It appears, however, that while those superior entities did not need physical forms, still they had a need to dominate physical beings. Thus responsibly, the Primal Father *Brahmā* took steps to establish guidelines for a reciprocal relationship between the administrators who used bodies of light and the physical beings on the earthly planet.

*Brahmā* was particular to explain that the supernatural people needed to be nourished by cooperative acts of sacrifice by the human beings. This suggests that if the human beings did not comply, an ensuing resentment from the supernatural people would convert into hardship for the human beings.

These are all facts today, even though modern civilizations do not heed this. A *yogin*, particularly a *brahma* yogin, gets rid of his tendency to dominate others. This occurs when one masters the appropriation energy in the psyche. This energy then diverts permanently into the chit akash, the sky of consciousness. As such it no longer finds expression for itself in this world. One no longer feels any resentment towards anyone who might disobey one's orders. This is total indifference to the affairs of this realm.

The *devas* are supernatural people using bodies of light, but they are affected by resentments when their wills are not executed. It is not that their ideas are harmful to one and all. In fact, their ideas are beneficial for material prosperity and social well-being *(śreyah)*. All the same, their tendency for dominance is a fault. Thus a student *brahma yogin* is advised not to aspire to become a deva. He should avoid that aspiration, staying on as a human being life after life, until he sheds the need for human opportunity and can become liberated. Liberation, however, occurs gradually in the sense that one develops the required detachment after long, long practice. Thus a *yogin* must patiently work with his faulty nature, until he can get every defective part of it purified.

*Śrī* Krishna did not at this stage in the conversation, advise Arjuna in *brahma yoga*. Instead he gave advice for *yajña kriyā*, which is ceremonial rites and cultural actions approved by the beings of light who are empowered to supervise human society. A *brahma yogin* has no use for such *yajña kriyā* but nevertheless he cannot avoid it totally. So long as he is in the social setting, he must adhere to a degree and he must be attuned to commands from those supervisors appointed by *Brahmā*. Failure to cooperate with such people would cause impediments in one's destiny. These would in turn slow down one's yoga practice.

Since a *yogin* uses this creation of *Brahmā*, he cannot afford to disrespect that authority or ignore the *devas* who function under *Brahmā*'s sovereignty. Thus one must learn well from *Śrī* Krishna in this holy discourse, how to cooperate with the *devas* and simultaneously advance in yoga.

इष्टान्भोगान्हि वो देवा
दास्यन्ते यज्ञभाविताः ।
तैर्दत्तानप्रदायैभ्यो
यो भुङ्क्ते स्तेन एव सः ॥३.१२॥

*iṣṭān — most desired; bhogān — enjoyable people and things; hi — indeed; vo = vaḥ — to you; devā — supernatural rulers; dāsyante — they will give; yajñabhāvitāḥ — manifested through prescribed austerity and religious ceremony; tair = taiḥ — by*

iṣṭānbhogānhi vo devā
dāsyante yajñabhāvitāḥ
tairdattānapradāyaibhyo
yo bhuṅkte stena eva saḥ
(3.12)

*those; dattān — given items; apradāyaibhyo = apradāya — not offering + ebhyaḥ — to them; yo = yaḥ — who; bhuṅkte — enjoys; stena — a thief; eva — only; saḥ — he*

**The supernatural rulers, being manifested through prescribed austerity and religious ceremony, will, indeed, give you the most desired people and things. Whosoever does not offer those given items to them, but who enjoys these, is certainly a thief. (3.12)**

***Siddha Swami's Commentary:***

It is claimed in the *Mahābhārata* and in the *Purāṇas*, that the *devas* can be seen by human beings on occasion. For instance, when King *Kansa* violently hurled the infant body of the Goddess *Durgā*, it is said that She appeared to him in a supernatural form and spoke of his foolishness in trying to kill her. She also informed him, that for certain, the child who would kill his body was born elsewhere. Apparently *Kansa* saw Her with physical eyes. Again it is said that Princess Damayanti saw the *devas* and sorted between some of them and her lover Nala.

However for the purpose of yoga, we accept that someone in a physical body can see supernaturally, not by physical vision but only by subtle vision of the subtle body which is interspaced in the physical one. Thus it must be that *Kansa* and Princess Damayanti experienced the perception of their subtle eyes while they were stationed in physical forms.

*Yajñabhāvitāh* means that through religious ceremony and prescribed austerity, the *devas* will be directly or indirectly perceived. Those who see through subtle forms even while using physical ones, will see them directly, just as Kansa and Princess Damayanti did, while others who are subtly blind, will only see the *devas* indirectly by becoming aware of positive results in their life after performing a sacrifice. Seeing such results, these persons will assume the existence of the supernatural people and will believe that whatever prosperity and physical well-being they experience, was bestowed by the *devas*.

The power of the *devas* over human beings is clearly indicated, by the term *bhogān*, which means: that which is to be enjoyed grossly by earthly creatures. Thus, if anyone got rid of the need to enjoy grossly, the power of the *devas* would be ineffective in the life of that person. In *brahma yoga*, one learns how not to enjoy in the material world. Thus one becomes progressively freed from this dominance. This causes one to become exempt from the religious ceremonies and the social participation which those ceremonies require. Consequently, one gains more time for practice.

On the other hand, however, human beings who take the enjoyments from the *devas* but fail to worship and comply with them, are checkmated by providence. Their lives become full of frustrations. Ultimately they are sent down the evolutionary levels to lower and lower species of life. This is because without the help of the *devas*, a human being cannot maintain his status in the human species. He or she will, of necessity, slide downwards.

In the beginning of this time cycle of human manifestation, *Brahmā* warned the first created human beings that anyone who neglected the *devas* would be regarded as a thief and would be dealt with in due course of time. Arjuna was also warned, in the sense that even though he had lofty aspirations and was a benevolent being, still he had to comply with the request of the *devas*. It was not just a matter of his own feelings or opinions, nor of selecting only palatable or pleasant assignments given by them.

This was the problem the Kurus had, which brought them to the brink of that civil war.

They were indifferent to the feelings of the *devas*. They wanted to service their dynasty without being accountable to the *devas*. Thus their ideas of social life were flawed. Arjuna had to comply with the *devas*, even in the matter of disciplining his own family and friends, otherwise Arjuna himself would be inconvenienced by the domineering empowered *devas*.

यज्ञशिष्टाशिनः सन्तो
मुच्यन्ते सर्वकिल्बिषैः ।
भुञ्जते ते त्वघं पापा
ये पचन्त्यात्मकारणात् ॥ ३.१३ ॥
yajñaśiṣṭāśinaḥ santo
mucyante sarvakilbiṣaiḥ
bhuñjate te tvaghaṁ pāpā
ye pacantyātmakāraṇāt (3.13)

*yajñaśiṣṭāśinaḥ = yajñaśiṣṭa — sanctified items used after a religious ceremony + āśinaḥ — utilizing; santo = santaḥ — virtuous souls; mucyante — they are released; sarvakilbiṣaiḥ — from all faults; bhuñjate — consume; te — they; tvaghaṁ = tv (tu) — but + aghaṁ — impurity; pāpā — wicked people; ye — who; pacantyātmakāraṇāt = pacanti — prepare + ātma — self + kāraṇāt — for the sake of*

**(Krishna continued): The virtuous people who utilize the items after they are sanctified by prescribed ceremony, are released from all faults. But the wicked ones who prepare for their own sake, consume their own impurity. (3.13)**

***Siddha Swami's Commentary:***

Items and people who are duly-sanctified in a Vedic religious ceremony, are released from faults, not by the mere performance of the ceremony alone, but also significantly by the pious activity which led up to the ceremony and which was conducted in all honesty with due respect to Vedic religious principles. It is not the ceremony which sanctifies the items and people but rather the events in acquirement of the commodities. The ceremony itself only underscores the means of acquirement. If the means were impious, the ceremony cannot sanctify the performer.

*Santah* are the virtuous people, who are piously-inclined and who live in a way which makes them compatible to the Universal Form of *Śrī* Krishna. The Kauravas who opposed Arjuna and his brothers also did Vedic religious ceremonies with meticulous care, but still their lifestyles were scarred with irreligious activities. This is why *Śrī* Krishna encouraged Arjuna to discipline them.

As *Śrī* Krishna stated, those living entities who do not comply with the stipulations of *Brahmā*, and who use up the creation without respect to the supernatural rulers, are in fact consuming their own impurity, despite their successes here and there.

Even though a human being may be successful for the time being, while he flouts the authority of the *devas*, still we have to keep in mind, that the supernatural people do have the upper hand, since all who use material bodies, cannot keep those forms forever. Sooner or later, one has to shift to the subtle plane, the place where the *devas* have full leverage. Understanding this, a *yogin* should know that he cannot effectively disrespect the *devas*.

अन्नाद्भवन्ति भूतानि
पर्जन्यादन्नसंभवः ।
यज्ञाद्भवति पर्जन्यो
यज्ञः कर्मसमुद्भवः ॥ ३.१४ ॥

*annād = annāt — from nourishment; bhavanti — are produced; bhūtāni — the creatures; parjanyād = parjanyāt — from rain clouds; anna — nourishment; saṁbhavaḥ — originated; yajñād = yajñāt — from prescribed austerity and religious*

annādbhavanti bhūtāni
parjanyādannasaṁbhavaḥ
yajñādbhavati parjanyo
yajñaḥ karmasamudbhavaḥ (3.14)

*ceremony; bhavati — exists; parjanyo = parjanyaḥ — rain; yajñaḥ — prescribed austerity and religious ceremony; karma — cultural action; samudbhavaḥ — is caused*

**The creatures are produced from nourishment. From rain clouds, nourishment originated. From prescribed austerity and religious ceremony, rain clouds are produced. And prescribed austerity and religious ceremony are caused by cultural activities. (3.14)**

***Siddha Swami's Commentary:***

*Śrī* Krishna graciously traced the connection between physical acts and the grace or disapproval of the *devas*. Our bodies are produced from nourishment. As it is right now, regardless of the past, we derive these bodies from the nourishment in the body of the father and mother. Of course, nourishment on an earthly planet hinges on moisture, which is produced mostly by rainfall and dewfall.

Rain arises from evaporated moisture and static electricity in the atmosphere. This electricity, manifested as lightning, comes from the resultant thoughts of the populace. Those thoughts are caused by the cultural activities which provoke them. From the effort of human beings, the endeavor to follow traditions and to make use of varying weather conditions, psychological reliance occurs. This reliance is normally experienced as faith in God. Through it, one develops the inclination to religion, from which one adheres to religious discipline and ceremony.

With tact and precision, *Śrī* Krishna informed Arjuna and every other person on that battlefield who could hear the speech, that a human being is not free to act, except with the approval of the *devas* who were appointed as superiors by *Brahmā*.

कर्म ब्रह्मोद्भवं विद्धि
ब्रह्माक्षरसमुद्भवम् ।
तस्मात्सर्वगतं ब्रह्म
नित्यं यज्ञे प्रतिष्ठितम् ॥३.१५॥
karma brahmodbhavaṁ viddhi
brahmākṣarasamudbhavam
tasmātsarvagataṁ brahma
nityaṁ yajñe pratiṣṭhitam (3.15)

*karma — cultural activity; brahmodbhavaṁ = brahma — the Veda + udbhavaṁ — produced; viddhi — be aware; brahmākṣarasamudbhavam = brahma — Supreme Spirit + akṣara — the unaffected spiritual reality + samudbhavam — produced; tasmāt — hence; sarvagataṁ — all-pervading; brahma — spirit person; nityaṁ — always; yajñe — in prescribed austerity and religious ceremony; pratiṣṭhitam — is situated*

**Cultural activity is produced from the Personified Veda. The Personified Veda comes from the unaffected Supreme Spirit. Hence the all-pervading Supreme Spirit is always situated in prescribed austerity and religious ceremony. (3.15)**

***Siddha Swami's Commentary***

Cultural activity in this world was begun by the First Being in the Creative Space. This person is the Primal Personality. In some Vedic literature, He is said to be the *Vedas* Personified while in others, He is adored as the Person who produced the *Vedas* Personified. Whosoever that Person may be, He produced the cultural activity. Thus He is in the best position to define what culture is and how it should be executed.

*Śrī* Krishna accredited that Person as coming from the Unaffected Supreme Spirit *(brahmākṣara)*. One should respect that Person even if He is outside the range of ordinary sense perception.

एवं प्रवर्तितं चक्रं
नानुवर्तयतीह यः ।
अघायुरिन्द्रियारामो
मोघं पार्थ स जीवति ॥३.१६॥

evaṁ pravartitaṁ cakraṁ
nānuvartayatīha yaḥ
aghāyurindriyārāmo
moghaṁ pārtha sa jīvati (3.16)

*evaṁ — thus; pravartitaṁ — perpetuated; cakraṁ — circular process; nānuvartayatīha = na — not + anuvartayati — cause to be perpetuated + iha — on earth; yaḥ — who; aghāyurindriyārāmo = aghāyurindriyārāmaḥ = aghāyuḥ — malicious + indriyārāmaḥ — sensually-happy person; moghaṁ — worthless; pārtha — son of Pṛthā; sa = saḥ — he; jīvati — lives*

**O son of Pṛthā, a person who does not cause this circular process to be perpetuated here on earth, lives as a malicious, sensually-happy and worthless person. (3.16)**

***Siddha Swami's Commentary:***

It is possible to live without recognizing the *devas*. Many persons do so and continue their existence on earth day after day until death. *Śrī* Krishna opined that such persons live a malicious, sensually-happy and worthless life, because they are not guided by the *devas*. The promotion of their status from human to celestial does not automatically take place, for without the disciplines imposed by the *Prajāpatih Brahmā*, no one can rise above the lower levels in material nature.

Positive reciprocal association with the *devas* in the circular process of honoring them as stipulated and receiving their approvals and benedictions, results in elevation to the realm of the *devas* after death of the physical body. There are many instances of great kings, who after living a life on earth which was approved by the *devas*, were transferred into their realm temporarily and enjoyed celestial status in a body of light similar to that of the *devas*. Others persons who deliberately or through mere ignorance ignore the *devas*, only take one physical body after another, in the human, animal or vegetation status, without any idea that there is a celestial world.

यस्त्वात्मरतिरेव स्याद्
आत्मतृप्तश्च मानवः ।
आत्मन्येव च संतुष्टस्
तस्य कार्यं न विद्यते ॥३.१७॥

yastvātmaratireva syād
ātmatṛptaśca mānavaḥ
ātmanyeva ca saṁtuṣṭas
tasya kāryaṁ na vidyate (3.17)

*yastvātmaratireva = yas (yaḥ) — who + tv (tu) — but + ātma — spiritual self + ratir (ratiḥ) — pleased + eva — surely; syāt — should be; ātmatṛptaśca = ātma — self + tṛptaḥ — satisfied + ca — and; mānavaḥ — a human being; ātmanyeva = ātmany (ātmani) — in the self + eva — only; ca — and; saṁtuṣṭaḥ — content; tasya — of him; kāryaṁ — cultural duty; na — no; vidyate — it is experienced*

**A person who is spiritually-pleased, self-satisfied and internally-content, has no cultural duties. (3.17)**

***Author's Commentary:***

This was the second *kriyā* in *kriyā yoga*. Siddha Swami asked me to seek an instruction from *Śrī Bābāji Mahāśaya*

***Śrī Bābāji Mahāśaya's Commentary:***

The first technique deals with separating the intellect from the sensuous energy and memory, as described in Chapter Two, text 52. The second technique is described in verse 55 of the second chapter. And now that same second procedure is described in greater depth in this verse 17 of Chapter Three. This development in the second technique occurs after practicing sincerely for a time. Then one begins to feed on the core self, and the self, as well as its attention, begins to get satisfaction from that mystic activity. Śrī Krishna stressed this condition as *ratih* (spiritually-pleased), *tṛptas* (self satisfied), and *samtuṣtah* (spiritual contentment). This stress is made since initially when a student practices, he may not become satisfied by it and his mind will of necessity, again link up with the intellect and look forward to its expression through the senses to get satisfaction. It feels relieved from the process of meditation which appeared to be dry and tasteless initially. When, however, the practice persists and the addiction to the senses and memory ceases, the self settles down and begins to relish its own existence.

In that state, only his core self and its attention energy seem to exist to the meditator. This attention energy is its sense of identity, also known as the *ahankāra*, the right and power to perform psychological actions in a limited way. This allows one to perform physical actions when one's psyche is housed in a physical body.

***Siddha Swami's Commentary:***

Anyone who masters this procedure of the *kriyā yoga* process gets some exemption from cultural duties. He does not get a full exemption but he gets a partial one, which in time becomes full. This is granted by the Universal Form of *Śrī* Krishna, on the basis of one's stance towards non-involvement in cultural affairs. At the time of the discourse, Arjuna wished that he had that waiver from cultural activities, but he did not. It is important to understand that even a person who is spiritually-pleased, self-satisfied, spiritually-content, and who mastered this skill, still there might be cultural duties to perform. Since, however, he is detached from his intellectual and sensual mechanisms, he performs cultural duties freely and their consequences do not adhere or stick to him as liabilities or benefits to be experienced at some future time, under normal laws of destiny.

***Śrī Bābāji Mahāśaya*** said that the meditation of such a yogi looks like this:

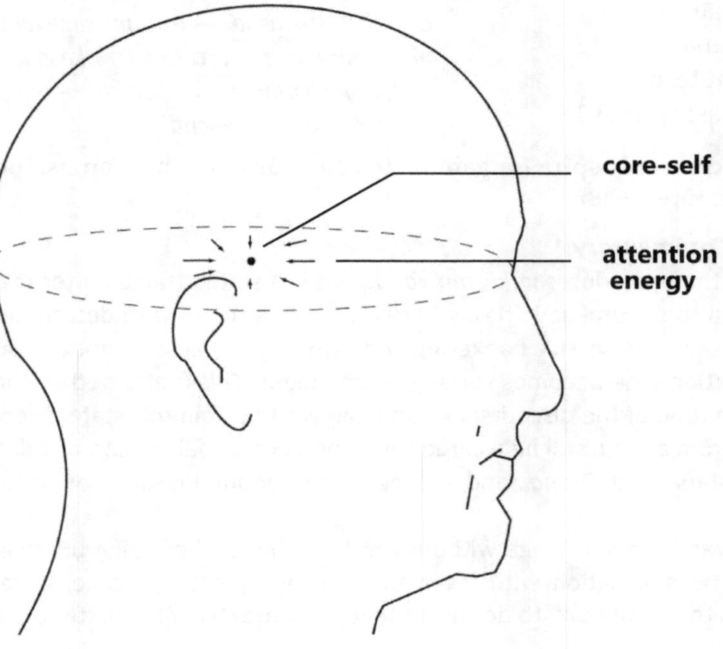

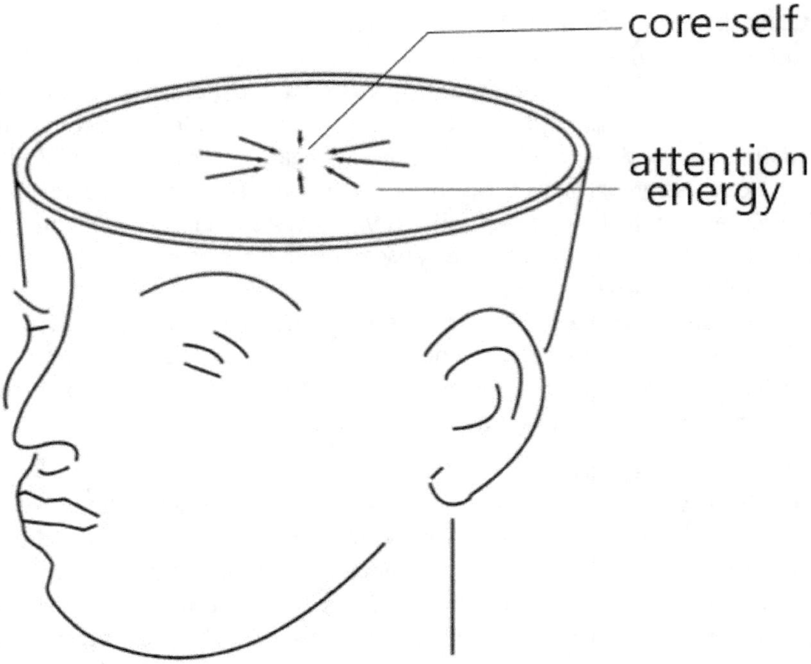


नैव तस्य कृतेनार्थो
नाकृतेनेह कश्चन ।
न चास्य सर्वभूतेषु
कश्चिदर्थव्यपाश्रयः ॥३.१८॥

naiva tasya kṛtenārtho
nākṛteneha kaścana
na cāsya sarvabhūteṣu
kaścidarthavyapāśrayaḥ (3.18)

*naiva = na — not + eva — indeed; tasya — regarding him; kṛtenārtho = kṛtena — with action + artho (arthaḥ) — gain; nākṛteneha = na — not + akṛtena — with non-action + iha — in this case; kaścana — anyone; na — not; cāsya = ca — and + asya — of him; sarvabhūteṣu — in all mundane creatures; kaścit — any; arthavyapāśrayaḥ = artha — purpose + vyapāśrayaḥ — depending*

**The person who does not aspire for gain in an action or in an inaction, is not reliant on any mundane creature. (3.18)**

***Siddha Swami's Commentary:***

This is one of the procedures in *karma yoga*. This is a state attained after mastering the application of yoga to cultural activities, where one is able to act with detachment because one's intellect ceased its obsessive hankering and planning. Because of not aspiring for gains in action or in inaction, one becomes socially independent. This is attained by the advanced *karma* yogi. At the time of the discourse, Arjuna had yet to attain this state. Even though he wanted to desist from action, still he aspired for gains, such as being liked by relatives, being approved by Bhishma and *Droṇa*, and feeling happy about his decision to spare them discipline.

One cannot practice higher yoga without reaching the level of being unreliant on other limited entities. The association with them takes away time to practice, because one is always required in their company to do this or that cultural activity for better or worse.

One must train the intellect to become specifically detached from both the sensual energy and the memory. Then one might be able to stop the intellect from its calculative obsessions, and one can stop aspiring for real or imagined benefits from particular types of associations and the related activities.

***Śrī Bābāji Mahāśaya's Commentary:***

The sensual energy is a mixed subtle force consisting of *praṇa* or subtle power, emotional feeling, and charged power emitted by the intellect. When this sensual energy is purified by kundalini yoga practice, one becomes freed from its dominance, and not otherwise. The memory is a botheration to all student yogis, but it is curbed by separation from the intellect. One must learn from within the mind, how to keep the intellect from supplying the memory with power to operate. If it gets no energy from the intellect, it cannot operate. Then it remains blank as if it were non-existent, and the yogi is free to practice *samādhi*. The intellect is located close to the core self, and the memory is between the intellect and the sensual orbs. The student yogi must meditate repeatedly and learn to locate where each of these subtle organs are located.

Here are diagrams:

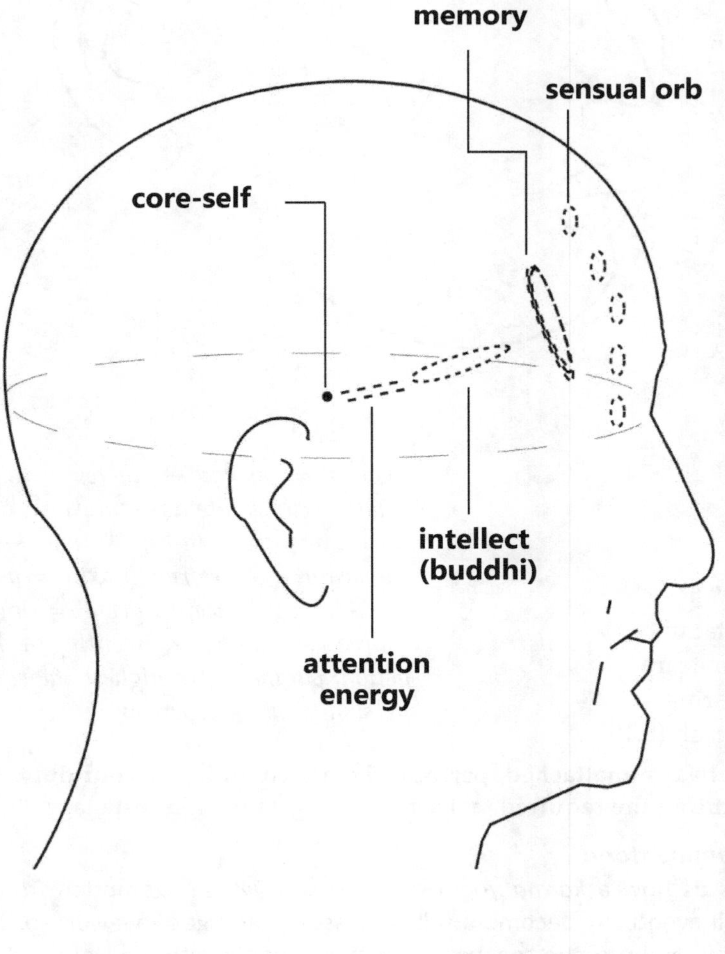

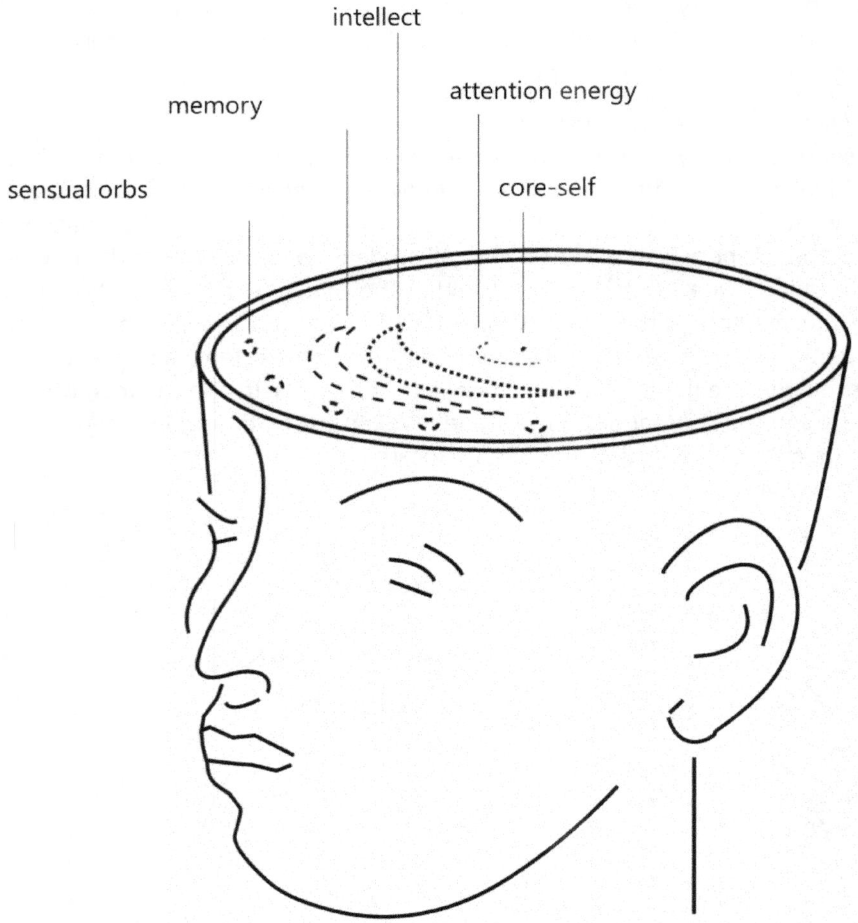


तस्मादसक्तः सततं
कार्यं कर्म समाचर ।
असक्तो ह्याचरन्कर्म
परमाप्नोति पूरुषः ॥३.१९॥
tasmādasaktaḥ satataṁ
kāryaṁ karma samācara
asakto hyācarankarma
paramāpnoti pūruṣaḥ (3.19)

*tasmād = tasmāt — therefore; asaktaḥ — unattached; satataṁ — always; kāryaṁ — duty, required tasks; karma — action; samācara — perform; asakto = asaktaḥ — unattached; hyācarankarma = hy (hi) — indeed + ācaran — executing + karma — action; param — the highest stage; āpnoti — gets; pūruṣaḥ — a person*

**Therefore, being always unattached, perform the action which is your duty. By being detached and executing the required tasks, a person gets the highest stage. (3.19)**

***Siddha Swami's Commentary:***

This verse tells us how a *karma* yogi ultimately will get an exemption from cultural activity, how he will eventually become a full time ascetic and get a waiver, so that he no longer has to be a cultural pawn in the world. He must comply with the Universal Form. He must do the duties assigned by that Lord. Then over time, by cultivating and applying detachment, when he is matured in the practice, he will get the highest stage *(param)*. This person must not give up yoga practice while performing social duties. He must continue the practice and make efforts to consistently apply himself in a detached manner, whenever involved in worldly acts. Then by repeated practice, he eventually gains the highest stage.

कर्मणैव हि संसिद्धिम्
आस्थिता जनकादयः ।
लोकसंग्रहमेवापि
संपश्यन्कर्तुमर्हसि ॥३.२०॥
karmaṇaiva hi saṁsiddhim
āsthitā janakādayaḥ
lokasaṁgrahamevāpi
saṁpaśyankartumarhasi (3.20)

*karmaṇaiva = karmaṇa — by cultural activities + eva — alone; hi — indeed; saṁsiddhim — perfection; āsthitā — attained; janakādayaḥ = janaka — Janaka + ādayaḥ — beginning with; lokasaṁgrahamevāpi = loka — world + saṁgraham — maintenance + eva – only + api — only; saṁpaśyan — seeing mentally; kartum — to act; arhasi — you should*

**Beginning with Janaka, perfection was attained by cultural activities alone. Seeing the necessity for world maintenance, you should act. (3.20)**

***Siddha Swami's Commentary:***

This perfection of *samsiddhim* is the perfection of acting in the world and being detached, acting in the world and not being tagged with liabilities for the involvement. This happens by virtue of coverage from the Universal Form of *Śrī* Krishna. This does not mean perfection of yoga. For perfection of yoga, one must eventually leave aside the *karma yoga* life and take to higher yoga or the highest stage.

Janak and others like him acted with the detachment gained through mastership of *karma yoga*, but later on in life, they assumed a fully detached life as *vanaprastha* ascetic retirees. Then they completed the higher yoga and became perfected. One does not attain full perfection by *karma yoga* but one gets an exemption from the same *karma yoga*, and through that waiver, one can dedicate fully to the higher yoga achievements. These have nothing to do with cultural acts of this world.

*Śrī* Krishna advised Arjuna that he should see the necessity for world maintenance *(lokasamgraham)* and should willingly help the Supreme Lord in that task; otherwise Arjuna ran the risk of disapproval from that God of the world and would then be subjected to the great fear mentioned before:

*nehābhikramanāśo'sti pratyavāyo na vidyate*
*svalpamapyasya dharmasya trāyate mahato bhayāt (2.40)*

***In this insight, no endeavor is lost nor is there any reversal. Even a little of this righteous practice protects from the great danger. (2.40)***

It may be added that one would be protected from the great danger of being rejected by *Śrī* Krishna, something a limited being cannot afford, as will be explained later in this discourse.

यद्यदाचरति श्रेष्ठस्
तत्तदेवेतरो जनः ।
स यत्प्रमाणं कुरुते
लोकस्तदनुवर्तते ॥३.२१॥

*yadyad — whatever; ācarati — does; śreṣṭhaḥ — the greatest; tattad = tad tad — this and that; evetaro (evetaraḥ) = eva — only + itaraḥ — the others; janaḥ — perform; sa = saḥ —*

yadyadācarati śreṣṭhas
tattadevetaro janaḥ
sa yatpramāṇaṁ kurute
lokastadanuvartate (3.21)

*he; yat — what; pramāṇaṁ — trend; kurute — establishes; lokastadanuvartate = lokaḥ — the world + tad — that + anuvartate — pursues*

**Whatever a great person does, for that only, others aspire. Whatever trend he establishes, the world pursues. (3.21)**

***Siddha Swami's Commentary:***

This explains a rule of responsibility for all leaders. Even if one refuses to be a leader, but others accept one as a leader, this rule will apply. One is accountable to the Supreme Being for whatever trends one sets in society and for whatever trends develop due to one's presence in the world. Even if one does not want to lead, if one happens to be an inspiration to others, one is held accountable for whatever impact one's presence has on others.

This ruling falls under the category of *karma yoga*, meaning that one should be aware of the views of the Universal Form of *Śrī* Krishna, and one should work to suit, so that one has His approval at all times. This means one has to be detached from one's nature.

The world will pursue whatever trend a great person established, due to the force of personality. Hence someone has to be responsible for that. God will not accept responsibility unless a great man does exactly what God dictates, and God will hold the liability only for particular acts of a great man, which were in fact inspired by the Supreme Being; otherwise a great personality is held accountable for his activities.

*Śrī* Krishna warned Arjuna that even if he left the battlefield, there would be repercussions, and those might not be to Arjuna's liking either. In addition, Arjuna would be responsible for anyone who followed his example and refused to act to protect *dharma* or righteous lifestyle. Thus Arjuna would not only be tagged for his disregard of the views of the Universal Form, but for that of any others who might follow him. He would then be responsible to reform any persons who took to his views or who used his views to strengthen their own resolves about not completing unpalatable duties.

Such repercussions are covered under the heading of the great fear of getting the disapproval of the Universal Form. Please study this verse:

*nehābhikramanāśo'sti pratyavāyo na vidyate*
*svalpamapyasya dharmasya trāyate mahato bhayāt (2.40)*

***In this insight, no endeavor is lost nor is there any reversal. Even a little of this righteous practice protects from the great danger. (2.40)***

न मे पार्थास्ति कर्तव्यं
त्रिषु लोकेषु किंचन ।
नानवाप्तमवाप्तव्यं
वर्त एव च कर्मणि ॥ ३.२२ ॥
na me pārthāsti kartavyaṁ
triṣu lokeṣu kiṁcana
nānavāptamavāptavyaṁ
varta eva ca karmaṇi (3.22)

*na — not; me — of me; pārthāsti = pārtha — O son of Pṛthā + asti — is; kartavyaṁ — should be done; triṣu — in the three divisions; lokeṣu — in the universe; kiṁcana — anything specific; nānavāptamavāptavyaṁ = na — not + anavāptam — not attained + avāptavyam — to be acquired; varta — I function; eva — yet; ca — and; karmaṇi — in cultural activities*

**For Me, O son of Pṛthā, there is nothing specific that must be done in the three divisions of the universe. And there is nothing that I have not attained or should acquire, and yet I function in cultural activities. (3.22)**

***Siddha Swami's Commentary:***

That God has all He ever could need and can produce effortlessly whatever He might want, and still He functions in the cultural activities of human beings, is an enigma, a puzzle. But the reason is simply this: All the beings who are involved in this world, have responsibilities. God is no exception to this. The mass of responsibilities are distributed among the individual living entities, and the Supreme Person is one of them. Thus if God is accountable, then what can be said of others?

यदि ह्यहं न वर्तेयं
जातु कर्मण्यतन्द्रितः ।
मम वर्त्मानुवर्तन्ते
मनुष्याः पार्थ सर्वशः ॥३.२३॥
yadi hyahaṁ na varteyaṁ
jātu karmaṇyatandritaḥ
mama vartmānuvartante
manuṣyāḥ pārtha sarvaśaḥ (3.23)

*yadi — if; hyahaṁ = hy (hi) — perchance + ahaṁ — I; na — not; varteyaṁ — should perform; jātu — ever; karmaṇyatandritaḥ = karmaṇy (karmaṇi) — in work + atandritaḥ — attentively; mama — of me, my; vartmānuvartante = vartma — pattern + anuvartante — they follow; manuṣyāḥ — human beings; pārtha — O son of Pṛthā; sarvaśaḥ — in all respects*

**If perchance, I did not perform attentively, then all human beings, O son of Pṛthā, would follow Me in all respects. (3.23)**

***Siddha Swami's Commentary:***

This is the world of responsible living, even for the Supreme Being. Responsibility wears out the living being and causes him to want liberation. Responsibility passes under the respectable name of *dharma*, which also means righteous living or being supervised by the Supreme Lord in all social dealings.

The Supreme Being feels responsible to live in a such a way as to lead the limited beings on the right path socially, so that eventually they would, one by one, attain liberation from material existence. The other aspect is this: The living beings do infringe on the lifestyles of each other. Thus there is need for justice. This is enforced by the Supreme Being, either directly as *Śrī* Krishna did during His life on earth, or indirectly through others like Arjuna who was empowered to discipline for *Śrī* Krishna. Since limited beings instinctively cry out to the Supreme Being when their rights are hampered by others, the Supreme Being becomes responsible to chastise those who bully others. And the Supreme Being, whenever He appears, must act in an exemplary way.

उत्सीदेयुरिमे लोका
न कुर्यां कर्म चेदहम् ।
संकरस्य च कर्ता स्याम्
उपहन्यामिमाः प्रजाः ॥३.२४॥
utsīdeyurime lokā
na kuryāṁ karma cedaham
saṁkarasya ca kartā syām
upahanyāmimāḥ prajāḥ (3.24)

*utsīdeyur = utsīdeyuh — would perish; ime — these; lokā — worlds; na — not; kuryāṁ — I should engage; karma — cultural activity; cedaham = cet — if + aham — I; saṁkarasya — of the social chaos; ca — and; kartā — producer; syām — I should be; upahanyām — I should destroy; imāḥ — these; prajāḥ — creatures*

**If I should not engage in cultural activity, these worlds would perish. And I would be a producer of social chaos. I would have destroyed these creatures. (3.24)**

***Siddha Swami's Commentary:***

This is the rationale behind the Supreme Being's reason for righteous action in this world. This explains His obligation. All others function under this reason for righteous lifestyle in cultural activities. The Supreme Being as the Universal Form displayed to Arjuna, is the functional basis for human society in this world.

सक्ताः कर्मण्यविद्वांसो
यथा कुर्वन्ति भारत ।
कुर्याद्विद्वांस्तथासक्तश्
चिकीर्षुर्लोकसंग्रहम् ॥ ३.२५ ॥
saktāḥ karmaṇyavidvāṁso
yathā kurvanti bhārata
kuryādvidvāṁstathāsaktaś
cikīrṣurlokasaṁgraham (3.25)

*saktāḥ — attached; karmaṇyavidvāṁso = karmaṇyavidvāṁsaḥ = karmaṇi — in activities + avidvāṁsaḥ — unintelligent; yathā — as; kurvanti — they act; bhārata — O son of the Bharata family; kuryād = kuryāt — he should perform; vidvāṁs — the wise person; tathāsaktaś = tathā — so + asaktaḥ — detached; cikīrṣur = cikīrṣuḥ — intending to do; lokasaṁgraham = loka — society + saṁgraham — maintenance*

**As the unintelligent people perform with attachment to cultural activity, O son of the Bharata family, so the wise person should act, but in a detached manner, for the maintenance of society. (3.25)**

***Siddha Swami's Commentary:***

This explains the difference between ordinary *karma* and *karma yoga*, between ordinary cultural activities and those which are regulated with the actor's yoga expertise. The difference is attachment or lack of it. An ordinary person is motivated naturally by attachment. He or she is pushed by moods which arise in the psyche, while the *karma* yogi ignores moods or eliminates them, and acts by the grace of the Supreme Person in the Universal Form. By the practice of *buddhi yoga*, one develops detachment from the sensual energies. This gives one the freedom to act under the influence of the Supreme Being. The attached person, the *kāmakāmī* (2.70), is also concerned with the maintenance of society but he or she is like Arjuna in the confused state described in Chapter One, whereby that person feels that society must be maintained to promote the family at all costs. The other person, the *samyamī* (Bg. 2.69), wants to maintain society as an agent of the Supreme Being. He acts in a manner that is detached from his family.

न बुद्धिभेदं जनयेद्
अज्ञानां कर्मसङ्गिनाम् ।
जोषयेत्सर्वकर्माणि
विद्वान्युक्तः समाचरन् ॥ ३.२६ ॥
na buddhibhedaṁ janayed
ajñānāṁ karmasaṅginām
joṣayetsarvakarmāṇi
vidvānyuktaḥ samācaran (3.26)

*na — not; buddhibhedaṁ = buddhi — intelligence + bhedaṁ — breaking (broken intelligence, indetermination); janayet — should produce; ajñānāṁ — of the simpletons; karmasaṅginām — of those attached to action; joṣayet — should inspire to be satisfied; sarvakarmāṇi — all actions; vidvān — the wise person; yuktaḥ — disciplined; samācaran — performing*

**One should not produce indetermination in the minds of the simpletons. A wise person should inspire them to be satisfied by action. The wise one should be disciplined in behavior. (3.26)**

***Siddha Swami's Commentary:***

Even though a *karma* yogi knows that the *kāmakāmī* sensuous-minded persons will be frustrated in time, still, he should advise them to act responsibly. By his example, he should inspire them to act in a righteous manner. This is his duty. He knows well that they are pathetic because they are motivated by the promise of results which they might never enjoy, but still he does not discourage them, because in one way or the other, the world should be maintained in righteous order.

The mistake of the sensuously-inclined persons is this: They feel that they will get just rewards for all pious acts. They do not understand the idea of working without expecting or desiring results. When no results are forth-coming, the sensuous persons become disappointed and suffer needlessly. Still, a knowledgeable person, who mastered *buddhi yoga* and who applies his psychological detachment to cultural activities, should not discourage others from working in the world, but should ask them to be industrious in righteous living.

प्रकृतेः क्रियमाणानि
गुणैः कर्माणि सर्वशः ।
अहंकारविमूढात्मा
कर्ताहमिति मन्यते ॥३.२७॥
prakṛteḥ kriyāmāṇāni
guṇaiḥ karmāṇi sarvaśaḥ
ahaṁkāravimūḍhātmā
kartāhamiti manyate (3.27)

*prakṛteḥ — of the primal mundane energy; kriyamāṇāni — performed; guṇaiḥ — by the variations; karmāṇi — actions; sarvaśaḥ — in all cases; ahaṁkāravimūḍhātmā = ahaṁkāra – falsely-asserted identity + vimūḍha — confused + ātmā — self; kartāham = kartā — performer + aham — I; iti — thus; manyate — he thinks*

**In all cases, actions are performed by variations of the primal mundane energy. But the identity-confused person thinks: "I am the performer." (3.27)**

***Siddha Swami's Commentary:***

By proximity to the Supreme Lord and to the limited spiritual individuals, the primal mundane energy operates by variations in itself to produce the material world. The rules for existence have much to do with the way that energy operates. The Supreme Personality knows the most efficient way to coordinate with the mundane potency. Thus He advises the limited persons to act in a way which would give them the maximum insight into material nature, and which would eventually cause them to gain liberation from its affiliation.

Because he uses psychological instruments which are fused into his energy, the limited entity feels that he is one with the subtle instruments, and thus he cannot sort between himself and his subtle or gross psychology. *Śrī* Krishna has, however, given the course for *buddhi yoga* so that the limited entity can sort himself, and in effect separate the core-self from the intellect. Once this is done, the entity can understand how he is influenced to consent to material nature's activities. Instead of feeling that he is the performer, the enlightened entity begins to understand that he was influenced by the intellect, memory, sensual energy and survival instinct to perform various activities, which were enacted by the variations of material nature. He can then detach himself and find out from the God of the world about his duty.

तत्त्ववित्तु महाबाहो
गुणकर्मविभागयोः।
गुणा गुणेषु वर्तन्त
इति मत्वा न सज्जते ॥३.२८॥
tattvavittu mahābāho
guṇakarmavibhāgayoḥ
guṇā guṇeṣu vartanta
iti matvā na sajjate (3.28)

*tattvavit — reality-perceiving person; tu — but; mahābāho — O powerful man; guṇakarmavibhāgayoḥ = guṇa – moods of nature + karma — action + vibhāgayoḥ — in two-fold basis; guṇa — the variation of material nature; guṇeṣu — in the variations of material nature; vartanta — they interact; iti — thus; matvā — having thought; na — no; sajjate — is attached*

**But, O powerful man, having considered that variations of material nature interact with variations of material nature, the reality-perceiving person is not attached to action. (3.28)**

***Siddha Swami's Commentary:***

The *tattvavit* is the masterful *buddhi* yogi. By direct mystic perception, he can see how the mind is altered and conditioned by the sensual energies. This causes him to become detached from the intellect, the subtle organ which intimidates the self and causes it to endorse ideas of the senses. One becomes very detached, once one sees in fact, how the intellect takes instructions from the memory and the sensual energy. Thus one does not habitually go along with the plans of one's psychology. At that stage of practice, one becomes submissive to higher personalities, who are near and dear to Lord Krishna.

प्रकृतेर्गुणसंमूढाः
सज्जन्ते गुणकर्मसु।
तानकृत्स्नविदो मन्दात्
कृत्स्नविन्न विचालयेत् ॥३.२९॥
prakṛterguṇasaṁmūḍhāḥ
sajjante guṇakarmasu
tānakṛtsnavido mandāt
kṛtsnavinna vicālayet (3.29)

*prakṛter = prakṛteḥ — of subtle material nature; guṇasaṁmūḍhāḥ = guṇa — variations of material nature + saṁmūḍhāḥ — deluded people; sajjante — they are attached; guṇakarmasu — in the mood-motivated activities; tān — them; akṛtsnavido = akṛtsnavidaḥ — partially-knowing; mandāt — foolish people; kṛtsnavin — the person who understands the whole reality; na — not; vicālayet — should unsettle*

**Those who are deluded by the variations of material nature are attached to mood-motivated activities. The person who understands the reality should not unsettle those foolish people who have partial insight. (3.29)**

***Siddha Swami's Commentary:***

This is a description of the *kāmakāmīs*. An advanced person should never laugh at or ridicule these sensuously-motivated persons, who feel that they should be getting something from material nature, and who think that the existence is here for their benefit. All the limited entities do initially look to material nature as their benefactor. This is natural. *Śrī* Krishna warned that the advanced persons and their students should not unsettle the sensuous souls.

The attachment to mood-motivated activities is the indication that these persons have not curbed their psychologies. They can do this if they take lessons from *Śrī* Krishna in *buddhi yoga* and then apply their psychological control to cultural activities, thus practicing *karma yoga*. When *buddhi yoga* is mastered and applied to cultural activities, it is called *karma yoga*. The second chapter of the *Bhagavad Gītā* is to be called *buddhi yoga*, for it is there that *Śrī* Krishna first gave details of that practice. This third chapter should be called *karma yoga*, for herein *Śrī* Krishna shows how to apply the psychological control one gains from *buddhi yoga*.

Those with little or no insight into these matters have no alternative but to be influenced by the various moods produced by their emotions. And thus they require social guidance, which they receive from more advanced souls. They learn mainly from the example of the great souls, and not so much from philosophical explanations.

मयि सर्वाणि कर्माणि
संन्यस्याध्यात्मचेतसा ।
निराशीर्निर्ममो भूत्वा
युध्यस्व विगतज्वरः ॥३.३०॥
mayi sarvāṇi karmāṇi
saṁnyasyādhyātmacetasā
nirāśīrnirmamo bhūtvā
yudhyasva vigatajvaraḥ (3.30)

*mayi — to me; sarvāṇi — all; karmāṇi — working power; saṁnyasyādhyātmacetasā = saṁnyasya — entrusting + adhyātmacetasā — by meditation on the Supreme Spirit; nirāśīr — from cravings; nirmamo = nirmamaḥ — indifferent to selfishness; bhūtvā — being; yudhyasva — do fight; vigatajvaraḥ = vigata — departed + jvaraḥ — feverish mood*

**All your working power should be entrusted to Me. On the Supreme Spirit, you should meditate. Being free from cravings, indifferent to selfishness, do fight. Be a man whose feverish mood has departed. (3.30)**

***Siddha Swami's Commentary:***

*Adhyātmacetasā* is a *brahma yoga* practice. This is not *buddhi yoga*. The particulars of how to do this will be explained elsewhere in the *Gītā*. Here the idea is being introduced by *Śrī* Krishna. One must first master *buddhi yoga* and then apply oneself to worldly life for *karma yoga*. Then one must master *kriyā yoga* followed by *brahma yoga*. *Kriyā yoga* includes kundalini yoga which is the curbing of the life force energy in the subtle body.

Even though *brahma yoga* practice is introduced by *Śrī* Krishna here, it cannot be practiced by anyone who has not mastered *buddhi yoga, karma yoga* and *kriyā yoga*. This will be evident as we proceed through the *Gītā*.

Meditation on the Supreme Spirit occurs by a focus of the spirit's attention outside of the psyche. One does this, however, from inside the psyche. One has to develop the *jñāna dīpah*, which Arjuna was bestowed with by *Śrī* Krishna in Chapter Eleven of this discourse. One can neither see the Supreme Spirit nor perceive Him through material senses. Thus one must develop the spiritual senses to perceive him. This development begins by becoming conscious of the sensual equipments in the higher subtle body.

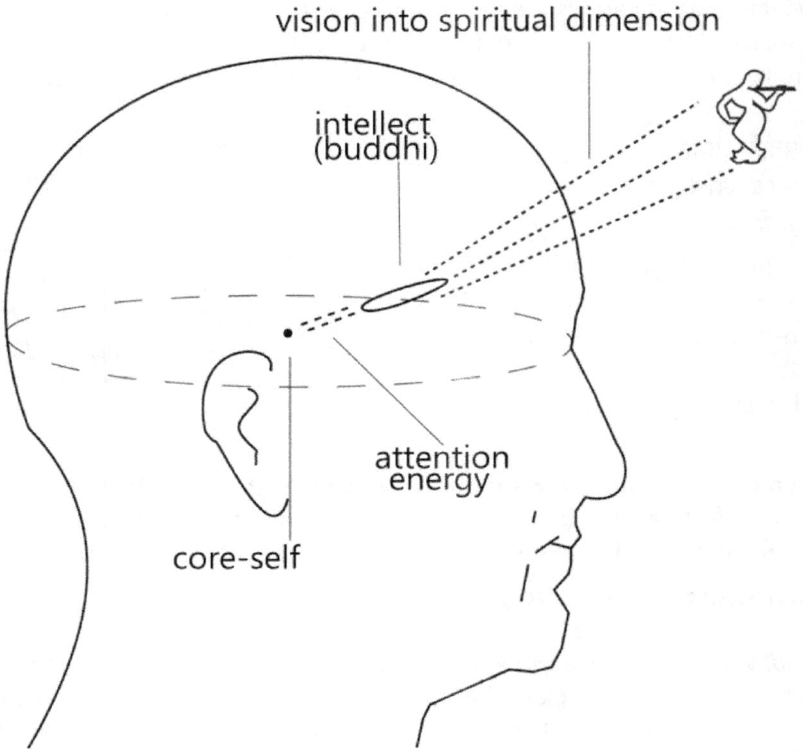


Here is a diagram:

**Perception of the Supreme Spirit**
**through the developed buddhi imagination orb**

One cannot meditate on something or someone, which or who, is not revealed. One must first get a revelation of the Supreme Spirit and then one may meditate upon Him provided the revelation was not a flash occurrence. Meditation upon an idea of the Supreme Spirit, or upon the Murti Form of the Supreme Spirit in the temple, is not what is meant by *adhyātmacetasā*. There must first be revelation. Then there must be revelation for a sufficient period of time, so that the meditator can locate how to reach the Supreme Spirit when the vision disappears. Then one can proceed with this technique of *brahma* yoga which is given by *Sri Krishna.* This meditation is not the Deity Worship procedure.

The surrender to *Śrī* Krishna instruction is given in this verse as *mayi sarvāṇi karmāṇi,* surrender of all one's working power to Him, for His usage, for His affairs which may or may not coincide with one's desire. Arjuna was ordered to do this. This is the culmination of *karma yoga*. The *buddhi yoga* mastership is mentioned as *nirāsīh nirmano bhūtvā*, freedom from cravings and indifferent to selfishness. One's feverish mood should have departed, due to not having the emotions convert into exciting or depressing feelings, which in turn prejudice the intellect and cause it to be adverse and judgmental towards to the supreme will.

ये मे मतमिदं नित्यम्
अनुतिष्ठन्ति मानवाः ।
श्रद्धावन्तोऽनसूयन्तो
मुच्यन्ते तेऽपि कर्मभिः ॥३.३१॥
ye me matamidaṁ nityam
anutiṣṭhanti mānavāḥ
śraddhāvanto'nasūyanto
mucyante te'pi karmabhiḥ (3.31)

*ye — whosoever; me — My; matam — idea; idam — this; nityam — constantly; anutiṣṭhanti — they apply; mānavāḥ — human beings; śraddhāvanto = śraddhāvantaḥ — having faith; 'nasūyanto = anasūyantaḥ — not complaining; mucyante — are freed; te — they; 'pi = api — also; karmabhiḥ — from the consequences of action*

**Those human beings, who believe My idea, constantly applying it, not complaining, are freed from the consequences of action. (3.31)**

***Siddha Swami's Commentary:***

If one is able to surrender to *Śrī* Krishna as dictated in the previous verse by entrusting all of one's working power to the Central Person in the Universal Form, then one would indeed be free from the consequences of action. There will be consequences regardless but those repercussions would go to the Central Figure in the Universal Form. If one received any as a primary agent of Him, then one would not take the brunt of that reactionary force, except as an agent of the Supreme with the power to cushion such energy.

The term *nityam*, which means constantly, is important. It implies that those human beings who surrender partially are protected partially, and those who surrender fully over time are protected completely. This concerns the practice of *karma yoga*, or disciplined activities in the cultural environment under the direct supervision of *Śrī* Krishna.

Some authorities do advocate this as a form of *bhakti yoga*. They say this is done by love of *Śrī* Krishna. However, this Chapter Three concerns *karma yoga* which has developed as a result of *buddhi yoga* as explained in Chapter Two.

ये त्वेतदभ्यसूयन्तो
नानुतिष्ठन्ति मे मतम् ।
सर्वज्ञानविमूढांस्तान्
विद्धि नष्टानचेतसः ॥३.३२॥
ye tvetadabhyasūyanto
nānutiṣṭhanti me matam
sarvajñānavimūḍhāṁstān
viddhi naṣṭānacetasaḥ (3.32)

*ye — who; tvetad = tv (tu) — but + etad — this; abhyasūyanto = abhyasūyantaḥ — discrediting; nānutiṣṭhanti = na — not + anutiṣṭhanti — they practice; me — My; matam — idea; sarvajñānavimūḍhāṁs = sarva — all + jñāna — insight + vimūḍhāṁs — muddled; tān — them; viddhi — know; naṣṭān — jinxed; acetasaḥ — senseless*

**Know that those who discredit this instruction and do not practice My ideas, being of muddled insight, are jinxed and senseless. (3.32)**

***Siddha Swami's Commentary:***

If one does not understand how the Universal Form operates, and how the liabilities for cultural activity are divested, one is bound to question *Śrī* Krishna's views. Such persons would be jinxed and their insight would be muddled. Being unconnected to the higher insight of the Supreme Being, such persons, no matter how well intended they are, would of necessity become confused and act in a detrimental way.

सदृशं चेष्टते स्वस्याः
प्रकृतेर्ज्ञानवानपि ।
प्रकृतिं यान्ति भूतानि
निग्रहः किं करिष्यति ॥३.३३॥
sadṛśaṁ ceṣṭate svasyāḥ
prakṛterjñānavānapi
prakṛtiṁ yānti bhūtāni
nigrahaḥ kiṁ kariṣyati (3.33)

*sadṛśam — according to; ceṣṭate — on acts; svasyāḥ — from one's own; prakṛter = prakṛteḥ — from material nature; jñānavān — wise man; api — also; prakṛtiṁ — material nature; yānti — they submit; bhūtāni — the creatures; nigrahaḥ — restraint; kiṁ — what; kariṣyati — will do*

**A human being, even a wise man, acts according to his material nature. The creatures submit to the material nature. What will restraint do? (3.33)**

***Siddha Swami's Commentary:***

Even though the creatures must submit to material nature, still the human beings must condition their movements to be coordinated with the Supreme Being. He has a method for handling material nature and causing it to be beneficial for the elevation of the human beings. It is known that animals have their own wild nature, and yet they are domesticated by human beings. A horse for example is used to help human beings for conveyance and hard labor. Similarly, the Supreme Lord *Śrī* Krishna causes material nature to assist in the development of the limited spirits. On their own, these spirits do try to exploit material nature, but usually their ideas cause deeper involvement and no spiritual clarity. Thus they need to take help from the Supreme Being in dealing with the material world.

Restraint only helps if it causes one to adopt higher habits and if it causes higher spiritual perceptions; otherwise it causes frustrations and deeper involvements in vices, which are ruinous to one and all. There is a constructive use for restraint. *Śrī* Krishna spoke of it in a previous verse:

*sukhaduḥkhe same kṛtvā lābhālābhau jayājayau*
*tato yuddhāya yujyasva naivaṁ pāpamavāpsyasi (2.38)*

***Having regarded happiness, distress, gains, losses, victory and defeat, as the same emotions, apply yourself to battle. Thus you will get no demerit. (2.38)***

This is the first technique in *buddhi yoga*. The idea is to restrain the emotions so that they are not converted into varying moods which prejudice the psyche. One should do one's duty in a sober mood and restrain one's feelings so that they are not allowed to form biases in the intellect.

इन्द्रियस्येन्द्रियस्यार्थे
रागद्वेषौ व्यवस्थितौ ।
तयोर्न वशमागच्छेत्
तौ ह्यस्य परिपन्थिनौ ॥३.३४॥
indriyasyendriyasyārthe
rāgadveṣau vyavasthitau
tayorna vaśamāgacchet
tau hyasya paripanthinau (3.34)

*indriyasyendriyasyārthe = indriyasya — of a sense organ + indriyasya – of a sense organ + arthe — in an attractive object; rāgadveṣau = rāga — the response of liking + dveṣau — the response of disliking; vyavasthitau — deep-seated; tayor = tayoḥ — of these two; na — not; vaśam — power; āgacchet — should be influenced; tau — two; hyasya = hy (hi) — indeed + asya — of him; paripanthinau — two hindrances*

**The response of liking or disliking that is felt between a sense and an attractive object, is deep-seated. One should not be influenced by the power of these two moods. They are hindrances. (3.34)**

***Siddha Swami's Commentary:***

This is the first objective of kundalini yoga. In such a practice, one learns how to surcharge the subtle body, particularly the life force energy in the subtle spinal passage, the *suśumnā nāḍi*. When this is done successfully, the deep-seated urges are eliminated. However, initially a student yogi must observe in his day-to-day dealings, as well as during his attempts at meditation, that the sensual energies and the life force fluctuate between moods of liking, disliking and indifference. These are hindrances because they prejudice the intellect, which in turn draws the attention of the spirit and causes it to endorse irrational views.

*Śrī* Krishna advised that we not be influenced by these moods. However, it is not just a matter of will power and human determination. One has to purify the sensual energy and life force. Then one can enforce the decision not to be influenced, otherwise one will be swerved from determination and will be forced to comply with what *Śrī* Krishna does not recommend.

श्रेयान्स्वधर्मो विगुणः
परधर्मात्स्वनुष्ठितात् ।
स्वधर्मे निधनं श्रेयः
परधर्मो भयावहः ॥३.३५॥
śreyānsvadharmo viguṇaḥ
paradharmātsvanuṣṭhitāt
svadharme nidhanaṁ śreyaḥ
paradharmo bhayāvahaḥ (3.35)

*śreyān — better; svadharmo = svadharmaḥ — one's righteous duty; viguṇaḥ — imperfect; paradharmāt — than the righteous duty of another; svanuṣṭhitāt = sv (su) — good, great + anuṣṭhitāt — than done; svadharme — in one's righteous duty; nidhanaṁ — death; śreyaḥ — it is better; paradharmo = paradharmaḥ — righteous duty of another; bhayāvahaḥ = bhaya — risk + āvahaḥ — bringing on*

**Better to do one's righteous duty imperfectly, than to do the duty of another with great efficiency. Death is better in the course of one's duty but the task of another is risky. (3.35)**

***Siddha Swami's Commentary:***

This concerns working under the supervision of the Universal Form of *Śrī* Krishna, Who is the on-going, moment-to-moment Supreme Spirit. Regardless of whether a person is aware of *Śrī* Krishna or not, if that man or woman were to comply with *Śrī* Krishna, he or she would graduate into a higher species of life and eventually get liberation from the material world; otherwise one may degrade into a lower species of life. The force that pulls a limited spirit up towards the divine existence, is this Supreme Spirit, *Śrī* Krishna. Acts which are hostile to Him, which contravene His desire and authority, cause a person to go downwards in the mundane evolutionary cycle.

*Śrī* Krishna defined duty as it was assigned to the individual by the Universal Form. As we heard in Arjuna's case, he wanted to free himself from the compulsion of duty but *Śrī* Krishna objected. On the other side of the war field, opposing Arjuna, were fellows who felt that opposing Arjuna and *Śrī* Krishna was their duty. Thus, duty in the *Bhagavad Gītā* does not mean a man's duty as he sees it, but rather a man's duty as *Śrī* Krishna would have assigned it. For this very reason, the opponents, the Kauravas who did not do their duty as *Śrī* Krishna dictated or considered it, would be disciplined by Arjuna.

Thus it is better to do one's righteous duty as assigned by *Śrī* Krishna, imperfectly, than to do the duty of any other person with great efficiency, no matter what that duty may be. As *Śrī* Krishna sees it, death is better in the course of the duty He assigns. To leave aside that assignment and take up the task of another person is risky in terms of the negative outcome resulting from His disapproval.

These are rules in the performance of *karma yoga*. Compliance with all this, makes for a successful *karma* yogi.

अर्जुन उवाच
अथ केन प्रयुक्तोऽयं
पापं चरति पूरुषः ।
अनिच्छन्नपि वार्ष्णेय
बलादिव नियोजितः ॥३.३६॥
arjuna uvāca
atha kena prayukto'yaṁ
pāpaṁ carati pūruṣaḥ
anicchannapi vārṣṇeya
balādiva niyojitaḥ (3.36)

*arjuna – Arjuna; uvāca — said; atha — then; kena — by what?; prayukto = prayuktaḥ — forced; 'yaṁ = ayam — this; pāpaṁ — evil; carati — commits; pūruṣaḥ — a person; anicchannapi = anicchan — unwilling + napi (api) — even; vārṣṇeya — family man of the Vṛṣṇis; balād = balāt — from force; iva — as if; niyojitaḥ — compelled*

**Arjuna said: Then explain, O family man of the Vṛṣṇis, by what is a person forced to commit an evil unwillingly, just as if he were compelled to do so? (3.36)**

(*Śrī Bābāji* commented on this and some of the following verses.)

***Śrī Bābāji Mahāśaya's Commentary:***

This question is asked by those who are about to take up the practice of *buddhi yoga*, which is the curbing of the intellect from its attachment to the senses. The objective in *buddhi yoga* is to curtail the dominance of the senses and the memories over the *buddhi*, so that the *buddhi* or intellect organ can be free to follow the needs of the spirit. When the intellect becomes a willing and able servant of the spirit, and when it no longer prefers the association of the sensual energies, memory, and life force, then *buddhi yoga* is mastered by the yogi.

A person who has not mastered *buddhi yoga*, is compelled by the sensual energy, the memories and the life force energies, to commit criminal acts or cultural moves which are ultimately not in his interest. It does not matter if he wants to do the act or not or even if he is determined to not perform it. If his intellect is pegged to the sensual energies, the memories and the life force, he will be compelled to act under their influence.

श्रीभगवानुवाच
काम एष क्रोध एष
रजोगुणसमुद्भवः।
महाशनो महापाप्मा
विद्ध्येनमिह वैरिणम् ॥३.३७॥
śrībhagavānuvāca
kāma eṣa krodha eṣa
rajoguṇasamudbhavaḥ
mahāśano mahāpāpmā
viddhyenamiha vairiṇam (3.37)

*śri bhagavān — the Blessed Lord; uvāca — said; kāma — craving; eṣa — this; krodha — anger; eṣa — this; rajoguṇasamudbhavaḥ = rajo (rajaḥ) — passion + guṇa — emotion + samudbhavaḥ — source; mahāśano (mahāśanaḥ) = mahā — great + aśana — consuming power; mahāpāpmā = mahā — much + pāpmā — damage; viddhyenam = viddhi — recognize + enam — this; iha — in this case; vairiṇam — enemy*

**The Blessed Lord said: This force is craving. This power is anger. The passionate emotion is the source. It has a great consuming power and does much damage. Recognize it as the enemy in this case. (3.37)**

***Śrī Bābāji Mahāśaya's Commentary:***

The force is craving, known to Hindus as *kāma*, but the energy of it is the sensual force intermixed with the life force. To master this force means to purify it by the practice of kundalini yoga, for an intake of fresh pranic energy and a change of diet. *Śrī* Krishna identified the source as *rajoguṇa*, the passionate emotion. This is the same sensual energy mixed with life force. It is experienced usually as one emotional force but it is in fact an admixture. This force can be converted into sensual pleasure, sensual frustration or anger, but it is the same force. This is why *Śrī* Krishna gave the first technique of *buddhi yoga* as follows:

*sukhaduḥkhe same kṛtvā lābhālābhau jayājayau*
*tato yuddhāya yujyasva naivaṁ pāpamavāpsyasi (2.38)*

***Having regarded happiness, distress, gains, losses, victory and defeat, as the same emotions, apply yourself to battle. Thus you will get no demerit.(2.38)***

For the purpose of *buddhi yoga*, one must keep this force clean and keep it from converting into craving. As *Śrī* Krishna stated, this passionate emotional force has great consuming power and does much damage. It consumes the attention of the spirit, which it receives through the *buddhi* intellect organ. In this case, it is the enemy, because the spirit becomes liable for the decisions it endorses under the influence of that sensual power. It damages the psyche by putting it in disorder, such that the spirit acts as a stooge for providing power for the decisions and actions the intellect makes, as suggested by the sensual energy, life force and memory.

धूमेनाव्रियते वह्निर्
यथादर्शो मलेन च ।
यथोल्बेनावृतो गर्भस्
तथा तेनेदमावृतम् ॥ ३.३८॥
dhūmenāvriyate vahnir
yathādarśo malena ca
yatholbenāvṛto garbhas
tathā tenedamāvṛtam (3.38)

*dhūmenāvriyate = dhūmena — by smoke + āvriyate — is obscured; vahnir = vahniḥ — the sacrificial fire; yathā — similarly; 'darśo = ādarśaḥ — mirror; malena — with dust; ca — and; yatholbenāvṛto = yatholbenāvṛtaḥ = yatho (yatha) — similarly + ulbena — by skin + āvṛtaḥ — is covered; garbhaḥ — embryo; tathā — so; tenedam = tena — by this + idam — this; āvṛtam — is blocked*

**As the sacrificial fire is obscured by smoke, and similarly as a mirror is shrouded by dust or as an embryo is covered by skin, so a man's insight is blocked by the passionate energy. (3.38)**

***Śrī Bābāji Mahāśaya's Commentary:***

Until one masters *buddhi yoga*, or alternately *kriyā yoga*, another name of the same discipline, one cannot experience the insight. Normally, a human being comes into this world with the muddled insight. Thus, many people assume that is the normal condition of mind. The passionate energy (*rajoguṇa* 3.37) sponsors the birth of material bodies, and generally its energy is considered to be the normal psychology. It takes the discipline of *buddhi yoga* to clear up the insight.

*Śrī* Krishna gave some fitting examples. In a sacrificial fire, there is supposed to be no smoke; the sacrificial performer is supposed to procure smokeless, dry, easy burning wood which would be consumed effortlessly by the fire god and his companion spirits. However, sometimes smoke still emerges. The smoke dampers the ceremony by irritating the eyes of the priest and the sacrificial performer. It causes their minds to shift to lower modes.

In the case of a mirror, one is supposed to see a clear image but often dust settles on a mirror. Then one gets a distorted image, just as when using the intellect if it is prejudiced by the sensual energy, memory and life force, one will misread reality.

For protection an embryo is covered by a membrane, but the same membrane which serves to isolate the fetus and protect it from bacteria, also restricts its vision. Similarly, the passionate energy fosters the subtle body of the limited spirit, but the same energy restricts and conditions the spirit, causing it to make decisions which are not in its long-ranged interest.

आवृतं ज्ञानमेतेन
ज्ञानिनो नित्यवैरिणा ।
कामरूपेण कौन्तेय
दुष्पूरेणानलेन च ॥३.३९॥
āvṛtaṁ jñānametena
jñānino nityavairiṇā
kāmarūpeṇa kaunteya
duṣpūreṇānalena ca (3.39)

*āvṛtam — is adjusted; jñānam — discernment; etena — by this; jñānino = jñāninaḥ — educated people; nityavairiṇā = nitya — eternal + vairiṇā — by the enemy; kāmarūpeṇa = kāma — yearning for various things + rūpeṇa — by the sense or form of; kaunteya — son of Kuntī; duṣpūreṇānalena = duṣpūreṇa — is hard to satisfy + analena — by fire; ca — and*

**The discernment of educated people is adjusted by their eternal enemy which is the sense of yearning for various things. O son of Kuntī, the lusty power, is as hard to satisfy as it is to keep a fire burning. (3.39)**

***Śrī Bābāji Mahāśaya's Commentary:***

*Kāmarūpa* is the sensuous energy in conjunction with the life force and memory. These allied forces are the real enemy of the spirit *(vairiṇā)*. Arjuna faced external enemies but his real problem was the internal force of passionate emotions.

For those who have not mastered *buddhi yoga*, this passionate emotion guides their every action, compelling them to act in favor of its biases. It demands continual satisfaction, or it reacts by inducing distressful states of mind. In this way it intimidates the spirit and causes the spirit to endorse its schemes for enjoyment.

One person may be educated *(jñānam)* but he may not have his intellect separated from the influence of this sensuous energy. Subsequently it will adjust his mentality and use his education to serve the sensuality.

इन्द्रियाणि मनो बुद्धिर्
अस्याधिष्ठानमुच्यते ।
एतैर्विमोहयत्येष
ज्ञानमावृत्य देहिनम् ॥३.४०॥
indriyāṇi mano buddhir
asyādhiṣṭhānamucyate
etairvimohayatyeṣa
jñānamāvṛtya dehinam (3.40)

*indriyāṇi — the senses; mano = manaḥ — the mind; buddhir = buddhiḥ — the intelligence; asyādhiṣṭhānam = asya — if this + adhiṣṭhānam — warehouse; ucyate — it is authoritatively stated; etair = etaiḥ — with these; vimohayatyeṣa = vimohayaty (vimohayati) — confuses + eṣa — this; jñānam — insight; āvṛtya — is shrouded; dehinam — embodied soul*

**It is authoritatively stated that the senses, the mind and the intelligence are the combined warehouse of the passionate enemy. By these faculties, the lusty power confuses the embodied soul, shrouding his insight. (3.40)**

***Siddha Swami's Commentary:***

This technique pertains to both *kriyā* and *brahma yoga*. In *kriyā yoga,* this procedure of the passionate energy is realized but the *yogin* tries to purify the mindal energy by kundalini yoga, by raising kundalini into the head of the subtle body. In *brahma yoga,* this *kriyā* is used in a mystic practice to keep the spirit separated from the influence of the intellect, so as not to give the intellect any power to persuade the self to follow the dictates of the senses.

***Śrī Bābāji Mahāśaya's Commentary:***

The senses which are in the subtle body and which are connected to the gross senses, plus the mind chamber with its sensitive energy, and the *buddhi* intellect organ which analyzes information; these are the combined repository of the passionate force, the emotions. *Śrī Patañjali Mahārṣi* in a detailed analysis of the psychology listed this differently as follows:

*vṛttayaḥ pañcatayyaḥ kliṣṭā akliṣṭāḥ*
*pramāṇa viparyaya vikalpa nidrā smṛtayaḥ*

***The vibrations in the mento-emotional energy are five-fold being agonizing or non-troublesome. They are correct perception, incorrect perception, imagination, sleep and memory. (Yoga Sūtra, 1.5-6)***

*Śrī Patañjali* listed these to show how the psychology functions. *Śrī* Krishna made His enumerations on the basis of *buddhi yoga* practice. In *buddhi yoga* one is first told to located the passionate energy which is in the senses, mind and intelligence. The student has to meditate repeatedly to discover this. Then he discusses the discovery with his teacher. At first one can locate the mind, but one is unable to locate the senses, other than their production as physical eyes, ears, nostrils, tongue and skin membrane. However, one has to go deeper in meditation to locate the sensual energy and the sensual orbs which are in the subtle body.

In looking for the internal enemy, the passionate force, one first discovers its hiding places in the psyche. Then one observes its tactics for influencing the mind and its contents. A student also observes how he is influenced by the lusty power. Everything which it motivates and operates must be observed in slow motion. Everyone has the spiritual insight, but most limited beings never use it because it is shrouded from the very beginning when one first received or assumed a subtle body. Only significant endeavor will remove the shrouding influence.

***Siddha Swami's Commentary:***

*Buddhi yoga* as taught in the *Bhagavad Gītā* by *Śrī* Krishna, beginning in Chapter Two, is the elementary meditational practice for *brahma yoga*. *Brahma yoga* begins when the spirit can distance itself from the *buddhi* organ. Once this is done, then the influences and feedback through that organ to the spirit, cease.

तस्मात्त्वमिन्द्रियाण्यादौ
नियम्य भरतर्षभ ।
पाप्मानं प्रजहिह्येनं
ज्ञानविज्ञाननाशनम् ॥ ३.४१ ॥

*tasmāt — thus; tvam — you; indriyāṇyādau = indriyāṇi — senses + ādau — initially; niyamya — regulating; bharatarṣabha — powerful man of the Bharata family; pāpmānaṁ — degrading power; prajahi — squelch, destroy; hyenaṁ = hy (hi) —*

tasmāttvamindriyāṇyādau
niyamya bharatarṣabha
pāpmānaṁ prajahihyenaṁ
jñānavijñānanāśanam(3.41)

*certainly + enaṁ — this; jñānavijñānanāśanam = jñāna — knowledge + vijñāna — discernment + nāśanam — ruining*

**Thus regulating the senses initially, you should, O powerful man of the Bharata family, squelch this degrading power which ruins knowledge and discernment. (3.41)**

***Śrī Bābāji Mahāśaya's Commentary:***

This is part of the second step in yoga which is *niyama*, observances to be made for the moral and righteous lifestyle of a yogi. *Śrī Patañjali Mahārṣi* defined *niyama* as consisting of the following:

*śauca saṅtoṣa tapaḥ svādhyāya īśvarapraṇidhānāni niyamāḥ*

***Purification, contentment, austerity and profound religious meditation on the Supreme Lord are the recommended behaviors. (Yoga Sūtra 2.32)***

*Ādau* means in the beginning or initially, when one first begins to practice yoga. At that time one is attracted to *yama* moral restraints and *niyama* behaviors. This is because at first one feels no need to do anything physical. Most people take up religion without doing any *āsana* postures or *prāṇāyāma* breath procedures. For them, regulating the senses are conducted by scriptural guidelines. Thus they control the senses initially by taking help from behavioral rules which are socially-approved in human society. *Śrī Patañjali* recommended purification but initially *(ādau)* this means external purification, while in the advanced stages it means purification of the subtle body, which is a mystic development, having little or nothing to do with bodily baths and the like.

*Śrī Patañjali* recommended contentment which initially *(ādau)* means to be satisfied with very little on the material level. At the advanced stages, this means to abandon the material level and to seek shelter in the spirit alone for satisfactions. *Patañjali Mahārṣi* spoke of austerity. Initially *(ādau)*, that means to leave aside pleasurable pursuits and make religious observances, like attending a temple function and fasting on a certain religious day. At the advanced level this means the austerities in yoga concerning *āsana* postures, *prāṇāyāma* breath techniques, *pratyāhār* sensual energy withdrawal, and *dhāranā* focusing of the attention on higher concentration forces or persons.

*Śrī Patañjali Mahāyogin* mentioned study of the psyche. This takes place in *kriyā yoga* practice at the advanced level but initially *(ādau)*, this takes place by hearing from yogic authorities, by studying the *Bhagavad Gītā* and by studying the Samkhya philosophy which is extensively quoted and referenced in the *Bhagavad Gītā* (*ucyate* 3.40)

The last feature of *niyama* given by *Śrī Patañjali* is the profound religious meditation on the Supreme Lord. This is initially done according to how one heard of the God from others and from scriptures. In the advanced stages, one meditates and reaches that Supreme Person in His superior domain, the *brahman* world.

Like this, if one initially applies the required restrictions on the senses (*yamah*) and direct the senses accordingly to what is recommended, then one will feel what it is like to squelch this degrading power which ruins knowledge and discernment. This squelching operation will be haphazard at first. Then, however, one will begin noticing which techniques are more effective. One will seek teachers who are proficient in the particular discipline one wishes to master.

इन्द्रियाणि पराण्याहुर्
इन्द्रियेभ्यः परं मनः ।
मनसस्तु परा बुद्धिर्
यो बुद्धेः परतस्तु सः ॥३.४२॥
indriyāṇi parāṇyāhur
indriyebhyaḥ paraṁ manaḥ
manasastu parā buddhir
yo buddheḥ paratastu saḥ (3.42)

*indriyāṇi — the senses; parāṇyāhur = parāṇi — are energetic + āhur (āhuḥ) — the ancient psychologists say; indriyebhyaḥ — the senses; paraṁ — more energetic; manaḥ — the mind; manasas — in contrast to the mind; tu — but; parā — more sensitive; buddhir = buddhiḥ — the intelligence; yo = yaḥ — which; buddheḥ — in reference to the intelligence; paratas — most sensitive; tu — but; saḥ — he, the spirit*

**The ancient psychologists say that the senses are energetic, but in comparison to the senses, the mind is more energetic. In contrast to the mind, the intelligence is even more sensitive. But in reference, the spirit is most elevated. (3.42)**

***Śrī Bābāji Mahāśaya's Commentary:***

This is to be realized in *kriyā yoga* practice, stage by stage, step by step. The confusion of identity or rather the fusion of identity of the core self with the intelligence, the mind compartment and the senses is removed by mystic clarity. It happens first by the energization of the subtle body through the kundalini yoga practice.

In normal existence, the core self mimics the senses because the self's energy is down-shifted or converted into a slower vibration. When, however, the self retracts from the sensual energies, it realizes itself as the general energy in the mind and then when it retracts further it feels as if it were the intellect organ. More progression inwards, leads it to know itself as its attention energy.

Yogis of the hoary past, before the time of *Śrī* Krishna, took notations on their practice of higher yoga. Some of these records are mentioned in the *Vālmīki Rāmāyaṇa* and in the Upanishads. By careful insight, they realized that the spirit itself was a higher reality than the intellect, which was higher than the mind chamber with its mixed subtle force, which in turn was higher than the subtle senses.

It is through intense *prāṇāyāma* practice, that one observes the various speeds at which the parts of subtle body operate. It is said that a chain is as strong as its weakest link, so the core self experiences itself as being identical with the slowest moving instrument in the subtle body. Thus, when by kundalini yoga practice one energizes the subtle body and accelerates the energy within it, one's core self shifts its dependence and takes shelter of higher pranic forces. The self then gets higher realization about the relative positions of the senses, mind chamber, intellect and attention energy.

एवं बुद्धेः परं बुद्ध्वा
संस्तभ्यात्मानमात्मना ।
जहि शत्रुं महाबाहो
कामरूपं दुरासदम् ॥३.४३॥
evaṁ buddheḥ paraṁ buddhvā
saṁstabhyātmānamātmanā
jahi śatruṁ mahābāho
kāmarūpaṁ durāsadam (3.43)

*evaṁ — thus; buddheḥ — than the intelligence; paraṁ — higher; buddhvā — having understood; saṁstabhyātmānamātmanā = saṁstabhya — keeping together + ātmānam — the personal energies + ātmanā — by the spirit; jahi — uproot; śatruṁ — enemy; mahābāho — O powerful man; kāmarūpaṁ — form of passionate desire; durāsadam — difficult to grasp*

**Thus having understood what is higher than intelligence, keeping the personal energies under control of the spirit, uproot, O powerful man, the enemy, the form of passionate desire which is difficult to grasp. (3.43)**

***Śrī Bābāji Mahāśaya's Commentary:***

*Ātmānam* in this verse means the attention of the core self. This attention is the power from which the mind chamber, intellect and sensual energies are created and to an extent are derived. Translating *ātmānam* as the personal energies is not wrong but it is not precise. For a precise translation, this would read that the *yogin* keeps his attention under the control of his core self. Now through that control of his attention, he will in turn, indirectly control the other parts of the psychology, because these other constituents cannot influence him except through their commandeering of his attention. When this same attention is commandeered by the other parts of the psyche, it is called *ahankār*, the sense of initiative to act in the material world.

***Śrī Bābāji Mahāśaya*** translated this verse as follows:

**Thus having understood what is higher than the intelligence, keeping the spiritual attention under control of the core self, root out, O powerful man, the enemy, the form of passionate desire which is difficult to commandeer.**

***He said:***

This is a technique for *buddhi* yogis. This occurs from a vigorous mystic practice, in recognizing and curbing the sensual energies in the psyche. It is mastered only after having vigorously practiced *prāṇāyāma* for kundalini yoga mastership. The sensuous energies, having a passionate motivation, are hard to commandeer by the self, because the self is related to that indirectly through the intellect, which is an unreliable agent. Being dependent on the senses for information and pleasurable indulgence, the intellect has no independence. Hence it is unreliable. It can be made into a fit and loyal servant, if the kundalini chakra is purified. When purified, this energy cooperates for the liberation of the spirit instead of working for its continued bondage in the subtle and gross material world.

As soon as kundalini chakra is purified, it cooperates with the spirit self, otherwise it does not, except for the practice of superficial, phony and go-no-where religions. Initially in *brahma yoga*, as we explained in *Bhagavad Gītā* 2.44, the self-focused intellect is experienced but eventually the ascetic comes to understand that he can exist without the intellect. Thus he no longer relies on its support. *Śrī Patañjali* called this stage of separation between the core self and the intellect, *kaivalyam*, which means the aloneness of the spirit self, being split off from reliance on the subtle psychology.

The passionate energy is experienced as one's sensuality and thus it is difficult to split off from it. In fact, many student ascetics complain bitterly that such a thing cannot be done, because they say that it is their very self. However, they can all rest assured that it is not. To realize this in fact, by mystic experience, one has to master kundalini shakti. That is the key to it. One must flush out the old pranic force and bring new and fresh pranic energy into the psyche. Then one can feel distinctly what is the self and what are its adjuncts.

# CHAPTER 4

## Bahuvidhā Yajñā

## Disciplines of Accomplishment*

*evaṁ bahuvidhā yajñā vitatā brahmaṇo mukhe*
*karmajānviddhi tānsarvān evaṁ jñātvā vimokṣyase (4.32)*

***Many types of disciplines of accomplishment were expounded in the mouth of the spiritual existence. Know them all to be produced from action. Realizing this, O Arjuna, you will be freed. (4.32)***

***Siddha Swami assigned this chapter title on the basis of verse 32 of this chapter.***

श्रीभगवानुवाच
इमं विवस्वते योगं
प्रोक्तवानहमव्ययम् ।
विवस्वान्मनवे प्राह
मनुरिक्ष्वाकवेऽब्रवीत् ॥४.१॥
śrībhagavānuvāca
imaṁ vivasvate yogaṁ
proktavānahamavyayam
vivasvānmanave prāha
manurikṣvākave'bravīt (4.1)

*śrī bhagavān – the Blessed Lord; uvāca — said; imaṁ — this; vivasvate — to Vivasvat; yogaṁ — yogic skill of controlling personal energies; proktavān — having explained; aham — I; avyayam — perpetual; vivasvān — Vivasvat; manave — to Manu; prāha — explained; manur = manuḥ — Manu; ikṣvākave — to Ikṣvāku; 'bravīt = abravīt — imparted*

**The Blessed Lord said: I explained to Vivasvat, this perpetual teaching of controlling the personal energies through yoga. Vivasvat explained it to Manu. Manu imparted it to Ikṣvāku. (4.1)**

***Siddha Swami's Commentary:***

This yoga taught to *Vivasvat*, the sun god, a supposedly mystical person, is the yoga described by *Śrī* Krishna as *jñāna yoga* and *karma yoga*. *Śrī* Krishna told us:

*śrībhagavānuvāca*
*loke'smindvividhā niṣṭhā purā proktā mayānagha*
*jñānayogena sāṁkhyānāṁ karmayogena yoginām (3.3)*

***The Blessed Lord said: In the physical world, a two-fold standard was previously taught by Me. O Arjuna, my good man. This was mind regulation by the yoga practice of the Sāṁkhya philosophical yogis and the action regulation by the yoga practice of the non-philosophical yogis. (3.3)***

This must be the complete yoga package given by the God to humanity. It cannot be otherwise. All the details may not be given in one verse or the other, but the complete teaching was given to those ancient students of the Supreme Lord. This is a perpetual teaching, remaining unchanged over centuries. It concerns the control of the personal energies through yoga and life under the supervision of the God of the creation.

एवं परंपराप्राप्तम्
इमं राजर्षयो विदुः ।
स कालेनेह महता
योगो नष्टः परंतप ॥४.२॥
evaṁ paraṁparāprāptam
imaṁ rājarṣayo viduḥ
sa kāleneha mahatā
yogo naṣṭaḥ paraṁtapa (4.2)

*evam — thus; paramparāprāptam = paramparā — a series of teachers + prāptam — received; imaṁ — this; rājarṣayo = rājarṣayaḥ — yogi kings; viduḥ — they knew; sa = saḥ — it; kāleneha = kālena — in time + iha — here on earth; mahatā — long; yogo = yogaḥ — yogic discipline; naṣṭaḥ — was lost; paraṁtapa — O burner of enemy forces*

**Thus, received through a series of teachers, the yogi kings knew this skill of controlling the personal energies. After a long time, here on earth, this yoga application was lost, O burner of enemy forces. (4.2)**

***Siddha Swami's Commentary:***

The *rājarśis* are the yogi kings, rulers who were proficient *karma* yogis. There also existed another group of students who were ascetics studying the Samkhya philosophy. It appears that even though the ascetics continued their study of Samkhya along with the practice of yoga disciplines, the rulers lost proficiency in *karma yoga*. *Śrī* Krishna confidentially told Arjuna that after a long time on earth, the yoga application to cultural activities had become unknown. Even persons like Bhishma and *Droṇa* did not exhibit the proficiency, even though they were to an extent masters of yoga. Thus the skill of yoga may only be applied to cultural activities by the special teaching of *Śrī* Krishna.

स एवायं मया तेऽद्य
योगः प्रोक्तः पुरातनः ।
भक्तोऽसि मे सखा चेति
रहस्यं ह्येतदुत्तमम् ॥४.३॥
sa evāyaṁ mayā te'dya
yogaḥ proktaḥ purātanaḥ
bhakto'si me sakhā ceti
rahasyaṁ hyetaduttamam (4.3)

*sa = saḥ — it; evāyaṁ = eva — indeed + ayam — this; mayā — by me; te — to you; 'dya = adya — today; yogaḥ — yoga technique; proktaḥ — is explained; purātanaḥ — ancient; bhakto = bhaktaḥ — devoted; 'si = asi — you are; me — of me; sakhā — friend; ceti = ca — and + iti — thus; rahasyaṁ — confidential teaching; hyetad = hi — truly + etad — this; uttamam — best*

**Today, this ancient yoga technique is explained to you by Me, since you are devoted to Me and are My friend. Indeed, this is confidential and is the best teaching. (4.3)**

***Siddha Swami's Commentary:***

*Śrī* Krishna was greatly relieved for the opportunity to again teach the *karma yoga* skill., As someone devoted and friendly to Krishna *(bhakto'si me sakhā)*, Arjuna was the right student for this teaching. We must therefore assume that the persons listed, namely *Vivasvat, Manu* and *Ikṣvāku*, were very dear and friendly to *Śrī* Krishna. It is not just the teaching being imparted but it is also the relationship between the student and teacher. It seems that *Śrī* Krishna could not teach the *karma yoga* skill to any ruler who was not dear and friendly in relation to Him.

For the sake of governing in this world, this is the most confidential teaching and the best instruction any ruler or any government agent can get, because it saves one from doing things which run contrary to the supreme will. It saves one from the great fear of being disapproved by the Supreme Person.

अर्जुन उवाच
अपरं भवतो जन्म
परं जन्म विवस्वतः ।
कथमेतद्विजानीयां
त्वमादौ प्रोक्तवानिति ॥४.४॥
arjuna uvāca
aparaṁ bhavato janma
paraṁ janma vivasvataḥ
kathametadvijānīyāṁ
tvamādau proktavāniti (4.4)

*arjuna — Arjuna; uvāca — said; aparaṁ — later; bhavato = bhavataḥ — Your Lordship; janma — birth; paraṁ — earlier; janma — birth; vivasvataḥ — Vivasvat; katham — how; etad — this; vijānīyāṁ — I should understand; tvam — you; ādau — in the beginning, before; proktavān — having explained; iti — thus*

**Arjuna said: Your Lordship's birth was later. The birth of Vivasvat was earlier. How should I understand that You explained this before? (4.4)**

***Siddha Swami's Commentary:***

Arjuna was so confused when confronting the Kurus, that he forgot the reality of reincarnation. Thus he contested *Śrī* Krishna's claim as the teacher of some ancient kings.

The basic question is: Why should anyone accept *Śrī* Krishna's claims?

श्रीभगवानुवाच
बहूनि मे व्यतीतानि
जन्मानि तव चार्जुन ।
तान्यहं वेद सर्वाणि
न त्वं वेत्थ परंतप ॥४.५॥
śrībhagavānuvāca
bahūni me vyatītāni
janmāni tava cārjuna
tānyahaṁ veda sarvāṇi
na tvaṁ vettha paraṁtapa (4.5)

*śrī bhagavān — the Blessed Lord; uvāca — said; bahūni — many; me — of Me; vyatītāni — transpired; janmāni — births; tava — your; cārjuna = ca — and + arjuna — Arjuna; tānyahaṁ = tāny (tāni) — them + aham — I; veda — I recall; sarvāṇi — all; na — not; tvaṁ — you; vettha — you remember; paraṁtapa — O scorcher of the enemies*

**The Blessed Lord said: Many of My births transpired, and yours, Arjuna. I recall them all. You do not remember, O scorcher of the enemies. (4.5)**

***Siddha Swami's Commentary:***

A distinction is made for *Śrī* Krishna's ability to recall past births. Arjuna, categorically, cannot have such recall.

The practice of yoga is meant to give a limited spirit the ability to recall births, perhaps not all births, but certainly the significant ones. The limited spirit has potential for recalling past births, and yoga may activate that recall.

Obviously *Śrī* Krishna does not need yoga to have unlimited recall because He is the Supreme Being. He is free from the constraints of the limited spirit and its shrouded insight:

*indriyāṇi mano buddhir asyādhiṣṭhānamucyate*
*etairvimohayatyeṣa jñānamāvṛtya dehinam (3.40)*

***It is authoritatively stated that the senses, the mind and the intelligence are the combined warehouse of the passionate enemy. By these facilities, the lusty power confuses the embodied soul, shrouding his insight. (3.40)***

Whatever insight a limited person has, is shrouded by the passionate force. Thus in yoga, the objective is to eliminate the effects of the passionate power. A limited being cannot at any time be as great as God, as *Śrī* Krishna, but that limited person may improve his lot by purification of the psyche, which is the main purpose for the practice of yoga.

अजोऽपि सन्नव्ययात्मा
भूतानामीश्वरोऽपि सन् ।
प्रकृतिं स्वामधिष्ठाय
संभवाम्यात्ममायया ॥४.६॥
ajo'pi sannavyayātmā
bhūtānāmīśvaro'pi san
prakṛtiṁ svāmadhiṣṭhāya
saṁbhavāmyātmamāyayā (4.6)

*ajo = ajaḥ — birthless; 'pi = api — even though; sann = san — being; avyayātmā = avyaya — imperishable + ātmā — person; bhūtānām — of the creatures; īśvaro = īśvaraḥ — Lord; 'pi = api — even; san — being; prakṛtiṁ — material energies; svām — my own; adhiṣṭhāya — controlling; saṁbhavāmyātmamāyayā = sambhavāmy (saṁbhavāmi) — I become visible + ātma — self + māyayā — by supernatural power*

**Even though I am birthless and My person is imperishable, and even though I am the Lord of the creatures, by controlling My material energies, I become visible by My supernatural power. (4.6)**

***Siddha Swami's Commentary:***

*Śrī* Krishna, as the Supreme Being, has His own arrangements which differ from those of limited entities like Arjuna. Despite similarities between *Śrī* Krishna and the other beings, one particularity in the Supreme Person separates him fron the limited entities. *Ajo (ajah)* means someone who is not caused to be in appearance by any other agency. While the limited beings are caused to be in this world, the Supreme Being, as their cause of appearance here, is not dominated by any other person or force. Thus He is not produced. This characteristic singles Him out from all others.

Since He is not subjected to memory lapses like others, *Śrī* Krishna's personality is constant. Thus it is said, even in the *Vedas* and the Upanishads, that His character is imperishable. It is not reliant on specific cultural conditions for its optimum functioning. And even though He is the Lord of all creatures, still He can become manifested among the creatures when He decides to use a form in any species of life. He is not pressured to do so as are many others, but rather He does that by choice *(ātma māyayā).*

These distinctions between a limited being and the Supreme Person are to be studied by the *brahma yogi* after having penetrated the chit akasha, the sky of consciousness. There he can observe many divine beings and discern by comparison which quality emanates from which personality.

यदा यदा हि धर्मस्य
ग्लानिर्भवति भारत ।
अभ्युत्थानमधर्मस्य
तदात्मानं सृजाम्यहम् ॥४.७॥
yadā yadā hi dharmasya
glānirbhavati bhārata
abhyutthānamadharmasya
tadātmānaṁ sṛjāmyaham (4.7)

*yadā yadā — whenever; hi — indeed; dharmasya — of righteousness; glānir = glāniḥ — decrease; bhavati — it is; bhārata — O son of the Bharata family; abhyutthānam — increasing; adharmasya — of unrighteousness, of wickedness; tadā — then; 'tmānaṁ = ātmānaṁ — My self; sṛjāmyaham = sṛjāmy (sṛjāmi) — show + aham — I*

**Whenever there is a decrease of righteousness, O son of the Bharata family, and when there is an increase of wickedness, then I show Myself. (4.7)**

***Siddha Swami's Commentary:***

Some believe and it is stated in some of the Vedic texts, that the Supreme Person appears in this world in a playful way, by *līlā*. The word *līlā* indicates something that is done for the fun of it. Thus some feel that the Supreme Being comes here for fun, and that His activities here are all a play. However in all seriousness, *Śrī* Krishna in explaining *karma yoga* to Arjuna, gave righteousness as the cause of His descent. Elsewhere, *Śrī* Krishna stressed this repeatedly. He indicated that He is not attracted to this world, since His own world is sufficient for His purposes.

It is appropriate that the Supreme Lord should come here to establish righteousness. In fact, if not for that, there might not be a *Bhagavad Gītā* discourse. He shows Himself in one way or the other, directly or indirectly, when there is a decrease of righteousness and an increase in irreligious lifestyle among the human beings, since under such condition their progression ceases and His investment of energy in this world is essentially squandered.

This brings to fore the importance of *karma yoga*. This is why *Śrī* Krishna identified that type of yoga as His particular type of discipline. It is because *karma yoga* assists Him in this establishment of righteousness, something which He considers to be His prime duty.

परित्राणाय साधूनां
विनाशाय च दुष्कृताम् ।
धर्मसंस्थापनार्थाय
संभवामि युगे युगे ॥४.८॥
paritrāṇāya sādhūnāṁ
vināśāya ca duṣkṛtām
dharmasaṁsthāpanārthāya
saṁbhavāmi yuge yuge (4.8)

*paritrāṇāya — to protect; sādhūnāṁ — of the saintly persons; vināśāya — to destruction; ca — and; duṣkṛtām — of the wicked people; dharmasaṁsthāpanārthāya = dharma — righteousness + saṁsthāpana — the establishing of + arthāya — for the sake of; saṁbhavāmi — I come into visible existence; yuge yuge —from era to era*

**To protect the saintly people, to destroy the wicked ones, and to establish righteousness, I come into the visible existence from era to era. (4.8)**

***Siddha Swami's Commentary:***

This is the main reason for the incarnation of Godhead. God and His parallel divinities also come into the world to show accelerated paths of salvation, which are even more important than *karma yoga* and which are taught through the *jñāna yoga* process mentioned in verse 3 of Chapter Three as *jñānayogena sāmkhyānām*. However, for the mass of humanity at any given stage, the process of *karma yoga* protects them from misguided leaderships. This in turn creates a religious atmosphere for appreciation of the austerities practiced in *jñāna yoga*. Thus *karma yoga* is supportive of *jñāna yoga*, which is higher and which is the direct means of salvation for those rare individuals who can work for it.

Kundalini yoga, *kriyā yoga* and *brahma yoga*, including paths which are known as *ātma* yoga, *ātma śuddha* yoga, and *rāja* yoga, are all included in the term *jñāna yoga*. In a *karma yoga* society, *jñāna* yogis can flourish because what they try to achieve is appreciated by the *karma* yogis.

It may be questioned as to why *bhakti yoga* is not mentioned as one of the methods taught to the ancient kings and ancient Samkhya yogis. The answer is this: *Bhakti yoga* is included in *karma yoga* and in *jñāna yoga*. It was not considered a completely separate path for male students. For them it was included in their apprenticeship to their teacher. This is why *Śrī* Krishna used the terms *bhakto* and *sakhā* to appraise Arjuna as qualified to be taught *karma yoga*. Unless one has devotion to *Śrī* Krishna and is friendly towards Him, one cannot be trained in *karma yoga*. The same goes for *jñāna yoga*. One was not even taught any of these yoga processes unless one was a devotee of *Śrī* Krishna and in friendly dealings with Him. Mostly in those times, the students were male. These boys were taught by their teachers on the basis of a student-teacher reciprocal relationship in which devotion and friendship were always present.

God is interested in a righteous political environment, because in such a society each person can progress at the appropriate rate according to evolutionary development. Those who were the most advanced studied *jñāna yoga*. Those just below these studied *karma yoga*, and the rest of the people were governed by the *karma* yogi administrators. This is the type of society that God Himself organized. The ideal *karma* yogi ruler was *Śrī Rāma*, the Divine Personality. When He shot Bāli, the unforgiving brother of Sugriva, he was asked the reason for wounding Bāli, even though Bāli had offered him no aggression. *Śrī Rāma* explained that as a representative of *dharma*, of righteous lifestyle, He had to chastize Bāli for committing acts hostile to a righteous lifestyle, and that He did so dispassionately. *Śrī Rāma* acted as the ideal *karma* yogi ruler, and he protected all those ascetics who practiced *jñāna yoga* in the forested areas near *Ayodhyā* and who were harassed and intimidated by *Rāvaṇa's* brothers, Khara and Dushana. This shows the relationship between the two paths, and how *bhakti yoga* is included in the relationship between the student and teacher.

जन्म कर्म च मे दिव्यम्
एवं यो वेत्ति तत्त्वतः ।
त्यक्त्वा देहं पुनर्जन्म
नैति मामेति सोऽर्जुन ॥४.९॥
janma karma ca me divyam
evaṁ yo vetti tattvataḥ
tyaktvā dehaṁ punarjanma
naiti māmeti so'rjuna (4.9)

*janma — visitation; karma — deed; ca — and; me — of me; divyam — supernatural; evaṁ — thus; yo = yaḥ — who; vetti — realizes; tattvataḥ — in truth; tyaktvā — abandoning; dehaṁ — body; punarjanma = rebirth; naiti = na — not + eti — goes; mām — to Me; eti — goes; so = saḥ — he; 'rjuna = arjuna — Arjuna*

**One who knows My supernatural visitation and deeds, who truly realizes this while abandoning his body, does not seek rebirth. He goes to Me, O Arjuna. (4.9)**

***Siddha Swami's Commentary:***

In the *Vālmīki Rāmāyaṇa*, the example of a person who understood this was Shabari, the female ascetic disciple of *Śrī* Matanga Rishi. This lady understood the mission of *Śrī Rāma*. She recognized His divinity. A student of that caliber does not go for rebirth haphazardly, rather that person goes to the Divine Lord or to His agents and gets directions on where to go in the next transmigration if there is to be one. Since that person is not focused on the materialistic lifestyle and is unattached to the social milieu of this world, he or she is freed from the natural process of human or animal birth in this world.

The ordinary person takes *prakṛtam* or natural births and actions, but *Śrī* Krishna and His agents do so supernaturally or *divyam*. This is another distinction between the Supreme Person and others.

After being accepted for studentship by *Śrī* Krishna, on the basis of being devoted and friendly towards Him, one develops faith in the teachings. Now obviously, one cannot do this directly if another person is one's teacher. In that case, one would develop faith in *Śrī* Krishna indirectly by being devoted and friendly towards the teacher. But if that person is indeed the agent of *Śrī* Krishna, one's faith in that person would gravitate towards *Śrī* Krishna, even at the time of abandoning the body.

When one knows for sure, both by faith and by experience of mystic and spiritual truths, that *Śrī* Krishna makes these supernatural visitations and deeds on the basis of His interest in maintaining righteousness and setting conditions for the soul's progression in yoga, either in *karma* or *jñāna yoga* as is suitable for the particular student, then one's spirit naturally will go to *Śrī* Krishna or to His agents after leaving the body, and one will not be attracted into another womb merely on the basis of familial feelings.

It is not true that every student with this faith in *Śrī* Krishna, will definitely go to *Śrī* Krishna's world after leaving the body. What is true is this: Every student will go to get direction on where he or she should go after leaving the body. Those who have to complete austerities will go to a place where they can achieve that. Only the purified ones may go to *Śrī* Krishna's domains, if He so desires for any of them.

Whatever influence was predominant in one's life, dictates one's rebirth. One gravitates naturally towards the predominant force which one was attracted to and which guided one here or there during one's life. As such, those who were under the guidance of *Śrī* Krishna directly, like Arjuna, or indirectly like the ascetic lady *Shabari*, who was guided by *Śrī* Matanga Rishi, will go to either *Śrī* Krishna or that agent of *Śrī* Krishna when the physical body is lost. Another person who was family-centered will again come back into the association of family members by the force of that attraction. When this force of attraction or relational energy is fused to *Śrī* Krishna or His agent, it is known as *bhakti* or devotion to the Divinity.

वीतरागभयक्रोधा
मन्मया मामुपाश्रिताः ।
बहवो ज्ञानतपसा
पूता मद्भावमागताः ॥४.१०॥
vītarāgabhayakrodhā
manmayā māmupāśritāḥ
bahavo jñānatapasā
pūtā madbhāvamāgatāḥ (4.10)

*vītarāgabhayakrodhā = vīta — gone + rāga — craving + bhaya — fear + krodhā — anger; manmayā — think of Me; mām — Me; upāśritāḥ — rely on; bahavo = bahavaḥ — many; jñānatapasā — by austerity/education; pūtā — purified; madbhāvam — my level of existence; āgatāḥ — attained*

**Many, whose cravings, fear and anger are gone, who are totally focused on Me, who are purified by austerity and education, attained My level of existence. (4.10)**

***Siddha Swami's Commentary:***

Without purification *(pūtā)*, no one can use *bhakti* or devotion and reach *Śrī* Krishna on His level of existence. In other words, no one can go to the divine world merely by being devoted to *Śrī* Krishna in any way except by full purity. By a careful study of this verse, one will get the idea of the requirements needed along with the devotion. Mastership of *buddhi yoga* is required. This is given in the words *vīta rāga bhaya krodhā*, the complete removal and non-recurrence of craving, fear and anger. If craving, fear and anger recur, then one does not qualify and it is only by mastership of *buddhi yoga* as explained primarily in Chapter Two, that one can eradicate this in the psyche.

Mastership of the student-teacher relationship is required. This might be termed *bhakti*. The relationship must be such that there are no misgivings. A complete focus on fulfilling the needs of that relationship is absolutely required. The student will find that gradually he is compelled more and more to live for the satisfaction of the teacher, and that this life consists of constant striving for purification by following the yoga disciplines. His associations with others should be reduced day after day such that he feels exempt from the routine affairs of this world.

If there is no *jñānatapasā*, then the *bhakti* or devotion is in question. This means that there must be austerity and education. Some teachers of *bhakti* belittle the attempt of *Śrī* Uddhava to instruct the gopis in austerity and education, but actually it is a requirement. It was a requirement for the ascetic lady Shabari in the *Vālmīki Rāmāyaṇa*.

It depends on what is desired by the devotee. Does the devotee want to attain *Śrī* Krishna's level of existence *(mad bhāvam āgatāh)?* If so, that person must gain the qualification mentioned in this verse. One does not have to qualify this much to be a devotee of *Śrī* Krishna. There are devotees of *Śrī* Krishna who have not attained His level of existence. Shabari wanted to go to the higher worlds where her spiritual master, *Śrī* Matanga Rishi, and his other students had journeyed. Thus she exerted herself in austerity and education to reach that place, and she was blessed by *Śrī Rāma* for that accomplishment, but specifically on the basis of her sincerity in endeavors. This should be noted.

ये यथा मां प्रपद्यन्ते
तांस्तथैव भजाम्यहम् ।
मम वर्त्मानुवर्तन्ते
मनुष्याः पार्थ सर्वशः ॥४.११॥
ye yathā māṁ prapadyante
tāṁstathaiva bhajāmyaham
mama vartmānuvartante
manuṣyāḥ pārtha sarvaśaḥ (4.11)

*ye — who; yathā — as; māṁ — me; prapadyante — they rely; tāṁs = tan — them; tathaiva = tathā — so + eva — indeed; bhajāmyaham = bhajāmy (bhajāmi) — relate to + aham — I; mama — my; vartmānuvartante = vartma — course of an action + anuvartante — are affected; manuṣyāḥ — human beings; pārtha — son of Pṛthā; sarvaśaḥ — everywhere*

**As they rely on Me, so I relate to them, O son of Pṛthā. All human beings, everywhere, are affected by My course of action. (4.11)**

***Siddha Swami's Commentary:***

A person's relationship with *Śrī* Krishna is important. The degree of devotion and friendliness to *Śrī* Krishna is a force to reckon with in any person's life. This may, however, happen indirectly through a spiritual teacher or through an inborn sense of kinship with the Lord. If there is a Supreme Being, then obviously, everyone everywhere would be affected by His course of action. Even physically, every creature is affected by the course of the sun. It cannot be avoided. If there is no sunshine, then there might be no heat and no vegetative growth for nutrition. Thus we can understand that if there is a Supreme Being, His existence would always affect our course of action.

*Brahma yoga* students endeavor to become more and more aware of the Supreme Being. They gravitate more and more towards the Supreme Lord, in compliance with these verses.

काङ्क्षन्तः कर्मणां सिद्धिं
यजन्त इह देवताः ।
क्षिप्रं हि मानुषे लोके
सिद्धिर्भवति कर्मजा ॥४.१२॥
kāṅkṣantaḥ karmaṇāṁ siddhiṁ
yajanta iha devatāḥ
kṣipraṁ hi mānuṣe loke
siddhirbhavati karmajā (4.12)

*kāṅkṣantaḥ — wanting; karmaṇām — of ritual action; siddhiṁ — success; yajanta — they worship; iha — here on earth; devatāḥ — supernatural authorities; kṣipraṁ — quickly; hi — indeed; mānuṣe — in the humans; loke — in the world; siddhir = siddhiḥ — fulfillment; bhavati — there is, comes to be; karmajā — produced of ritual action*

**Wanting their ritual action to succeed, people in the world, worship the supernatural authorities. Quickly in this human world, there is fulfillment which comes from ritual action. (4.12)**

***Siddha Swami's Commentary:***

This means that most people are not concerned specifically with the Supreme Being. Most are concerned with results for the fulfillment of desires in family life. These persons are involved in cultural activities *(karmaṇām)* on a superstitious basis *(yajanta devatāḥ)*. They think that they should submit to the supernatural supervisors in order to get what they want for the well-being of their families. This type of thinking is against the thinking described in the previous verses, where the person focuses on *Śrī* Krishna or on His agent.

The natural system, however, is to work for family improvement and to use the connection with the demigods for that purpose only. And it does work, even though it may frustrate a person from time to time. *Śrī* Krishna even said that it works quickly *(kṣipram)*.

Even though *Brahmā* wanted the human beings to work as stipulated by the supernatural rulers, still the natural system as dictated by the attachment energy in their psyches, causes the human beings to try to use the demigods for family progression over others. Thus it is necessary to master *buddhi yoga*, so that one can supersede the natural physiology and psychology.

In all cases there will be a relationship with the supernatural people but in the case of wanting only one's family to benefit, one will have a relationship of wanting to use the demigods to get favors. This type of devotion to the demigods is perverse and will cause reversals as was the case for the Kurus whom Arjuna confronted.

चातुर्वर्ण्यं मया सृष्टं
गुणकर्मविभागशः ।
तस्य कर्तारमपि मां
विद्ध्यकर्तारमव्ययम् ॥४.१३॥
cāturvarṇyaṁ mayā sṛṣṭaṁ
guṇakarmavibhāgaśaḥ
tasya kartāramapi māṁ
viddhyakartāramavyayam (4.13)

*cāturvarṇyaṁ — the four career categories; mayā — by me; sṛṣṭaṁ — instituted; guṇa — habit; karma — work tendency; vibhāga — distribution; śaḥ — by; tasya — of it; kartāram — creator; api — also; mām — me; viddhyakartāram = viddhy (viddhi) — know + akartāram — one not required to act; avyayam — eternal*

**According to the distribution of habits and work tendencies, the four career categories were instituted by Me. Know that I am never required to participate. (4.13)**

***Siddha Swami's Commentary:***

This explains that even though there is one Supreme Being governing the world, still the limited entities in the various life forms are categorized differently according to their habits and work tendencies *(guṇakarma)*. The Supreme Lord however is not limited. He can freely choose to enter any category. He may set an example for any of the higher or lower life forms. Even though there are four career categories *(cāturvarṇyam)*, still there are numerous subdivisions within each grouping, all depending on the proportion of habits and work tendencies. Each person requires minute adjustments for elevation, just as different patients get different dosages of the same or different medicines according to the type and stage of disease each possesses.

A *brahma yogi* does side-step these work categories. He is ready to do anything, to serve in anyway, because he acknowledges destiny as his master. To him a higher or lower, weaker or stronger, greater or lesser occupation, is irrelevant. It has nothing to do with spiritual status and cannot in any way help discover the spiritual body.

न मां कर्माणि लिम्पन्ति
न मे कर्मफले स्पृहा ।
इति मां योऽभिजानाति
कर्मभिर्न स बध्यते ॥४.१४॥
na māṁ karmāṇi limpanti
na me karmaphale spṛhā
iti māṁ yo'bhijānāti
karmabhirna sa badhyate (4.14)

*na — not; māṁ — me; karmāṇi — actions; limpanti — they entrap; na — not; me — of me; karmaphale — in a pay-off; spṛhā — desire; iti — thus; māṁ — me; yo = yaḥ — who; 'bhijānāti = abhijānāti — understands; karmabhir = karmabhiḥ — by actions; na — not; sa = saḥ — he; badhyate — is entrapped*

**Actions do not entrap Me. The desire for payoff is not in Me. The person who understands this is not entrapped by action. (4.14)**

***Siddha Swami's Commentary:***

To transcend material existence, one must appreciate the Supreme Being. One must first admire God's immunity from these material worries and their constraints. The desire for a payoff is not in the Supreme Being, but it is in others. These others should appreciate the Supreme Lord for what He is, for the difference between Him and themselves. From such appreciation comes a proximity to Him, and from that comes an elevation, which ultimately results in the promotion to His level of existence (*mad bhāvam āgatāh* Bg. 4.10).

A limited being, by proximity to the Supreme Person, attains some divine attributes, just as by closeness to material nature, the limited spirit feels affected. To get coverage from the Supreme Being, a limited being must serve as an agent for that Supreme Lord. By himself or herself the limited person cannot get the immunity from entrapment in material nature. This goes back to the mastership of *buddhi yoga*. Such mastership when applied in cultural activities, makes a person a proficient *karma* yogi, free from taints and liabilities.

एवं ज्ञात्वा कृतं कर्म
पूर्वैरपि मुमुक्षुभिः ।
कुरु कर्मैव तस्मात्त्वं
पूर्वैः पूर्वतरं कृतम् ॥४.१५॥
evaṁ jñātvā kṛtaṁ karma
pūrvairapi mumukṣubhiḥ
kuru karmaiva tasmāttvaṁ
pūrvaiḥ pūrvataraṁ kṛtam (4.15)

*evaṁ — thus; jñātvā — having understood; kṛtaṁ — done; karma — functional work; pūrvair = pūrvaih — by the ancient rulers like Janaka; api — even; mumukṣubhiḥ — by those who desire liberation; kuru — perform; karmaiva = karma — cultural acts + eva — indeed; tasmāt — therefore; tvaṁ — you; pūrvaiḥ — by the yogi kings like Janaka; pūrvataraṁ — before; kṛtam — performed*

**Having understood this conclusion, functional work was done, even by the yogi kings who desired liberation. Therefore you should perform cultural acts, just as it was done before. (4.15)**

***Siddha Swami's Commentary:***

Since one must act in the world, since one is accountable for the type of action performed and even for indifference and non-action, it is best that one act under the supervision of the Divine Lord, since one then avoids liabilities and gains divine approval. This is why the yogi kings who desired liberation performed functional work for a righteous lifestyle in this world.

किं कर्म किमकर्मेति
कवयोऽप्यत्र मोहिताः ।
तत्ते कर्म प्रवक्ष्यामि
यज्ज्ञात्वा मोक्ष्यसेऽशुभात् ॥४.१६॥
kiṁ karma kimakarmeti
kavayo'pyatra mohitāḥ
tatte karma pravakṣyāmi
yajjñātvā mokṣyase'śubhāt (4.16)

*kiṁ — what; karma — action; kiṁ — what; akarmeti = akarma — no action + iti — thus; kavayo = kavayaḥ — eloquent philosophers; 'py = api — even; atra — in this matter; mohitāḥ — confused; tat — this; te — to you; karma — action; pravakṣyāmi — I will discuss; yaj = yad — which; jñātvā — knowing; mokṣyase — you will be freed; aśubhāt — from undesirable circumstances*

**What is action? What is not an action? Even eloquent philosophers are confused on this subject. I will discuss the subject of action with you. Knowing this, you will be freed from undesirable circumstances. (4.16)**

***Siddha Swami's Commentary:***

The question of what to do and what not to do, is ever before a human being, day after day as he or she confronts various situations. Each person wants to act in his interest to get positive results, to be able to live comfortably and in an advantageous position, to be liked and honored. The eloquent philosophers *(kavayah)* ponder over what is right and what is wrong, what is in the long-range interest and what would benefit immediately and be detrimental eventually. Yet, none of them have the supreme insight. That is reserved for the Supreme Being. Thus one has to link up with the opinion of the Supreme Lord to find out which act is appropriate in any given circumstance. There is absolutely no way a limited entity with a limited intellect can determine what is appropriate, because such a being cannot perfectly assess the past and the future. Only the Supreme Person is capable of that. In His association, one may get the correct view.

कर्मणो ह्यपि बोद्धव्यं
बोद्धव्यं च विकर्मणः ।
अकर्मणश्च बोद्धव्यं
गहना कर्मणो गतिः ॥४.१७॥
karmaṇo hyapi boddhavyaṁ
boddhavyaṁ ca vikarmaṇaḥ
akarmaṇaśca boddhavyaṁ
gahanā karmaṇo gatiḥ (4.17)

*karmaṇo = karmaṇah — of action; hyapi = hy (hi) — indeed + api — also; boddhavyaṁ — should be known; boddhavyaṁ — should be recognized; ca — and; vikarmaṇaḥ — inappropriate action; akarmaṇaś = akarmaṇaḥ — no action + ca — and; boddhavyaṁ — should be understood; gahanā — difficult to comprehend; karmaṇo = karmaṇaḥ — of action; gatiḥ — the course*

**Indeed, appropriate action should be known and one should also recognize the inappropriate type. The effect of no action should be understood. The course of action is difficult to comprehend. (4.17)**

***Siddha Swami's Commentary:***

Since the human being is a rational creature, it is expected that he would know the appropriate type of action, and he should know what the consequences would be for him if he does not act. The animals are not expected to understand this. Still, even though the human being has much rational power, he is limited and the course of action *(karmaṇo gatih)* is difficult for him to comprehend. A human being can certainly calculate his limitation is that he gains access to a limited amount of information. Thus his reasoning is ever prone to error.

कर्मण्यकर्म यः पश्येद्
अकर्मणि च कर्म यः ।
स बुद्धिमान्मनुष्येषु
स युक्तः कृत्स्नकर्मकृत् ॥४.१८॥
karmaṇyakarma yaḥ paśyed
akarmaṇi ca karma yaḥ
sa buddhimānmanuṣyeṣu
sa yuktaḥ kṛtsnakarmakṛt (4.18)

*karmaṇyakarma = karmaṇy (karmaṇi) — in performance + akarma — non-action; yaḥ — who; paśyed = paśyet — he should see; akarmaṇi — in non-action; ca — and; karma — action; yaḥ — who; sa = saḥ — he; buddhimān — wise person; manuṣyeṣu — of human beings; sa = saḥ — he; yuktaḥ — skilled in yoga; kṛtsnakarmakṛt = kṛtsna – all + karmakṛt — action performance*

**He who perceives the non-acting factor in a performance and sees an acting factor when there is no action, is the wise person among human beings. He is skilled in yoga and can perform all actions. (4.18)**

***Siddha Swami's Commentary:***

This type of perception is gained by one who mastered *buddhi yoga,* to become detached from moods and to cause his nature not to convert into exciting or depressing attitudes. Due to soberness, he possesses detachment which allows him to be sensitive to the view of the Supreme Being. It is not that he can have infallible perception, but rather he can be in touch with the Supreme Being who has such vision.

A limited being can be expert in performing all actions only when he is totally surrendered to the Supreme Being as described in Chapter Three, text 30:

*mayi sarvāṇi karmāṇi saṁnyasyādhyātmacetasā*
*nirāśīrnirmamo bhūtvā yudhyasva vigatajvaraḥ (3.30)*

***All your working power should be entrusted to Me. On the Supreme Spirit, you should meditate. Being free from cravings, indifferent to selfishness, do fight. Be a man whose feverish mood has departed. (3.30)***

Such a person being detached from his own nature, can see when an action is really no action at all, and when a refusal to participate would significantly impact a circumstance. Being detached, he or she would be inclined only to what the Supreme Being desires. This is a description of the expert *karma* yogi, who mastered *buddhi yoga* and applies it to his day to day activities.

यस्य सर्वे समारम्भाः
कामसंकल्पवर्जिताः ।
ज्ञानाग्निदग्धकर्माणं
तमाहुः पण्डितं बुधाः ॥४.१९॥
yasya sarve samārambhāḥ
kāmasaṁkalpavarjitāḥ
jñānāgnidagdhakarmāṇaṁ
tamāhuḥ paṇḍitaṁ budhāḥ (4.19)

*yasya — one whom; sarve — all; samārambhāḥ — endeavors; kāmasaṁkalpa varjitāḥ = kāma — desire + saṁkalpa — intention + varjitāḥ — not mixed into; jñānāgni dagdha karmāṇaṁ = jñāna — knowledge + āgni — fiery force + dagdha — burnt, destroyed + karmāṇaṁ — reactionary work; tam — him; āhuḥ — call; paṇḍitaṁ — learned man; budhāḥ — wise man*

**He for whom desires and intentions are not mixed into his endeavors, who destroyed reactionary work by the fiery force of his knowledge, he, the wise men call a pandit or learned man. (4.19)**

***Siddha Swami's Commentary:***

This is another detailed description of the application of *buddhi yoga* expertise to cultural life. In the mind of a *buddhi* yogi, the desires which arise from the *citta,* the mento-emotional energy, and the intentions which form in the *buddhi* organ are effectively suppressed. Thus he is free to work under the direction of higher personalities who are connected into the energy circuit of the Supreme Spirit. Due to control of the emotional energy and the analytical intellect, that *yogin* no longer performs reactionary work. He avoids it. He does participate in worldly life as induced by providence, but his involvement is trouble-free. Such a person is rated by *Śrī* Krishna as a *budha* or a pandit, a truly learned personality.

***Śrī Bābāji Mahāśaya's Commentary:***

The desires lay dormant in the general mind space as mental and emotional energies.

Minute parts of these energies convert into full blown ideas when they enter into the intellect organ housed in the mind compartment. They enter into the imagination faculty of the intellect and convert into mental pictures, sounds, odors, feelings and flavors. Most of these are converted into pictures and sounds only. These audio and visual images stimulate the attention. From such stimulation, the spirit is induced to endorse plans for action. All of these actions come about by operating the appropriation or grabbing ability of the self, but this grabbing ability is experienced as a sense of identity or familiarity with the said images.

It is very important to become detached from the mento-emotional energy *(citta).* As *Śrī Patañjali Mahārṣi* suggested, all yogis must work to stop the operations in the *citta* force, since these destroy one's ability to be successful in *samādhi* practice. The intellect should not be allowed to analyze everything it encounters or everything presented to it by the senses and memory. It should ignore most of the impressions sent by the sensual energy and memory chamber. That gives the yogi the required detachment needed to give up the impulsive need to mix his intentions into obligations.

Even though a mailman needs money, he should not check the mail of citizens to determine the contents of envelopes. He should desist from that; otherwise his need for money will get mixed into his duty of mail delivery and he will open certain mail articles to pilfer funds. Similarly, a *yogin* should act for the Supreme Spirit without trying to get a benefit for himself from such activity. This requires control of the internal nature, the *antah karaṇa*, the psychology.

The desires, many millions of them, are laying dormant in the mental space in the emotional energy. Any of these may burst out in the imagination. If the attention is attached to the imagination, the core self will be forced to endeavor for their fulfillment. He will then use every opportunity perversely for satisfactions. Thus he will incur demerits and gain disfavor with the Supreme Person. One must therefore meditate in the *buddhi yoga* practice, given by *Śrī* Krishna in this *Bhagavad Gītā* discourse, and gain a resistance to the emotional energy. One must stop its communication with the imagination, so that the desire energies remain dormant and do not convert. This is part of *pratyāhār* practice. It is the same *buddhi yoga* but it is listed as the 5$^{th}$ step in the *aṣṭanga* yoga techniques, given by *Śrī Patañjali.*

Conversely, a person whose desire and intention are mixed into his endeavors is not suitable to serve the Supreme Person. He is bound to resist the will of the Lord on occasion, when his nature does not find the instructions to be palatable and useful for desire fulfillments.

*Śrī* Krishna described this desire and intentional energy as *kāmarūpa*, the sense of yearning for various things (3.39). Those who are under its power are not free to help the Supreme Being establish righteousness, but they do from time to time, when convenient, cooperate with Him. A *karma yogin*, however, is inclined to cooperate with the Supreme Person at all times, even when the instructions are unpalatable, and even when they seem to make no sense or serve no rational purpose. This comes from a confidence in the Supreme Being as having infallible vision.

That confidence arises out of the original student-to-teacher relationship whereby the student is devoted and loyal to the spiritual teacher who is serviceable to *Śrī* Krishna *(bhakto' si me sakhā).*

In the *kriyā yoga* system, which I teach, this is the training given during the first technique, explained by *Śrī* Krishna as follows:

*yadā te mohakalilaṁ buddhirvyatitariṣyati*
*tadā gantāsi nirvedaṁ śrotavyasya śrutasya ca (2.52)*

***When from your delusion-saturated mind, your discrimination departs, you will become disgusted with what is to be heard and what was heard. (2.52)***

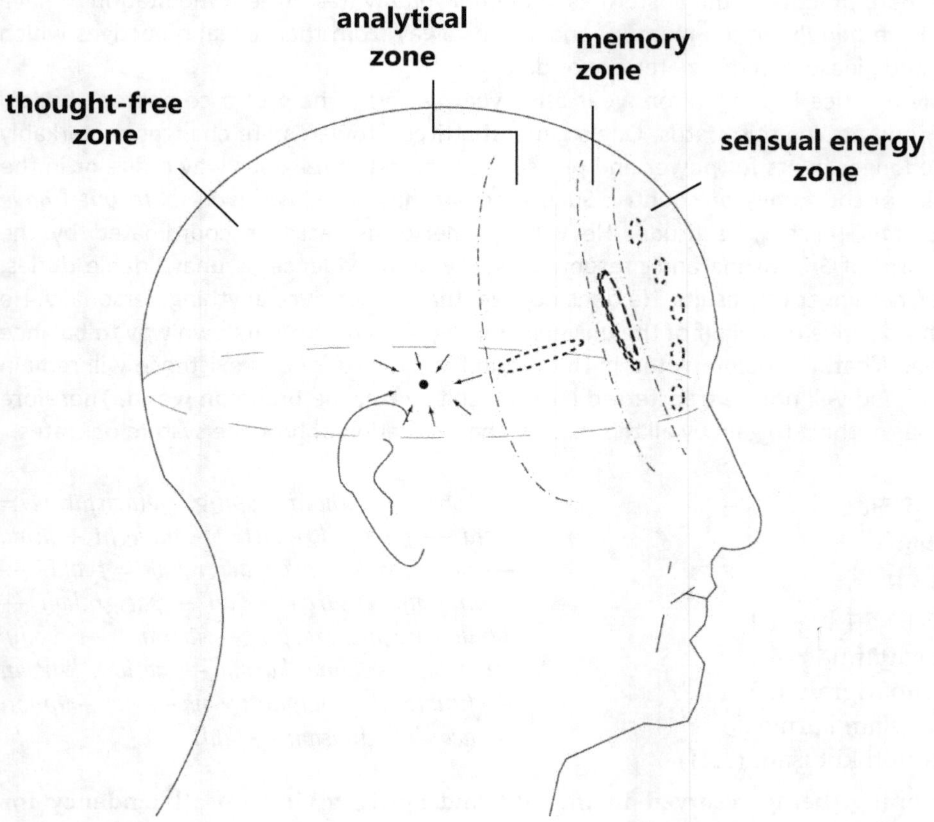


The sensual energy, memory and intellect should not be allowed to inter-mix or to communicate haphazardly or impulsively. This practice of *kriyā yoga* can be mastered by the meditation practice with guidance from a more advanced yogi. We call this *kriyā yoga* but *Śrī* Krishna originally presented this as *buddhi yoga*.

त्यक्त्वा कर्मफलासङ्गं
नित्यतृप्तो निराश्रयः ।
कर्मण्यभिप्रवृत्तोऽपि
नैव किंचित्करोति सः ॥४.२०॥
tyaktvā karmaphalāsaṅgaṁ
nityatṛpto nirāśrayaḥ
karmaṇyabhipravṛtto'pi
naiva kiṁcitkaroti saḥ (4.20)

*tyaktvā — given up; karmaphalāsaṅgaṁ = karma — action + phala — pay-off + āsaṅgaṁ — attachment, quest; nityatṛpto (nityatṛptaḥ) = nityaḥ — always + tṛptaḥ — satisfied; nirāśrayaḥ — not dependent; karmaṇy = karmaṇi — in performance; abhipravṛtto = abhipravṛttaḥ — proceeding, functioning; 'pi = api — even; naiva = na — not + eva — indeed; kiṁcit — anything; karoti — does; saḥ — he*

**Giving up the quest for a payoff from actions, being always satisfied, not depending on anything, he does nothing at all even while performing. (4.20)**

***Śrī Bābāji Mahāśaya's Commentary:***

This pertains to the changed psyche of the proficient *buddhi* yogi. This is not a mental state of resolve or determination to be detached and to not be result-oriented. This comes about after hard practice in the austerities of *buddhi yoga* with sufficient meditation to have re-oriented the *buddhi* organ, memory and senses away from their usual objectives which are power and pleasure in the material world.

By daily practice in meditation, year after year, with the help of a competent *buddhi yoga* guru, one attains this status. One's general attitude towards life changes remarkably and one no longer hunts for power and pleasure either in the religious way of life or in the social affairs of the family or country. Such a person has an, *"I will work here but I have nothing to gain thereby,"* attitude. He willingly performs tasks as coordinated by the Universal Form of *Śrī* Krishna and presented usually by providence as unavoidable duties, but he does not linger for results. He does not feel that he achieves anything personally. He feels that he is active on behalf of the universal energy, which acts in its own way to balance the creation. Whatever is completed in this world for the sake of this existence will remain in this world and will not be transferred into the chit akash, the brahman world. Therefore one really has nothing to gain by all this, except the realization of how the system operates.

निराशीर्यतचित्तात्मा
त्यक्तसर्वपरिग्रहः ।
शारीरं केवलं कर्म
कुर्वन्नाप्नोति किल्बिषम् ॥४.२१॥
nirāśīryatacittātmā
tyaktasarvaparigrahaḥ
śārīraṁ kevalaṁ karma
kurvannāpnoti kilbiṣam (4.21)

*nirāśīr — without hoping; yatacittātmā = yata — reserved + citta — thought + ātmā — spirit; tyaktasarvaparigrahaḥ = tyakta — giving up + sarva — all + parigrahaḥ — tendency for grasping; śārīraṁ — body; kevalaṁ — alone; karma — action; kurvan —functioning; nāpnoti = na — not + āpnoti — acquire; kilbiṣam —fault*

**Without hoping, being reserved in thought and spirit, giving up all tendency for grasping, using the body effectively for action, he does not acquire a fault. (4.21)**

***Śrī Bābāji Mahāśaya's Commentary:***

This is another description of a technique given in Chapter Two:

*traiguṇyaviṣayā vedā nistraiguṇyo bhavārjuna*
*nirdvaṁdvo nityasattvastho niryogakṣema ātmavān (2.45)*

***Three moody phases are offered by the Vedas. Be without the three modes, O Arjuna. Be without the moody fluctuations. Be always anchored to reality. Be free from grasping and possessiveness. (2.45)***

When one has advanced to *brahma yoga* from the rigors of mystic practice in *kriyā yoga*, one is introduced to the appropriation energy. This energy comes out of the sense of initiative *(ahankāra)* which is experienced by the self as its attention. The habit, and the only habit of the attentive power, is the appropriating or taking of subtle information from the intellect. The intellect in turn takes or accepts projections which are offered to its imagination faculty by the memory and the senses. These faculties work in tandem and influence the core self to accept liabilities for gross or subtle actions. Those who have gross bodies become involved in physical movements. Those who have only subtle forms are restricted to mystic activity, but for them such mystic acts are reality, just as in the physical world, a physical movement is a solid fact which affects those in the environment.

One should take note of the term *kevalam*, which means: alone or in isolation, without admixtures. Referring to text 19 of this chapter, we hear of not mixing the desires and intentions into the endeavors *(samārambhāh kāma samkalpa varjitāh)*. When this is done, the body becomes isolated from the personal psychology of sensual energy and mentality. It is freed from the influence of desires and intentions. Thus the spirit is free to respond favorably to demands of the Supreme Spirit.

In my example of a mailman, he can deliver a letter without interference if he does not keep his financial needs in mind and if he has no intentions of interfering in the lives of others. But in his case, he will fall short of his objectives and interfere from time to time, because mere determination is insufficient to curb the nature. One must curb it by changing its tendencies through mystic methods in *kriyā yoga* and *brahma yoga*, or as *Śrī* Krishna named it, in *buddhi yoga*. Determination is good for ordinary religion but in yoga it has no place, because it is unreliable and haphazard and it gives way to certain emotions which entice it and weaken resolve.

A person who follows ordinary religion does not accept the weakness of his determination, and thus he has no use for yoga. When, however, he considers the matter seriously and really becomes determined for full success, he takes up yoga practice in earnest. Then he takes *Śrī* Krishna seriously. Those who feel that they will be determined by grace, either by grace of the Supreme Being or by grace of their spiritual master, are being rather foolish and naive.

If we take this verse part by part, we will see that this is only possible in *brahma yoga* practice, the advanced level of *kriyā yoga*. At first *Śrī* Krishna said *nirāśīr* which means without hoping. This is only possible when the spirit has broken off from its psychology, which is the intellect and the sensing mechanisms of the mind. *Śrī Patañjali Mahārṣi* calls this *kevala* or *kaivalyam*, which is the aloneness of the spirit, its isolation from the influence of its psychology. This is the result of a mystic act. It does not comes about by wishing for it or by the grace of anybody. It is the power of a particular spirit to separate its core-self from its psychology. Why is this necessary? It is because the psychology is prejudiced to the sensual energy and the memory. No amount of hoping will change the nature of it. Only the discipline of depriving it of the power of the core self can change it and this can only be done by mystic means in higher meditation.

*Yatacittātma* means being reserved or disciplined *(yata)* in thought *(citta)* and spirit *(ātma)*. *Śrī Patañjali Mahārṣi* dismissed the *citta* energy, the mental and emotional force, as a total nuisance to the *yogin*. He advised the complete stoppage of its operations and influences. One cannot reserve one's *ātma* from one's intellect and the mental-emotional mechanism, unless one uses yoga. It is not possible by other means. If an easier method were possible, *Śrī* Krishna would not have bothered to cite the special method of *buddhi yoga* taught to the ancient kings who were devoted and friendly towards Him.

*Tyakta sarva parigrahah* means giving up all tendency for grasping. This is not easy. This can only be achieved when one mastered the *kriyā yoga* practice proficiently. This is because the tendency for grasping comes out at first from the attention of the core self. This was explained by *Śrī* Krishna differently when he discussed the fact that the limited spirits, His dependents, do draw to themselves the senses, of which the mind may be regarded as the sixth detection device. That indicates that the grasping tendency is precursory to the mind. It existed before the mind came into being. This is why we have put that practice into the realm of *brahma yoga*, even though *Śrī* Krishna initially taught it as *buddhi yoga*. We did that because technically speaking the control of the grasping tendency or appropriation-taking tendency is not in the realm of the *buddhi* organ. It is in the realm of controlling the attention of the spirit, its raw energy. That is *ātma* yoga or *brahma yoga*. Actually later in Chapter Six, *Śrī* Krishna listed it as *ātma viśuddha* yoga.

Everything is mastered step by step in the right order, scientifically, from lower organ to higher organ. Since the grasping appropriation tendency comes from the sense of attention, it follows that it can only be controlled after one has controlled the life force, the sensual energy, the memory and the intellect. Each is controlled one after the other. First there is kundalini yoga, for controlling the life force and for energizing the sensual energy, then there is *kriyā yoga* for the final control of the sensual energy and the regulation of the memory. And then there is *buddhi yoga* or higher *kriyā yoga* for controlling the intellect and its delicate and super sensitive instruments. Then at last one can control the attention of the core self by *brahma yoga*.

When the attention is controlled and freed from its impulsion for grasping, then one can use the body effectively for action without behaving in a prejudiced manner under the influences of the desires and intentions. Hereby, one acquires no fault. One's subtle body remains unblemished.

यदृच्छालाभसंतुष्टो
द्वंद्वातीतो विमत्सरः ।
समः सिद्धावसिद्धौ च
कृत्वापि न निबध्यते ॥४.२२॥
yadṛcchālābhasaṁtuṣṭo
dvaṁdvātīto vimatsaraḥ
samaḥ siddhāvasiddhau ca
kṛtvāpi na nibadhyate (4.22)

*yadṛcchā — by chance; lābha — benefit; saṁtuṣṭaḥ — satisfied; dvandvātīto (dvandvātītaḥ) = dvandva — likes and dislikes + atītaḥ — ignoring; vimatsaraḥ — free from envy; samaḥ — even — minded; siddhāv = siddhau — in success; asiddhau — in failure; ca — and; kṛtvā — having performed; 'pi = api — also; na — no; nibadhyate — is implicated*

**Being satisfied by benefit which comes by chance, ignoring likes and dislikes, being free from envy, even-minded in success and failure, and having performed, a man is still not implicated. (4.22)**

***Siddha Swami's Commentary:***

It is very interesting that *Śrī* Krishna expected Arjuna to be that advanced so that Arjuna would be a masterful *buddhi* yogi and then apply that expertise in the cultural field in day to day life as a government administrator. This means that *Śrī* Krishna taught the ancient *karma* yogis how to live in the world and be His agents perfectly. He wanted Arjuna to demonstrate this.

Unless one's intellect is in agreement, one cannot be satisfied with benefits which come by chance. This is because the intellect has a tendency to want to create or participate in providence. Under normal conditions of psychology, the intellect will work for results and will not be satisfied to be inactive, just taking what comes by chance *(yadṛcchālābha)*.

To bring the intellect into agreement with this idea on a consistent and permanent basis, reflexively, one has to master *buddhi yoga*, to cut the power of the intellect by separating the attention energy from it. This must be done internally by mystic methods in long hours of meditation practice.

*Dvamdvātīto* or the ignoring of likes and dislikes happens consistently only when the intellect is segregated from the memory and sensual energies which usually prejudice its selections and make it subordinate to desires for pleasure. This is a part of *kriyā yoga* practice but it also involves kundalini yoga techniques.

*Vimatsarah* or freedom from envy comes about by the segregation of the *buddhi* intellect from the memory and sensual energy. If the *buddhi* is allowed to be fused with the memory and sensual energy, it will have to envy this or that because of the prejudices of the memory and sensual powers.

*Samah siddhau asiddhau* or even-mindedness in success and failure, is a result of kundalini yoga practice, whereby the lower sensual energies are energized sufficiently, whereby the senses no longer have need for lower gratifications. This is part of *pratyāhār* practice in *kriyā yoga,* but *Śrī* Krishna considered it as part of *buddhi yoga*.

With such accomplishments, a person who performs in the cultural field, would not be implicated. It would be impossible to pin him down with liabilities, because he is free from limitations, through his surrender to the Supreme Being.

गतसङ्गस्य मुक्तस्य
ज्ञानावस्थितचेतसः ।
यज्ञायाचरतः कर्म
समग्रं प्रविलीयते ॥४.२३॥
gatasaṅgasya muktasya
jñānāvasthitacetasaḥ
yajñāyācarataḥ karma
samagraṁ pravilīyate (4.23)

gatasaṅgasya = gata — gone + saṅgasya — of attachment; muktasya — of the liberated person; jñānāvasthitacetasaḥ = jñāna — knowledge + avasthita — established + cetasaḥ — of an idea; yajñāyācarataḥ = yajñāya — for austerity and religion + ācarataḥ — doing; karma — action; samagraṁ — completely; pravilīyate — cancels

**Concerning a person whose attachment is finished, who is liberated, whose idea is established in knowledge, any of his action which is done solely for austerity and religion, does cancel completely. (4.23)**

***Siddha Swami's Commentary:***

*Śrī* Krishna already described this world as being for the most part action-bound, unless one acts for the sake of religious fulfillment and ceremony:

*yajñārthātkarmaṇo'nyatra loko'yaṁ karmabandhanaḥ*
*tadarthaṁ karma kaunteya muktasaṅgaḥ samācara (3.9)*

***Besides action for religious fulfillment and ceremony, this world, is action-bound. Act for the sake of religious fulfillment and ceremony, O son of Kuntī. Be free from attachment. Act promptly. (3.9)***

This means that unless one acts to please the supervising supernatural personalities, one will be bound by liabilities. All the same, when acting for the supervisors, one should do so with detachment or one will be bound up nevertheless.

The limited being has an attachment within his mind and emotions. Thus, unless he gets rid of that, he will be bound up even if he acts for the supervisors, because his own nature will cause him to be blighted with the liabilities. To get rid of the attachment *(gatasaṅgasya)* one has to practice higher yoga. One has to develop the ability for himself or herself. Then from that liberation, which is a liberation from being bound to one's intellect, memory and senses, one will be isolated from the reactions which occur in the material world. It is not the physical reactions, but rather the emotional and sensual reactions which occur on the psychological level.

If in the cultural field, one acts only as stipulated by the supervisors and if one pursues spiritual disciplines in one's spare time, then one will be exempt from the hassles of this world.

ब्रह्मार्पणं ब्रह्महविर्
ब्रह्माग्नौ ब्रह्मणा हुतम् ।
ब्रह्मैव तेन गन्तव्यं
ब्रह्मकर्मसमाधिना ॥४.२४॥
brahmārpaṇaṁ brahmahavir
brahmāgnau brahmaṇā hutam
brahmaiva tena gantavyaṁ
brahmakarmasamādhinā (4.24)

*brahmārpaṇaṁ = brahma — spiritual existence + arpaṇam — ceremonial articles; brahma — spiritual existence; havir = haviḥ — sacrificial ingredients, ghee; brahmāgnau = brahma — spiritual existence + agnau — in fire; brahmaṇā — by the qualified brahmin priest; hutam — offering oblations; brahmaiva = brahma — spiritual existence + eva — indeed; tena — by him; gantavyaṁ — to be attained; brahmakarmasamādhinā = brahma — spiritual existence + karma — activity + samādhinā — by meditative contact*

**Spiritual existence is the basis of his ceremonial articles. It is the foundation of sacrificial ingredients. The perceptive priest pours the stipulated items into the fiery splendor of spiritual existence. It is the spiritual existence which is attained by a person who keeps contact with the spiritual level while acting. (4.24)**

***Siddha Swami's Commentary:***

The disengagement of the spirit self from its psychological equipments causes the spirit to be solely and only in the spiritual existence, in *brahman*. Then if such a liberated (*muktasya*, 4.23) spirit still applies himself or herself to the material world, that application occurs in detachment without the psychic equipments domineering the actions of his or her body.

Thus, as stated even before the time of *Śrī* Krishna by the sages who wrote the Upanishads, that person is spiritual existence, and whatever he or she does is also the spiritual existence.

This is done by meditative contact, by *samādhi*. It is done because the ascetic is so practiced at *samādhi*, the final stage of yoga, that he remains in a residual status of *samādhi* even when he acts culturally.

दैवमेवापरे यज्ञं
योगिनः पर्युपासते ।
ब्रह्माग्नावपरे यज्ञं
यज्ञेनैवोपजुह्वति ॥४.२५॥
daivamevāpare yajñaṁ
yoginaḥ paryupāsate
brahmāgnāvapare yajñaṁ
yajñenaivopajuhvati (4.25)

*daivam — to a supernatural authority; evāpare = eva — indeed + apare — some; yajñaṁ — austerity and religious ceremony; yoginaḥ — yogis; paryupāsate — practice; brahmāgnāv = brahmāgnau — in the fiery brilliance of spiritual existence; apare — others; yajñaṁ — austerity and religious ceremony; yajñenaivopajuhvati = yajñena — by austerity and religious ceremony + eva — indeed + upajuhvati — they offer*

**Some yogis perform austerity and religious ceremony in relation to a supernatural authority. Others offer austerity and religious ceremony as the sacrifice into the fiery brilliance of spiritual existence. (4.25)**

***Siddha Swami's Commentary:***

Some persons who take up yoga, the same yoga practice described by *Śrī* Krishna as *buddhi yoga*, do so with motives which are not in agreement with *Śrī* Krishna's intention for teaching yoga. *Śrī* Krishna listed his intention as twofold. Thus anyone who takes up the practice and uses yoga in any other way, is in effect, in opposition to *Śrī* Krishna. However, *Śrī* Krishna gave a synopsis of the various ways this yoga practice may be used or applied by those who are in agreement with Him and by those who oppose Him. In the previous verse, He summarized the ultimate objective of yoga according to how He intended it. Review now the two-fold intention of *Śrī* Krishna:

*śrībhagavānuvāca*
*loke'smindvividhā niṣṭhā purā proktā mayānagha*
*jñānayogena sāṁkhyānāṁ karmayogena yogināṁ (3.3)*

***The Blessed Lord said: In the physical world, a two-fold standard was previously taught by Me. O Arjuna, my good man. This was mind regulation by the yoga practice of the Sāṁkhya philosophical yogis and the action regulation by the yoga practice of the non-philosophical yogis. (3.3)***

Even though the yoga was originally invented by *Śrī* Krishna, still there are others who have independently taught it. Yoga, like everything else that is possible in any of the existences, is latent within that existence and may be discovered by anyone besides the Supreme Lord. Even if one person discovers something, others might get possession of it and use it in their own way. Thus some persons in the past who performed yoga, took to religious ceremony and austerities in relation to a supernatural authority, without regard for *Śrī* Krishna. This is because some persons are more attracted to other superior souls than they are to *Śrī* Krishna, even though He is the Supreme Lord. The persons who performed yoga and then used their psychological expertise to finetune their attraction to a supernatural authority, irrespective of *Śrī* Krishna, were different to modern worshipers of the supernatural people. Most of the modern worshippers do not master *buddhi yoga*. *Śrī* Krishna described persons prior to and in his own time, persons who mastered the *buddhi yoga* to a greater degree but who did not care about His intention for the use and application of the practice.

There were others too, who mastered *buddhi yoga* to a greater extent and who did not adhere themselves to *Śrī* Krishna or to any supernatural personality. Instead they adhered to or made attempts to adhere to the fiery brilliance of spiritual existence, *brahmāgnau*, the spiritual existence at large. These persons felt no compulsion to align themselves to any personality. In the yogic history of India, there were many such persons and many more are to come. We may question, however, if they had any need for *bhakti* and *sakhā*, devotion and friendliness. The answer is that if there is *bhakti* and *sakhā* in the nature of everyone, then these persons are no exception. Hence they were devoted to a teacher perhaps, and were friendly to him, or they discovered the *buddhi yoga* process all by themselves and became devoted and endearing to the spiritual effulgence at large. This happened in the lives of many ascetics in India.

श्रोत्रादीनीन्द्रियाण्यन्ये
संयमाग्निषु जुह्वति ।
शब्दादीन्विषयानन्ये
इन्द्रियाग्निषु जुह्वति ॥४.२६॥
śrotrādīnīndriyāṇyanye
saṁyamāgniṣu juhvati
śabdādīnviṣayānanye
indriyāgniṣu juhvati (4.26)

*śrotrādīnīndriyāṇy = śrotrādīnīndriyāṇi = śrotra — hearing + ādīni — and related aspects + indriyāṇi — senses; anye — others; saṁyamāgniṣu = saṁyama — restraint + agniṣu — in the fiery power; juhvati — they offer; śabdādīn = śabda — sound + ādīn — and so on; viṣayān — sensual pursuits; anye — others; indriyāgniṣu — in the fiery energy of sensuality; juhvati — they offer*

**Other yogis offer hearing and other sensual powers into the fiery power of restraint. Some offer sound and other sensual pursuits into the fiery sensual power. (4.26)**

***Siddha Swami's Commentary:***

These are two procedures in *kriyā yoga*. These are preliminary in that practice. Seek a commentary from *Śrī Bābāji Mahāśaya*.

***Śrī Bābāji Mahāśaya's Commentary:***

These are indeed preliminary steps in *kriyā yoga*. In the system of *buddhi yoga*, taught by *Śrī* Krishna, this is elementary. Students who could not do *buddhi yoga* outright initially, did these elementary processes. In the first, a student who has an over-grown, out-reached sense or senses, made efforts at *pratyāhār* to curb that elongated mystic psychic appendage. He restrained it by using the same power it used to attract the objects.

This concerns the anatomy of the subtle body. If for instance, the subtle ear was elongated, then the person would try to pull it in, to shorten it. He would have to restrain himself from hearing certain sounds and would limit its auditory intake to only certain sounds which were mantras given to him by the teacher. Each student yogi must discover or be shown which of his senses are elongated or extended too far out from his subtle body. Then he has to pull that sense in, retract it, by restraining it for some time, long enough for it to shrink inwards. When it is shrunk inwards, that particular sense no longer procures certain lower objects.

An example of the physical body may be given to understand this. In infancy, male children are unable to drink alcohol. Their tasting sense being very short, does not have the variety of needs which an adult male might have. A child likes milk but abhors alcohol. Later, however, his tasting sense grows out further and becomes divested to the extent that it might dislike milk and prefer alcohol. Thus if that sense is again pulled in, it would not exhibit the need for strong flavors like alcohol. This actually takes place when the adult male leaves his gross body. His subtle body goes through a shrinkage and its variety of tastes are again decreased considerably, such that as a baby, its tongue cannot tolerate alcohol.

In *aṣṭanga* yoga, the 5$^{th}$ development is *pratyāhār*. This is the process of pulling in the senses so that they do not crave such a variety of attractive objects for enjoyments. Persons like *Vivasvat, Manu* and *Ikṣvāku* were so advanced as students that they did not need to do anything like *pratyāhār*, which is required nowadays. *Śrī Patañjali* mentioned it; therefore it was required in his time too. To *Śrī* Krishna it was extra practice for certain persons who attempted *buddhi yoga* but who were not qualified as students of the practice, when they first approached a teacher to learn of it.

This is factual, for in the *Mahābhārata*, when *Śrī* Krishna as a student performed austerities, He did not do any preliminary practice. He did *samādhi* practice only. He did not have to do any remedial course or anything to subsidize any ignorance or deficiency in the learning.

The second type of yogis mentioned in this verse are those who are so weak in psychological control, that they begin the *kriyā yoga* mostly by chanting mantras. They offer the sound of the mantra into their physical ears. After practicing a long time like this they are able to internalize. These persons come to do yoga, but since they are extroverted by nature, strongly and impulsively so, they are unable to do the *pratyāhār*, *dhāranā*, *dhyāna* and *samādhi*. They do not understand any of this and feel it is impossible. They consider themselves to be physical beings mostly. They have no idea of a psychic physiology. These persons start the process at an elementary stage by offering a physical sound or a physical object into the corresponding physical sense of their body.

To such a person spiritual discipline begins with physical objects of some sort. They cannot perceive of anything which is not physically present. However, such a person might have a strong belief in the supernatural and spiritual nonetheless, but they have no direct perception of the same. Their psyche is habituated to the physical world only and initially it has to be turned away from that existence by elementary austerities.

Usually such persons attempt *buddhi yoga,* and then after a time, not getting results, they become disheartened and go away. They usually stick to a physical religion only.

सर्वाणीन्द्रियकर्माणि
प्राणकर्माणि चापरे ।
आत्मसंयमयोगाग्नौ
जुह्वति ज्ञानदीपिते ॥४.२७॥
sarvāṇīndriyakarmāṇi
prāṇakarmāṇi cāpare
ātmasaṁyamayogāgnau
juhvati jñānadīpite (4.27)

*sarvāṇīndriyakarmāṇi = sarvāṇi — all + indriyakarmāṇi — sensual actions; prāṇakarmāṇi = prāṇa — breath function + karmāṇi — activities; cāpare = ca — and + apare — some; ātmasaṁyamayogāgnau = ātmasaṁyama — self-restraint + yogāgnau — in fiery yoga austerities; juhvati — they offer; jñānadīpite = jñāna — experience + dīpite — illuminated*

**Some ascetics subject the sensual actions and the breath function to self-restraint by fiery yoga austerities, which are illuminated by experience. (4.27)**

***Siddha Swami's Commentary:***

This is a general description of the *kriyā yoga* which *Śrī Bābāji Mahāśaya* taught. Let him comment on this.

***Śrī Bābāji Mahāśaya's Commentary:***

The objective of *kriyā yoga* is to develop *jñānadīpa*, which is the spiritual eye. Once this is developed, the yogi stays on course all by himself. He is able to see into the chit akasha, the sky of consciousness. By contact with supernatural and divine personalities, he gets whatever instruction he needs to finish the austerities.

This verse is indeed a general description of the *kriyā* practice I introduced. Take note of the term *ātmasamyama*. This is the focusing of the self on itself by the process of *samyama*, which is the development from *dhāraṇā* to *dhyāna* to *samādhi*. A yogi has to learn how to do this. The sensual actions must definitely be curtailed and one must become introverted. The senses mislead the self to go outwards into concerns of the material world and its allied subtle counterpart. Thus the senses must be curtailed. The breath function, *prāṇakarmāṇi*, must be curtailed as well since it dictates the life urges and causes the life force to remain bound in creature survival when it has a material body and in creature body acquirement when it does not have a body. If these two facilities are curtailed, namely the sensual actions and the breath function, then one can effectively internalize. One can then study the physiology of the subtle form and plan how to bring it under control for self realization.

Even though *Vivasvat, Manu* and *Ikṣvāku* did the *karma yoga* practice easily and did not have to do these elementary practices, still modern people must take up these basic disciplines because they do not have the gifted self control of those great personalities. Modern persons will have to gain much mystic experience before they develop the required confidence and mastership of the *buddhi yoga* practices described by *Śrī* Krishna.

द्रव्ययज्ञास्तपोयज्ञा
योगयज्ञास्तथापरे ।
स्वाध्यायज्ञानयज्ञाश्च
यतयः संशितव्रताः ॥४.२८॥
dravyayajñāstapoyajñā
yogayajñāstathāpare ।
svādhyāyajñānayajñāśca
yatayaḥ saṁśitavratāḥ (4.28)

*dravya — property; yajñās — austerity and religious ceremony; tapo (tapaḥ) — self denial; yajñā — austerity and religious ceremony; yoga –eight-part yoga process; yajñāḥ — austerity and religious ceremony; tathāpare = tathā — as well as + apare — some others; svādhyāyajñānayajñāśca = svādhyāya — study of the Veda + jñāna – knowledge + yajñāḥ — austerity and religious ceremony + ca — and; yatayaḥ — ascetics; saṁśitavratāḥ = saṁśita — strict + vratāḥ — vows*

**Persons whose austerity and religious ceremony involve the control of material possession, those whose austerity and religious life involve some self-denial, as well as some others whose penance and religious procedure is the eight-part yoga discipline, and those whose austerity and religious ceremony is the study of the Veda and the acquirement of knowledge, all these are regarded as ascetics with strict vows. (4.28)**

***Siddha Swami's Commentary:***

There are many types of ascetics and the yogis are one type. Generally, the ascetics are known as *yatis*. *Śrī* Krishna lists off the general categories of such individuals. Some people feel that religious ceremony and related austerities like fasting, attending temple functions, dressing in a certain way, following certain moral principles, are sufficient as the way of perfection. They feel that one will attain spiritual experience in that way, so they perform recommended austerities which come down to them from religious leaders and through scriptures. Some of these people feel that it is adequate if one makes money and offers it for a religious cause, especially if one gives to the poor in charity. Some others feel that self denial is the way to spiritual perfection. They do some haphazard method of keeping themselves restrained from eating or drinking at certain times of the year and they feel this is perfection.

There are also those of us who are convinced of the yoga process which was described by *Śrī* Krishna. This process consists of eight parts, but *Śrī* Krishna discussed it so far as a process of *buddhi yoga* in application to cultural activities or in application to self knowledge and to a relationship to the Supreme Being, *Śrī* Krishna Himself.

Others believe only that one should study the *Vedas*. They feel that merely by studying the *Vedas* one will graduate to the world of *Brahmā*, the master of the *Vedas*. All these persons are categorized by *Śrī* Krishna as ascetically-inclined persons with strict vows *(vratāh).*

अपाने जुह्वति प्राणं
प्राणेऽपानं तथापरे ।
प्राणापानगती रुद्ध्वा
प्राणायामपरायणाः ॥४.२९॥

*apāne — in exhalation; juhvati — they offer; prāṇam — inhalation; prāṇe — in inhalation; 'pānaṁ = apāṇaṁ — in exhalation; tathāpare = tathā — similarly + apare — others; prāṇāpāna gatī = prāṇa — energizing air + apāna — de-*

apāne juhvati prāṇaṁ
prāṇe'pānaṁ tathāpare
prāṇāpānagatī ruddhvā
prāṇāyāmaparāyaṇāḥ (4.29)

*energizing air + gatī — channel; ruddhvā — restraining; prāṇāyāmaparāyaṇāḥ = prāṇa — inhaling + āyāma — regulating + parāyaṇāḥ — intent*

**Some offer inhalation into the exhalation channels; similarly others offer the exhalation into the inhalation channels, thus being determined to regulate the channels of the energizing and de-energizing airs. (4.29)**

***Śrī Bābāji Mahāśaya's Commentary:***

This concerns mastery over kundalini shakti, the power in the subtle spine. This has to do with curbing the life force, so that it does not drive the psyche into being attached to material bodies any longer. There are variations in this practice, depending on the stage of the yogi involved. This is known as *prāṇāyāma*, but it is mentioned in verse 27 of this chapter as *prāṇakarmāṇi*.

Even though one may attempt to control the sensual energies, if one does not at first adjust the breath mechanism and the intake of food, the digestion, one will not be successful. One must master kundalini yoga before one can complete the sensual energy restraint which is *pratyāhār* practice. This is why in the eight-part yoga process one is advised to master prana before one does *pratyāhār* or sensual energy restraint. So long as kundalini chakra is unclean and wayward, one's attempts at sense mastery will be a failure, since the kundalini power will undermine one's effort to control the senses.

As the attention is attached to the *buddhi* intellect, so that intellect is attached to the memory, which is attached to the sensual energies, which in turn is attached to the life force or kundalini energy. Thus an ascetic must curb these step by step beginning with the lowest energy.

अपरे नियताहाराः
प्राणान्प्राणेषु जुह्वति ।
सर्वेऽप्येते यज्ञविदो
यज्ञक्षपितकल्मषाः ॥४.३०॥
apare niyatāhārāḥ
prāṇānprāṇeṣu juhvati
sarve'pyete yajñavido
yajñakṣapitakalmaṣāḥ (4.30)

*apare — others; niyatāhārāḥ — persons restrained in diet; prāṇān — fresh air; prāṇeṣu — into the previous inhalations; juhvati — impel; sarve — all; 'pyete (apyete) = apy (api) — also + ete — these; yajñavido = yajñavidaḥ — those who know the value of an act of sacrifice; yajñakṣapitakalmaṣāḥ = yajña — austerity and religious ceremony + kṣapita — destroyed, removed + kalmaṣāḥ — impurities*

**Others who were restrained in diet, impel fresh air into the previously inhaled air. All these ascetics whose impurities were removed by austerity and religious ceremony understand the value of an act of sacrifice. (4.30)**

***Śrī Bābāji Mahāśaya's Commentary:***

*Apare niyatāhārāh prāṇānprāṇeṣu juhvati* is also a procedure in elementary *buddhi yoga* process. The gross body is controlled by restraint in diet and by āsana postures, but one finds that to seal this control one has to do *prāṇāyāma*. Thus Rishi Gorakshnatha did stress these austerities for all neophyte yogins. However, as Śrī Krishna states, if one's impurities are removed by one's austerity and religious ceremony, then it is understood that one has a valid process. The whole idea is to remove the impurities *(kalmasāh)* and to finally clear off the shrouded insight:

*indriyāṇi mano buddhir asyādhiṣṭhānamucyate*
*etairvimohayatyeṣa jñānamāvṛtya dehinam (3.40)*

***It is authoritatively stated that the senses, the mind and the intelligence are the combined warehouse of the passionate enemy. By these facilities, the lusty power confuses the embodied soul, shrouding his insight. (3.40)***

यज्ञशिष्टामृतभुजो
यान्ति ब्रह्म सनातनम्।
नायं लोकोऽस्त्ययज्ञस्य
कुतोऽन्यः कुरुसत्तम ॥४.३१॥
yajñaśiṣṭāmṛtabhujo
yānti brahma sanātanam
nāyaṁ loko'styayajñasya
kuto'nyaḥ kurusattama
(4.31)

*yajñaśiṣṭāmṛtabhujo = yajñaśiṣṭāmṛtabhujaḥ = yajñaśiṣṭa — the physical result of a sacrifice + amṛta — the psychological enjoyment + bhujaḥ — enjoying; yānti — they go; brahma — to the spiritual region; sanātanam — primeval; nāyaṁ = na — not + ayam — this; loko = lokaḥ — world; 'sty = asty (asti) — is (properly utilized); ayajñasya — of a person who performs no austerity or religious ceremony; kuto = kutaḥ — how can it be?; 'nyaḥ = anyaḥ — other; kurusattama — best of the Kurus*

**Those who enjoy the physical and psychological results of a sacrifice, go to the primeval spiritual region. This world is not properly utilized by those who do not perform austerity or religious ceremony. How then can the other world be, O best of the Kurus? (4.31)**

***Commentary:***

*Śrī Bābāji Mahāśaya* asked Yogi *Madhvācārya* to clarify the meaning of *yajñaśiṣṭāmṛta* as follows:

***Yajna is the proper sacrificial procedure as ordained in the Vedic literature. Śiṣṭa is the remnants or remains of such a sacrifice which is perceived on the physical level while amṛta is what is perceived on the psychic or supernatural planes. Anyone who does as ordained by Śrī Krishna or alternately by a great personality like Lord Brahmā, the Prajāpatih mentioned previously by Śrī Krishna, could safely enjoy the results of their efforts after these were approved by divine authority. Both the physical and psychic results can be enjoyed safely by the worshipper, provided there is approval.***

*Śrī Bābāji Mahāśaya* indicated that if everything goes right for yoga practice, from start to finish, then one may assume that one will be elevated to the primeval spiritual region when one leaves the material body *(yānti brahma sanātanam).*

Conversely, a person who does not adhere to the Vedic process cannot utilize this world as it was intended by *Śrī* Krishna and so he cannot flourish in the hereafter either. Those whose lives are partially successful will reap partial benefits after leaving their bodies and they will be given the opportunity to complete their obligation to *Śrī* Krishna.

एवं बहुविधा यज्ञा
वितता ब्रह्मणो मुखे ।
कर्मजान्विद्धि तान्सर्वान्
एवं ज्ञात्वा विमोक्ष्यसे ॥४.३२॥

*evaṁ — thus; bahuvidhā — many types; yajñā — disciplines of accomplishment; vitatā — expounded; brahmaṇo = brahmaṇaḥ — of spiritual existence; mukhe — in the mouth; karmajān — action-produced; viddhi*

evaṁ bahuvidhā yajñā
vitatā brahmaṇo mukhe
karmajānviddhi tānsarvān
evaṁ jñātvā vimokṣyase (4.32)

*— know; tān — them; sarvān — all; evaṁ — thus; jñātvā — having realized; vimokṣyase — you will be freed*

**Many types of disciplines of accomplishment were expounded in the mouth of the spiritual existence. Know them all to be produced from action. Realizing this, O Arjuna, you will be freed. (4.32)**

***Siddha Swami's Commentary:***

The mouth of the spiritual existence, *brahmaṇah mukhe*, is *Brahmā*, the Procreator Lord. In the beginning he began a discourse with his mind-born sons, telling them of the need to expand the creation and to inaugurate *yajña* or disciplines of accomplishment. Yet, it was all motivated, for the most part, by passionate energy. When *Śrī* Krishna spoke in detail to Uddhava, there was mention of the *sūtram*, the emotionally-charged force. That is the power which drives this creation; the full capacity for expression lies within the range of the *sūtram* force.

More or less, *Śrī* Krishna informed Arjuna that action is mandatory in the material world. The whole basis of the creation is action-energy. Thus Arjuna need not think that he could desist completely from action. There are many disciplines of accomplishment such as the *yajña* expounded by *Brahmā*, those discovered by others, and those which have yet to be discovered. Thus this creation is surcharged for action.

श्रेयान्द्रव्यमयाद्यज्ञाज्
ज्ञानयज्ञः परंतप ।
सर्वं कर्माखिलं पार्थ
ज्ञाने परिसमाप्यते ॥४.३३॥
śreyāndravyamayādyajñāj
jñānayajñaḥ paraṁtapa
sarvaṁ karmākhilaṁ pārtha
jñāne parisamāpyate (4.33)

*śreyān — better; dravyamayād = dravyamayāt — than property; yajñāj = yajñāt — than control and ritual regulation; jñānayajñaḥ = jñāna — theoretical knowledge and primitive practical knowledge + yajñaḥ — control and ritual regulation; paraṁtapa — scorcher of the enemy; sarvaṁ — all; karmākhilaṁ = karma — activity + akhilaṁ — without exception; pārtha — son of Pṛthā; jñāne — as conclusion; parisamāpyate — is realized completely*

**Better than property control and its ritual regulation is knowledge control and its ritual regulation, O scorcher of the enemy. Every activity without exception, O son of Pṛthā, is realized as a conclusion in the final analysis. (4.33)**

***Siddha Swami's Commentary:***

*Śrī* Krishna, after recognizing the materialistic, psychological and spiritual forms of sacrifice, now down-rates the materialistic type, the *dravyayajñāt* (Bg. 4.28). Materialistic religion is the least of the processes of salvation and is ineffective to change the inner psyche. In the final analysis, it is realized experience on the psychological and spiritual levels which counts and which will give freedom from the unwanted features of any existence.

Every activity, be it physical, psychological, spiritual, or any combination of these, is realized eventually as a conclusion about the beneficial or degrading aspects yielded. In this way, a person selects the path he or she will take.

तद्विद्धि प्रणिपातेन
परिप्रश्नेन सेवया ।
उपदेक्ष्यन्ति ते ज्ञानं
ज्ञानिनस्तत्त्वदर्शिनः ॥४.३४॥
tadviddhi praṇipātena
paripraśnena sevayā
upadekṣyanti te jñānaṁ
jñāninastattvadarśinaḥ (4.34)

*tad — this; viddhi — know; praṇipātena — by submitting as a student; paripraśnena — by asking questions; sevayā — by serving as requested; upadekṣyanti — they will teach; te — you; jñānaṁ — knowledge; jñāninaḥ — those who know; tattvadarśinaḥ — perceptive reality-conversant sages*

**This you ought to know. By submitting yourself as a student, by asking questions and by serving as requested, the perceptive reality-conversant teachers will teach you the knowledge. (4.34)**

***Siddha Swami's Commentary:***

This was the standard procedure for entry into the training of *buddhi yoga* and *karma yoga*. One had to submit to an authority who was in the disciplic succession from *Śrī* Krishna. One first learned *buddhi yoga* and then if one were to become a government official, one took up a position for administration and was trained in *karma yoga*. Those who were inclined to the Samkhya philosophy learned *jñāna yoga* and did not take the study of *karma yoga*, namely the application of *buddhi yoga* to cultural life in day to day worldly affairs.

To become a student, one had to have *bhakti*, to be devoted to the teacher, and one had to be friendly *(sakhā)* to the teacher. This is what is meant by submitting oneself as a student *(paripraśnena)*. One required an aptitude for the *buddhi yoga* practice; this is explained by the word *paripraśnena*. One had to serve the teacher as requested, having a willingness to comply for menial services or for anything the teacher required *(sevayā)*. This relational connection with the teacher was cultivated throughout the period of studentship.

Each student stayed with a teacher until the particular skill was gained. A student might go to various teachers or might stay with one teacher throughout.

यज्ज्ञात्वा न पुनर्मोहम्
एवं यास्यसि पाण्डव ।
येन भूतान्यशेषेण
द्रक्ष्यस्यात्मन्यथो मयि ॥४.३५॥
yajjñātvā na punarmoham
evaṁ yāsyasi pāṇḍava
yena bhūtānyaśeṣeṇa
drakṣyasyātmanyatho mayi (4.35)

*yaj = yad — which; jñātvā — having known; na — not; punar — again; moham — delusion; evaṁ — thus; yāsyasi — you succumb; pāṇḍava — O son of Pāndu; yena — by which; bhūtāny = bhūtāni — living beings; aśeṣeṇa — without exception, all; drakṣyasy = drakṣyasi — you will perceive; ātmany = ātmani — in the self; atho — then; mayi — in me*

**Having known that experience, you will never again succumb to delusion, O son of Pāndu. By that experience, you will perceive all beings in relation to yourself and then in relation to Me. (4.35)**

***Siddha Swami's Commentary:***

This is a *brahma yoga* technique. It is a transitional *samādhi* from *ātma yoga* to *adhyātma yoga*. This relates specifically to the *Sat Puruṣa*, the God of the world. In this *samādhi* practice, one first sees one's own spirit in relation to other beings in the existential environment and then one sees all those spirits and oneself, a limited being as well, in relation to the God of the environment. He is the *Sat Puruṣa*.

*Śrī* Krishna attests to the fact that when one completed the training of *buddhi yoga* as He taught it, and *karma yoga* or alternately *jñāna yoga*, then one reaches a stage of perceiving spiritually the relationship between oneself and other limited spirits, as well as the relationship between all those limited ones and the *Sat Puruṣa*, the God of the world.

When that experience is ongoing, the *yogin* never succumbs to delusion, because he never again connects intimately with his intellect organ in the subtle body and so he never again becomes victimized by the prejudices of the sensual energies. He remains under the influence of kindred realized spirits and the *Sat Puruṣa*. Even his mundane existence becomes cleaned up, free from the taints of *kāmarūpah*, the passionate energy.

अपि चेदसि पापेभ्यः
सर्वेभ्यः पापकृत्तमः ।
सर्वं ज्ञानप्लवेनैव
वृजिनं संतरिष्यसि ॥४.३६॥
api cedasi pāpebhyaḥ
sarvebhyaḥ pāpakṛttamaḥ
sarvaṁ jñānaplavenaiva
vṛjinaṁ saṁtariṣyasi (4.36)

*api — even; ced — if; asi — you are; pāpebhyaḥ — of the culprits; sarvebhyaḥ — of all; pāpakṛttamaḥ — most wicked; sarvaṁ — all; jñānaplavenaiva = jñāna — experience + plavena — by conveyance + eva — indeed; vṛjinaṁ — bad tendencies; saṁtariṣyasi — you will overcome*

**Even if you were the most wicked of the culprits, you will overcome all bad tendencies by the conveyance of this experience. (4.36)**

***Siddha Swami's Commentary:***

This pertains to persons who lived an irreligious life, doing things which are against the grain of righteousness. These persons were hostile to the divine will, hostile to the Universal Form of *Śrī* Krishna. If any such person is able to get the spiritual experience of their relationship to other limited spirits and to the Supreme Being, then that experience would cause their transformation, such that all bad tendencies would be overcome in due course. This is because such a person would, after the experience, begin gravitating to the divine will. He or she would lose those prejudices which were hostile to *Śrī* Krishna and would aspire to be a servant of the Lord.

This sort of life is *sadhu saṅga*, the association of the saintly persons. However, it is precisely the association of the Supreme Spirit, and the experience of the spiritual connection between oneself and the other limited spirits using subtle and material bodies. Thus when one experiences that connection, one no longer stresses one's family. Then one sees the spiritual family and not the family of the present material body, even though convention dictates that one should function in the biological family.

*Śrī* Krishna freed Arjuna from the limitation of the family consciousness, so that Arjuna could experience the spiritual family which is explained in the previous verse. It is not a theoretical analysis. It is an actual experience which comes from mastery of *buddhi yoga*, when one's emotional energy is no longer converted into many bewildering moods, and when one's sensual energy and memory are no longer able to influence the intellect.

यथैधांसि समिद्धोऽग्निर्
भस्मसात्कुरुतेऽर्जुन ।
ज्ञानाग्निः सर्वकर्माणि
भस्मसात्कुरुते तथा ॥४.३७॥

*yathaidhāṁsi = yathā — as + idhāṁsi (edhāṁsi) — firewood; samiddho = samiddhaḥ — set on fire; 'gnir = agnir — fire; bhasmasāt kurute — it reduces to ashes; 'rjuna (arjuna) = Arjuna; jñānāgniḥ = jñāna — realized knowledge + agniḥ*

yathaidhāṁsi samiddho'gnir
bhasmasātkurute'rjuna
jñānāgniḥ sarvakarmāṇi
bhasmasātkurute tathā (4.37)

*— fiery potency; sarvakarmāṇi = sarva — all + karmāṇi — actions; bhasmasāt kurute — it reduces to nothing; tathā — so*

**As when wood is set on fire, it is reduced to ashes, O Arjuna, so the fiery potency of realized knowledge reduces all actions to nothing. (4.37)**

***Siddha Swami's Commentary:***

This does not apply to knowledge of this in the mind based only on hearing from the *Bhagavad Gītā* or a realized soul. The person must hear of this and also experience this for himself or herself. A person hearing of this from a realized soul will not be able to consistently act on this. He would act from time to time in a synchronization with this, but he will of necessity deviate, because his basic consciousness is outside of this experience.

Thus the analogy of the fire applies to him only partially. Only part of his actions would be liability free, only that part which was conducted when he happened to be under the influence of the Supreme Spirit. Only those who have this spiritual experience continuously would have all their liabilities for cultural involvement cancelled completely.

न हि ज्ञानेन सदृशं
पवित्रमिह विद्यते ।
तत्स्वयं योगसंसिद्धः
कालेनात्मनि विन्दति ॥४.३८॥
na hi jñānena sadṛśaṁ
pavitramiha vidyate
tatsvayaṁ yogasaṁsiddhaḥ
kālenātmani vindati (4.38)

*na — nothing; hi — indeed; jñānena — with direct experience; sadṛśaṁ — compared with; pavitram — purifier; iha — in this world; vidyate — is relevant; tat — that realization; svayaṁ — himself; yogasaṁsiddhaḥ = yoga — yoga practice + saṁsiddhaḥ — perfected; kālenātmani = kālena — in time + ātmani — in the self; vindati — he locates*

**Nothing, indeed, can be compared with direct experience. No other purifier is as relevant in this world. That man who himself is perfected in yoga practice, will in time, locate the realization in himself. (4.38)**

***Siddha Swami's Commentary:***

Direct experience is the ultimate purifier. Each religious person only becomes fully realized by direct experience. Faith in a religion or in a person like *Śrī* Krishna, Who made these declarations, remains subject to change until there is direct sensual experience of the facts mentioned. A person becomes convinced by direct experience only. In fact, religion is solidified by direct experience, even though persons usually pursue it on the basis of faith.

Sooner or later, a person will, in this life or in some other, leave aside a religion if he does not get a sensual spiritual experience of the Deity of that faith. All religious beliefs are ultimately tested by direct experience which must be sensual and spiritual.

Normally one experiences the sensual and material, but in religious matters, one has to experience the sensual and spiritual. Here *Śrī* Krishna appraised yoga as the means of acquiring the direct sensual and spiritual experience *(yogasamsiddhah)*.

One must locate the experience in or through his soul *(ātmani)*, not by the mere testimony of another. Then one sees spiritually for himself or herself.

श्रद्धावाँल्लभते ज्ञानं
तत्परः संयतेन्द्रियः ।
ज्ञानं लब्ध्वा परां शान्तिम्
अचिरेणाधिगच्छति ॥४.३९॥
śraddhāvāṁllabhate jñānaṁ
tatparaḥ saṁyatendriyaḥ
jñānaṁ labdhvā parāṁ śāntim
acireṇādhigacchati (4.39)

*śraddhāvān — one who has faith; labhate — he gets; jñānaṁ — the experience; tatparaḥ = tad — that + paraḥ — being devoted to; saṁyatendriyaḥ = saṁyata — restraining + indriyaḥ — sensual energy; jñānaṁ — experience; labdhvā — having acquired; parāṁ — supreme; śāntim — peace; acireṇādhigacchati = acireṇa — quickly + adhigacchati — goes*

**One who has faith, gets the experience. Being devoted to restraining the sensual energy, having acquired the experience, he goes quickly to the supreme peace. (4.39)**

***Siddha Swami's Commentary:***

Faith is required but faith is the beginning. The sensual and spiritual experience which follows, seals or destroys a person's faith. This faith is based on the devotedness and friendliness a student has in relation to the teacher. This was described of Arjuna previously:

*sa evāyaṁ mayā te'dya yogaḥ proktaḥ purātanaḥ*
*bhakto'si me sakhā ceti rahasyaṁ hyetaduttamam (4.3)*

***Today, this ancient yoga technique is explained to you by Me, since you are devoted to Me and are My friend. Indeed, this is confidential and is the best teaching. (4.3)***

Out of devotion and friendliness *(bhaktah sakhā)* comes the development of faith in what the teacher says. From such faith comes the will to practice the disciplines through which one gets the direct sensual and spiritual experience. Even though initially, the experience is in the true teacher *(sat guru),* it is felt also in the sincere student who completes the disciplines. If yoga was not the requirement, *Śrī* Krishna would not have said *yogasamsiddhah*. It is through yoga that one gets purity of the psyche as will be explained in Chapter Six.

The restraining of the sensual energy *(samyatendriyah)* is part of the *buddhi yoga* process which *Śrī* Krishna laid out in the previous chapter. By consistently doing such practices, one masters this. Then quietly, as the Lord states, one goes to the supreme peace.

अज्ञश्चाश्रद्दधानश्च
संशयात्मा विनश्यति ।
नायं लोकोऽस्ति न परो
न सुखं संशयात्मनः ॥४.४०॥
ajñaścāśraddadhānaśca
saṁśayātmā vinaśyati
nāyaṁ loko'sti na paro
na sukhaṁ saṁśayātmanaḥ (4.40)

*ajñaścāśraddadhānaśca = ajñaḥ — ignorant person + ca — and + aśraddadhānaḥ — faithless person + ca — and; saṁśayātmā = saṁśaya — doubtful + ātmā — self; vinaśyati — is degraded; nāyaṁ = na — not + ayam — this; loko = lokaḥ — world; 'sti = asti — is; na — not; paro = paraḥ — beyond the physical world; na — not; sukhaṁ — in happiness; saṁśayātmanaḥ = saṁśaya — doubting + ātmanaḥ — for the self*

**The ignorant person, the faithless one who is doubtful, is degraded. Neither this physical world, nor the dimensions beyond this, nor happiness, is for the person who is doubtful. (4.40)**

***Siddha Swami's Commentary:***

This is related to the requirement for devotedness and friendliness to the teacher. If one does not have these, one will be initially doubtful. Some may come with devotedness and friendliness and then develop doubts afterwards. When doubts are developed, one loses confidence in the teacher. One who does not get the sensual and spiritual experience, is bound to develop doubts, because that person remained ignorant of what was described by the teacher. Since it was not revealed in actuality, it is reasonable that he or she should have doubts.

Assuming that *Śrī* Krishna is the Supreme Spirit, doubts about what He says would imply that the doubter was lost to the actual facts of this life as well as any life hereafter. Such a person would be unable to use this physical world or the subtle world for his benefit in real terms, because he would not have the insight in the proper usages of these dimensions. Thus as *Śrī* Krishna indicated, such a person is to a degree condemned, because a limited being needs to supplement his ignorance with advice from the Supreme Person. Without that counsel, he probably cannot make decisions which are actually in his interest.

योगसंन्यस्तकर्माणं
ज्ञानसंछिन्नसंशयम् ।
आत्मवन्तं न कर्माणि
निबध्नन्ति धनंजय ॥४.४१॥
yogasaṁnyastakarmāṇaṁ
jñānasaṁchinnasaṁśayam
ātmavantaṁ na karmāṇi
nibadhnanti dhanaṁjaya (4.41)

*yogasaṁnyastakarmāṇaṁ = yoga — yoga technique + saṁnyasta — renounced + karmāṇaṁ — action; jñānasaṁchinnasaṁśayam = jñāna — realized knowledge + saṁchinna — removed + saṁśayam — doubt; ātmavantaṁ — self-composed; na — no; karmāṇi — cultural activities; nibadhnanti — they bind; dhanaṁjaya — O conqueror of wealthy countries*

**Cultural activities do not implicate a person whose actions are renounced through techniques developed in yoga practice, whose doubt is removed by realized knowledge and who is self-composed, O conqueror of wealthy countries. (4.41)**

***Siddha Swami's Commentary:***

As stated before, *karma yoga* is *buddhi yoga* expertise applied in the cultural field, in day to day affairs as one is duty-bound. There can be no *karma yoga* as meant in the *Bhagavad Gītā* without the *buddhi yoga* practice and expertise. The actions which are renounced *(samnyastakarmāṇam)* must be done through techniques developed in yoga practice, in *buddhi yoga* practice, in curbing the intellect from its servitude to the memory and sensual energies. This is explained by the term *yogasamnyastakarmāṇam*.

Doubts can be removed by higher yoga, to see into the spiritual dimensions and to verify or deny by actual experience what the teacher said. It does not matter if the teacher is *Śrī* Krishna or some other person. One should enter into the spiritual dimension to verify what the teacher said, or to deny it and find out the actual situation.

The student must also become self-composed *(ātmavantam)*. This comes about by getting the experience of the spiritual dimensions. Once he or she knows this firsthand, that person develops a maturity and a self-confidence, along with an increased faith in the spiritual dimensions, which before were vague or non-existent.

तस्मादज्ञानसंभूतं
हृत्स्थं ज्ञानासिनात्मनः ।
छित्त्वैनं संशयं योगम्
आतिष्ठोत्तिष्ठ भारत ॥४.४२॥

*tasmād = tasmāt — therefore; ajñānasaṁbhūtaṁ = ajñāna — ignorance + saṁbhūtaṁ — produced by; hṛtsthaṁ — lodged in your being; jñānāsinā = jñāna — realized knowledge + asinā — by the cutting effect; 'tmanaḥ = ātmanaḥ — of yourself; chittvainaṁ =*

| | |
|---|---|
| tasmādajñānasaṁbhūtaṁ<br>hṛtsthaṁ jñānāsinātmanaḥ<br>chittvainaṁ saṁśayaṁ yogam<br>ātiṣṭhottiṣṭha bhārata (4.42) | *chittva — having severed entirely + enam — this; saṁśayam — doubt; yogaṁ — to yogic technique; ātiṣṭhottiṣṭha = ātiṣṭha — resort to + uttiṣṭha — make a stand; bhārata — man of the Bharata family* |

**Therefore having severed entirely, with the cutting instrument of realized knowledge, this doubt that comes from the ignorance, lodged in your being, resort to yogic technique and make a stand, O man of the Bharata family! (4.42)**

***Siddha Swami's Commentary:***

Doubts are removed only by sensual and spiritual experience. We have no doubts about the material world which is before us, this is because we have sensual and physical contact with it. Thus, to remove our doubts about the supposed spiritual world or spiritual truths, we have to experience these individually.

*Śrī* Krishna required Arjuna to do this instantly, but only because Arjuna was a proficient yogi, who already knew *buddhi yoga*. Arjuna knew the practice but he did not understand how to apply it. *Śrī* Krishna prompted Arjuna to apply the yoga expertise to day to day life, rather than keep yoga as a separate practice which did not apply to worldly duties. *Śrī* Krishna ordered Arjuna to resort to yogic technique and make a stand on that war field *(yogam ātiṣṭhottiṣṭha bhārata)*.

# CHAPTER 5

## Brahma Yoga Yukta Ātmā

## Linking the Spirit to the Spiritual Plane through Yoga*

*bāhyasparśeṣvasaktātmā vindatyātmani yatsukham*
*sa brahmayogayuktātmā sukhamakṣayamaśnute (5.21)*

***The person who is not attached to the external sensations, who finds happiness in the spirit, whose spirit is linked to the spiritual plane through yoga process, makes contact with the non-fluctuating happiness. (5.21)***

***Siddha Swami assigned this chapter title on the basis of verse 21 of this chapter.**

अर्जुन उवाच
संन्यासं कर्मणां कृष्ण
पुनर्योगं च शंससि ।
यच्छ्रेय एतयोरेकं
तन्मे ब्रूहि सुनिश्चितम् ॥५.१॥

arjuna uvāca
saṁnyāsaṁ karmaṇāṁ kṛṣṇa
punaryogaṁ ca śaṁsasi
yacchreya etayorekaṁ
tanme brūhi suniścitam (5.1)

*arjuna — Arjuna; uvāca — said; saṁnyāsaṁ — renunciation of involvement; karmaṇām — of social activity; kṛṣṇa — Krishna; punar — again; yogaṁ — the application of yoga austerities to worldly life; ca — and; śaṁsasi — you approved; yacchreya = yad — which + chreya (śreyaḥ) — better; etayor = etayoḥ — of these two; ekaṁ — one; tan — this; me — to me; brūhi — tell; suniścitam — with certainty*

**Arjuna said: You approved renunciation of social activity and also mentioned the application of yoga to worldly life. Which one of these is better? Tell me this with certainty. (5.1)**

***Siddha Swami's Commentary:***

Up to this point, *Śrī* Krishna did not approve renunciation of social activity. Thus it is obvious that Arjuna misunderstood what *Śrī* Krishna explained. Arjuna's mind is prejudiced by emotional energy. He is still unable to apply his *buddhi yoga* expertise to stop his emotional energy from converting into moods. In addition, his intellect was not isolated or separated from the sensual energies which prejudiced it. Thus Arjuna heard whatever *Śrī* Krishna had to say, but he heard it and processed it to suit his desire and intentions. He did not exhibit the standard of a pandit or learned man:

*yasya sarve samārambhāḥ kāmasaṁkalpavarjitāḥ*
*jñānāgnidagdhakarmāṇaṁ tamāhuḥ paṇḍitaṁ budhāḥ (4.19)*

***He for whom desires and intentions are not mixed into his endeavors, who destroyed reactionary work by the fiery force of his knowledge, he, the wise men call a pandit or learned man. (4.19)***

In text 41 of the previous chapter, *Śrī* Krishna spoke of a person whose actions are renounced through techniques developed in yoga practice. He stated that cultural activities do not implicate such a person. Here is that verse:

*yogasaṁnyastakarmāṇaṁ jñānasaṁchinnasaṁśayam*
*ātmavantaṁ na karmāṇi nibadhnanti dhanaṁjaya (4.41)*

***Cultural activities do not implicate a person whose actions are renounced through techniques developed in yoga practice, whose doubt is removed by realized knowledge and who is self-composed, O conqueror of wealthy countries. (4.41)***

Thus *Śrī* Krishna recommended renounced actions by someone who developed detachment through *buddhi yoga* practice. Apparently Arjuna misunderstood this. To Arjuna, one either has to act in the world or not act at all, either to be involved or not be involved at all. *Śrī* Krishna, however, spoke of being involved in a detached manner on the basis of expertise in the *buddhi yoga* practice. Such activities are termed *karma yoga*. In any case, as a student of *Śrī* Krishna, Arjuna had every right to ask for clarification.

श्रीभगवानुवाच
संन्यासः कर्मयोगश्च
निःश्रेयसकरावुभौ ।
तयोस्तु कर्मसंन्यासात्
कर्मयोगो विशिष्यते ॥५.२॥
śrībhagavānuvāca
saṁnyāsaḥ karmayogaśca
niḥśreyasakarāvubhau
tayostu karmasaṁnyāsāt
karmayogo viśiṣyate (5.2)

*śrī-bhagavān — the Blessed Lord; uvāca — said; saṁnyāsaḥ — total renunciation of social opportunities; karmayogaśca = karmayogaḥ — disciplined use of social opportunities by a yogi + ca — and; niḥśreyasakarāv = niḥśreyasa — ultimate happiness + karāv (karau) — leading to; ubhau — both; tayos — of the two; tu — but; karmasaṁnyāsāt — than the renunciation of cultural activity; karmayogo = karmayogaḥ — disciplined use of social opportunities by a yogi; viśiṣyate — is better*

**The Blessed Lord said: Both methods, the total renunciation of social opportunities and the disciplined use of opportunities by a yogi, lead to ultimate happiness. But of the two aspects, the disciplined use of opportunities in a yogic mood is better than total renunciation of cultural activity. (5.2)**

***Siddha Swami's Commentary:***

*Śrī* Krishna graciously follows with Arjuna's line of reasoning, in accepting that there is a course for the total renunciation of social opportunities, even though he was not recommending Arjuna for that. In fact, He deliberately steered Arjuna away from that, since that was not in Arjuna's interest at the time.

Even though both methods, that of totally leaving aside social opportunities and that of using society in a detached manner under God direction, are valid, still one should take the method which is appropriate to one's status in life. For Arjuna it was inappropriate for him to leave aside the social opportunities.

There is a clear distinction between *karmasamnyāsa* and *karma yoga*. *Karmasamnyāsa* means the total renunciation of cultural activity, while *karma yoga* means the performance of cultural activity with yogically developed detachment. These two paths are distinct. One is taken by the *karma* yogi and the other by the *jñāna* yogi. When the *karma* yogi has advanced, he becomes a *jñāna* yogi, and if the *jñāna* yogi retrogresses or fails to complete his practice, he falls back to the status of a *karma* yogi. Both of these are required to have *bhaktah*, devotion, and *sakhā*, friendly attitude, to *Śrī* Krishna and to the teacher who represents the Lord.

ज्ञेयः स नित्यसंन्यासी
यो न द्वेष्टि न काङ्क्षति ।
निर्द्वंद्वो हि महाबाहो
सुखं बन्धात्प्रमुच्यते ॥५.३॥
jñeyaḥ sa nityasaṁnyāsī
yo na dveṣṭi na kāṅkṣati
nirdvaṁdvo hi mahābāho
sukhaṁ bandhāt pramucyate (5.3)

*jñeyaḥ — to be known; sa = saḥ — he; nityasaṁnyāsī = nitya — consistent + saṁnyāsī — a renouncer of social opportunities; yo = yaḥ — who; na — not; dveṣṭi — dislikes; na — not; kāṅkṣati — craves; nirdvandvo = nirdvandvaḥ — indifferent to opposite features; hi — indeed; mahābāho — O strong-armed man; sukhaṁ — easily; bandhāt — from implication; pramucyate — is freed*

**Indeed, a person who neither dislikes nor craves, who is indifferent to opposite features, should be recognized as a consistent renouncer, O strong-armed man. He is easily freed from implication. (5.3)**

***Siddha Swami's Commentary:***

The *nityasamnyāsī*, the consistent renouncer, may be a *karma* yogi or a *jñāna* yogi, all depending on the supreme will. In either case, he will be recognized by his usual indifference to opposite features *(nirdvamdvo).* Such a person, if directed, can act culturally can do so and still be easily free from implications. This is because he remains uninvolved.

सांख्ययोगौ पृथग्बालाः
प्रवदन्ति न पण्डिताः ।
एकमप्यास्थितः सम्यग्
उभयोर्विन्दते फलम् ॥५.४॥
sāṁkhyayogau pṛthagbālāḥ
pravadanti na paṇḍitāḥ
ekamapyāsthitaḥ samyag
ubhayorvindate phalam (5.4)

*sāṁkhyayogau = sāṁkhya — Sāṁkhya ideas + yogau — and yoga practices; pṛthagbālāḥ — simple-minded people; pravadanti — they describe; na — not; paṇḍitāḥ — the perceptive speakers; ekam — one; apy = api — even; āsthitaḥ — practiced; samyag — correctly; ubhayor = ubhayoḥ — of either; vindate — one gets; phalam — result*

**It is the simple-minded people, not the perceptive speakers, who say that Sāṁkhya ideas and yoga practices are separate. Even if one method is practiced correctly, the practitioner gets the result of either. (5.4)**

***Siddha Swami's Commentary:***

It is an age-old misunderstanding that yoga is hostile to social life and that social life cannot be coordinated with yoga. *Śrī* Krishna, the God of the world, explained a yoga system which was compatible to social affairs. That is the *karma yoga* discipline used by Janak and other yoga-conversant rulers.

It is an innate fear of yoga which causes childish people to think that anywhere yoga is practiced, social life cannot flourish. It appears that Arjuna had also picked up on these conventional opinions about yoga. Some people are of the view that Samkhya is a philosophical system only and is not connected to yoga austerities. These are misunderstandings. In any case, *Śrī* Krishna attested that if one studied the Samkhya philosophy, one would eventually complete it in such a way as to get the same result gained by those who practice yoga austerities. Of course, people usually feel that the result of yoga austerities is mystic *siddhi* perfections or absolute exit of one's spirit from the material existence, while they feel that one who masters the philosophy will become a learned speaker, giving advice to human society in how to develop determination to live out philosophical ideas.

यत्सांख्यैः प्राप्यते स्थानं
तद्योगैरपि गम्यते ।
एकं सांख्यं च योगं च
यः पश्यति स पश्यति ॥५.५॥
yatsāṁkhyaiḥ prāpyate sthānaṁ
tadyogairapi gamyate
ekaṁ sāṁkhyaṁ ca yogaṁ ca
yaḥ paśyati sa paśyati (5.5)

*yat — whatever; sāṁkhyaiḥ — by the Sāṁkhya experts; prāpyate — is attained; sthānaṁ — the level; tad — that; yogair = yogaiḥ — by the yogis; api — also; gamyate — is reached; ekaṁ — one; sāṁkhyaṁ — Samkhya; ca — and; yogaṁ — yoga; ca — and; yaḥ — who; paśyati — perceived; sa = saḥ — he; paśyati — sees*

**The level obtained by the Sāṁkhya experts is also reached by the yogis. Sāṁkhya and yoga are essentially one. He who perceives that really sees. (5.5)**

***Siddha Swami's Commentary:***

Samkhya as *Śrī* Krishna originally taught it in the *jñāna yoga* system instituted by Him, included yoga practice. But in the process of time, by the advent of Lord Krishna, there developed split systems whereby Samkhya was seen as a process of taking knowledge about the cosmology of the world and the theoretical layout of our place in it. Yoga was seen as a process for austerities only, without application to social life and without coordination with the Samkhya ideas.

The real Samkhya experts practiced yoga, so the level reached by them was also attained by those who did yoga and who did not specifically study or become conversant with the Samkhya theories of existence.

The two systems are one, because if one has a theoretical idea of the existential layout of reality, then by practicing yoga he will see the practical aspects of those diagrams. Conversely if one does not have the Samkhya knowledge and one sincerely practices yoga, one will see the existential situation firsthand by mystic and spiritual perception. Thus the two systems are not opposed to each other.

A man who studies the geography of a foreign land, will see that place firsthand if he travels there, while another man who has no geographical knowledge, will also view the foreign surroundings if he relocates there. Only those who feel that Samkhya begins and ends with a theoretical study, become misled into thinking that Samkhya and yoga are contrary.

संन्यासस्तु महाबाहो
दुःखमाप्तुमयोगतः ।
योगयुक्तो मुनिर्ब्रह्म
नचिरेणाधिगच्छति ॥५.६॥
saṁnyāsastu mahābāho
duḥkhamāptumayogataḥ
yogayukto munirbrahma
nacireṇādhigacchati (5.6)

*saṁnyāsaḥ — renunciation of opportunity; tu — indeed; mahābāho — O mighty man; duḥkham — difficulty; āptum — to obtain; ayogataḥ — without yoga-proficiency; yogayukto = yogayuktaḥ — yoga-proficient; munir = muniḥ — sage; brahma — spiritual level; nacireṇādhigacchati = nacirena — in no span of time + adhigacchati — reaches*

**Renunciation of opportunities is difficult to attain without yoga practice, O mighty man. In the nick of time, a yoga-proficient sage reaches the spiritual plane. (5.6)**

***Siddha Swami's Commentary:***

Those who advocated that *karma yoga* has little or nothing to do with yoga and that it is merely based on a detached attitude from the results of action, should pay close attention to this verse, where *Śrī* Krishna declared the possibility of *karma yoga* practice without yoga but with a restriction, stating that it is difficult. *Ayogatah* means without yoga proficiency, and this indicated that even in the time of *Śrī* Krishna, there were persons of the view that they could be *karma* yogis even without practicing yoga. They felt they could do just as well as Janak and the other yoga-proficient *(yogatah)* rulers. Generally, however, persons who advocate *karma yoga* without yoga are lazy people who are afraid of the pains and aches of a yoga practice. These are people who want the benefit of *karma yoga* without following in the footsteps of Janak and other rulers.

One might occasionally behave like a true *karma* yogi, like the fabled King Janak, in the cultural field or in association in a religious society where one is given an opportunity to demonstrate such behavior, but one will go no further; one may not develop into *samnyāsa*. And we find that generally those who want to do *karma yoga* without yoga, do in their old age stay on as such *karma* yogis in their selected religious societies and never graduate to *samnyāsa*. This happens because even though one might take pride in renouncing some fruits of one's action, still one can hardly renounce the actions themselves unless one has the expertise in yoga, in *buddhi yoga*.

It is one thing to be a successful professional with a worldly education and a privileged status in society while giving part of one's income or pension to religious societies, and it is entirely different to leave aside one's status and live without any social opportunities and recognition whatsoever. To complete that, one must do yoga. Indeed, a yoga-proficient sage or a yoga-proficient *karma* yogi like Janak, will reach the spiritual plane (*brahma*) in the nick of time, near the end of his body, because he practiced the *buddhi yoga* all along, and by that time had developed proficiency to master higher yoga in terms of *dhyāna* and *samādhi*.

योगयुक्तो विशुद्धात्मा
विजितात्मा जितेन्द्रियः ।
सर्वभूतात्मभूतात्मा
कुर्वन्नपि न लिप्यते ॥५.७॥
yogayukto viśuddhātmā
vijitātmā jitendriyaḥ
sarvabhūtātmabhūtātmā
kurvannapi na lipyate (5.7)

*yogayukto = yogayuktaḥ — one proficient in yoga; viśuddhātmā — one of purified self; vijitātmā — one who is self-controlled; jitendriyaḥ — one who has conquered his senses; sarvabhūtātmabhūtātmā = sarva — all + bhūta — being + ātma — self + bhūta — being + ātmā — self (sarvabhūtātmabhūtātmā — one who feels related to all beings); kurvan — acting; api — even; na — not; lipyate — is implicated*

**A person who is proficient in yoga, whose soul is purified, who is self-controlled, who conquered his senses, whose self feels related to all beings, is not implicated when acting. (5.7)**

***Siddha Swami's Commentary:***

*Śrī* Krishna's stress on yoga speaks for itself. Repeatedly in verse after verse, He spoke of the value and He insisted on its practice. This is a description of a *brahma yogi*, for it described a person who is proficient in yoga, who completed *ātma śuddha* yoga, whose psyche operates through *buddhi yoga* and who conquered the senses through kundalini and *kriyā yoga*.

This person feels related to all beings because he experienced the spiritual family connection on the transcendental plane by mastery of *ātma śuddha* yoga and *adhyātma* yoga. When he acts in the world, he is not implicated like others and he does not pretend to be renounced or to have abandoned the results of actions.

This verse describes the condition of a person who mastered the stabilization of the higher meditation, *samādhi* practice. This takes years of repeated effort at higher meditation so that the effects are sustained in one's psyche even while being involved in the social field. Such yogis come out of isolation and mix with worldly people freely and easily. Sometimes they are not recognized as advanced souls.

नैव किंचित्करोमीति
युक्तो मन्येत तत्त्ववित् ।
पश्यञ्शृण्वन्स्पृशञ्जिघ्रन्
अश्नन्गच्छन्स्वपञ्श्वसन् ॥५.८॥

*naiva = na — not + eva — indeed; kiṁcit— anything; karomīti = karomi — initiate + iti — thus; yukto = yuktaḥ — proficient in yoga; manyeta — he thinks; tattvavit — knower of reality; paśyañśṛṇvan = paśyan — seeing + śṛṇvan —*

naiva kiṁcitkaromīti
yukto manyeta tattvavit
paśyañśṛṇvanspṛśañjighrann
aśnangacchansvapañśvasan (5.8)

*hearing; spṛśañjighrann = spṛśan — touching + jighran — smelling; aśnan — eating; gacchan — walking; svapañśvasan = svapan — sleeping + śvasan — breathing*

प्रलपन्विसृजन्गृह्णन्
उन्मिषन्निमिषन्नपि ।
इन्द्रियाणीन्द्रियार्थेषु
वर्तन्त इति धारयन् ॥५.९॥
pralapanvisṛjangṛhṇann
unmiṣannimiṣannapi
indriyāṇīndriyārtheṣu
vartanta iti dhārayan (5.9)

*pralapan — talking; visṛjan — evacuating; gṛhṇan — holding; unmiṣan — opening the eyelids; nimiṣan — closing the eyelids; api — also; indriyāṇīndriyārtheṣu = indriyāṇi — senses + indriyārtheṣu — in the attractive objects; vartanta — interlock; iti — thus; dhārayan — considers*

**"I do not initiate anything." Being proficient in yoga, this is what the knower of reality thinks. While seeing, hearing, touching, smelling, eating, walking, sleeping and breathing, (5.8)**

**...while talking, evacuating, holding, opening and closing the eyelids, he considers, "The senses are interlocked with the attractive objects." (5.9)**

***Siddha Swami's Commentary:***

In yoga parlance, we call this power to act in the subtle material world, *cittih*. This is Chitti *Devī*, a goddess. She is greatly admired and respected by the advanced yogins. She is otherwise known as *Yogamāyā*. For purposes of realization in yoga, she is known as Chitti *Devī* because it is through her that all the psychic actions take place. One must bow to this goddess. In fact, anyone who uses a subtle body bows to this goddess day and night and depends on her entirely.

It is a wonderful observation, when one can see that the psychic actions are taking place by the grace of the *citta* energy. *Śrī Patañjali* alerted that for success in yoga, one has to gain distance from this energy, so that her enticing movements may stop.

Even though the *citta* energy is vast, cosmic, and infinite, still one must distance the spirit from one's touch point with it. If one can accomplish this, it would be a major breakthrough for one in particular, even though thereafter others will remain hypnotized to be entertained and to be the power supply of this *citta* mento-emotional, creative, ideational potency.

The senses and their attractive objects *(indriyāṇīndriyārtheṣu)* do interlock but the *yogin* has to distance himself from that by buddhi yoga to separate the buddhi from the sensual energies and memory. At any moment when the spirit cannot keep those psychic components separated, they will interact and the spirit will serve as the power supply for whatever transactions may take place. Still one should not become offended by this. One should keep striving for a final separation from it.

ब्रह्मण्याधाय कर्माणि
सङ्गं त्यक्त्वा करोति यः ।
लिप्यते न स पापेन
पद्मपत्रमिवाम्भसा ॥५.१०॥

*brahmaṇy = brahmaṇi — on the spiritual level; ādhāya — putting on, focused on; karmāṇi — actions; saṅgaṁ — attachment; tyaktvā — having discarded; karoti — he acts; yaḥ — who; lipyate — affected; na — not; sa = saḥ — he;*

brahmaṇyādhāya karmāṇi
saṅgaṁ tyaktvā karoti yaḥ
lipyate na sa pāpena
padmapatramivāmbhasā (5.10)

*pāpena — by necessary violence; padmapatram = padma — lotus + patram — leaf; ivāmbhasā = iva — just as + ambhasā — by water*

**Being focused on the spiritual level, discarding attachments, his acts are not defiled by necessary violence, just as a lotus leaf is not affected by water. (5.10)**

***Siddha Swami's Commentary:***

Any type of action in the material world is an act of violence in one way or the other, since in all activity, some energy and some living being, however microscopic or psychic, is displaced. Even if one sits still and does not move as some yogins do for hours, days or weeks, still it causes problems for some living entities who might prefer that one move from a location or that one act in a way to facilitate their living circumstance.

In *brahma yoga*, a yogi loses concern for these displacements in the material world. He stops being responsible or he stops pretending that he is, can be or is not responsible for what takes place as a result of his existence here. Being focused on the spiritual level *(brahmaṇi),* and discarding the intimate connection with his intellect which usually picks up the attachments of the sensual energy and memory, whatever he does or appears to do, whatever takes place as a result of the movement of his gross or subtle body, does not defile his consciousness. The sensual energy is no longer empowered to imprint itself with the reactions which come from the mundane environments.

Even though *Śrī* Krishna is essentially giving Arjuna the course in *karma yoga*, this verse in particular and many other verses throughout pertain to the higher practice of *brahma yoga*. These should not be mistaken for *karma yoga*, because these occur in the life of a more advanced ascetic.

कायेन मनसा बुद्ध्या
केवलैरिन्द्रियैरपि ।
योगिनः कर्म कुर्वन्ति
सङ्गं त्यक्त्वात्मशुद्धये ॥५.११॥
kāyena manasā buddhyā
kevalairindriyairapi
yoginaḥ karma kurvanti
saṅgaṁ tyaktvātmaśuddhaye (5.11)

*kāyena — with the body; manasā — with the mind; buddhyā — with the intellect; kevalair = kevalaiḥ — alone; indriyair = indriyaiḥ — by the senses; api — even; yoginaḥ — yogis; karma — cultural activity; kurvanti — they perform; saṅgaṁ — attachment; tyaktvā — having discarded; 'tmaśuddhaye = ātmaśuddhaye = ātma — self + śuddhaye — towards purification*

**With the body, mind and intelligence, or even with the senses alone, the yogis, having discarded attachment, perform cultural acts for self-purification. (5.11)**

***Siddha Swami's Commentary:***

This is done by the *brahma yogi*s mostly and by others, either yogis or ordinary ascetics *(yatis)* who come under the divine influence. The *brahma yogi*s who mature in practice, do this continually. Others, either *brahma yogi*s, ordinary yogis or religious people, may do this from time to time, periodically, when they fall under the divine influence. This verse describes an advanced condition of the *brahma yoga* technique given in texts 8 and 9 of this chapter.

It so happens that even a person proficient in *brahma yoga* may have to go back into society to perform certain cultural acts for final purification, as insisted by the Supreme Being. Then going back into the world and either starting a religious mission or doing ordinary cultural activities, the yogi may direct his body, mind and intelligence to do whatever is stipulated for him by providence. Sometimes the yogi engages his senses only, without involving his intellect in an act. This frees his intellect from being conditioned by the sensual energies and leaves him with a clean intellect to complete *samādhi* practice.

Once the intellect is weaned from attachments to the sensual energies and memory, a yogi again becomes particular about indulging the intellect. Thus when he acts in the world, he painstakingly keeps his intellect isolated. Otherwise the intellect which was converted into *jñāna-dīpa*, the spiritual eye, may be re-converted into ordinary imaginations and considerations. Thus a yogi avoids that re-conversion, so as to avoid repeated regulatory austerities. This is why *Śrī* Krishna stated that the yogis may act even with the senses alone *(kevalaih indriyaih)*.

A yogi, a *brahma yogi* specifically, will only perform the cultural acts which are mandatory for him and which are indicated by providence. These help to bring on full purification by making him act in a way that compensates for irresponsible acts in his past lives and to let him complete duties which he avoided before but which were compulsory for him as stipulated by the Universal Form of *Śrī* Krishna.

Even though a yogi may shun society for the sake of doing his austerities efficiently, without social interference, still he might have to return to worldly life again in order to clear some liabilities and do what he is assigned by the supreme will.

युक्तः कर्मफलं त्यक्त्वा
शान्तिमाप्नोति नैष्ठिकीम् ।
अयुक्तः कामकारेण
फले सक्तो निबध्यते ॥५.१२॥
yuktaḥ karmaphalaṁ tyaktvā
śāntimāpnoti naiṣṭhikīm
ayuktaḥ kāmakāreṇa
phale sakto nibadhyate (5.12)

*yuktaḥ — proficient in yoga; karmaphalaṁ — reward of cultural activity; tyaktvā — having abandoned; śāntim — peace; āpnoti — obtains; naiṣṭhikīm — steady; ayuktaḥ — a person not proficient in yoga; kāmakāreṇa — by action which is motivated by desire; phale — in result; sakto = saktaḥ — attached; nibadhyate — is bound*

**The person who is proficient in yoga, and who abandons the rewards of cultural activity, obtains steady peace. The person who is not proficient in yoga, being attached to results, is bound by desire-motivated action. (5.12)**

***Siddha Swami's Commentary:***

The proper definition of *śāntīm*, a popular Sanskrit and Hindi word, is given by *Śrī* Krishna as the existential state of a proficient yogi who abandons the rewards of cultural activity. In such a state of mind, there is a consistent link with the absolute, with the Supreme Being. The yo-yo, swing-here swing-there, moody state of ordinary persons goes away from a yogi whose emotions are not converted into moods, as *Śrī* Krishna stated in Chapter Two initially.

*sukhaduḥkhe same kṛtvā lābhālābhau jayājayau*
*tato yuddhāya yujyasva naivaṁ pāpamavāpsyasi (2.38)*

***Having regarded happiness, distress, gains, losses, victory and defeat, as the same emotions, apply yourself to battle. Thus you will get no demerit. (2.38)***

सर्वकर्माणि मनसा
संन्यस्यास्ते सुखं वशी ।
नवद्वारे पुरे देही
नैव कुर्वन्न कारयन् ॥५.१३॥
sarvakarmāṇi manasā
saṁnyasyāste sukhaṁ vaśī
navadvāre pure dehī
naiva kurvanna kārayan (5.13)

*sarvakarmāṇi = sarva — all + karmāṇi — actions; manasā — with the mind; saṁnyasyāste = saṁnyasy (saṁnyasi) — renouncing + āste — he sits; sukhaṁ — happily; vaśī — director; navadvāre = nava — nine + dvāre — in the gate; pure — in the city; dehī — the embodied soul; naiva = na — not + eva — indeed; kurvan — acting; na — nor; kārayan — causing activity*

**Renouncing all action with the mind, the embodied soul resides happily within as the director in the nine-gated city, neither acting nor causing activity. (5.13)**

***Siddha Swami's Commentary:***

Even though there is a formal renunciation, still the real renunciation is an introverted condition whereby the person may or may not act culturally, but remains detached mentally when acting. The renunciation, for it to have impact, must be committed in the psyche by disconnecting the intellect from the domineering senses and memory. This was described before in the *buddhi yoga* discipline taught by *Śrī* Krishna to those ancient yogi kings and then to Arjuna.

*Sukham* or happiness, *śānti* or peace of mind, comes to a person who ordered his psyche, so that his intellect is not prejudiced by the memory and senses. The nine-gated city is this body, which has nine openings, two for hearing, two for seeing, one for speaking and tasting, two for smelling, one for evacuating solids and one for evacuating liquids.

The limited spirit does not act, nor can he cause someone else to act. He can, however, be used as a power-supply for action of his own or of another's body, but that brings to him certain costly liabilities.

न कर्तृत्वं न कर्माणि
लोकस्य सृजति प्रभुः ।
न कर्मफलसंयोगं
स्वभावस्तु प्रवर्तते ॥५.१४॥
na kartṛtvaṁ na karmāṇi
lokasya sṛjati prabhuḥ
na karmaphalasaṁyogaṁ
svabhāvastu pravartate (5.14)

*na — not; kartṛtvaṁ — means of action; na — nor; karmāṇi — actions; lokasya — of the creatures; sṛjati — he creates; prabhuḥ — the Lord; na — nor; karmaphalasaṁyogaṁ = karma — action + phala — consequence + saṁyogaṁ — cyclic connection; svabhāvaḥ — inherent nature; tu — but; pravartate — it causes*

**The Lord does not create the means of action, nor the actions of the creatures, nor the action-consequence cycle. But the inherent nature causes this. (5.14)**

***Siddha Swami's Commentary:***

This is a realization in *brahma yoga*, coming from direct mystic perception into the component parts of any activity, the potential *(svabhāvah)* of the components and random energies involved. Even though the limited spirits and the Supreme Spirit are in proximity to material nature, still the real cause of the interactions is the material energy itself.

Religious persons usually tag God with all liability. They feel that God personally causes this entire universe to operate on an action-consequence cycle *(karmaphalasamyogam)*, but in fact, the Lord is only indirectly responsible by virtue of proximity to the mundane energy. Even though *Śrī* Krishna, the Supreme Being, takes responsibility for everything, still He does so as a matter of connection to the involved limited spirits and not because He personally operates the interactions. These changes occur by their own potency, which is activated by the presence of the spirits and the Supreme Lord.

नादत्ते कस्यचित्पापं
न चैव सुकृतं विभुः ।
अज्ञानेनावृतं ज्ञानं
तेन मुह्यन्ति जन्तवः ॥५.१५॥
nādatte kasyacitpāpaṁ
na caiva sukṛtaṁ vibhuḥ
ajñānenāvṛtaṁ jñānaṁ
tena muhyanti jantavaḥ (5.15)

*nādatte = na — not + ādatte — perceives; kasyacit — of anyone; pāpaṁ — evil consequence; na — not; caiva = ca — and + eva — indeed; sukṛtaṁ — good reaction; vibhuḥ — the Almighty God; ajñānenāvṛtaṁ = ajñānena — by ignorance + avṛtam — shrouded; jñānaṁ — knowledge; tena — through which; muhyanti — they are deluded; jantavaḥ — the people*

**The Almighty God does not receive from anyone, an evil consequence or a good reaction. The knowledge of this is shrouded by ignorance through which the people are deluded. (5.15)**

***Siddha Swami's Commentary:***

The people cannot see the truth because their insight is shrouded by the sensual energies which dictate to them certain untruths as if such ideas were actual facts. Naturally, a limited being trapped in the material world in some body, especially in a human form, would appeal to the Supreme Being for assistance, and would believe that He would remove problems and accept from them their good wishes and creature affections. However, all this is for the most part fictitious, for the Supreme Being can hardly relate to the people who are conditioned in this world.

The material world, its gross forms and its subtle energies are a complete outfit, a complete cosmos in which there is a balance of the energies enclosed. The Supreme Person does not and cannot adjust the energies because they are self constrained and react accordingly. What the Supreme can and does do periodically is regulate some of the movement of the mundane energy, but regulation of a force is not the same as full adjustment. The energies have their inherent nature (*svabhāvah* Bg. 5.14); there is a limit to what the Supreme Person or anyone else may do to adjust them. Thus the Lord invites the limited entities to make an exit from this environment if they really want a trouble-free existence.

When a person comes to understand through direct mystic perception, that the Supreme Being is detached from whatever may occur here, that person no longer follows superficial religions. He no longer begs God for this or that in terms of the material existence, either its gross or subtle phases. Once you see that the mundane potency can give you whatever you may desire from it, if you work within its scope; then there is no need to beg anything from the God. The real requirement is the association of the Supreme Spirit. All other needs are superficial.

ज्ञानेन तु तदज्ञानं
येषां नाशितमात्मनः ।
तेषामादित्यवज्ज्ञानं
प्रकाशयति तत्परम् ॥५.१६॥

*jñānena — by experience; tu — however; tad — this; ajñānaṁ — ignorance; yeṣāṁ — of whom; nāśitam — removed; ātmanaḥ — of the self; teṣām — of them; ādityavaj = ādityavat — like the sun; jñānam —*

jñānena tu tadajñānaṁ
yeṣāṁ nāśitamātmanaḥ
teṣāmādityavajjñānaṁ
prakāśayati tatparam (5.16)

*revelation; prakāśayati — causes to appear; tat – that; param — Supreme Truth (explained in two previous verses)*

**However, for those, in whose souls the ignorance is removed by experience, that revelation of theirs, will cause the Supreme Truth to appear distinctly like the sun. (5.16)**

***Siddha Swami's Commentary:***

Clarity on the mystic and spiritual planes comes about by higher yoga, not otherwise. Through that spiritual perception, one begins to perceive life on the spiritual plane, which before was just darkness. It is an apt comparison made by *Śrī* Krishna, that for such an advanced *yogin* the spiritual reality is clear, just as for a human being, the sun in the sky is very clear and distinct.

In materialistic life without spiritual perception, one has vague ideas about spiritual reality, all based on sensual needs and on what one heard from scriptures and religious authorities. These are conceptions only and not actual vision on the spiritual plane. When by higher yoga, one develops the spiritual eyesight, one sees into the spiritual level just as clearly as one normally sees on the material plane. As one developed physical vision in the mother's womb, so by the yoga practice, one gradually develops the spiritual perception, *jñāna dīpah*.

तद्बुद्धयस्तदात्मानस्
तन्निष्ठास्तत्परायणाः ।
गच्छन्त्यपुनरावृत्तिं
ज्ञाननिर्धूतकल्मषाः ॥५.१७॥
tadbuddhayastadātmānas
tanniṣṭhāstatparāyaṇāḥ
gacchantyapunarāvṛttiṁ
jñānanirdhūtakalmaṣāḥ (5.17)

*tadbuddhayaḥ — those whose intellects are situated in that supreme truth; tadātmānaḥ — those whose spirits are focused on that supreme truth; tanniṣṭhāḥ — those whose reference is that supreme truth; tatparāyaṇāḥ — those who aspire to that supreme truth as the highest reality; gacchanty (gacchanti) — go + apunar – never again + āvṛttim — rebirth; jñana — experience + nirdhūta — removed + kalmaṣāḥ — faults*

**Those whose intellects are situated in that Supreme Truth, whose souls are focused on it, whose basic reference is that, whose faults are removed by the experience, who aspire to that as the highest reality, never go again to rebirth. (5.17)**

***Siddha Swami's Commentary:***

This describes the status of a *brahma yogi*, an ascetic who developed the spiritual perception and who earned the right not to take rebirth in the material world, even rebirth for the purpose of doing righteous acts for the benefit of society. Such a person has split off from the concerns of this world, and having the permission of the Supreme Spirit, he or she departed, never to return again. It is no loss to the world however, because others will perform whatever tasks those great souls did or could do if they had remained here.

विद्याविनयसंपन्ने
ब्राह्मणे गवि हस्तिनि ।
शुनि चैव श्वपाके च
पण्डिताः समदर्शिनः ॥५.१८॥

*vidyāvinayasampanne = vidyā — learning + vinaya — trained + sampanne — accomplished; brāhmaṇe — in a brahmin; gavi — in a cow; hastini — in an elephant; śuni — in a dog; caiva*

vidyāvinayasaṁpanne
brāhmaṇe gavi hastini
śuni caiva śvapāke ca
paṇḍitāḥ samadarśinaḥ (5.18)

*= ca — and + eva — indeed; śvapāke — in a dog-flesh eater; ca — and; paṇḍitāḥ — scripturally-conversant mystic seers; samadarśinaḥ = sama — common factor + darśinaḥ — observing*

**In a learned, trained, accomplished brahmin, in a cow, an elephant, a dog, or a dog-flesh eater, the scripturally-conversant mystic seers observe a common factor. (5.18)**

***Siddha Swami's Commentary:***

Each of the material forms used by human beings or animals is powered in the same way, by a limited spirit in conjunction with the Supreme Spirit. Elsewhere in the *Bhagavad Gītā, Śrī* Krishna explained this when He spoke of the *kṣetrajña*. He will describe the limited knower who is aware of a body and the unlimited person who is aware of all bodies. In each body, in each subtle and gross form, there is a limited spirit and there is the Supreme Spirit as well. While the limited spirit is constrained by his individual body, the Supreme Spirit inhabits all the bodies alongside the limited souls.

Thus the observation is that these bodies are powered and regulated by a limited spirit in conjunction with the Supreme Being. This must be seen on the spiritual plane. At first one will only see a limited spirit of a similar type in each of the bodies. When one advances further in *brahma yoga* meditation practice, one will begin to see the Supreme Spirit alongside a limited soul in each of the forms. This is not the same as the conception of this in the mind for understanding and explanation purposes. This is an actual vision, a spiritual perception seen by the spirit itself after developing spiritual vision through higher yoga practice.

इहैव तैर्जितः सर्गो
येषां साम्ये स्थितं मनः ।
निर्दोषं हि समं ब्रह्म
तस्माद्ब्रह्मणि ते स्थिताः ॥५.१९॥
ihaiva tairjitaḥ sargo
yeṣāṁ sāmye sthitaṁ manaḥ
nirdoṣaṁ hi samaṁ brahma
tasmādbrahmaṇi te sthitāḥ (5.19)

*ihaiva = iha — here in this world + iva (eva) — indeed; tair = taiḥ — by those; jitaḥ — conquered; sargo = sargaḥ — birth; yeṣāṁ — of whom; sāmye — in impartiality; sthitaṁ — established; manaḥ — mind; nirdoṣaṁ — faultless; hi — indeed; samaṁ — equally disposed; brahma — pure spirit; tasmāt — therefore; brahmaṇi — on the pure spiritual plane; te — they; sthitāḥ — established*

**Here in this world, birth is conquered by those whose minds are established in impartiality. Indeed, pure spirit is faultless and equally disposed. Therefore they are established on the pure spiritual plane. (5.19)**

***Siddha Swami's Commentary:***

This has to do with the same *buddhi yoga* practice, which *Śrī* Krishna explained in Chapter Two and He continued to teach in many other verses so far. The pure spirit, brahma, is faultless and is equally disposed to all facets of material existence, but when that spirit takes on a subtle body, it is inclined to the prejudices of the subtle psychology. To go upward and to realize itself, the spirit has to adopt an impartial mood to the various pairs of opposites like heat and cold, happiness and distress, profit and loss. However in *buddhi yoga*, one is trained in how to separate one's *buddhi* organ from the sensual and recollective influences.

न प्रहृष्येत्प्रियं प्राप्य
नोद्विजेत्प्राप्य चाप्रियम् ।
स्थिरबुद्धिरसंमूढो
ब्रह्मविद्ब्रह्मणि स्थितः ॥५.२०॥
na prahṛṣyetpriyaṁ prāpya
nodvijetprāpya cāpriyam
sthirabuddhirasaṁmūḍho
brahmavidbrahmaṇi sthitaḥ
(5.20)

*na — not; prahṛṣyet — should become excited; priyaṁ — dear item or favorable circumstance; prāpya — having attained; nodvijet = na — no + udvijet — should detest; prāpya — having obtained; cāpriyam = ca — and + apriyam — something unpleasant; sthira — stable; buddhiḥ — intelligent; asaṁmūḍho = asammūḍhaḥ — without confusion; brahmavid — a person who continually experiences the spiritual reality; brahmaṇi — on the spiritual plane; sthitaḥ — situated*

**Having attained a desired item or favorable circumstance, a person should not become excited. Having attained something unpleasant, he should not detest it. With stable intelligence, without confusion, a person who continually experiences the spiritual reality, remains situated on the spiritual plane. (5.20)**

***Siddha Swami's Commentary:***

*Buddhi yoga* begins by external efforts to control the behavior of one's body. Then later, one moves internally to control the various parts of the psyche. *Śrī* Krishna gave the preliminary part of the basic practice which he gave in Chapter 2, texts 38 and 39. An effort is made to control the body's behavior. This has an effect on the subtle form. It is not a full effect because sometimes the subtle form, being impulsive and more powerful than the gross one, will overcome the gross one and cause it to behave improperly even if the person prefers the higher culture.

The practice begins by training oneself not to be excited when one receives a desired item or finds oneself in a favored circumstance. Then, even if one has some excitement in the mental and emotional feelings, still one should restrain that and not exhibit any of it. One does the same restraint in reference to detestable feelings when one is confronted by unpleasant circumstances. After practicing this mood suppression for some time, one may become expert at it. Then after long sincere practice, one will advance to understand that one needs to work only with the internal psychology rather than become preoccupied with adjusting the behavior of the gross body.

This adjusting of the gross body in the social environment falls under the 1st and 2nd stages of yoga, namely, *yama* prohibitions and *niyama* observances. It is elementary religion and is the starting point for most people. A *buddhi* yogi also follows these rules but he does so on the basis of psychological rather than physical control. His intelligence becomes stable because he makes it immune to the influences of the senses and the probing reactive memory. Since he puts his *buddhi* intellect organ at a distance from the sensual energies and memories, it remains stable and is not prejudiced by various feelings and notions. From this expertise he becomes *brahmavid*, a person who continually experiences the spiritual reality.

बाह्यस्पर्शेष्वसक्तात्मा
विन्दत्यात्मनि यत्सुखम् ।
स ब्रह्मयोगयुक्तात्मा
सुखमक्षयमश्नुते ॥५.२१॥

*bāhya — external; sparśeṣv (sparśeṣu) — sensation; asakta — not attachéd; ātmā — soul; vindatyātmani = (vindati) — finds + ātmani — in the spirit; yat — who; sukham — happiness; sa = saḥ — he; brahmayogayuktātmā = brahma — spiritual plane +*

bāhyasparśeṣvasaktātmā
vindatyātmani yatsukham
sa brahmayogayuktātmā
sukhamakṣayamaśnute (5.21)

*yoga — yoga process; yukta — linked + ātmā — spirit; sukham — happiness; akṣayam — non-fluctuating; aśnute — makes contact with*

**The person who is not attached to the external sensations, who finds happiness in the spirit, whose spirit is linked to the spiritual plane through yoga process, makes contact with the non-fluctuating happiness. (5.21)**

***Siddha Swami's Commentary:***

*Bāhyasparśeṣu*, external sensations, apply in two ways, physically and psychically, so that these sensations fuse into the gross or subtle body from outside either of those forms. Emotions, for instance, which are in the subtle body of one person might fuse into and then affect another person's subtle form. Similarly, sensation detected by the gross body of a man, might come from that of another person in the physical world. External may mean what is outside a physical body or it might mean what is outside a subtle form.

*Vindatyātmani* means finding happiness in the spirit. This does not mean in the psychology of mental and emotional makeup of that spirit, but it means in the core spirit itself, without reference to the selections that person would make if he were under the influence of varying moods. He must be detached from his own intellect, which is detached from the memory and sensual energy.

*Brahmayogayuktātma* means a person whose spirit *(ātma)* is linked *(yukta)* to the spiritual plane *(brahma)* through the yoga process *(yoga)*. If we subtract yoga, we are not speaking of the same linkage. The particular happiness is the *sukham akṣayam*, the non-fluctuating type which is on the spiritual plane. The *buddhi* yogi, when he masters the practice, reaches that spiritual environment and shares in that consciousness.

ये हि संस्पर्शजा भोगा
दुःखयोनय एव ते ।
आद्यन्तवन्तः कौन्तेय
न तेषु रमते बुधः ॥५.२२॥
ye hi saṁsparśajā bhogā
duḥkhayonaya eva te
ādyantavantaḥ kaunteya
na teṣu ramate budhaḥ (5.22)

*ye — which; hi — indeed; saṁsparśajā — coming from sensual contact; bhogā — pleasures; duḥkhayonaya = duḥkha — pain + yonayaḥ — sources; eva — indeed; te — they; ādyantavantaḥ = ādy (ādi) — beginnings + anta — ending + vantaḥ — possessed with; kaunteya — O son of Kuntī; na — never; teṣu — in them; ramate — delights; budhaḥ — a wise person*

**The pleasures that come from sensual contacts are sources of pain. They have a beginning and ending, O son of Kuntī. A wise person never delights in them. (5.22)**

***Siddha Swami's Commentary:***

Pleasures come from sensual contact because the spirit invested attention into the senses. If there were no investment of attention, no person would feel any sort of pleasure or pain from the external physical or psychic environments. The investment is made automatically because a limited being is naturally fused into his psychology and endures the contacts which come to it or which it pursues. Still, the material world is so designed and so created, that any contact is altered, and the investment of energy is not efficiently utilized. In advanced *buddhi yoga* practice, one sees how the energies operate and one makes a decision to not try to enjoy them any longer.

The material energy is always canted towards the balance of power in the material world, and so it has little or no regard for needs of the spirit who wants eternal happiness. Thus the only solution is to break contact with the mundane energy. That requires mastership of higher yoga.

शक्नोतीहैव यः सोढुं
प्राक्शरीरविमोक्षणात् ।
कामक्रोधोद्भवं वेगं
स युक्तः स सुखी नरः ॥५.२३॥
śaknotīhaiva yaḥ soḍhuṁ
prākśarīravimokṣaṇāt
kāmakrodhodbhavaṁ vegaṁ
sa yuktaḥ sa sukhī naraḥ (5.23)

*śaknotīhaiva = śaknoti — can + iha — here on earth + iva (eva) — indeed; yaḥ — who; soḍhuṁ — to endure; prāk — before; śarīravimokṣaṇāt = śarīra — body + vimokṣaṇāt — from leaving; kāmakrodhodbhavaṁ = kāma — craving + krodha — anger + udbhavaṁ — basis; vegaṁ — impulsion; sa = saḥ — he; yuktaḥ — discipline; sa = saḥ — he; sukhī — happy; naraḥ — human being*

**The person who, before leaving the body, endures the craving-based, anger-based impulsions, is disciplined. He is a happy human being. (5.23)**

***Siddha Swami's Commentary:***

*Prāk śarīravimokṣaṇāt* means before leaving the material body, at the death of that form. If one practices and masters *buddhi yoga* before that occurrence, then one is truly a happy human being, having come in contact consistently with the unfluctuating happiness (*sukham akṣayam* Bg. 5.21).

At a certain stage of *buddhi yoga* practice, the craving-based and anger-based impulsions remain but since the ascetic distanced his intellect from the memory and sensual energies, those impulsions are unable to bring the intellect under their control. This technique was described before:

*yadā te mohakalilaṁ buddhirvyatitariṣyati*
*tadā gantāsi nirvedaṁ śrotavyasya śrutasya ca (2.52)*

***When from your delusion-saturated mind, your discrimination departs, you will become disgusted with what is to be heard and what was heard. (2.52)***

योऽन्तःसुखोऽन्तरारामस्
तथान्तर्ज्योतिरेव यः ।
स योगी ब्रह्मनिर्वाणं
ब्रह्मभूतोऽधिगच्छति ॥५.२४॥
yo'ntaḥsukho'ntarārāmas
tathāntarjyotireva yaḥ
sa yogī brahmanirvāṇaṁ
brahmabhūto
'dhigacchati (5.24)

*yo = yaḥ — who; 'ntaḥsukho = antahsukhaḥ — he who is happy within; 'ntarārāmas = antarārāmas — he who is spiritually delighted; tathāntarjyotir (tathāntarjyotiḥ) = tathā — as a result + antarjyotiḥ — he who has brilliant consciousness within; eva — indeed; yaḥ — who; sa = saḥ — he; yogī — yogi; brahmanirvāṇaṁ — stoppage of disturbing sensuality and attainment of constant spirituality; brahmabhūto = brahmabhūtaḥ — absorption on the spiritual plane; 'dhigacchati = adhigacchati — he attains*

**The person who is happy within, who is spiritually delighted and as a result, experiences the brilliant consciousness, he, that yogi, experiences the stoppage of disturbing sensuality and attains constant spirituality in absorption on the spiritual plane. (5.24)**

***Siddha Swami's Commentary:***

This is a *brahma yoga technique*, but *Śrī* Krishna gave this to Arjuna as the *buddhi yoga* process which was taught to the ancient *karma* yogis and *jñāna* yogis. Many persons studied this verse, but few notice the term *tathāntarjyotih*. When broken into individual words, this means *tathā* or as a result, *antar* or within the psyche, within the subtle body, and *jyotih* or supernatural and spiritual light. Usually a human being has only visual darkness within the mind, with flashes of ideas from the memory and imagination.

However, as a result of advanced *buddhi yoga*, one develops light, *jyotih*, in the subtle body, both in the head of it and elsewhere in the kundalini-*nāḍi* system. *Śrī Patañjali Mahārṣi* has called the disturbing sensuality, *cittavṛtti*, and he recommends that one bring its movements and interaction to a complete halt. When this is done, then that state is real yoga, called *brahmanirvāṇam* by *Śrī* Krishna.

*Antarjyotih* or the brilliant consciousness within the psyche comes after completion of joint practice in kundalini yoga, *kriyā yoga* and *brahma yoga*. This may be called *rāja* yoga, but the title is not as important as the process. Kundalini yoga brings about *antar jyotih* or brilliances within the subtle spine and within its extensions, the tiny and large nadis which exist all over the subtle body. When the kundalini energy changes color and becomes like white light, then it is in the category of *antar jyotih*. In *kriyā yoga*, one works specifically on the head of the subtle body, to clear up its chakras. Mainly, there are two chakras, one between the eyebrows and one at the crown of the head. Other minor ones exist at the top front of the forehead, the top back of the head, the lower center back of the head, and the right ear, as well as two at each of the temple indentations. These are chakras of the subtle body and they are purified to make them brilliant in terms of having clear subtle light. Mastery of this is elementary *kriyā yoga*.

In advanced *kriyā yoga*, one no longer bothers with the kundalini chakra, as it becomes purified and no longer expresses a negative influence. One with a sickness will take medicine. As soon as the sickness is cured, he no longer takes it. If the ascetic can clear kundalini and maintain it through the proper yoga lifestyle, he does not have to continue the strenuous endeavors at *haṭha* yoga practice with various bandhas or bodily locks and mudras or bodily restrictions of energy flow.

In advanced *kriyā yoga* the ascetic focuses on what *Śrī* Krishna called *buddhi yoga*, to separate his intellect from the sensual energies and the memory. When completed, this separation causes the intellect to become brilliant in the head of the subtle body. A dull light which does not get sufficient current to keep it well lit, will increase in brilliance if it has a steady, sufficient power supply. As soon as the intellect is no longer being drained by its involvements with the sensual energies and the memory, it will gradually, over a time of consistent practice, increase in brilliance.

Higher yet, is the process of splitting off the *buddhi* organ from the attention energy. This energy is the focus of the spirit itself. When that is separated from the intellect, then the *yogin*'s spirit self becomes stabilized and is able to keep in touch with the naad spiritual sound which comes into the right ear of the subtle body. From this stability, light develops all around. This all surrounding light is called *antar jyotih*.

The mere fact that *Śrī* Krishna spoke of the attainment of constant spirituality on the basis of absorption on the spiritual plane, *brahmabhuto*, means clearly that it is based on *brahma yoga samādhi* practice. *Śrī* Krishna did not speak of any other process and it is quite unfair to tell an audience that this means something else. The Sanskrit is very clear on this. If it is not important to meditate and if meditation is not part of the Krishna conscious process, then what is the significance of the *antar jyotih?* Why did *Śrī* Krishna even bother to mention it and to conduct a discourse which developed into recognition of it?

लभन्ते ब्रह्मनिर्वाणम्
ऋषयः क्षीणकल्मषाः ।
छिन्नद्वैधा यतात्मानः
सर्वभूतहिते रताः ॥५.२५॥
labhante brahmanirvāṇam
ṛṣayaḥ kṣīṇakalmaṣāḥ
chinnadvaidhā yatātmānaḥ
sarvabhūtahite ratāḥ (5.25)

*labhante — they attain; brahmanirvāṇaṁ — cessation of material existence and a simultaneous absorption in spirituality; ṛṣayaḥ — the seers; kṣīṇakalmaṣāḥ = kṣīṇa – terminates + kalmaṣāḥ — sins, faults; chinnadvaidhā = chinna — removed + dvaidhā — doubts; yatātmānaḥ = yata – restrained + ātmānaḥ — souls; sarvabhūtahite = sarva – all + bhūta — creatures + hite — in welfare; ratāḥ — joy*

**Those seers whose sins and faults are terminated, whose doubts are removed, whose souls are restrained, who find joy in regarding the welfare of the creatures, attain a cessation of their material existence and a simultaneous absorption in spirituality. (5.25)**

***Siddha Swami's Commentary:***

Their sins and faults were terminated, not by performing pious activity or doing deity worship *pūja*, but by cleaning up their psychology in *buddhi yoga* practice. It is because their psychology became removed from the mundane energy and not because it handled the energy in a religious or sacred way. Their doubts were removed by mystic experiences of the spiritual truths discussed by *Śrī* Krishna, not by their intellectual or emotional acceptance of this *Bhagavad Gītā* discourse. Their souls were restrained *(yatātmānah)* by the elementary *buddhi yoga* practice, which *Śrī* Krishna explained in detail.

They find joy *(ratāh)* in the welfare of the creatures, not by trying to do good and to demonstrate non-violence and kindness, but through spiritual contact with the other limited spirits and with the Supreme Soul. Subsequently they are in *brahmanirvāṇam* which is being repeatedly mentioned by *Śrī* Krishna. *Nirvāṇam* is the cessation of material existence, for those particular persons who mastered the *buddhi yoga* practice as taught by *Śrī* Krishna to *Vivasvat, Manu, Ikṣvāku, Janaka* and also Arjuna. It is no other system or teaching.

कामक्रोधवियुक्तानां
यतीनां यतचेतसाम् ।
अभितो ब्रह्मनिर्वाणं
वर्तते विदितात्मनाम् ॥५.२६॥
kāmakrodhaviyuktānāṁ
yatīnāṁ yatacetasām
abhito brahmanirvāṇaṁ
vartate viditātmanām (5.26)

*kāmakrodhaviyuktānāṁ = kāma — desire + krodha — anger + viyuktānāṁ — of the separation from; yatīnāṁ — of the ascetics; yatacetasām — of those whose thinking is restrained; abhito = abhitaḥ — very close; brahmanirvāṇaṁ — cessation of material existence, assumption of enlightened spirituality; vartate — it is; viditātmanām — of those who understand the spiritual self*

**The cessation of material existence and assumption of enlightened spirituality is soon to be attained by those ascetics whose thinking is restrained and who understand the spiritual self. (5.26)**

***Siddha Swami's Commentary:***

*Śrī Patañjali Mahārṣi* gave different words for the same process of *yatacetasām*. This *cetasām* is the mental and emotional energy in the psyche. In *Patañjali*'s time, yogis called this *cittavṛtti*. *Patañjali* said it should be fully restrained but he called the restraint *nirodha*. Any ascetic who can restrain that energy, the mental and emotional forces which affect the mind, and who understands that the spirit self is usually fused into the mind with the intellect, memory and sensual energy, will in time attain the *brahmanirvāṇam* condition. *Śrī*

Krishna stated this to assure ascetics from various groups that if they are able to restrain their mental and emotional energies, they will in time, attain the spiritual state of full absorption in spirituality and the termination of material existence.

Even if one discovers it or learns it from someone other than *Śrī* Krishna, even someone who does not know Krishna or who never heard of Him or met Him, one would attain the *brahmanirvāṇam*. There is no restriction for a person who practices and masters the *buddhi yoga* process.

स्पर्शान्कृत्वा बहिर्बाह्यांश्
चक्षुश्चैवान्तरे भ्रुवोः ।
प्राणापानौ समौ कृत्वा
नासाभ्यन्तरचारिणौ ॥५.२७॥
sparśānkṛtvā bahirbāhyāṁś
cakṣuścaivāntare bhruvoḥ
prāṇāpānau samau kṛtvā
nāsābhyantaracāriṇau (5.27)

*sparśān — sensual contact; kṛtvā — having done; bahir = bahiḥ — external; bāhyāṁś = bāhyān — excluded; cakṣuścaivāntare = cakṣuś — visual focus + ca — and = eva — indeed + antare — in between; bhruvoḥ — of the two eyebrows; prāṇāpānau — both inhalation and exhalation; samau — in balance; kṛtvā — having made; nāsābhyantaracāriṇau = nāsa — nose + abhyantara — within + cāriṇau — moving*

**Excluding the external sensual contacts, and fixing the visual focus between the eyebrows, putting the inhalation and exhalation in balance, moving through the nose, (5.27)**

Siddha Swami referred to *Śrī Bābāji Mahāśaya* for this comment.

***Śrī Bābāji Mahāśaya's Commentary:***

This is the first and most elementary technique of the *kriyā yoga* system which I introduced. This may be called the first of the reference *kriyās*. From this basic *kriyā*, a *yogin* researches into the length and breadth, formulation and possible disintegration of his psyche. For success with this, one should practice *prāṇāyāma* to put the inhalation and exhalation in balance. Nowadays this has come to signify an even flow between the two channels, the right side and left side of the nostrils. It really means that the nadī on the left of the spine is cleared as well as the right channel. When the two are sufficiently cleared, a switching mechanism causes the energy to flow through the central channel without obstruction. This produces a stability for the intellect organ, the *buddhi*.

*Śrī* Krishna used the term *bahih* which means external. At first this means what is external to the material body. To retreat from what is external to the material body, one must go into isolation. Yoga practice has solitude as one of its requirements. Once the person gains some isolation, he can try to internalize the attention. This attention is, for a beginner, his mental force and his emotional interest combined. Later on as he advances, he gets clarity and can sort between mental force for analysis and emotional force for sensing and enjoying. Once the external world is kept away, the senses will relax themselves and give the beginner a chance to check within his nature, to make the detailed observations necessary to begin the process of *buddhi yoga*, as *Śrī* Krishna originally intended.

In order to trap the mind and cause the attention to be restricted, one should focus between the eyebrows (*bhruvoh*). The term *cakṣus* indicates a visual focus. The visual sense is the first sense to be conserved and restricted in this practice. Here the focus is on a location between the eyebrows. It is not a sound to be repeated. As the ascetic does this, he will from time to time have difficult and easy phases, but the main development is what he observes and what his teacher discusses with him about his experiences while trying to keep his attention between his eyebrows.

Higher yoga practice evolves naturally from this basic mid-eyebrow focus. Each student develops in a way that suits one's evolutionary status. Each must work within his or her limitations, along with guidance from a senior *yogin*.

Eventually in this practice, a query arises as to who is focusing and what sort of power is being directed through or into the mid eyebrows. What do I see in the middle of it? How often am I distracted? What force distracts me and then entertains me with thoughts, pictures, and sounds? What is between the observer and the point between the mid-eyebrows? This is then discussed with the teacher.

यतेन्द्रियमनोबुद्धिर्
मुनिर्मोक्षपरायणः ।
विगतेच्छाभयक्रोधो
यः सदा मुक्त एव सः ॥५.२८॥
yatendriyamanobuddhir
munirmokṣaparāyaṇaḥ
vigatecchābhayakrodho
yaḥ sadā mukta eva saḥ (5.28)

*yatendriyamanobuddhir = yata — controlled + indriya — sensual energy + mano (manaḥ) — mind + buddhiḥ — intelligence; munir = muniḥ — wise person; mokṣaparāyaṇaḥ — one who is dedicated to achieving liberation; vigatecchābhayakrodho = vigata — gone away + icchā — desire + bhaya — fear + krodho (krodhaḥ) — anger; yaḥ — who; sadā — always; mukta — liberated; eva — indeed; saḥ — he*

**...the wise man, who is dedicated to achieving liberation, whose sensual energy, mind and intellect are controlled, whose desire, fear and anger are gone, is liberated always. (5.28)**

***Siddha Swami's Commentary:***

*Mokṣaparāyaṇah* is another term with very clear meaning, since *mokṣa* means liberation from the material energy in any of its forms or dimensions. One who is dedicated to achieving liberation, will work to get just that. He will never give up. Whatever it might take in terms of austerities, he will painstakingly perform without complaint or petition for an easier process. Of course if one controlled the sensual energy (*indriya*), mind (*manah*) and intellect (*buddhih*), and if one's desire, fear and anger are gone from one's nature, then one would definitely have the power to strive for and attain full liberation *(brahmanirvāṇam)*.

भोक्तारं यज्ञतपसां
सर्वलोकमहेश्वरम् ।
सुहृदं सर्वभूतानां
ज्ञात्वा मां शान्तिमृच्छति ॥५.२९॥
bhoktāraṁ yajñatapasāṁ
sarvalokamaheśvaram
suhṛdaṁ sarvabhūtānāṁ
jñātvā māṁ śāntimṛcchati (5.29)

*bhoktāraṁ — enjoyer; yajñatapasāṁ — of the religious ceremonies and austerities; sarvalokamaheśvaram = sarva – all entire + loka — world + maheśvaram — Supreme God; suhṛdaṁ — friend; sarvabhūtānāṁ — of all creatures; jñātvā — recognizing; māṁ — me; śāntim — spiritual peace; ṛcchati — attains*

**Recognizing Me, as the enjoyer of religious ceremonies and austerities, the Supreme God of the entire world, the friend of the creatures, he attains spiritual peace. (5.29)**

***Siddha Swami's Commentary:***

Realization of the Supreme Person, the *bhoktāram*, supreme enjoyer of the religious ceremonies and austerities, God of the entire world, *sarvalokamaheśvaram*, comes about fully at the culmination of higher yoga. It is not an easy achievement. Ordinary faith in God is not the same as this realization on the spiritual plane of consciousness. *Śrī* Krishna is not achieved easily by anyone.

It is essential that the initial devotedness and friendliness towards *Śrī* Krishna and towards the teacher who taught on His behalf, evolve into the recognition of Him as the *suhṛdam*, friend of all creatures.

This verse describes another technique of *brahma yoga* given in this discourse of the holy, sacred, very pure and true *Bhagavad Gītā*. Just as one realizes that one is neither the material body, nor the mind, nor emotions, nor the life energy, that he is neither the subtle body, nor the causal form, so one must recognize the Supreme Being, *Śrī* Krishna,. This is the science of *brahma* yoga.

# CHAPTER 6

# Yogam Ātma Viśuddhaye

# Purity of the Psyche Yoga *

*tatraikāgraṁ manaḥ kṛtvā yatacittendriyakriyāḥ*
*upaviśyāsane yuñjyād yogamātmaviśuddhaye (6.12)*

***...being there, seated in a posture, having the mind focused, the person who controls his thinking and sensual energy, should practise the yoga discipline for self-purification. (6.12)***

****Siddha Swami assigned this chapter title on the basis of verse 12 of this chapter.***

श्रीभगवानुवाच
अनाश्रितः कर्मफलं
कार्यं कर्म करोति यः ।
स संन्यासी च योगी च
न निरग्निर्न चाक्रियः ॥ ६.१ ॥
śrībhagavānuvāca
anāśritaḥ karmaphalaṁ
kāryaṁ karma karoti yaḥ
sa saṁnyāsī ca yogī ca
na niragnirna cākriyāḥ (6.1)

*śrī bhagavān — the Blessed Lord; uvāca — said; anāśritaḥ — not relying on; karmaphalaṁ — result of an action; kāryaṁ — obligation; karma — action; karoti — he fulfills; yaḥ — who; sa = saḥ — he; saṁnyāsī — renouncer; ca — and; yogī — yogi; ca — and; na — not; niragnir = niragniḥ — without a fire ceremony; na — nor; cākriyaḥ = ca — and + akryaḥ — lacking physical activities*

**The Blessed Lord said: A person who fulfills obligatory action, without depending on the result of the action, is a renouncer, and a yogi, not the one who is without a fire ceremony or who lacks physical activity. (6.1)**

***Siddha Swami's Commentary:***

*Śrī* Krishna in the *Bhagavad Gītā* insisted on defining a *sannyāsi*, a renouncer, in terms of the person's psychological stance rather than his physical culture. This is because the physical acts of a man might conceal his contrary psychic activity. His internal posture must be gauged before he can be rated properly. For Arjuna, the implications are clear that *Śrī* Krishna did not mind him renouncing the results of actions at *Kurukṣetra*, but He objected to an actual evasion in Arjuna of the duties assigned by King Yudhishthira.

A person who could not detach his or her self from the results of action, could not in fact be a full time *sannyāsi* who renounces cultural actions altogether. And a person who in fact could renounce for the proper reason, while approved by *Śrī* Krishna, would readily return to cultural work if that was the desire of *Śrī* Krishna.

Renunciation is not earmarked by a person's refusal to participate in fire ceremonies or religious performances or by refusal to engage in social or political activity. It is earmarked by the internal posture of the person. *Śrī* Krishna made this clear for all to see.

यं संन्यासमिति प्राहुर्
योगं तं विद्धि पाण्डव ।
न ह्यसंन्यस्तसंकल्पो
योगी भवति कश्चन ॥ ६.२ ॥
yaṁ saṁnyāsamiti prāhur
yogaṁ taṁ viddhi pāṇḍava
na hyasaṁnyastasaṁkalpo
yogī bhavati kaścana (6.2)

*yaṁ — that which; saṁnyāsam — renunciation; iti — thus; prāhur = prāhuḥ — the authorities define; yogaṁ — applied yoga; taṁ — it; viddhi — know; pāṇḍava — Arjuna Pandava; na — not; hy = hi — indeed; asaṁnyastasaṁkalpo = (asaṁnyastasaṁkalpaḥ) = asaṁnyasta — without renunciation + saṁkalpaḥ — intention; yogī — yogi; bhavati — becomes; kaścana — anyone*

**That which the authorities define as renunciation, know it as applied yoga, O Arjuna Pandava. Indeed, no one becomes a yogi without an intention for renunciation. (6.2)**

***Siddha Swami's Commentary:***

The license for yoga practice is the intention for renunciation, not the development of mystic powers for political and charismatic purposes. In the past, many persons were successful in being admitted to yoga teachings but their motives dealth with glamour and power. In the *Purāṇas* such persons were called *asuras*, indicating that they had wicked intentions and wanted to subvert the administration of the Supreme Being, *Śrī* Krishna.

In the field of religious ceremony and general disciplines, one may have intentions *(samkalpah)* for charisma and power, but in the field of yoga, one requires renunciation of benefits in this world as the main motive. However, some persons managed to fool able gurus and were taught yoga even though their motives were improper. Even *Karṇa* fooled Lord *Paraśurāma* and was cursed when he was discovered. And Kacha fooled Shukracharya but was subsequently cursed by Shukracharya's daughter. Anyone who manages to fool a yoga teacher and is taught the science, becomes ruined in the course of time when he tries to apply the technique to acquire popularity or political power. Such persons are called *ku*-yogis or badly-motivated ascetics. The real yogis begin the practice with an intention for renunciation as defined in the previous verse.

Even if one begins yoga practice with a bad motive or with no particular purpose in mind, if one listens to the teacher with a devoted attitude and with a friendly demeanor (*bhakto'si me sakhā*, 4.3), one will give up the bad motive, namely the lack of intention to serve the Supreme Being and the teacher (*sevayā,* 4.34). One will develop the renounced attitude required, just by their association.

Upon careful study of this verse, one will understand that renunciation comes only after the application of *buddhi yoga* expertise in cultural life. In other words, renunciation is first developed when practicing *karma yoga* as originally taught by Krishna to those famous yogi kings.

आरुरुक्षोर्मुनेर्योगं
कर्म कारणमुच्यते ।
योगारूढस्य तस्यैव
शमः कारणमुच्यते ॥६.३॥
āruruksormuneryogaṁ
karma kāraṇamucyate
yogārūḍhasya tasyaiva
śamaḥ kāraṇamucyate (6.3)

*āruruksor = āruruksoḥ — of one who strives; muner = muneḥ — of a philosophical man; yogaṁ — yoga expertise; karma — cultural activity; kāraṇam — the means; ucyate — it is recommended; yogārūḍhasya — of one who mastered yoga; tasyaiva = tasya — of him + iva (eva) — indeed; śamaḥ — tranquil method; kāraṇam — the means; ucyate — it is recommended*

**For a philosophical man who strives for yoga expertise, cultural activity is recommended. For one who has mastered yoga already, the tranquil reserved method is the means. (6.3)**

***Siddha Swami's Commentary:***

If not philosophically inclined, one is unlikely to develop the correct motive of renunciation for doing yoga. This is why in the history of yoga, most of the successful ascetics were philosophers, persons who studied the Samkhya philosophy. However initially, any such person would be required to do certain duties, cultural acts. And so as *Śrī* Krishna emphasized, cultural activity is recommended while the person learns *buddhi yoga* practice. All the same, for a person who mastered yoga, the tranquil reserved method *(śamah)* is the means, because he can forego opportunities for cultural life. Exempt from cultural acts, he can devote himself fully to the practice of higher yoga.

यदा हि नेन्द्रियार्थेषु
न कर्मस्वनुषज्जते ।
सर्वसंकल्पसंन्यासी
योगारूढस्तदोच्यते ॥६.४॥

*yadā — when; hi — indeed; nendriyārtheṣu = na — not + indriyārtheṣu — in attractive objects; na — not; karmasv = karmasu — in performance; anuṣajjate — feels attached; sarvasaṁkalpasaṁnyāsī = sarvasaṁkalpa — all*

yadā hi nendriyārtheṣu
na karmasvanuṣajjate
sarvasaṁkalpasaṁnyāsī
yogārūḍhastadocyate (6.4)

*motivations + saṁnyāsī — discarding; yogārūḍhas — proficient in yoga practice; tadocyate = tada — then + ucyate — it is said*

**Indeed, when having discarded all motivations, a person feels no attachment to attractive objects nor to performance, he is said to be proficient in yoga practice. (6.4)**

***Siddha Swami's Commentary:***

*Yogāruḍhah* is a term signifying a person who mastered *buddhi yoga* practice and who is resistance to the subtle and gross material world. Somehow or the other, that type of ascetic has lost his or her attraction to this world. Such a person might be compared to the Supreme Being, who described Himself in Chapter Four:

*na māṁ karmāṇi limpanti na me karmaphale spṛhā*
*iti māṁ yo'bhijānāti karmabhirna sa badhyate (4.14)*

***Actions do not entrap Me. The desire for payoff is not in Me. The person who understands this about Me is not entrapped by action. (4.14)***

The discarding of all motivations *(sarvasankalpa samnyāsī)* is not a mental procedure of determination to be free from impulsions and devious designs; it is actually based on freeing the *buddhi* intellect organ from the sensual promptings and the memory prejudices within the mind. Once done, the nature of the individual becomes purified. Mere determination will merely create sporadic detachment. A *sannyāsi* should feel no attachment to attractive objects or to performance, but he should be willing to perform if requested by the Supreme Being or an agent of the Lord. For his own purposes, he should have genuinely lost interest in the affairs of this world. *Dharma* or righteous lifestyle should be promoted by any *sannyāsi* whenever in vicinity of human society or when others appeal for an opinion in their dealings, but he should know that *dharma* is the business of God and not that of a mere sannyāsi. Proficiency in yoga practice is thereby demonstrated. It comes about naturally in the course of learning and practicing higher yoga.

उद्धरेदात्मनात्मानं
नात्मानमवसादयेत् ।
आत्मैव ह्यात्मनो बन्धुर्
आत्मैव रिपुरात्मनः ॥६.५॥
uddharedātmanātmānaṁ
nātmānamavasādayet
ātmaiva hyātmano bandhur
ātmaiva ripurātmanaḥ (6.5)

*uddhared = uddharet — should elevate; ātmanā — by the self; 'tmānaṁ = ātmānam — the self; nātmānam = na — not + ātmānam — the self; avasādayet — should degrade; ātmaiva = ātmā — self + eva — only; hyātmano = hyātmanaḥ = hy (hi) — indeed + ātmanaḥ — of the self; bandhur = bandhuh — friend; ātmaiva = ātmā — self + eva — as well; ripur = ripuḥ — enemy; ātmanaḥ — of the self*

**One should elevate his being by himself. One should not degrade the self. Indeed, the person should be the friend of himself. Or he could be the enemy as well. (6.5)**

***Siddha Swami's Commentary:***

These are the general directions for *ātma-viśuddha* yoga, the purification by mystic process of the subtle environment within the mind of a limited being. All sorts of endeavor are made by a living entity in this creation, but usually people expect that God will singlehandedly cause spiritual purification as an act of grace in liberating the faithful follower. However, any person with a reasonable relationship to God understands that the endeavoring capacity of the living limited being should be exerted for his psychological purification mostly and not for anything else. Even cultural activities should be performed under the direction of the Supreme Person, for the purpose of purification only. Remember a verse from the previous chapter as follows:

*kāyena manasā buddhyā kevalairindriyairapi*
*yoginaḥ karma kurvanti saṅgaṁ tyaktvātmaśuddhaye (5.11)*

***With the body, mind and intelligence, or even with the senses alone, the yogis, having discarded attachment, perform cultural acts for self-purification. (5.11)***

The psychology or being of the self becomes the enemy of the self when the nature falls under the influence of the passionate emotional force. This was explained previously:

*āvṛtaṁ jñānametena jñānino nityavairiṇā*
*kāmarūpeṇa kaunteya duṣpūreṇānalena ca (3.39)*

***The discernment of educated people is adjusted by their eternal enemy which is the sense of yearning for various things. O son of Kuntī, the lusty power, is as hard to satisfy as it is to keep a fire burning. (3.39)***

The force of *kāmarūpa*, the lusty energy which promotes impulsion and passion, is the power which disrupts spiritual satisfaction and motivates the psyche to perform irresponsible acts. One has to control this by monitoring external behavior, as well as by restricting the various parts of the psyche from interacting with each other haphazardly and impulsively. To be friendly to oneself, one must master *buddhi yoga*, as *Śrī* Krishna taught it, to restrict the intellect so that it does not succumb to the influence of the sensual energies and memory.

बन्धुरात्मात्मनस्तस्य
येनात्मैवात्मना जितः ।
अनात्मनस्तु शत्रुत्वे
वर्तेतात्मैव शत्रुवत् ॥६.६॥
bandhurātmātmanastasya
yenātmaivātmanā jitaḥ
anātmanastu śatrutve
vartetātmaiva śatruvat (6.6)

*bandhur = bandhuḥ — friend; ātmā — personal energies; 'tmanas = ātmanas — of the self; tasya — of him; yenātmaivātmanā = yena — by whom + ātmā — self + eva — indeed + ātmanā — by the self; jitaḥ — subdued; anātmanas — of one who is not self-possessed; tu — but; śatrutve — in hostility; vartetātmaiva = varteta — it operates + ātmā — self + eva — indeed; śatruvat — like an enemy*

**The personal energies are the friend of the person by whom those energies are subdued. But for one whose personality is not self-possessed, the personal energies operate in hostility like an enemy. (6.6)**

***Siddha Swami's Commentary:***

*Anātmanah* means that the psyche operates in reverse, whereby the intellect, memory and sensual energies work in tandem to control the spirit which is supposed to direct these. In such a life of sensual indulgence, the sensual energies are the director of affairs. These take help from the memory in keeping the intellect subdued and cooperative, while the spirit stays privy to the intellect and is prejudiced by it.

Siddha Swami advised that *Śrī Bābāji Mahāśaya* give a comment to this verse.

***Śrī Bābāji Mahāśaya's Commentary:***

Even though in theory, the spirit directs the psyche to get valuable experiences in the subtle and gross material world, what happens in fact is this: The spirit is directed by the psyche. In fact, the psyche has components which connect in a particular way for operation. When these components become defective or get connected in an improper order, we say that a certain individual is crazy. Actually nearly everyone in the material world is crazy, because nearly every person is dominated by sensual urges. When someone is rationally-inclined, we say that person is intelligent, and when someone else is emotionally-inclined, we say that person is full of sentiment. Those who are rational take more to scientific and philosophical discourses. The emotional persons take more to affection and devotion. Some are equally attracted to philosophy and devotion.

In the subtle body the senses out-grow from the edge of the mind chamber. These senses are the first psychic components which make contact with the subtle world. When a material body is developed, it mimics the subtle system. It too, develops senses, and they in turn make contact with the external world. Thus the spirit has a tendency to rely on the senses, come what may, even if they prove to be in error. The senses of the subtle body do not reach in to give information directly to the spirit. These senses convert their information into impressions. The impressions are sent into the memory which is a sensitive compartment. The impressions are also sent to the intellect, which is a subtle mechanism much like modern electronic equipment. Once the impressions strike the intellect, they are converted into images. These images are shown to the spirit in the imagination chamber of the intellect.

The spirit can see these imaginations only through the attention energy, which serves as a light to display the images in the imagination chamber. Some refer to this imagination as the mind, but the mind is really the whole chamber which houses the self, attention, intellect, memory and sensual energy. For the purpose of *buddhi yoga*, one should study the components and plan how to subdue them, while taking help from higher yogis and even from *Śrī* Krishna.

Since the senses are designed mostly for extroverted or external probing, they have a tendency to not be submissive to the self. They instinctively take energy from the intellect and memory and probe into the external world irrespective of what the self might desire. This instinct should be changed by regulating the amount of energy which the memory and intellect give to the senses. Even though the senses desire to turn their backs on the self and to ignore the self, still the self may force the senses to be submissive. This occurs by limiting the energy flow through the attention from the self. If enemy soldiers cannot grow food in their own country and must purchase grain from a king whom they continually threaten, then that king may subdue them easily by depriving them of the grain. Instead of trying to control them by negotiating or by engaging in battles he could simply cut off their grain supply. Similarly, instead of trying to reason with one's senses or to effect certain behavior, one should merely restrict the energy supply.

Here are two diagrams:

**Attention energy flowing to the senses unrestrictedly**

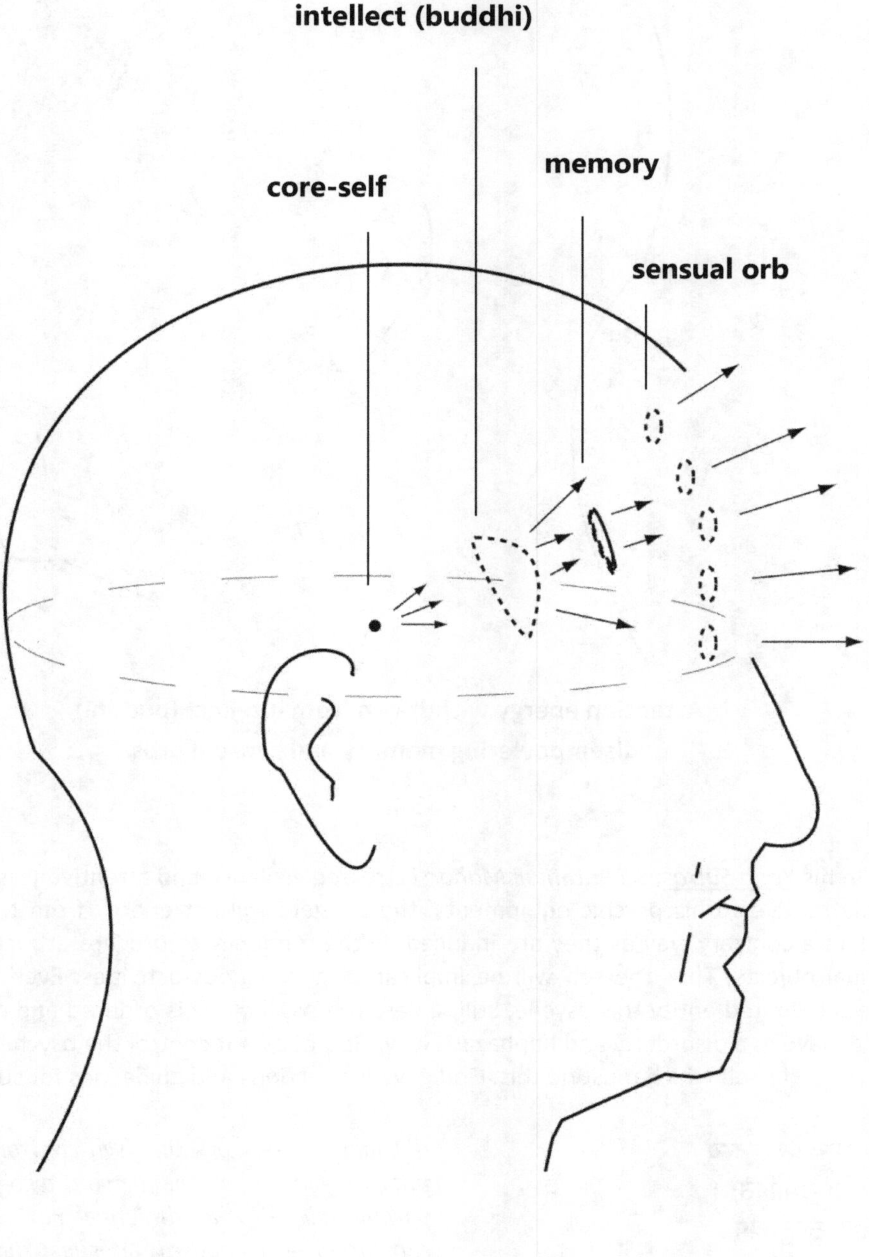

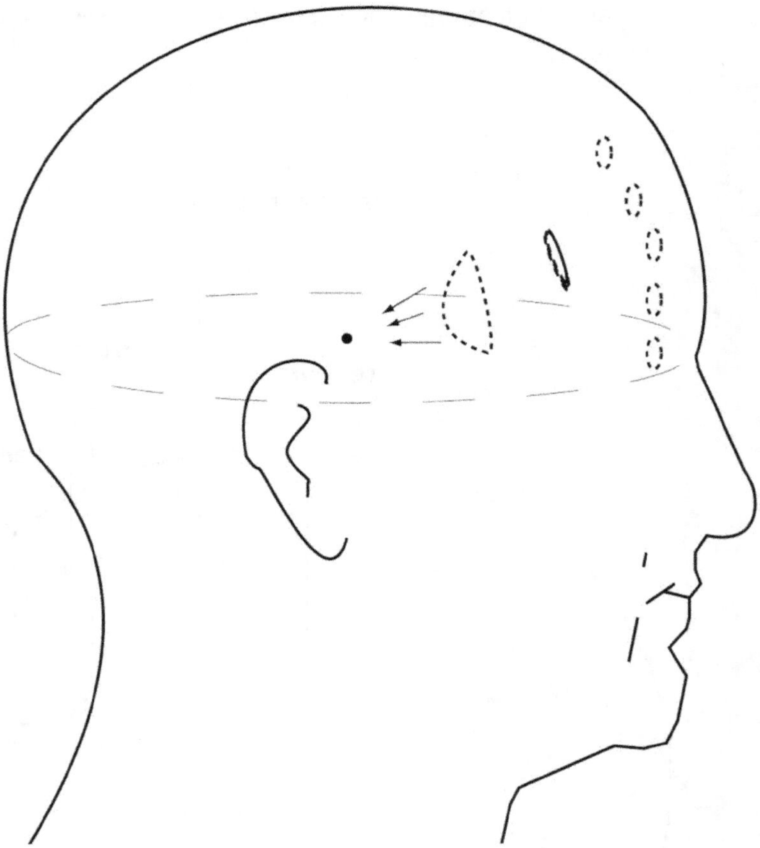

**Attention energy withdrawn from intellect (buddhi), disempowering memory and sensual orbs**

In his Yoga Sūtras, *Śrī Patañjali Mahārṣi* stressed vigilance and attentiveness. If the spirit is unattentive to his psychic equipments, the gadgets will get energy from the spirit and work in a contrary way as they are induced by the tendency to procure attractive gross or sensual objects. Thus the self will be implicated in irreligious activities. Even though God gave the limited entity this psyche, still, unless the psychology is ordered and controlled, it will behave in a disorderly and haphazard way. God does not control the psyche for the self; it is the self itself which must do this. God gave instructions and guidelines for such control.

जितात्मनः प्रशान्तस्य
परमात्मा समाहितः ।
शीतोष्णसुखदुःखेषु
तथा मानावमानयोः ॥६.७॥

*jitātmanaḥ — of the self-controlled person; praśāntasya — of the person who is peaceful; paramātmā — the directive part of the self; samāhitaḥ — composed; śītoṣṇasukhaduḥkheṣu = śīta — cold + uṣṇa — heat + sukha — pleasure +*

jitātmanaḥ praśāntasya
paramātmā samāhitaḥ
śītoṣṇasukhaduḥkheṣu
tathā mānāvamānayoḥ (6.7)

*duḥkheṣu — in pain; tathā — also; mānāvamānayoḥ = māna — honor + avamānayoḥ — in dishonor*

**The directive part of a self-controlled, peaceful person remains composed in the cold, heat, pleasure, pain, and also in honor and dishonor. (6.7)**

***Śrī Bābāji Mahāśaya's Commentary:***

*Paramātma* in this verse does not mean the Supreme Spirit who is in the psyche alongside the limited spirit. *Paramātma** in this verse uses a rare meaning for that word, which is the directive part of the limited self. It is the same limited self, the *ātma*, and he or she has not become God or become the *Paramātma* Supreme Spirit, but rather has discovered or repossessed its own honor and acts as it should have in the first place.

It is the same limited self who was confused about his identity before, but now after completing yoga disciplines, it becomes exalted or higher than before *(param).* The passive, directive part which before was entertained, amused and fooled by the intellect, memory and sensual energy, now no longer accepts those directions. By the psychological strength it gained from *buddhi yoga* practice, it can now remain isolated from the intellectual, recollective and sensual influences. Thus it remains composed even in cold, heat, pleasure, pain, honor and dishonor.

Even if the mental and emotional energies and psychic equipments go through their agitations, the spirit in this case, remains without moody variations, just as *Śrī* Krishna requested in Chapter Two when He first began to describe *buddhi yoga* practice.

ज्ञानविज्ञानतृप्तात्मा
कूटस्थो विजितेन्द्रियः ।
युक्त इत्युच्यते योगी
समलोष्टाश्मकाञ्चनः ॥६.८॥
jñānavijñānatṛptātmā
kūṭastho vijitendriyaḥ
yukta ityucyate yogī
samaloṣṭāśmakāñcanaḥ (6.8)

*jñānavijñānatṛptātmā = jñāna — knowledge + vijñāna — realized experience + tṛpta — content + ātmā — self; kūṭastho = kūṭasthaḥ — stable; vijitendriyaḥ = vijita — subdued + indriyaḥ — sensual energy; yukta — disciplined in yoga; ityucyate = ity (iti) — thus + ucyate — is called; yogī — yogi; samaloṣṭrāśmakāñcanaḥ = sama — same + loṣṭra — lump of clay + aśma — stone + kāñcanaḥ — gold*

**The yogi who is satisfied with knowledge and realized experience, who is stable and who has conquered his sensual energy, who regards a lump of clay, a stone or gold in the same way, is said to be disciplined in yoga. (6.8)**

* Of all the translations and commentaries, perhaps Mr. Winthrop Sargeant's translation gave an exact meaning for ***paramātma*** within the context of the other Sanskrit words in this verse, as ***the self which was exalted by yoga practice***.

***Śrī Bābāji Mahāśaya's Commentary:***

*Śrī* Krishna stressed again that one should judge the spiritual advancement of a person by his internal posture and not merely by his external actions. He indicated to Arjuna, that for all practical purposes, Arjuna should exhibit the internal discipline of yoga, but should do his physical duty regardless. One does not have to reject physical duties to complete yoga expertise; one has to do the duties, while using yoga to become detached from the various values human beings place on the different materials in material existence. Even though acting in the material world, an expert yogi remains satisfied with the realized experience he gained by mystic insight through higher yoga.

One does not find the non-fluctuating happiness by enjoying subtle and gross sense objects. One finds it by conquering the sensual energy, to remain at bay from those influences which use up spiritual power and draw one into liabilities.

सुहृन्मित्रार्युदासीन
मध्यस्थद्वेष्यबन्धुषु ।
साधुष्वपि च पापेषु
समबुद्धिर्विशिष्यते ॥६.९॥
suhṛnmitrāryudāsīna
madhyasthadveṣya bandhuṣu
sādhuṣvapi ca pāpeṣu
samabuddhirviśiṣyate (6.9)

*suhṛnmitrāryudāsīna = suhṛn (suhṛd) — friend + mitra — acquaintance + ary (ari) — enemy + udāsīna — indifferent; madhyasthadveṣyabandhuṣu = madhyastha — evenly disposed + dvesya — enemy + bandhuṣu — to kinsmen; sādhuṣv = sādhuṣu — in saintly people; api — also; ca — and; pāpeṣu — in sinful people; samabuddhir = samabuddhiḥ — one who exhibits balanced judgment; viśiṣyate — be regarded with distinction*

**A person who is indifferent to friend, acquaintance, and enemy, who is evenly-disposed to enemies and kinsmen, who exhibits balanced judgment towards saintly people or sinful ones, is to be regarded with distinction. (6.9)**

***Śrī Bābāji Mahāśaya's Commentary:***

This gives some idea of how a self-realized person acts and relates to others when he interacts in human society. We find that he is impartially-inclined even to enemies and he is not partially-disposed to relatives. It is as if everyone were his close relative indeed. This is because of the spiritual insight into the relationship between the spirits, one to another, regardless of the family of birth. Such a person, a saint, a sadhu, should be regarded with distinction as having attained spiritual realization.

Arjuna was biased towards relatives and thus *Śrī* Krishna upbraided Arjuna in the beginning of this conversation, stating that Arjuna mourned for that which should not be regretted and still expressed intelligent statements (2.11). If Arjuna were truly elevated and realized in scriptural truths, he would have qualified as a person with balanced judgment *(samabuddhih)*. He would not have singled out relatives and elders for pardon.

योगी युञ्जीत सततम्
आत्मानं रहसि स्थितः ।
एकाकी यतचित्तात्मा
निराशीरपरिग्रहः ॥६.१०॥
yogī yuñjīta satatam
ātmānaṁ rahasi sthitaḥ
ekākī yatacittātmā
nirāśīraparigrahaḥ (6.10)

*yogī — yogi; yuñjīta — should concentrate; satatam — constantly; ātmānam — on the self; rahasi — in isolation; sthitaḥ — situated; ekākī — alone; yatacittātmā = yata — controlling + citta — thinking + ātmā — self; nirāśīr — without desire; aparigrahaḥ — without possessions*

**In isolation, the yogi should constantly concentrate on the self. Being alone, he should be of controlled thinking and subdued self without desire and without possessions. (6.10)**

***Śrī Bābāji Mahāśaya's Commentary:***

Repeated attempts must be made to concentrate on the core self, in the middle of the mind chamber. At first one may not locate or perceive the various psychic components in the mind, but after steady practice for a time, there comes clarity, and then one can perceive the parts, one by one. One has to be in isolation *(rahasi),* otherwise one will be distracted continually and will be forced into the same normal pattern of psychic confusion and sensual endorsements. To separate the core self from the intellect, memory and sensual energy, one requires isolation, at least initially. Formerly, this isolation was maintained by yogis even in the advanced stages. There is sufficient evidence of this in the stories told in the Upanishads and the *Purāṇas* and elsewhere in the Vedic text like *Vālmīki Rāmāyaṇa* and *Mahābhārata*.

An ascetic yogi is required to be alone, even if he lives at the ashram, the school of the teacher's residence. Yoga practice is not collective religion. It is individual practice. This is necessary because each student is at a different stage. Each has to practice alone after receiving lessons and instructions on how to proceed.

During meditations or during introspective observations, one should be of controlled thinking. One may use a mantra, a repetitive meaningful sound, but one may not be required to do this. Ashram or hermitage life automatically means very little in the form of possessions and desires. This is the only way one can take up a serious yoga practice. Whatever one may gain in the material world will always be there, somewhere on some planet, in some dimension now and in the future, so when at the ashram, one should cast aside desires for worldly things and focus on the teachings and practice.

शुचौ देशे प्रतिष्ठाप्य
स्थिरमासनमात्मनः ।
नात्युच्छ्रितं नातिनीचं
चैलाजिनकुशोत्तरम् ॥६.११॥
śucau deśe pratiṣṭhāpya
sthiramāsanamātmanaḥ
nātyucchritaṁ nātinīcaṁ
cailājinakuśottaram (6.11)

*śucau — in clean; deśe — in place; pratiṣṭhāpya — fixing; sthiram — firm; āsanam — seat; ātmanaḥ — of his self; nātyucchritaṁ = na — not + atyucchritaṁ — too high; nātinīcam = na — not + atinīcam — too low; cailājinakuśottaram = caila — cloth + ajina — antelope skin + kuśa — kusha grass + uttaram — underneath*

**In a clean place, fixing for himself a firm seat which is not too high, not too low, with a covering layer of cloth, antelope skin and kusha grass underneath, (6.11)**

***Śrī Bābāji Mahāśaya's Commentary:***

This is the classic material environment for the practice of yoga austerities which include āsana, *prāṇāyāma, pratyāhār, dhāranā, dhyāna* and *samādhi*. The student yogi requires a small hut or room in the hermitage. The place needs to be clean. There should be a place where he would sit in yoga posture for meditation. This place is usually the same location where he would lie to sleep, even though it might be a different spot in the room. Formerly it was routine to have a covering of cotton or silk cloth, an antelope skin and kusha grass.

तत्रैकाग्रं मनः कृत्वा
यतचित्तेन्द्रियक्रियः ।
उपविश्यासने युञ्ज्याद्
योगमात्मविशुद्धये ॥६.१२॥
tatraikāgraṁ manaḥ kṛtvā
yatacittendriyakriyāḥ
upaviśyāsane yuñjyād
**yogamātmaviśuddhaye** (6.12)

*tatraikāgraṁ = tatra — there + ekāgram — single-focused; manaḥ — mind; kṛtvā — having made; yatacittendriyakriyaḥ = yata — controlled + citta — thought + indriyakriyaḥ — sense energy; upaviśyāsane = upaviśya — seating himself + āsane — in a posture; yuñyād = yuñyāt — should practice; yogamātmaviśuddhaye = yogam — to yoga discipline + ātma — self + viśuddhaye — to purification*

**...being there, seated in a posture, having the mind focused, the person who controls his thinking and sensual energy, should practice the yoga discipline for self-purification. (6.12)**

***Śrī Bābāji Mahāśaya's Commentary:***

Yoga practice, higher yoga in terms of *pratyāhār, dhāranā, dhyāna* and *samādhi,* is for self purification primarily. The student requires a single focus *(ekāgram)*. This is given to him by the advanced yoga teacher or he may select this for himself as he is inspired according to the level of practice. Such a single focus may change as he progresses through the course of yoga. Thinking must be stopped. Sensual energy must be disciplined, so that it does not induce the intellect to scheme up designs in the imagination faculty.

The student must sit for long periods, observing the workings of the various components of consciousness, until he can get all of them ordered and make the intellect capable of supernatural vision.

समं कायशिरोग्रीवं
धारयन्नचलं स्थिरः ।
संप्रेक्ष्य नासिकाग्रं स्वं
दिशश्चानवलोकयन् ॥६.१३॥
samaṁ kāyaśirogrīvaṁ
dhārayannacalaṁ sthiraḥ
saṁprekṣya nāsikāgraṁ svaṁ
diśaścānavalokayan (6.13)

*samam — balanced; kāyaśirogrīvaṁ = kāya — body + śiro (śiraḥ) — head + grīvam — neck; dhārayan — holding; acalam — without movement; sthiraḥ — steady; saṁprekṣya — gazing at; nāsikāgraṁ = nāsikā — nostril + agram — tip; svam — own; diśaścānavalokayan = diśaḥ — the directions + ca — and + anavalokayan — not looking*

**Holding the body, head and neck in balance, steady without movement, gaze at the tip of the nose, not looking in any other direction. (6.13)**

***Śrī Bābāji Mahāśaya's Commentary:***

*Samam kāyaśirogrīvam dhārayan acalam sthirah* is the age-old requirement for holding the body, head and neck in balance. This was found to be the most ideal posture for practicing meditation. Other postures for holding the body may be used, and particular individuals may find such other poses to be adequate, but this age-old recommendation was used by ancient yogis because they got the most success in that posture. It is the posture in which the force of gravity is centralized on the spinal column, passing through the column pulling downwards to the base of the spine. The same force of gravity exists in the subtle world, since those physical objects, from which gravity is derived, have a subtle counterpart.

*Nāsikāgrama* means the tip end of the nose, but some yogis say that it means the top tip of the bridge of the nose. Note the two positions as follows.

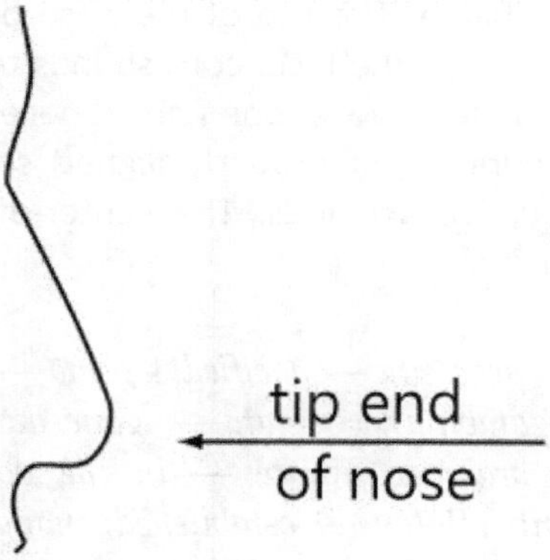


For student yogins, the tip of the nose, the most protruding point, is the initial focusing point. This is because such yogins have to purify the kundalini chakra. This point is the coordinate point with the base chakra. More advanced yogis whose kundalini chakras are purified, meditate at the brow chakra, which is a classic meditation point. These two points and others may be termed as location mantras rather than sound mantras, which are repeated orally or mentally. Location mantra focusing points are vital in *kriyā* practice.

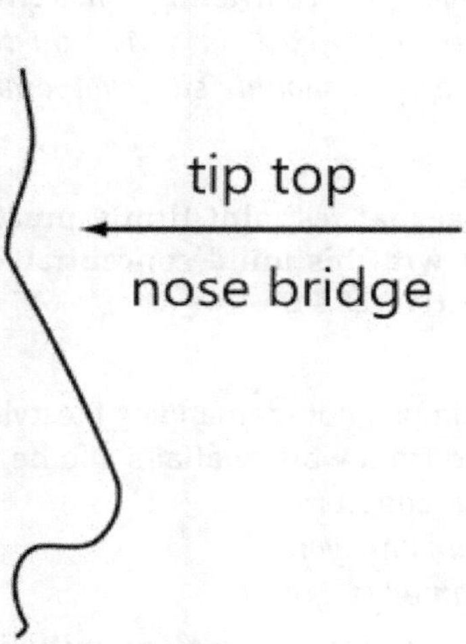


*Śrī* Krishna used the term *svam* which means your own. This makes it clear that the *yogin* has to practice for himself. He cannot use the practice of a more advanced *yogin*. He must progress through the stages of yoga by himself and advance quickly or slowly according to individual capacity. The teacher's advancement is not the student's credit and he cannot use that or bypass any stage. Everything depends on individual aptitude and rate of practice.

*Anavalokayan* means not looking in any other direction or thinking of anything else (*yatacitta,* 6.10). Thus if the student finds that he cannot help but look elsewhere and that he must think of one thing or another, either something sacred or profane, then it means that he must make a more detailed study of the components of consciousness, the various parts of the mind, to see what causes the diversions and to see why he unwillingly pursues the distractions. This is the beginning of *kriyā yoga* in earnest. The student must himself research this and discuss his problems with the teacher who is more advanced.

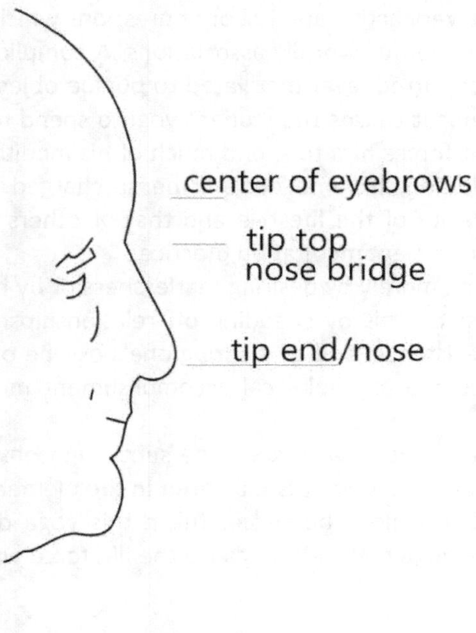


*Kriyā yoga* means direct control of the components in the mind. For mastership one must give up props including mantras, and whatever else is used in religious societies to pacify the unruly mind. For the purpose of yoga, the mind must be brought under tight and absolute control.

*Śrī* Krishna did not in the discourse give the reason for meditation at the tip end of the nose. However in the history of yoga, especially in *Śrī* Gorakshnatha's sect, there were many yogis who focused on the tip end of the nose. From our research, apart from what is written in small yoga journals like the <u>*Haṭha Yoga Pradīpika*</u>, we found that the tip end of the nose corresponds to the base chakra on the spine, the *mūlādhāra* or root chakra. The top of the nose bridge which is the highest point on the nose where it contours into the face, corresponds to the sex chakra, the *svādhiṣṭhāna* chakra. When practicing kundalini yoga, one finds it necessary to meditate on these points in order to get the chakras purified and properly aligned, so that they no longer influence the body in yogically-destructive activities. The center-of-the-eyebrows chakra is a different focusing point.

प्रशान्तात्मा विगतभीर्
ब्रह्मचारिव्रते स्थितः ।
मनः संयम्य मच्चित्तो
युक्त आसीत मत्परः ॥६.१४॥
praśāntātmā vigatabhīr
brahmacārivrate sthitaḥ
manaḥ saṁyamya maccitto
yukta āsīta matparaḥ (6.14)

*praśāntātmā = praśānta — pacified + ātmā — self; vigatabhīr (vigatabhīḥ) = vigata — gone away + bhīḥ — fear; brahmacārivrate — in the vow of sexual restraint; sthitaḥ — established; manaḥ — mind; saṁyamya — controlling; maccitto = maccittaḥ — though fixed on Me; yukta — disciplined; āsīta — should sit; matparaḥ — devoted to Me*

**With a pacified self, free from fears, with a vow of sexual restraint firmly practiced, with mind controlled and having Me in his thought with his mind concentrated, he should sit, being devoted to Me as the Supreme Objective. (6.14)**

***Śrī Bābāji Mahāśaya's Commentary:***

*Praśāntātmā*, a pacified self, happens by virtue of a simple, non-demanding lifestyle and high association with retired yogis. These must be retired from worldly affairs and be using the tranquil, reserved method mentioned in verse 3 of this chapter:

*āruruksormuneryogaṁ karma kāraṇamucyate*
*yogārūḍhasya tasyaiva śamaḥ kāraṇamucyate (6.3)*

***For a philosophical man who strives for yoga expertise, cultural activity is recommended. For one who has mastered yoga already, the tranquil reserved method is the means. (6.3)***

One who is not simple in lifestyle cannot successfully practice *buddhi yoga* or *kriyā yoga*, but such a person may practice anyway, without expecting rapid advancement. A complicated lifestyle causes the memory to be very active and full of impressions which are counterproductive to yoga and which foster numerous worldly associations. A complicated lifestyle causes the sensual energies to be ever stirred, ever motivated to pursue objects in the external subtle and gross environment. Thus it causes the student yogi to spend much time quelling and suppressing the sensuality. It forces him to spend much of his meditation time considering sensual impressions. In addition, his intellect will be surcharged with schemes and plans for supporting the complexity of the lifestyle and that of others with whom he associates. All this will cause a very inefficient meditation practice.

One cannot be *vigatabhīr* or free from fears, merely by desiring fearlessness or by being determined to challenge hardships. One must do this by shedding off relationships with persons who are involved in the struggle for existence, and by clearing one's psyche of the need for participating in such a struggle. This is a psychological accomplishment mostly, attained in the practice of *buddhi yoga*.

*Brahmacārivrate* means the vow of celibacy, the vow to keep the subtle and physical bodies without sexual polarity. This is vital in *buddhi yoga*. It is mastered in the elementary stages when one practices kundalini yoga. One cannot be successful in this yoga of *Śrī* Krishna if one does not become celibate by the yoga methods, because the life force will be needlessly dissipated by sexual involvements either on the subtle or gross levels or on both.

*Śrī* Krishna requested that every yogi be devoted to Him *(matparah)*. This was explained in the verse where *Śrī* Krishna appraised Arjuna's devotedness and friendliness:

*sa evāyaṁ mayā te'dya yogaḥ proktaḥ purātanaḥ*
*bhakto'si me sakhā ceti rahasyaṁ hyetaduttamam (4.3)*

***Today, this ancient yoga technique is explained to you by Me, since you are devoted to Me and are My friend. Indeed, this is confidential and is the best teaching. (4.3)***

In cases where someone practices *buddhi yoga* but has not heard of *Śrī* Krishna, and receives a valid practice from a teacher who did not hear of *Śrī* Krishna but who discovered the practice or was taught by a discoverer of the same, that student should be devoted and friendly to the teacher. We have to assume that even if someone has not heard of *Śrī* Krishna or if someone discovered the practice, then still, ultimately, *Śrī* Krishna is the origin of the teaching.

Everyone reading this translation and commentary, should heed this instruction of *Śrī* Krishna to be dear and friendly to Him, so as to stay in His confidence ever. *Śrī* Krishna recommended that the yogi should fix the mental and emotional energy on Krishna Himself as the Supreme Objective *(maccitta)*. This is not an ordinary request. It is extraordinary, because one has to first know Krishna before one can do this in fact. One gets to know *Śrī* Krishna by hearing of His lectures and reading of His pastimes or *līlās*. One must do this with faith. Gradually, as one masters *buddhi yoga*, one may reach Krishna outside of this subtle and gross material world, reaching Him in His spiritual domains. And that is the ultimate objective of this *buddhi yoga* practice, which is explained in the holy *Bhagavad Gītā*.

युञ्जन्नेवं सदात्मानं
योगी नियतमानसः ।
शान्तिं निर्वाणपरमां
मत्संस्थामधिगच्छति ॥६.१५॥
yuñjannevaṁ sadātmānaṁ
yogī niyatamānasaḥ
śāntiṁ nirvāṇaparamāṁ
matsaṁsthāmadhigacchati (6.15)

*yuñjan — disciplining; evaṁ — as described; sadā — continuously; 'tmānaṁ = ātmānam — himself; yogī — yogi; niyatamānasaḥ — one who has a subdued mind; śāntiṁ — spiritual security; nirvāṇaparamāṁ = nirvāṇa — extinction of mundane affinity + paramām — highest living state; matsaṁsthām — existentially positioned with Me; adhigacchati — achieves*

**Disciplining himself continuously as described, the yogi who has a subdued mind, experiences spiritual security. He achieves the extinction of mundane affinity as he simultaneously attains the highest living state. He achieves an existential position with Me. (6.15)**

### *Śrī Bābāji Mahāśaya's Commentary:*

*Matsamsthām* means to be existentially positioned with *Śrī* Krishna, to have one's existence relocated in focus out of this world, into the spiritual provinces. One can do this, only when one's attention is completely lifted from this world. This is beyond *karma yoga*. In *karma yoga* one's attention is lifted from personal needs and family interests, and shifts over to the priorities of *Śrī* Krishna's Universal Form. Hereby, one can perform duties which support a righteous lifestyle for all concerned, either willingly or being imposed by force, as Arjuna was requested to do at *Kurukṣetra*. In *ātma-viśuddha yoga* as explained in this chapter, one moves beyond that, so that one's attention is lifted from the concerns for this world, even from the concerns about righteousness or *dharma*. One relocates all of one's interest into the spiritual place where *Śrī* Krishna resides. That is the highest living state, the *paramām*, attained due to extinction of mundane affinity, *nirvāṇam*.

By a thorough discipline of the components of the mind *(niyatamānasah)*, by limiting the mind's access to the spirit's attention, the *yogin* experiences spiritual security due to not having to lean on the intellect, memory and senses for information and directions in what to sanction and what to prohibit. This verse describes a *brahma yoga* accomplishment.

नात्यश्नतस्तु योगोऽस्ति
न चैकान्तमनश्नतः ।
न चातिस्वप्नशीलस्य
जाग्रतो नैव चार्जुन ॥६.१६॥
nātyaśnatastu yogo'sti
na caikāntamanaśnataḥ
na cātisvapnaśīlasya
jāgrato naiva cārjuna (6.16)

*nātyaśnatas = na — not + atyaśnatas — of too much eating; tu — but; yogo = yogaḥ — yoga; 'sti = asti — it is; na — not; caikāntam = ca — and + ekāntam — solely; anaśnataḥ — of not eating at all; na — not; cātisvapnaśīlasya = ca — and + atisvapna — too much sleeping + śīlasya — of habit; jāgrato = jāgrataḥ — of staying awake; naiva = na — nor + eva — indeed; cārjuna = ca — and + arjuna — Arjuna*

**But Arjuna, yoga practice does not consist of eating too much. And it is not the practice of not eating at all, nor the habit of sleeping too much or staying awake either. (6.16)**

***Siddha Swami's Commentary:***

Yoga practice is something precise. Stage by stage, it is accomplished. It is not a matter of depriving anyone of food or sleep or anything else. It must be done in due consideration to the person's complexities. The austerities are to be performed with due regard to the physiology and psychology of the gross body and the subtle system.

Certainly yoga practice has nothing to do with over-eating but all the same it has nothing to do with eating so little that one becomes imbalanced in nutrition and disturbed mentally. It is not about over-sleeping and it does not eliminate the need for the sleep of the gross body and the proper rest of the subtle psychology.

Eating and sleeping are reduced considerably in yoga, but only as one masters the *āsana* postures and the *prāṇāyāma* methods which change one's lifestyle so that one does not require to over-eat or over-sleep. There is much resting of the psychology in yoga. Through resting one sets the mind away from anxieties and is able to detach the attention from the problems which stir up memories. This is all part of *buddhi yoga*, or as we sometimes call it, *kriyā yoga*.

युक्ताहारविहारस्य
युक्तचेष्टस्य कर्मसु ।
युक्तस्वप्नावबोधस्य
योगो भवति दुःखहा ॥६.१७॥
yuktāhāravihārasya
yuktaceṣṭasya karmasu
yuktasvapnāvabodhasya
yogo bhavati duḥkhahā (6.17)

*yuktāhāravihārasya = yukta — regulated + āhāra — eating + vihārasya — of leisure; yuktaceṣṭasya = yukta — disciplined + ceṣtasya — of endeavor; karmasu — in duties; yuktasvapnāvabodhasya = yukta — disciplined + svapna — sleep + avabodhasya — of waking; yogo = yogah — yoga practice; bhavati — is; duḥkhahā — distress-removing*

**For a person who is regulated in eating and in leisure, who is disciplined in the endeavor of duties, who is moderate in sleeping and waking, for him, the yoga practice is a distress-remover. (6.17)**

***Śrī Bābāji Mahāśaya's Commentary:***

*Śrī* Krishna attests that yoga practice is a distress remover. Yoga is for self purification and that entails removing whatever causes distress *(duhkhahā)*. In this verse *Śrī* Krishna listed five potential causes for distress, namely eating, leisure, endeavor of duties, sleeping and waking. These five ways of spending time, if not moderated properly and regulated efficiently, will cause distress. Yoga is designed to get these under control for their efficient usage.

यदा विनियतं चित्तम्
आत्मन्येवावतिष्ठते ।
निःस्पृहः सर्वकामेभ्यो
युक्त इत्युच्यते तदा ॥६.१८॥
yadā viniyataṁ cittam
ātmanyevāvatiṣṭhate
niḥspṛhaḥ sarvakāmebhyo
yukta ityucyate tadā (6.18)

*yadā — when; viniyataṁ — tightly controlled; cittam — thought; ātmany = ātmani — in the spiritual core self; evāvatiṣṭhate = eva — alone + avatiṣṭhate — is attentive; niḥspṛhaḥ — free from desire; sarvakāmebhyo (sarvakāmebhyaḥ) = sarva — all + kāmebhyaḥ — from cravings; yukta — proficient in yoga; ity = iti — thus; ucyate — is said; tadā — then*

**When with tightly controlled thought, he is attentive to his spiritual core self alone, being freed from desires and from all cravings, he is said to be proficient in yoga. (6.18)**

***Author's Commentary:***

Śrī *Bābāji Mahāśaya* suggested that this verse be translated as follows:

**When with tightly controlled mental and emotional energy, he is attentive to his spiritual core self alone, being freed from desires and from all cravings, he is said to be proficient in yoga.**

He suggested that the word *cittam* be translated, not as thought but as mental and emotional energy. He said this includes the sensual energy force. As far as thoughts are concerned, he stated that thoughts or ideas are included in *citta* but it means more than just thoughts. The ability to stop or even to greatly slow down the occurence of thoughts and ideas indicates that the *citta* mento-emotional forces are curbed, at least for the duration.

This verse describes an *ātma* yoga technique. This was explained by *Śrī* Krishna in different words in Chapter Two and Chapter Three as follows:

*śrībhagavānuvāca*
*prajahāti yadā kāmān sarvānpārtha manogatān*
*ātmanyevātmanā tuṣṭaḥ sthitaprajñastadocyate (2.55)*

***The Blessed Lord said: When someone abandons all cravings, O son of Pṛthā, and escapes from mental dominance, being self content, then that person is identified as one with steady insight. (2.55)***

*yastvātmaratireva syād ātmatṛptaśca mānavaḥ*
*ātmanyeva ca saṁtuṣṭas tasya kāryaṁ na vidyate (3.17)*

***A person who is spiritually-pleased, self-satisfied and spiritually-content, has no cultural duties. (3.17)***

***Sri Bābāji Mahāśaya stated:***

When a *yogin* becomes attentive to his spiritual core self alone, he is transferred to a *brahma yogin* teacher to begin a new set of disciplines. Some student yogis stop doing āsana and *prāṇāyāma* at this stage, but there is no harm in the continuation of those two disciplines.

यथा दीपो निवातस्थो
नेङ्गते सोपमा स्मृता ।
योगिनो यतचित्तस्य
युञ्जतो योगमात्मनः ॥६.१९॥
yathā dīpo nivātastho
neṅgate sopamā smṛtā
yogino yatacittasya
yuñjato yogamātmanaḥ (6.19)

*yathā — as; dīpo = dīpaḥ — lamp; nivātastho (nivātasthaḥ) = nivāta — windless + sthaḥ — situated; neṅgate = na — not + ingate — flickers; sopamā = so (sāḥ) — this + upamā — in comparison; smṛtā — recalled; yogino = yoginaḥ — of the yogi; yatacittasya — of a person whose thinking is restrained; yuñjato = yuñjataḥ — of practicing; yogam — yoga; ātmanaḥ — of the self*

**This comparison is recalled: A lamp in a windless place which does not flicker, and a yogi of controlled thought who performs disciplines in relation to the spiritual self. (6.19)**

***Author's Commentary:***

*Śrī Bābāji Mahāśaya* reminds yogins to translate *citta* as mental and emotional energy, not just as thoughts or ideas. The entire mental and emotional energies must be restrained for success in yoga meditation, otherwise the effort at stillness will be a farce.

He stated that this comparison is rather appropriate, since in the mind space, the self must be able to focus on itself without being distracted by the mental and emotional force, or by the mental components which use such energy for their operations. These components are the intellect, the memory and the senses. He said that the intellect has mainly two parts to it; one is the analytical switching device and the other is the imagination orb. This imagination orb functions also as a visualization instrument to create images and pictures in the minds of human beings.

यत्रोपरमते चित्तं
निरुद्धं योगसेवया ।
यत्र चैवात्मनात्मानं
पश्यन्नात्मनि तुष्यति ॥६.२०॥
yatroparamate cittaṁ
niruddhaṁ yogasevayā
yatra caivātmanātmānaṁ
paśyannātmani tuṣyati (6.20)

*yatroparamate = yatra — where + uparamate — it stops; cittaṁ — thinking; niruddhaṁ — restraint; yogasevayā = yoga – yoga discipline + sevayā — by practice; yatra — where; caivātmanā = ca — and + eva — indeed + ātmanā — by the self; 'tmānaṁ = ātmānam — the self; paśyan — seeing; ātmani — in the self; tuṣyati — is satisfied*

**At the place where being restrained by yoga practice, thinking stops, and at the place where the yogi perceives the self by the self, he is satisfied in the self. (6.20)**

***Author's Commentary:***

Thinking is not *citta* but rather thinking is one of the functions or operations of *citta*. According to *Śrī Patañjali Mahārṣi*, thinking is merely a *vṛtti* of the *citta*. Thinking is one of the five mental operations which *Śrī Patañjali* stated must cease for the perfection of yoga.

***Śrī Bābāji Mahāśaya's Commentary:***

*Yatra* as the beginning word in both of the Sanskrit sentences of this verse, has much significance in *kriyā yoga* or *buddhi yoga*. This is because of the introduction to the student yogi of a location mantra, instead of a sound repeating focus. The *yogin* focuses on a location.

The two locations mentioned are different places in the mind environment. The place where thinking ceases, where the mental and emotional energy ceases fluctuations, and the place where the self is perceived by itself without the aid of the intellect or the sensual energies which surround the mind, are two different locations. These must be discovered by the student yogi. He should discuss this with a teacher who is a more advanced *yogin*. This verse explains two *kriyā*s of the *kriyā* and *buddhi yoga* process. Here are diagrams:

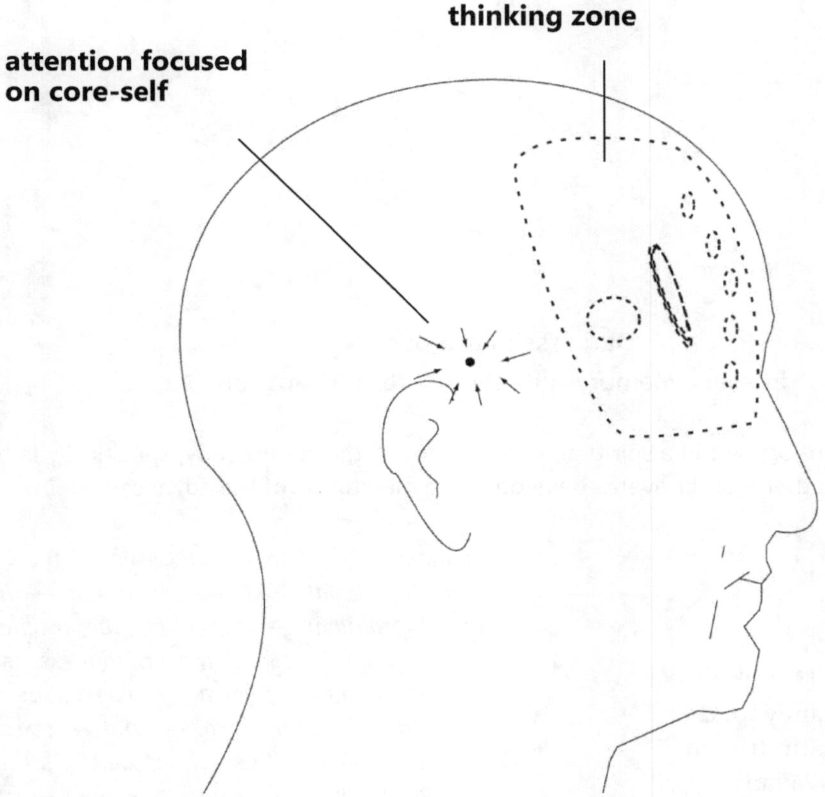


Thinking zone consists of intellect, memory and sensual orbs.

When attention is focused on core-self, thinking zone is disempowered.

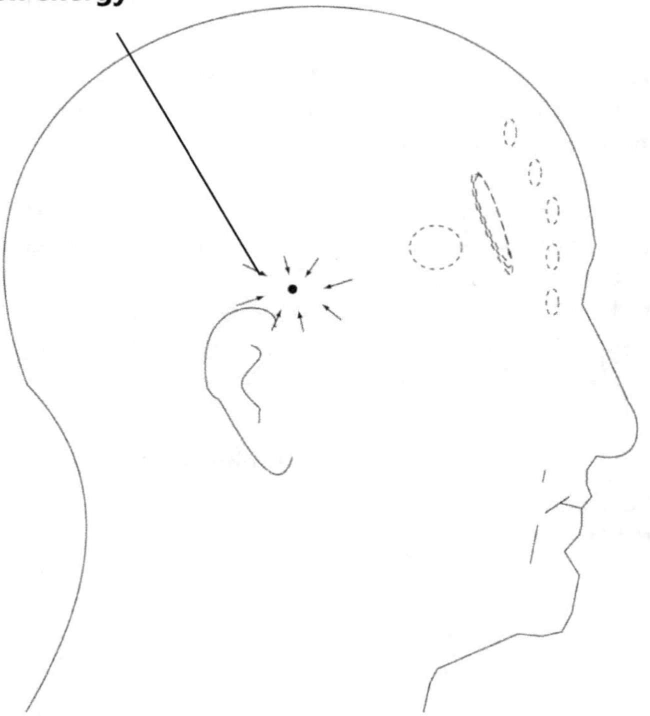


During self-absorption,
intellect, memory and sensual orbs remain silent

These locations are not in a spiritual world but are in the subtle body, specifically in the subtle head. From there, other events develop in the meditation of the advanced *yogin*.

सुखमात्यन्तिकं यत्तद्
बुद्धिग्राह्यमतीन्द्रियम् ।
वेत्ति यत्र न चैवायं
स्थितश्चलति तत्त्वतः ॥६.२१॥
sukhamātyantikaṁ yattad
buddhigrāhyamatīndriyam
vetti yatra na caivāyaṁ
sthitaścalati tattvataḥ (6.21)

*sukham — happiness; ātyantikaṁ — continuous; yat = yad — which; tad — this; buddhigrāhyam — grasp by the intellect; atīndriyam — beyond the mundane senses; vetti — he knows; yatra — whereabout; na — not; caivāyam = ca — and + eva — indeed + ayam — this; sthitaścalati = sthitaḥ — established + calati — he shifted; tattvataḥ — the reality*

**He knows the whereabouts of that continuous happiness, which is grasped by the intellect and which is beyond the mundane senses. And being established, he does not shift from that reality. (6.21)**

***Śrī Bābāji Mahāśaya's Commentary:***

This is in reference to the *antarjyotih* brilliant consciousness which was given in

*Bhagavad Gītā*, 5.24. This technique of the *kriyā yoga* process is a development which occurs after long sincere practice in isolation.

*yo'ntaḥsukho'ntarārāmas tathāntarjyotireva yaḥ*
*sa yogī brahmanirvāṇaṁ brahmabhūto'dhigacchati (5.24)*

***The person who is happy within, who is spiritually delighted and as a result, experiences the brilliant consciousness, he, that yogi, experiences the stoppage of disturbing sensuality and attains constant spirituality in absorption on the spiritual plane. (5.24)***

*Śrī* Krishna was specific in mentioning that this is grasped by the intellect but it is beyond the usual sensual energies. In other words, the intellect is able to enjoy something that transcends the normal sensual perception. And being established in this type of *samādhi* trance consciousness, the yogi does not shift from that reality. This confirms that the imagination orb of the intellect does transform into a spiritual eye with which to see into the chit akasha, the spiritual sky. This is done without the use of the subtle senses and without the use of the memory. It involves the spirit, his attention energies and the detached, highly energized, transformed intellect organ of the subtle body.

Having broken the link between the intellect and the memory, as well as the connection between the intellect and the sensual energy, the *yogin* holds the intellect in a voidal condition without ideas being derived from the memory or sensual energy. Then after some time, the intellect evolves into a transcendental sense and can perceive reality in the spiritual places. This is a supernatural vision. The spiritual vision of the spiritual body is higher yet, but this supernatural vision is preliminary in the course of realizing the spiritual form with limbs and senses.

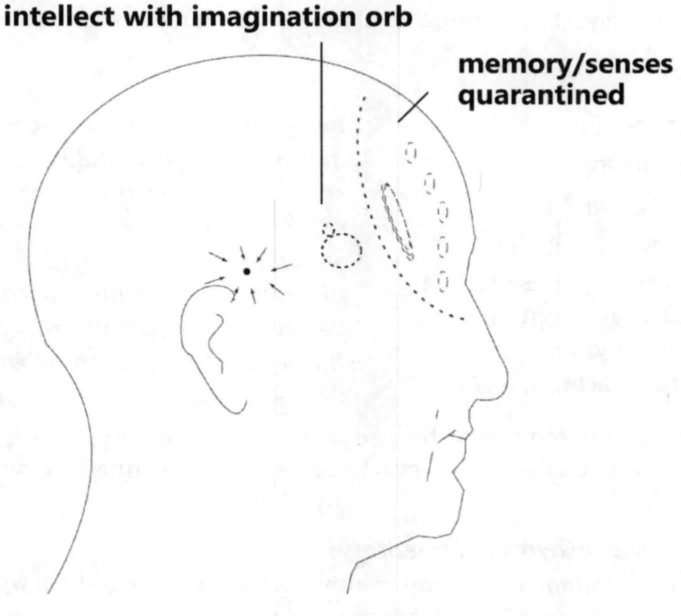


When memory and sensual orbs are quarantined,
the intellect manifests a separate imagination orb
which affords supernatural perception

यं लब्ध्वा चापरं लाभं
मन्यते नाधिकं ततः ।
यस्मिन्स्थितो न दुःखेन
गुरुणापि विचाल्यते ॥६.२२॥
yaṁ labdhvā cāparaṁ lābhaṁ
manyate nādhikaṁ tataḥ
yasminsthito na duḥkhena
guruṇāpi vicālyate (6.22)

*yaṁ — which; labdhvā — having attained; cāparaṁ = ca — and + aparaṁ — other; lābhaṁ — attainment; manyate — he thinks; nādhikam = na — not + adhikam — greater; tataḥ — than that; yasmin — which; sthito = sthitaḥ — established; na — not; duḥkhena — by distress; guruṇāpi = guruṇā — by deep + api — also; vicālyate — is drawn away*

**And having attained that, he thinks there is no greater attainment. Being established in that, he is not drawn away, even by deep distress. (6.22)**

***Śrī Bābāji Mahāśaya's Commentary:***

It is a great relief for the yogi when the imagination orb of the *buddhi* organ converts into supernatural vision to see into the chit akash. This is because the suspension of the intellect's relationship with the memory and sensual energies causes the meditation to be tedious on occasion. Many student yogins turned away from yoga after becoming frightened, disgusted or dried out by the lack of sensual interplay, when the intellect is effectively cut off from the memory and senses. Thus, when at last there develops supernatural vision, the *yogin* is relieved. Attaining that, as *Śrī* Krishna stated, the *yogin* thinks that there is no greater attainment *(lābham manyate nādhikam tatah)*. Some student yogins practice for years and due to faults in practice, never attain this stage. They eventually become disheartened and become very adverse to all types of existence, since they assume that there must not be any other varied reality except this subtle and gross material energy. It is because of flaws in their practice and due to a lack of competent teachers.

तं विद्यादुःखसंयोग -
वियोगं योगसंज्ञितम् ।
स निश्चयेन योक्तव्यो
योगोऽनिर्विण्णचेतसा ॥६.२३॥
taṁ vidyādduḥkhasaṁyoga-
viyogaṁ yogasaṁjñitam
sa niścayena yoktavyo
yogo'nirviṇṇacetasā (6.23)

*tam — this; vidyād = vidyāt — let it be understood; duḥkhasaṁyoga = duḥkha — emotional distress + saṁyoga — emotional identity with; viyogaṁ — separation; yogasaṁjñitam = yoga — mastery of yoga + saṁjñitam — recognized as; sa = saḥ — this; niścayena — with determination; yoktavyo = yoktavyaḥ — to be practiced; yogo = yogah — yoga; 'nirviṇṇacetasā (anirviṇṇacetasā) = anirviṇṇa — not depressed + cetasā — with thought*

**Let it be understood, that this separation from emotional distress is the mastery of yoga. This yoga is to be practiced with determination and without depressing thought. (6.23)**

***Śrī Bābāji Mahāśaya's Commentary:***

What *Śrī Patañjali* declared in other words, was stated by *Śrī* Krishna in a completely different way. *Śrī Patañjali Mahārṣi* stated that the mastery of yoga is denoted by stoppage of the *cittavṛtti*, the operations of the mental and emotional energies in the mind chamber. *Śrī* Krishna put it differently, describing that mastery from another angle. He acclaimed it as separation from emotional distress, *duhkhasamyogaviyogam*. In the *buddhi yoga* system, which *Śrī* Krishna originally introduced, this translated into the intellect organ being weaned completely from its dependence on and attachment to the memory and sensual energies.

*Śrī* Krishna stated tacitly that this yoga should be practiced with determination and without depressing feelings. This verse should be translated as:

**Let it be understood, that this separation from emotional distress is the mastery of buddhi yoga. This yoga is to be practiced with determination and without depressing feelings. (6.23)**

If there are depressing feelings, if the yogi gets bored in the practice, it is because he did not use the naad special sound which comes in through the right ear. This sound is expressly used as a focus until the intellect is transformed into supernatural vision to peer into spiritual dimensions. Even though the naad sound was not mentioned in the *Bhagavad Gītā* discourse to Arjuna, it was given to Uddhava as the *ghoṣa* subtle sound. It needs be practiced. Some student yogins who are lucky, progress quickly into the supernatural vision which is yielded by the blank intellect which was separated from the memory and ordinary sensual energy.

संकल्पप्रभवान्कामांस्
त्यक्त्वा सर्वानशेषतः ।
मनसैवेन्द्रियग्रामं
विनियम्य समन्ततः ॥६.२४॥
saṁkalpaprabhavānkāmāṁs
tyaktvā sarvānaśeṣataḥ
manasaivendriyagrāmaṁ
viniyamya samantataḥ (6.24)

*saṁkalpaprabhavān = saṁkalpa — motive + prabhavān — produced; kāmāṁs — cravings; tyaktvā — having abandoned; sarvān — all; aśeṣataḥ — without exception; manasaivendriyagrāmaṁ = manasā — by mind + eva — indeed + indriyagrāmaṁ — the total sensual energy; viniyamya — controlling; samantataḥ — completely*

**Abandoning without exception, all desires which are produced from motivation, and completely restraining the total sensual energy by the mind, (6.24)**

***Śrī Bābāji Mahāśaya's Commentary:***

This is evidence that the system of yoga codified by *Śrī Patañjali Mahārṣi* was valid and precise. *Cittavritti* in the *Patañjali* nomenclature is given here as *indriyagrāmam*, the aggregate of the senses, the total sensual energy. This is the mental and emotional energy in the psyche. *Patañjali* instructed that it be completely restrained *(niroḍha),* which is what *Śrī* Krishna also advised long before:

*yatroparamate cittaṁ niruddhaṁ yogasevayā*
*yatra caivātmanātmānaṁ paśyannātmani tuṣyati (6.20)*

***At the place where being restrained by yoga practice, the mental and sensual energy stops operating, and at the place where the yogi perceives the self by the self, he is satisfied in the self. (6.20)* (Sri Bābāji Mahāśaya's translation)**

*Manasā* means by the mind or by the arranged order of the components in the mind. Due to this arrangement whereby the *yogin* can enforce his will in the mind, the intellect is no longer prejudiced by the memory and sensual energy. The sensual energy remains but it numerous transformations whereby it bewitches and engages the intellect and thus misleads the attention of the spirit. This brings on a certain yogic order in the mental chamber. This is the objective of *buddhi yoga*, as *Śrī* Krishna originally taught it.

शनैः शनैरुपरमेद्
बुद्ध्या धृतिगृहीतया ।
आत्मसंस्थं मनः कृत्वा
न किंचिदपि चिन्तयेत् ॥ ६.२५ ॥
śanaiḥ śanairuparamed
buddhyā dhṛtigṛhītayā
ātmasaṁsthaṁ manaḥ kṛtvā
na kiṁcidapi cintayet (6.25)

*śanaiḥ śanair (śanaiḥ) — little by little; uparamed = uparamet — should withdraw from sensual activity; buddhyā — by intelligence; dhṛtigṛhītayā = dhṛti — firmness + gṛhītayā — grasped; ātmasaṁsthaṁ = ātma — spiritual self + saṁsthaṁ — fixed; manah — mind; kṛtvā — having made; na — not; kiṁcit — anything; api — even; cintayet — should think*

**...little by little, with a firm grasp by the intelligence, he should withdraw from sensual activity. Having made his mind to be fixed on the spiritual self, he should not think of anything. (6.25)**

***Author's Commentary:***

*Śrī Bābāji Mahāśaya* translated this verse as follows:

**...little by little, with a firm grasp by the intellect, he should withdraw from sensual activity. Having made his mind to be fixed on the spiritual self, he should not focus on anything else.(6.25)**

He changed the word *think* to *focus* and the word *intelligence* to *intellect.*

***Śrī Bābāji Mahāśaya's Commentary:***

Little by little means over a long period, practicing day after day steadily, until one masters the *buddhi yoga kriyā* to control the intellect. The intellect is then made to control the memory and sensual energies, so that these subtle instruments do not dominate the psychology. They are gradually and surely subdued by the *buddhi yoga* or *kriyā yoga* introspective process done under the direction of *Śrī* Krishna or His able agent.

The instruments in the mind are made to focus on the self but if any of them are unable to do so, they are left dormant without activity, so that they do not interfere with self-focus. It is necessary to withdraw backwards in the head of the subtle body, in order to disempower the intellect. Once done consistently, the intellect becomes subdued, even though for some careless students, the intellect may again build up its alliance with the memory and senses and conjointly fight the self to dominate it, rather than to be subdued.

यतो यतो निश्चरति
मनश्चञ्चलमस्थिरम् ।
ततस्ततो नियम्यैतद्
आत्मन्येव वशं नयेत् ॥ ६.२६ ॥
yato yato niścarati
manaścañcalamasthiram
tatastato niyamyaitad
ātmanyeva vaśaṁ nayet (6.26)

*yato yato = yataḥ yataḥ — wherever; niścarati — wanders away; manaścañcalam = manas — mind + cañcalam — drifting; asthiram — unsteady; tatastato = tatastataḥ — from there; niyamyaitad = niyamya — restrain + etad — it; ātmany (ātmani) — in the self; eva — indeed; vaśam — control; nayet — should direct*

**To wherever the unsteady, drifty mind wanders, from there he should restrain it. He should direct the mind to control it in the self. (6.26)**

***Śrī Bābāji Mahāśaya's Commentary:***

In attaining salvation or liberation, a limited entity cannot avoid controlling his mind. He must bring the mind under subjugation or he will continue onwards in the haphazard transmigrations. This does not mean that the mind is one thing or one component. It consists of several components which are the intellect, the memory and the sensual energies. Each of these is subdued by different methods because each has different ways of operation. The mind is the chamber which houses the sensual energy, memory, intellect, attention of the spirit and the spirit itself. The nature of the mind, its convention, is to drift from topic to topic and to stall sometimes on nothingness. The self has to force the mind to remain on one topic, on one focus and to go back to that focus if it drifts off by its wandering habit.

The mind is powered by *praṇa* or subtle material energy. This is sometimes called shakti or *cittavṛtti*. Thus a student yogi finds it necessary to study how the mind ingests and consumes pranic energy and how higher grades of such energy affect the instruments of the mind.

प्रशान्तमनसं ह्येनं
योगिनं सुखमुत्तमम् ।
उपैति शान्तरजसं
ब्रह्मभूतमकल्मषम् ॥ ६.२७॥
praśāntamanasaṁ hyenaṁ
yoginaṁ sukhamuttamam
upaiti śāntarajasaṁ
brahmabhūtamakalmaṣam (6.27)

*praśāntamanasaṁ = praśānta — psychologically pacified + manasaṁ — mind; hyenaṁ = hy (hi) — indeed + enam — him; yoginaṁ — yogi; sukham — happiness; uttamam — superior; upaiti — experiences; śāntarajasaṁ = śānta — calmed + rajasam — emotion; brahmabhūtam — spiritual level; akalmaṣam — free from bad tendencies*

**Indeed, being psychologically pacified, the yogi, whose emotions are calmed, who is on the spiritual plane, who is free from bad tendencies, experiences superior happiness. (6.27)**

***Śrī Bābāji Mahāśaya's Commentary:***

Until a *yogin* reaches the superior happiness, *sukham uttamam*, he cannot be certain about practice. Thus many students go away from yoga because of not linking into the plane of consciousness where this happiness emanates. But one must be freed from bad tendencies *(akalmaṣam)*, before one can get that superior joy. Otherwise, if one does not continue yoga practice, and if one does not succeed at it, one must go back to the material world and take up a religion that allows one to be satisfied with a happiness in the normal mind-set.

Arjuna was devoted and friendly towards *Śrī* Krishna, as the Lord proclaimed in Chapter Four *(bhakto'si me sakhā,* 4.3), and still Arjuna was not situated in the superior happiness at *Kurukṣetra*. It is hard to attain this, even for such dear devotees of the Lord. One's emotions must be calmed by the *buddhi yoga* mastership, and one must be freed from the bad tendencies which are dictated into the mind compartment by the unruly senses and memory which dominate the intellect, which in turn causes the self to be liable for irresponsible activities which contravene the divine will.

युञ्जन्नेवं सदात्मानं
योगी विगतकल्मषः ।
सुखेन ब्रह्मसंस्पर्शम्
अत्यन्तं सुखमश्नुते ॥ ६.२८॥
yuñjannevaṁ sadātmānaṁ
yogī vigatakalmaṣaḥ
sukhena brahmasaṁsparśam
atyantaṁ sukhamaśnute (6.28)

*yuñjan — applying yoga disciplines; evaṁ — thus; sadā — constantly; 'tmānaṁ = ātmānam — the self; yogī — yogi; vigatakalmaṣaḥ — free from faults; sukhena — easily; brahmasaṁsparśam — contacting the spiritual plane; atyantaṁ — endless; sukham — happiness; aśnute — attains*

**Applying the yoga disciplines constantly to the self, the yogi being freed from faults, easily contacting the spiritual plane, attains endless happiness. (6.28)**

***Śrī Bābāji Mahāśaya's Commentary:***

People sometimes wonder why there is so much fuss about *samādhi* practice. A hint is given here by *Śrī* Krishna. As the *atyantam sukham*, the endless happiness that is felt on the spiritual plane, *brahmasamsparśam*. Once the student yogi reaches this, he shifts off permanently from the material social scene, both from its gross and subtle levels. The only thing which might cause a *yogin* to return to social concerns in this world is the stipulation of his guru or of *Śrī* Krishna or a need he might feel to share his realization with others. All stress of the self is removed when one reaches that endless happiness on the spiritual plane.

सर्वभूतस्थमात्मानं
सर्वभूतानि चात्मनि ।
ईक्षते योगयुक्तात्मा
सर्वत्र समदर्शनः ॥६.२९॥
sarvabhūtasthamātmānaṁ
sarvabhūtāni cātmani
īkṣate yogayuktātmā
sarvatra samadarśanaḥ (6.29)

*sarvabhūtastham — existing in all mundane creature forms; ātmānaṁ — spirit; sarvabhūtāni — all creatures; cātmani = ca — see + ātmani — in the self; īkṣate — he sees; yogayuktātmā — one who is proficient in yoga; sarvatra — in all cases; samadarśanaḥ — seeing the same*

**With a spirit existing in every creature, and with every creature based on a spirit, a person who is proficient in yoga, perceives the same existential arrangement in all cases. (6.29)**

***Siddha Swami's Commentary:***

This is *brahma yoga* realization. It is the most basic experience in the *brahma yoga* accomplishments. One sees that in every case of a creature form, there is a predominant limited spirit. In each of these gross forms, there is interlocked into it, a subtle body. In each of the subtle bodies there is an intellect, a memory and a sensual energy. This pertains to all the creature forms. Animals and vegetation have this as well, but in the human form, a spirit finds that he has a wider usage and application of the psychic tools in the mind. The same subtle body is used by a spirit no matter what gross form develops for him or her, but that same subtle body is restricted or given facility according to the specific form acquired.

A *brahma yogi* who has this vision, does not underrate any other limited spirit, even if that spirit might be in a lower form. He knows that the spirits are, for the most part, of equal potential but they are restricted according to the type of form they acquire as they transmigrate. There are grades of spirit, according to their relative existential powers. For instance, *Śrī* Krishna is a spirit but He is the supreme spirit and His powers are unlimited. Then there are spirits who have just a little less power than *Śrī* Krishna. Those are His parallel divinities. These are rated as incarnations of Godhead, as *Avatārs* in the Vedic texts. But besides these, there are numerous other grades of spirit. Still, in each case the rating should be given, not on the basis of the subtle or gross body, but on the spirit itself, because the subtle and gross forms may attenuate the power of a spirit insofar as that power can be manifested in a particular environment through a certain type of body.

One should rate a spirit by his existential powers on the spiritual plane, and not by the attenuated display of potency which is exhibited through a particular gross body. This is the training given in *brahma yoga* austerities.

This verse described a *brahma yoga kriyā* technique.

यो मां पश्यति सर्वत्र
सर्वं च मयि पश्यति ।
तस्याहं न प्रणश्यामि
स च मे न प्रणश्यति ॥६.३०॥
yo māṁ paśyati sarvatra
sarvaṁ ca mayi paśyati
tasyāhaṁ na praṇaśyāmi
sa ca me na praṇaśyati (6.30)

*yo = yaḥ — who; mām — me; paśyati — sees; sarvatra — in all forms; sarvam — all creatures; ca — and; mayi — in Me; paśyati — sees; tasyāham = tasya — his + aham — I; na — never; praṇaśyāmi — I am out of range; sa = saḥ — he; ca — and; me — my; na — never; praṇaśyati — he is out of view*

**To him who sees Me in all forms and who sees all creatures in reference to Me, I am never out of range, and he is never out of My view. (6.30)**

***Siddha Swami's Commentary:***

This is not a physical vision. This does not pertain to the physical Deity Murti in the temple. This occurs after the student yogi reaches the spiritual level and begins to perceive light there. This is the brilliant consciousness *antarjyoti*. When one practices to become stable in meditation on this light, then one begins to see the divine beings one by one. When one looks back into the material world, one sees clusters of spirits who, though they took material bodies, are still clustered-together as spiritual lights near spiritual lights, closely existing side by side on all sides together.

The Supreme Being is also seen as the most brilliant of these lights, as the ultimate attractor. This vision stays with the *yogin*, even when he moves about in the material world, perceiving in the conventional way through a material body. But others do not know that he or she sees more than just the material objects normally perceived by everyone.

सर्वभूतस्थितं यो मां
भजत्येकत्वमास्थितः ।
सर्वथा वर्तमानोऽपि
स योगी मयि वर्तते ॥६.३१॥
sarvabhūtasthitaṁ yo māṁ
bhajatyekatvamāsthitaḥ
sarvathā vartamāno'pi
sa yogī mayi vartate (6.31)

*sarvabhūtasthitam — existentially situated in all creatures; yo = yaḥ — who; māṁ — Me; bhajaty = bhajati — he honors; ekatvam — in harmony; āsthitaḥ — established; sarvathā — in various circumstances; vartamāno = vartamānaḥ — existentially situated; 'pi = api — although; sa = saḥ — he; yogī — yogi; mayi — in Me; vartate — he remains in touch*

**Although moving in various circumstances, the yogi who is established in that harmony, who honors Me as being existentially situated in all creatures, remains in touch with Me. (6.31)**

***Siddha Swami's Commentary:***

This is the *brahma yoga* technique which is the same technique and accomplishment denoted in the previous verse. The material world is very complicated. Social actions are very intertwining and cannot be deciphered by a limited being. Only the Supreme Person can know perfectly what should or should not be done. Thus it is important to link up with Him, to be informed by Him on the right course of action in any dimension or place.

आत्मौपम्येन सर्वत्र
समं पश्यति योऽर्जुन ।
सुखं वा यदि वा दुःखं
स योगी परमो मतः ॥६.३२॥

*ātmaupamyena = ātma — self + aupamyena — by reference; sarvatra — in all cases; samaṁ — similarity; paśyati — he sees; yo = yaḥ — who; 'rjuna = arjuna — Arjuna; sukhaṁ — pleasurable*

ātmaupamyena sarvatra
samaṁ paśyati yo'rjuna
sukhaṁ vā yadi vā duḥkhaṁ
sa yogī paramo mataḥ (6.32)

*sensations; vā — or; yadi — regardless; vā — or; duḥkhaṁ — painful sensations; sa = saḥ — he; yogī — yogi; paramo = paramaḥ — highest; mataḥ— considered as*

**He who, in reference to himself, sees the same facilities in all cases, regardless of pleasure or painful sensations, he, O Arjuna, is considered as the highest yogi. (6.32)**

***Siddha Swami's Commentary:***

This is the *brahma yoga technique* described in text 29 of this chapter. A student yogi must learn from a senior ascetic about the introspective process through which one begins to see objectively in the subjective energy of the self. Though subjective from the physical view point, the psychology of the self has distinct parts. One should accept a *brahma yoga* teacher and begin the practice in earnest, so as to realize all this in fact, on the mystic levels of consciousness.

अर्जुन उवाच
योऽयं योगस्त्वया प्रोक्तः
साम्येन मधुसूदन ।
एतस्याहं न पश्यामि
चञ्चलत्वात्स्थितिं स्थिराम् ॥६.३३॥
arjuna uvāca
yo'yaṁ yogastvayā proktaḥ
sāmyena madhusūdana
etasyāhaṁ na paśyāmi
cañcalatvātsthitiṁ sthirām (6.33)

*arjuna — Arjuna; uvāca — said; yo = yah – who; 'yaṁ = ayaṁ — this; yogas — yoga practices; tvayā — by you; proktaḥ — explained; sāmyena — by comparative similarity; madhusūdana — O slayer of Madhu; etasyāhaṁ = etasyā — of this + aham — I; na — not; paśyāmi — see; cañcalatvāt — due to shiftiness; sthitiṁ — position; sthirām — standard*

**Arjuna said: O slayer of Madhu, due to a shifty vision, I do not see this standard position of a comparatively similar view which is yielded by this yoga practice, declared by You. (6.33)**

***Śrī Bābāji Mahāśaya's Commentary:***

One cannot usually see this but one can understand it in theory and can imagine it. Arjuna, being a seasoned mystic, a yogi of worth, was not satisfied with the mere understanding after hearing from *Śrī* Krishna. Arjuna wanted to see in fact with spiritual vision. Even though a devotee of *Śrī* Krishna, a dear and friendly devotee in fact, still Arjuna did not achieve that technique of *brahma yoga*, whereby one can see spiritually, to perceive the existential relationship between the limited spirits and between those and the Supreme Person, spirit to spirit, without respect to the positions or status of the material bodies which were used by such persons. Arjuna particularly wanted the vision which was yielded by the yoga practice, declared by *Śrī* Krishna. That is the *buddhi yoga* technique.

चञ्चलं हि मनः कृष्ण
प्रमाथि बलवद्दृढम् ।
तस्याहं निग्रहं मन्ये
वायोरिव सुदुष्करम् ॥६.३४॥

*cañcalam — unsteady; hi — indeed; manaḥ — the mind; kṛṣṇa — Krishna; pramāthi — troubling; balavat — impulsive; dṛḍham — resistant; tasyāham = tasya — of it + aham — I; nigraham — controlling; manye — I think; vāyor = vāyoḥ — of*

cañcalaṁ hi manaḥ kṛṣṇa
pramāthi balavaddṛḍham
tasyāhaṁ nigrahaṁ manye
vāyoriva suduṣkaram (6.34)

*the wind; iva — compared to; suduṣkaram — very difficult to accomplish*

**Unsteady indeed is my mind, O Krishna. It is troublesome, impulsive and resistant. I think that controlling it is comparable to controlling the wind. It is very difficult to accomplish. (6.34)**

***Śrī Bābāji Mahāśaya's Commentary:***

One cannot achieve yoga unless one separates the intellect from the memory and sensual energy. Without accomplishing that, one cannot experience what is described by *Śrī* Krishna as the results of a consistent *buddhi yoga* practice. Being a devotee of *Śrī* Krishna is not the sole qualification of this success; otherwise Arjuna, who *Śrī* Krishna acclaimed as being devoted and friendly, would have experienced the brahman vision of the spirits in their relationship to each other and to the Supreme Lord.

An unsteady mind which is troublesome, impulsive and resistant, and which is unruly and haphazard like the wind, cannot ever grasp the spiritual reality, which is at all times, off limits to it. The issue here is mind component control, not devotedness to *Śrī* Krishna. Trapping the unruly mind into doing many chores on *Śrī* Krishna's behalf is not the same as rigid mind control attained by mastery of *buddhi yoga*.

श्रीभगवानुवाच
असंशयं महाबाहो
मनो दुर्निग्रहं चलम्।
अभ्यासेन तु कौन्तेय
वैराग्येण च गृह्यते ॥६.३५॥
śrībhagavānuvāca
asaṁśayaṁ mahābāho
mano durnigrahaṁ calam
abhyāsena tu kaunteya
vairāgyeṇa ca gṛhyate (6.35)

*śrībhagavān — the Blessed Lord; uvāca — said; asaṁśayam — undoubtedly; mahābāho — O powerful man; mano = manah — the mind; durnigraham — difficult to control; calam — unsteady; abhyāsena — by practice; tu — however; kaunteya — O son of Kuntī; vairāgyena — by the indifference to response; ca — and; gṛhyate — it is restrained*

**The Blessed Lord said: Undoubtedly, O powerful man, the mind is difficult to control. It is unsteady. By practice, however, O son of Kuntī, by indifference to its responses, also, it is restrained. (6.35)**

***Śrī Bābāji Mahāśaya's Commentary:***

Here the solution is given as practice, *abhyāsena*. What practice is this? It is the practice of *buddhi yoga* disciplines. It is that kind of service to *Śrī* Krishna, the service of yoga practice as taught by *Śrī* Krishna to *Vivasvat, Manu, Ikṣvāku* and others. There must be indifference to the mind's responses, an indifference which comes by detaching the intellect from the memory and sensual energies. The mind components are restrained by indifference because by that, the spirit's energy of attention, does not reach the components to empower them to act in impulsive ways. Being deprived of power supply, the components then act in a humble way. Their power of command over the spirit is broken and they are compelled by the spirit to act in a way that is expedient for spiritual advancement.

असंयतात्मना योगो
दुष्प्राप इति मे मतिः ।
वश्यात्मना तु यतता
शक्योऽवाप्तुमुपायतः ॥ ६.३६ ॥
asaṁyatātmanā yogo
duṣprāpa iti me matiḥ
vaśyātmanā tu yatatā
śakyo'vāptumupāyataḥ (6.36)

*asaṁyatātmanā = asaṁyata — undisciplined + ātmanā — by the self; yogo = yogaḥ — yoga; duṣprāpa — difficult to master; iti — thus; me — my; matiḥ — opinion; vaśyātmanā = vaśya — disciplined + ātmanā — by the self; tu — however; yatatā — by endeavor; śakyo = śakyaḥ — possible; 'vāptum = avāptum — to acquire; upāyataḥ — by effective means*

**For the undisciplined person, yoga is difficult to master. This is My opinion. For the disciplined one, however, by endeavor, it is possible to acquire the skill by an effective means. (6.36)**

***Śrī Bābāji Mahāśaya's Commentary:***

Arjuna was a devotee of *Śrī* Krishna, and still he complained about the difficulty of mind control. It means therefore that merely being a devoted student and a friendly one, is not sufficient for mastering the psychology. One has to practice the *buddhi yoga* discipline originally taught by *Śrī* Krishna.

अर्जुन उवाच
अयतिः श्रद्धयोपेतो
योगाच्चलितमानसः ।
अप्राप्य योगसंसिद्धिं
कां गतिं कृष्ण गच्छति ॥ ६.३७ ॥
arjuna uvāca
ayatiḥ śraddhayopeto
yogāccalitamānasaḥ
aprāpya yogasaṁsiddhiṁ
kāṁ gatiṁ kṛṣṇa gacchati (6.37)

*arjuna – Arjuna; uvāca — said; ayatiḥ — indisciplined person; śraddhayopeto = śraddhayopetaḥ = śraddhayā — by faith + upetaḥ — has got; yogāccalitamānasaḥ = yogāc (yogāt) — from yoga practice + calita — deviated + mānasaḥ — mind; aprāpya — not attain; yogasaṁsiddhiṁ — yoga proficiency; kāṁ — what; gatiṁ — course; kṛṣṇa — Krishna; gacchati — he goes*

**Arjuna said: What about the undisciplined person who has faith? Having deviated from yoga practice, having not attained yoga proficiency, what course does he take, O Krishna? (6.37)**

***Śrī Bābāji Mahāśaya's Commentary:***

This faith, *śraddhaya*, is the confidence in *Śrī* Krishna which is a requirement for studentship. But this faith is not itself the disciplinary attitude required for the practice of yoga. Arjuna asked an important question to find out the relationship between having faith in *Śrī* Krishna and deserving special concern from the Blessed Lord. It is important to obtain this special interest of *Śrī* Krishna or of His agent. Without it, many would never perfect the *buddhi yoga* practice.

Arjuna indicated that a devotee with strong faith might still lack the self discipline required to complete the *buddhi yoga* practice. What then would be the outcome of such a devotee of the Lord? What allowances would be given to that devotee? And how would divine grace be effective in his life?

कच्चिन्नोभयविभ्रष्टश्
छिन्नाभ्रमिव नश्यति ।
अप्रतिष्ठो महाबाहो
विमूढो ब्रह्मणः पथि ॥६.३८॥
kaccinnobhayavibhraṣṭaś
chinnābhramiva naśyati
apratiṣṭho mahābāho
vimūḍho brahmaṇaḥ pathi (6.38)

*kaccin = kaccid — is he; nobhayavibhraṣṭaś = na — not + ubhaya — both + vibhraṣṭaḥ — lost out; chinnābhram = chinna — faded + abhram — cloud; iva — like; naśyati — lost; apratiṣṭho = apratiṣṭhaḥ — without foundation; mahābāho — O Almighty Kṛṣṇa; vimūḍho = vimūḍhaḥ — baffled; brahmaṇaḥ — of the spirituality; pathi — on the path*

**Is he not like a faded cloud, lost from both situations, like being without a foundation? O Almighty Krishna, he is baffled on the path of spirituality. (6.38)**

***Śrī Bābāji Mahāśaya's Commentary:***

This query of Arjuna pertained to himself and to others as well, persons who were devoted and friendly to *Śrī* Krishna, who developed faith in what the Lord explained, but who were unable to gain mastery of the *buddhi yoga* practice. Such persons, it seemed to Arjuna, lost both cultural and spiritual attainments. They could neither practice *karma yoga* perfectly nor do *jñāna yoga* and leave aside the cultural opportunities. Their lives were full of uncertainty.

एतन्मे संशयं कृष्ण
छेत्तुमर्हस्यशेषतः।
त्वदन्यः संशयस्यास्य
छेत्ता न ह्युपपद्यते ॥६.३९॥
etanme saṁśayaṁ kṛṣṇa
chettumarhasyaśeṣataḥ
tvadanyaḥ saṁśayasyāsya
chettā na hyupapadyate (6.39)

*etan = etad — this; me — of mine; saṁśayam — doubt; kṛṣṇa — Krishna; chettum — remove; arhasy = arhasi — you can; aśeṣataḥ — without reminder, fully; tvadanyaḥ = besides you; saṁśayasyāsya = saṁśayasya — of doubt + asya — of this; chettā — remover of doubt; na — not; hy (hi) — indeed; upapadyate — he exists*

**You can, O Krishna, remove this doubt of mine fully. Besides You, no other remover of doubt exists here. (6.39)**

***Śrī Bābāji Mahāśaya's Commentary:***

It is essential that one's doubts be removed by the Supreme Lord or by His agent, the teacher who mastered the *buddhi yoga* practice; otherwise one will not adhere to the path. Still ultimately, one's confidence becomes permanent only when one has gained transcendental experience.

श्रीभगवानुवाच
पार्थ नैवेह नामुत्र
विनाशस्तस्य विद्यते ।
न हि कल्याणकृत्कश्चिद्
दुर्गतिं तात गच्छति ॥६.४०॥
śrībhagavānuvāca
pārtha naiveha nāmutra
vināśastasya vidyate
na hi kalyāṇakṛtkaścid
durgatiṁ tāta gacchati (6.40)

*śrībhagavān — the Blessed Lord; uvāca — said; pārtha — O son of Pṛthā; naiveha = na — either + eva — indeed + iha — here on earth; namutra = na — nor + amutra — above in the celestial regions; vināśaḥ — loss; tasya — his; vidyate — it is realized; na — not; hy (hi) — indeed; kalyāṇakṛt — performer of pious acts; kaścid — anyone; durgatiṁ — into misfortune; tāta — O ideal one; gacchati — goes down permanently*

**The Blessed Lord said: O son of Pṛthā, it is realized that neither here on earth nor above in the celestial regions, does the unaccomplished yogi lose his skill. Indeed, O dear Arjuna, no performer of virtuous acts goes down permanently into misfortune. (6.40)**

***Śrī Bābāji Mahāśaya's Commentary:***

Take note of the word *kalyāṇakṛt*, performer of pious acts. Such a person does not go down permanently into misfortune, though he or she may endure hellish life from time to time. Arjuna asked about the undisciplined person who did not attain yoga proficiency, but *Śrī* Krishna answered the question in a much broader way, covering all persons who were performers of pious acts. These persons were addressed as yatis or ascetics in Chapter Four:

*dravyayajñāstapoyajñā yogayajñāstathāpare*
*svādhyāyajñānayajñāśca yatayaḥ saṁśitavratāḥ (4.28)*

***Persons whose austerity and religious ceremony involve the control of material possession, those whose austerity and religious life involve some self-denial, as well as some others whose penance and religious procedure is the eight-part yoga discipline, and those whose austerity and religious ceremony is the study of the Veda and the acquirement of knowledge, all these are regarded as ascetics with strict vows. (4.28)***

प्राप्य पुण्यकृताँल्लोकान्
उषित्वा शाश्वतीः समाः ।
शुचीनां श्रीमतां गेहे
योगभ्रष्टोऽभिजायते ॥ ६.४१ ॥
prāpya puṇyakṛtāṁllokān
uṣitvā śāśvatīḥ samāḥ
śucīnāṁ śrīmatāṁ gehe
yogabhraṣṭo'bhijāyate (6.41)

*prāpya — obtaining; puṇyakṛtām — of the performer of virtuous acts; lokān — celestial places; uṣitvā — having lived; śāśvatīḥ — many, many; samāḥ — years; śucīnām — of the purified person; śrīmatām — of the prosperous person; gehe — in the social circumstance; yogabhraṣṭo = yogabhraṣṭaḥ — fallen from yoga; 'bhijāyate = abhijāyate — is born*

**After obtaining the celestial places where the virtuous souls go, having lived there for many, many years, the fallen yogi is born into the social circumstances of the purified and prosperous people. (6.41)**

***Śrī Bābāji Mahāśaya's Commentary:***

*Śrī* Krishna addressed only the fallen yogis, *yogabhraṣṭah*. These persons who fell from the practice of *buddhi yoga*, will get their just reward after leaving their material bodies. Due to practice while the physical body was used, they will gravitate towards places in the hereafter where the virtuous souls reside. And having lived there according to the equivalency of their yoga practice on earth, they would leave such exalted places and return to the earth for birth in social circumstances of purified and prosperous persons.

अथ वा योगिनामेव
कुले भवति धीमताम् ।
एतद्धि दुर्लभतरं
लोके जन्म यदीदृशम् ॥ ६.४२ ॥
atha vā yogināmeva
kule bhavati dhīmatām
etaddhi durlabhataraṁ
loke janma yadīdṛśam (6.42)

*atha vā — alternately; yoginām — of the yogi; eva — indeed; kule — in the family situation; bhavati — is born; dhīmatām — of the enlightened people; etad — this; dhi = hi — indeed; durlabhataram — difficult to attain; loke — in this world; janma — birth; yad — which; īdṛśam — such*

**Alternately, he is born into a family of enlightened people. But such a birth is very difficult to attain in this world. (6.42)**

***Śrī Bābāji Mahāśaya's Commentary:***

This type of birth is very rare, due to the scarcity of accomplished householders. The three important terms are two from the previous verse and one from this verse, namely, *śucīnām*, *śrīmatām* and *dhīmatām*. *Śucīnām* indicates persons whose subtle existence is cleaned up because they maintain a righteous lifestyle and are not stained by criminal acts in irreligious life. Such persons are expert at following *dharma* or righteous responsible lifestyle.

*Śrīmatām* means those who are prosperous materially such that they do not have to endeavor much for a livelihood. Material nature is gracious to them and the Goddess of fortune seems to live with them. Such persons do not acquire wealth by exploitive means.

*Dhīmatām* refers to those enlightened persons who mastered the *buddhi yoga* practice and developed supernatural and spiritual vision. These are the highest of the human beings. Whether such persons are rich or poor is irrelevant. Their asset is spiritual insight into spiritual dimensions. These are expert at higher yoga meditation.

तत्र तं बुद्धिसंयोगं
लभते पौर्वदेहिकम् ।
यतते च ततो भूयः
संसिद्धौ कुरुनन्दन ॥६.४३॥
tatra taṁ buddhisaṁyogaṁ
labhate paurvadehikam
yatate ca tato bhūyaḥ
saṁsiddhau kurunandana (6.43)

*tatra — there; tam — it; buddhisaṁyogam — cumulative intellectual interest; labhate — inspired with; paurvadehikam — from a previous birth; yatate — he strives; ca — and; tato = tataḥ — from that time; bhūyaḥ — again; saṁsiddhau — to perfection; kurunandana — O dear son of the Kurus*

**In that environment, he is inspired with the cumulative intellectual interest from a previous birth. And from that time, he strives again for yoga perfection, O dear son of the Kurus. (6.43)**

***Śrī Bābāji Mahāśaya's Commentary:***

Any advanced yogi who again takes on another body, will sooner or later in that body, realize his former endeavors in the spiritual quest. Then he will again take up the practice in earnest. It is best if one could take birth in a family of great yogins, since then one gets an early start and will be provided with all the encouragement needed, right from the onset of taking that new body from the yogi-parents.

However, in cases where a yogi does not get such a body and instead takes a body from parents who have no interest in yoga, even then, due to the force of his former practice in a past life, he would again feel the need to practice, and will in time seek out the teaching and try to reinstate himself in the practice.

पूर्वाभ्यासेन तेनैव
ह्रियते ह्यवशोऽपि सः ।
जिज्ञासुरपि योगस्य
शब्दब्रह्मातिवर्तते ॥६.४४॥

*pūrvābhyāsena = pūrva — previous + abhyāsena — by practice; tenaiva = tena — by it + eva — indeed; hriyate — he is motivated; hy (hi) — indeed; avaśo = avaśaḥ — without conscious desire; 'pi = api — even; saḥ — he;*

pūrvābhyāsena tenaiva
hriyate hyavaśo'pi saḥ
jijñāsurapi yogasya
śabdabrahmātivartate (6.44)

*jijñāsuḥ — persistently inquiring; api — even; yogasya — of yoga; śabdabrahmātivartate = śabda – spoken description + brahma — spiritual reality + ativartate — instinctively sees beyond (śabdabrahma — Vedas)*

**Indeed, by previous practice, he is motivated, even without conscious desire. He who persistently inquires of yoga, instinctively sees beyond the Veda, the spoken description of the spiritual reality. (6.44)**

***Śrī Bābāji Mahāśaya's Commentary:***

Every living entity transmigrates on the basis of past lives in conjunction with the opportunities afforded in the social world. Each person is motivated without conscious desire, to do what was done before and to complete whatever experience one had an interest in but did not completely understand or benefit from before. But yogis have the special facility to see beyond the *Veda*, the spoken description of the spiritual reality. They get spiritual vision to see the spiritual world.

प्रयत्नाद्यतमानस्तु
योगी संशुद्धकिल्बिषः ।
अनेकजन्मसंसिद्धस्
ततोयाति परां गतिम् ॥६.४५॥
prayatnādyatamānastu
yogī saṁśuddhakilbiṣaḥ
anekajanmasaṁsiddhas
tatoyāti parāṁ gatim (6.45)

*prayatnāt — from steady effort; yatamānaḥ — consistently controlled; tu — but; yogī — yogi; saṁśuddha — thoroughly cleansed; kilbiṣaḥ — bad tendencies; anekajanmasaṁsiddhas = aneka — not one + janma — birth + saṁsiddhaḥ — perfected; tato = tataḥ — from then onwards; yāti — reaches; parāṁ — supreme; gatim — goal*

**From a steady effort and a consistently controlled mind, the yogi who is thoroughly cleansed of bad tendencies, who is perfected in many births, reaches the supreme goal. (6.45)**

***Śrī Bābāji Mahāśaya's Commentary:***

Undoubtedly yoga practice takes many births to perfect, because of the necessity for the removal of bad tendencies *(kilbiṣah)*. These are mostly flaws in the intellect, the memory process and the sensual operations. When these are put in order by *buddhi yoga* practice, the yogi makes rapid advancement, all by the grace of *Śrī* Krishna. Still, it may take many births. Only a person who is really serious about spiritual life, about removing bad tendencies, will reach the perfection described in this chapter on purity of the psyche yoga, *ātmaviśuddha* (Bg. 6.12).

तपस्विभ्योऽधिको योगी
ज्ञानिभ्योऽपि मतोऽधिकः ।
कर्मिभ्यश्चाधिको योगी
तस्माद्योगी भवार्जुन ॥६.४६॥
tapasvibhyo'dhiko yogī
jñānibhyo'pi mato'dhikaḥ
karmibhyaścādhiko yogī
tasmādyogī bhavārjuna (6.46)

*tapasvibhyo = tapasvibhyaḥ — to the other types of ascetics; 'dhiko = adhikaḥ — is superior; yogī — yogi; jñānibhyo = jñānibhyaḥ — to the masters of the philosophical theory; 'pi = api — also; mato = mataḥ — is considered to be; 'dhikaḥ = adhikaḥ — is superior; karmibhyaḥ — to the ritual performers; cādhiko (cādhikaḥ) = ca — and + adhikaḥ — is better than; yogī — yogi; tasmād = tasmāt — hence; yogī — yogi; bhavārjuna = bhava — be + arjuna — Arjuna*

**The yogi is superior to other types of ascetics; he is also considered to be superior to the masters of philosophical theory, and the yogi is better than the ritual performers. Hence, be a yogi, Arjuna. (6.46)**

***Śrī Bābāji Mahāśaya's Commentary:***

*Śrī* Krishna named the various ascetics in Chapter Four. Then He declared that the yogi was superior to all other types of ascetics. He is superior to the masters of philosophical theory, the *jñānis*. He is better than the ritual performers, the *karmis*. Everyone who is dear to *Śrī* Krishna and who is devoted to the Lord, may take the same advice given to Arjuna, to be a yogi, *tasmāt yogī bhava*.

योगिनामपि सर्वेषां
मद्गतेनान्तरात्मना ।
श्रद्धावान्भजते यो मां
स मे युक्ततमो मतः ॥ ६.४७॥
yoginām api sarveṣāṁ
madgatenāntarātmanā
śraddhāvānbhajate yo māṁ
sa me yuktatamo mataḥ (6.47)

*yoginām — of the yogis; api — also; sarveṣāṁ — of all these; madgatenāntarātmanā = madgatena — attracted to me + antarātmanā — with his soul; śraddhāvān — full of faith; bhajate — worships; yo = yaḥ — who; mām — me; sa = saḥ — he; me — to me; yuktatamo = yuktatamaḥ — most devoted; mataḥ — is regarded*

**Of all yogis, the one who is attracted to Me with his soul, who worships Me with full faith, is regarded as being most devoted to Me. (6.47)**

***Śrī Bābāji Mahāśaya's Commentary:***

This is the description of the highest yogi. He must be a person whose soul is attracted internally to *Śrī* Krishna. This is an attraction to *Śrī* Krishna in the spiritual places, not so much to *Śrī* Krishna's idol in the temple or to *Śrī* Krishna's physical appearance for establishing righteousness on earthly planets. This is a direct attraction internally, seeing internally through the supernatural and spiritual vision to peer upon the divine *Śrī* Krishna with spiritual vision alone, without using the perception of a physical body or a lower subtle form. This is the significance of *antar ātmanā*, being attracted to *Śrī* Krishna from within *(antar)* the *ātma* or spirit itself, and not having to go through the material body, not having to rely on that body for worshipping or seeing physical manifestations of *Śrī* Krishna.

# Special Notation:

At the end of this 6th chapter of the holy *Śrīmad Bhagavad Gītā*, **Śrīpad Yogiraja Swami Kṛpalvānānda** asked me to make a statement on his behalf as follows:

*"Yoga operates on two hinges, namely the grace of the Almighty God and the endeavor of the yogin. Both of these are necessary. If one has the grace of God in fact, one will be motivated to endeavor for the spiritual perfection. And if one endeavors, then more divine grace will be forthcoming.*

*"It is similar to agriculture. Aborigines may not cultivate the land in a systematic way and still they survive but on bare subsistence. They get the grace of God without being attentive to God. But a farmer uses the same weather pattern in a more efficient way by organized agriculture. Similarly, a yogin who endeavors in the proper way, by the methods recommended by Śrī Krishna and by Śrīmad Patañjali Maharṣi, will get much benefit, because of using both the grace of God and personal endeavor. A yogin gets more from spiritual practice as compared to persons who do not endeavor strenuously and steadily. This is because of being submissive to both the mercy energy and the directive energy which comprise the grace of God. A person who only uses the mercy energy cannot advance as quickly, because he or she was unable to submit to the directive part of the divine grace.*

*"One must learn in higher yoga, how to curtail the attentive energy, for by doing this one cuts short the influence of the buddhi, memory and sensual energy. And this accelerates practice."*

# CHAPTER 7

# Vijñānam

# The Experience*

*jñānaṁ te'haṁ savijñānam idaṁ vakṣyāmyaśeṣataḥ*
*yajjñātvā neha bhūyo'nyaj jñātavyamavaśiṣyate (7.2)*

***I will explain the information and give the experience to you without deleting anything. Having known that, no other experience would be left to be discovered in this world. (7.2)***

****Siddha Swami assigned this chapter title on the basis of verse 2 of this chapter.***

**श्रीभगवानुवाच**
**मय्यासक्तमनाः पार्थ**
**योगं युञ्जन्मदाश्रयः ।**
**असंशयं समग्रं मां**
**यथा ज्ञास्यसि तच्छृणु ।७.१॥**
śrībhagavānuvāca
mayyāsaktamanāḥ pārtha
yogaṁ yuñjanmadāśrayaḥ
asaṁśayaṁ samagraṁ māṁ
yathā jñāsyasi tacchṛṇu (7.1)

*śrībhagavān — the Blessed Lord; uvāca — said; mayy = mayi — in Me; āsaktamanāḥ — attention absorbed in; pārtha — O son of Pṛthā; yogam — yoga; yuñjan — practicing; madasrayah = mad — on me + āśrayah — being dependent; asaṁśayaṁ — without doubt; samagraṁ — fully; māṁ — Me; yathā — as; jñāsyasi — you will know; tac = tad — this; chṛṇ = śṛṇu — hear*

**The Blessed Lord said: With attention absorbed in Me, O son of Pṛthā, practicing yoga, being dependent on Me, you will know of Me fully without a doubt. Hear of this. (7.1)**

***Siddha Swami's Commentary:***

This is the *brahma yoga technique* which allows the practicing yogi to see, in *samādhi*, the divine Lord in the spiritual sky. This happens after the spiritual eyes open by a consistent *buddhi yoga* practice. *Yogam yuñjan* means practicing yoga directly. That is higher yoga.

After having such spiritual visions of *Śrī* Krishna in the spiritual world, one becomes fully dependent on Him. This is spiritual dependence. Everyone is dependent on the Supreme Being, but not everyone realizes that. Those who know of it are mostly persons who heard of it from others and who believed it and have faith in that knowledge. But those who see the spiritual connection between the limited spirits, and between those and the Supreme Being, have a stronger reliance on the Supreme Lord. It is not a reliance for bread and butter, or for conquering enemies, or even for suppressing religious opponents, but it is in relationship to the spiritual connection with the Lord.

**ज्ञानं तेऽहं सविज्ञानम्**
**इदं वक्ष्याम्यशेषतः ।**
**यज्ज्ञात्वा नेह भूयोऽन्यज्**
**ज्ञातव्यमवशिष्यते ॥७.२.**
jñānaṁ te'haṁ savijñānam
idaṁ vakṣyāmyaśeṣataḥ
yajjñātvā neha bhūyo'nyaj
jñātavyamavaśiṣyate (7.2)

*jñānam — information; te — to you; 'ham = aham — I; savijñānam — with experience; idam — this; vakṣyāmy (vakṣyāmi) — I will explain; aśeṣataḥ — without deleting anything; yaj = yad — which; jñātvā — having known; neha = na — not + iha — in this world; bhūyo = bhūyaḥ — further; 'nyaj = anyat — other; jñātavyam — to be discovered; avaśiṣyate — is left*

**I will explain the information and give the experience to you without deleting anything. Having known that, no other experience would be left to be discovered in this world. (7.2)**

***Siddha Swami's Commentary:***

One requires both the information *(jñānam)* and the experience *(vijñānam)* which verifies that knowledge once and for all. *Śrī* Krishna promised to give Arjuna both. Obviously, if one acquired such information and experience, there would be nothing more to be known.

मनुष्याणां सहस्रेषु
कश्चिद्यतति सिद्धये ।
यततामपि सिद्धानां
कश्चिन्मां वेत्ति तत्त्वतः ॥७.३॥
manuṣyāṇāṁ sahasreṣu
kaścidyatati siddhaye
yatatāmapi siddhānāṁ
kaścinmāṁ vetti tattvataḥ (7.3)

*manuṣyāṇām — of human beings; sahasreṣu — in thousands; kaścid — someone; yatati — strives; siddhaye — to psychological perfection; yatatām — of those who endeavor; api — even; siddhānām — of those who are perfected; kaścin = kaścid — someone; mām — me; vetti — comprehends; tattvataḥ — in truth*

**Someone, in thousands of human beings, strives for psychological perfection. Of those who endeavor, even of those who are perfected, someone knows Me in truth. (7.3)**

***Śrī Bābāji Mahāśaya's Commentary:***

There are many, many siddhas in the astral worlds in certain dimensions. Many of them are still trying to perfect certain disciplines. Being convinced in one way or another that the gross material existence is needlessly troublesome, these ascetics aspire for liberation from material affiliation. But few of these people know who the Supreme Being is in fact. The Supreme Person is disinclined to forcing Himself on any and everyone, even upon those who attain some mystic or spiritual perfection *(siddhānām)*.

Perfection is the right of any living being who may aspire in an effective way for it. Thus one may become perfected and not even be aware of the Supreme Being, or not even realize who that person is. The Supreme Person is not knocking on every door proclaiming His glories and accepting obeisances from others.

भूमिरापोऽनलो वायुः
खं मनो बुद्धिरेव च ।
अहंकार इतीयं मे
भिन्ना प्रकृतिरष्टधा ॥७.४॥
bhūmirāpo'nalo vāyuḥ
khaṁ mano buddhireva ca
ahaṁkāra itīyaṁ me
bhinnā prakṛtiraṣṭadhā (7.4)

*bhūmir = bhūmiḥ — solid substance; āpo = āpaḥ — liquid substance; 'nalo = analaḥ — flames; vāyuḥ — gas; kham — space; mano = manaḥ — mindal energy; buddhir = buddhiḥ — intelligence; eva — indeed; ca — and; ahaṁkāra — initiative; itīyam = iti — thus + iyam — this; me — My; bhinnā — apportioned; prakṛtir = prakṛtiḥ — mundane energy; aṣṭadhā — eight-sectioned*

**Solid substance, liquid substance, flame, gas, space, mindal energy, intelligence, and initiative are My apportioned, eight-sectioned mundane energy. (7.4)**

***Śrī Bābāji Mahāśaya's Commentary:***

The cultural personality consists of these eight substances along with a limited spirit. Thus by convention, the personality is partially material. However, for the purposes of yoga we accept what *Śrī* Krishna stated, that the mindal energy, the intelligence and the sense of initiative are all material energy. These are energies which comprise the subtle body. The gross form consists of solid substances, liquids, heat, gas and space.

***Siddha Swami's Commentary:***

In the *brahma yoga* practice, the training is designed for dismantling the cultural personality, so that the limited spirit is sorted or separated from the other components. *Śrī Patañjali Mahārṣi* speaks of *kevalam* and *kaivalyam* which means separating the limited spirit from his subtle body, from his psyche, from his means of seeing into the gross and subtle material world.

*tad abhāvāt saṁyogā abhāvaḥ hānaṁ taddṛśeḥ kaivalyam*

***The elimination of the conjunction which results from the elimination of that spiritual ignorance is the withdrawal that is the total separation of the perceiver from the mundane psychology. (Yoga Sūtra 2.25)***

Mathematically, this means that the human personality minus the cultural identities developed through the subtle body, equals to the eternal spirit.

अपरेयमितस्त्वन्यां
प्रकृतिं विद्धि मे पराम् ।
जीवभूतां महाबाहो
ययेदं धार्यते जगत् ॥७.५॥
apareyamitastvanyāṁ
prakṛtiṁ viddhi me parām
jīvabhūtāṁ mahābāho
yayedaṁ dhāryate jagat (7.5)

*apareyam = apara — inferior + iyam — this; tv = tu — but; anyām — another; prakṛtiṁ — energy; viddhi — know; me — of Me; parām — higher; jīvabhūtām — the hosts of individual spirits; mahābāho — O strong man; yayedam = yaya — through which + idam — this; dhāryate — is sustained; jagat — universe*

**That is inferior. But, O strong man, know of My other higher energy which consists of the hosts of individual spirits, through which this universe is sustained. (7.5)**

***Siddha Swami's Commentary:***

*Prakṛtim* usually means material nature, either the subtle or gross aspects of it. But in this verse, *prakṛtim* is used as energy, otherwise *Śrī* Krishna would have contradicted Himself. The hosts of the individual limited spirits *(jīvabhūtām)* do sustain *(dhāryate)* the universe. They act as a power supply for its mobility and emotional movement or flux. In the instruction to Uddhava, *Śrī* Krishna called the cosmic energy, the *sūtram*.

In *brahma yoga*, one learns that liberation comes about when one stops being a power supply for material nature. But if one limited entity ceases to function in that role, the others continue as usual.

एतद्योनीनि भूतानि
सर्वाणीत्युपधारय ।
अहं कृत्स्नस्य जगतः
प्रभवः प्रलयस्तथा ॥७.६॥
etadyonīni bhūtāni
sarvāṇītyupadhāraya
ahaṁ kṛtsnasya jagataḥ
prabhavaḥ pralayastathā (7.6)

*etadyonīni = etad — this + yonīni — multiple origins; bhūtāni — the creatures; sarvāṇīty = sarvāṇi — all + ity (iti) — thus; upadhāraya — understand; aham — I; kṛtsnasya — of the entire; jagataḥ — of the universe; prabhavaḥ — cause of production; pralayaḥ — cause of the destruction; tathā — as well*

**This higher energy functions as the multiple origins of all creatures. Understand this. I am the cause of production as well as destruction of the entire universe. (7.6)**

***Siddha Swami's Commentary:***

Without the higher energy, without the limited spirits, there would be no creature forms in the material world. The limited spirits form the basis for the origin of the varied creature forms. Material nature by itself, the lower energy by itself, cannot produce the creature forms. Since these mixings between material nature and the limited spirits occur under the supervision and protection of the Supreme Being, He is said to be the cause of production as well as of destruction of it all.

Some ascetics, some *mahāyogīns*, are of the opinion that all this occurred spontaneously by the proximity of *brahman* to the *prakṛti* material energy. They do not regard any Supreme Person as being the Primal Cause. They attest to this based on transcendental experiences in which they found no evidence of a Supreme Person. But *Śrī* Krishna admitted in verse 3 of this chapter, that of the perfected souls, some know Him but not everyone recognizes Him. And He does not blacklist such persons.

मत्तः परतरं नान्यत्
किंचिदस्ति धनंजय ।
मयि सर्वमिदं प्रोतं
सूत्रे मणिगणा इव ॥७.७॥
mattaḥ parataraṁ nānyat
kiṁcidasti dhanaṁjaya
mayi sarvamidaṁ protaṁ
sūtre maṇigaṇā iva (7.7)

*mattaḥ — than myself; parataram — higher; nānyat = na — not + anyat — other; kiṁcid — anything; asti — is; dhanaṁjaya — O conqueror of rich countries; mayi — on Me; sarvam — all; idam — this; protam — strong; sūtre — on a thread; maṇigaṇā — pearls; iva — like*

**O conqueror of rich countries, no other reality is higher than Myself. All this existence relies on Me, like pearls strung on a string. (7.7)**

***Siddha Swami's Commentary:***

If as *Śrī* Krishna declared, He is the cause of production as well as destruction of the entire universe, then there is no other reality higher than Himself. Everything would be reliant on Him, like pearls strung on a string. In the *brahma yoga* process, a *yogin* is expected to research this, either to affirm or deny it in transcendental experience.

A student yogi should not doubt anything that *Śrī* Krishna declared about Himself. The student should believe this with full faith, but he should also strive to gain direct mystic and spiritual experiences to confirm this. Belief in *Śrī* Krishna is only the start of spiritual life. One has to go further to get the relevant experiences which verify this.

रसोऽहमप्सु कौन्तेय
प्रभास्मि शशिसूर्ययोः ।
प्रणवः सर्ववेदेषु
शब्दः खे पौरुषं नृषु.॥७.८॥
raso'hamapsu kaunteya
prabhāsmi śaśisūryayoḥ
praṇavaḥ sarvavedeṣu
śabdaḥ khe pauruṣaṁ nṛṣu (7.8)

*raso = rasaḥ — taste; 'ham = aham — I; apsu — in water; kaunteya — O son of Kuntī; prabhāsmi = prabhā — light + asmi — I am; śaśisūryayoḥ — of the sun and moon; praṇavaḥ — of the sacred syllable Om; sarvavedeṣu — in all the Vedas; śabdaḥ — sound; khe — in the atmosphere; pauruṣam — manliness; nṛṣu — in men*

**I am represented as taste in water, O son of Kuntī. I am signified as light in the moon and sun, as the sacred syllable *Om* in all the *Vedas*, as the sound in the atmosphere, as the manliness in men. (7.8)**

***Siddha Swami's Commentary:***

This is the initial instruction on developing faith in *Śrī* Krishna, in the Supreme Being, from the materialistic view point. If one has no mystic or spiritual insight or vision, then one should still have faith in the God. This is developed by perceiving the effects of God's overall influence in the world. In the *Bhagavad Gītā* here and elsewhere, *Śrī* Krishna gave directions on how to acquire such confidence in God.

Generally, when a child is born, he has no other idea except his existence as a physical body. This is because his energies, his spiritual attention, are efficiently used to manufacture the body while it forms in the parent forms. And because his energy was fully invested in that formation of a new material form, he tends to identify not with his attention but with what his attentive powers developed.

Thus for most people, religion begins in childhood, as an idea about creation of material objects. This is explained by teachers who state that this world was created by God. The next stage is to show how God created the world by showing God's effects in the world. Since God is not physically present, teachers can do nothing besides point to various physical objects like the sun, moon and the earth, and state that these were created by God. This is how religion begins.

After childhood, one subjects whatever one hears to reason. Thus one is apt to reject much of what one was told by elders, unless it sounds reasonable or can be proven physically. The elders explain that God created the most essential and most desirable features of anything.

*Śrī* Krishna presented such teachings to Arjuna, beginning with a basic feature of infant life which is taste. A child is very sensitive about taste, and taste is the child's approach to life, because it is through tasting and its corollary, eating, that the child's body grows. Since the child mistakes himself or herself for his or her physical form, tasting and eating are very dominant in the child's mind. The most basic necessity in terms of tasting is water. The secondmost is milk from the mother's breast. All other foods are representative of water and milk. Water represents the liquids and milk represents the solid type of food. Milk unlike water, converts into curd in the stomach of the child This is a solid.

From the onset, the parents, especially the mother, should instruct the child that God is present as the taste of water. God is to be appreciated just as one appreciates the taste of pure water.

The next feature presented by *Śrī* Krishna concerns vision. It is by vision that the child gets the most information to discern one thing from another. He or she recognizes his mother or father, mostly by vision, except of course for child with blind or defective eyes. The first teaching for the child is that Krishna is signified as the light of the sun and the moon.

The next feature presented by *Śrī* Krishna concerns hearing. Hearing is very important for the education of the child, because the parents and teachers cannot present everything physically to the child. Thus the child has to learn by hearing of something which is not physically present, something which cannot be perceived immediately. In the Vedic religion in the time of *Śrī* Krishna, *Om* was the most important sound to be made. The parents and teachers are to equate *Śrī* Krishna with that sound, so that the child would develop respect and veneration for that sacred sound, equating that with the Supreme Being. In general sound which travels easily through the air is to be equated with God also.

The next feature relates to the sense of touch. *Śrī* Krishna said that He was represented by the manliness in male human beings. Human society is dependent on this manliness as well as on the femininity of women.

पुण्यो गन्धः पृथिव्यां च
तेजश्चास्मि विभावसौ ।
जीवनं सर्वभूतेषु
तपश्चास्मि तपस्विषु ॥७.९॥

*puṇyo (puṇyaḥ) — wholesome; gandhaḥ — odor; pṛthivyām — in the earth; ca — and; tejaḥ — brilliance; cāsmi = ca — and + asmi — I am; vibhavasau — in the sun; jīvanam — life; sarvabhūteṣu — in all creatures;*

puṇyo gandhaḥ pṛthivyāṁ ca
tejaścāsmi vibhāvasau
jīvanaṁ sarvabhūteṣu
tapaścāsmi tapasviṣu (7.9)

*tapaścāsmi = tapaḥ — austerity + ca — and + asmi — I am; tapasviṣu — in the ascetics*

**I am represented as wholesome odor in the earth. I am sensed by the brilliance in the sun, by the life in all creatures. I am indicated by the austerity of the ascetics. (7.9)**

***Siddha Swami's Commentary:***

The next feature concerns the sense of smell. This is the most basic sense. In animal forms, smell is very important to determine what to eat and what not to eat. A cow, for instance, will not taste anything unless its sense of smell verified that the item smells edible. The atmosphere is mostly odorless, except for pleasing or noxious odors which come out of the earth. One should consider that the wholesome odor of the earth is representative of the Supreme Being. The shining brilliance of the sun is to be appreciated in a theistic way. There would be no life on earth, if it were not for sunshine. Thus God is indicated by the sun's rays.

The next feature, something dear to all creatures, is life in a material form, *jīvanam*. No one likes a dead body. Thus we should appreciate the Supreme Being by understanding that He is behind the animation which we consider to be life. The austerity of the ascetic is important, for through penance in one form or another, a person elevates himself above mere animal considerations.

बीजं मां सर्वभूतानां
विद्धि पार्थ सनातनम् ।
बुद्धिर्बुद्धिमतामस्मि
तेजस्तेजस्विनामहम् ॥७.१०॥
bījaṁ māṁ sarvabhūtānāṁ
viddhi pārtha sanātanam
buddhirbuddhimatāmasmi
tejastejasvināmaham (7.10)

*bījam — primary cause; mām — Me; sarvabhūtānām — of all creatures; viddhi — know; pārtha — O son of Pṛtha; sanātanam — primeval; buddhir = buddhiḥ — intelligence; buddhimatām — of the geniuses; asmi — I am; tejaḥ — splendor; tejasvinām — of the splendrous things; aham — I*

**Know me as the primeval, primary cause of all creatures, O son of Pṛthā. I can be inferred as the intelligence of the geniuses and glimpsed by the splendor of the splendrous things. (7.10)**

***Siddha Swami's Commentary:***

The Supreme Being must be such a person, that He would have started this creation and can by His omnipotence easily conclude it. He must be very near to this creation and very, very far also, as the origin of it, the primeval primary cause of all the creatures who surfaced in this existence, and through these gross forms, came to realize themselves as existences.

One who can neither see nor meet that Supreme Person, can deduce God's existence by observing the intelligence of the geniuses and the splendor of the splendorous things. *Śrī Patañjali Mahārṣi* described Him like this:

*kleśa karma vipāka āśayaiḥ aparāmṛṣṭaḥ puruṣaviśeṣaḥ īśvaraḥ*
*tatra niratiśayaṁ sarvajñabijam*
*sa-eṣaḥ pūrveṣām api guruḥ kālena anavacchedāt*
*tasya vācakaḥ praṇavaḥ*

***The Supreme Lord is that special person Who is not affected by troubles, actions, developments or by subconscious motivations.***

***There, in Him, is found the unsurpassed origin of all knowledge.***

***He, this particular person, being unconditioned by time is the guru even of the ancient teachers, the authorities from before.***

***Of Him, the sacred syllable auṁ (Oṁ) is the designation.( Yoga Sūtra 1.24-27)***

बलं बलवतां चाहं
कामरागविवर्जितम् ।
धर्माविरुद्धो भूतेषु
कामोऽस्मि भरतर्षभ ॥७.११॥
balaṁ balavatāṁ cāhaṁ
kāmarāgavivarjitam
dharmāviruddho bhūteṣu
kāmo'smi bharatarṣabha (7.11)

*balam — strength; balavatām — of the strong; cāham = ca — and + aham — I; kāmarāgavivarjitam = kāma — selfish desires + rāgavivarjitam — free from passionate urges; dharmāviruddho = dhārmaviruddhaḥ = dharma — Vedic rules of morality + aviruddhaḥ — not opposed to; bhūteṣu — in creatures; kāmo = kāmaḥ — romance; 'smi = asmi — I am; bharatarṣabha — powerful son of the Bharatas*

**I am indicated as the strength of the strong, which is free from selfish desire and passionate urges. I am supportive of romance which is not opposed to the Vedic rules of morality, O powerful son of the Bharata family. (7.11)**

***Siddha Swami's Commentary:***

*Kāmarāga*, lusty energy and passionate urge, comprises the two forces in the mental and emotional energy which spell doom for a limited entity. But if by chance, or by divine grace, one can be freed from that energy, one becomes liberated. *Śrī* Krishna identified Himself with the strength of the strong which is free from such passionate content. In the material world, He does in His Universal Form use the non-passionate strength of strong men, in *karma yoga* activities for the good of the world.

Though *kāmarūpah*, the form of passionate desire for lusty purposes, is troublesome to one and all in material existence, *Śrī* Krishna identified with it when regulated by *dharma* or responsible life style according to Vedic rules of morality. By this lusty power, new human bodies are produced in this creation.

ये चैव सात्त्विका भावा
राजसास्तामसाश्च ये ।
मत्त एवेति तान्विद्धि
न त्वहं तेषु ते मयि ॥७.१२॥
ye caiva sāttvikā bhāvā
rājasāstāmasāśca ye
matta eveti tānviddhi
na tvahaṁ teṣu te mayi (7.12)

*ye — which; caiva — and indeed; sāttvikā — perceptive clarity; bhāvā — states of being; rājasāḥ — enthusiasm; tāmasāśca = tāmasāḥ — depression + ca — and; ye — which; matta — from Me; eveti = eva — indeed + iti — thus; tān — them; viddhi — know; na — not; tv = tu — but; aham — I; teṣu — in them; te — they; mayi — on Me*

**Regarding the states of being, which are perceptive clarity, enthusiasm, and depression, know that they are produced by Me. But I am not based in them. They are dependent on Me. (7.12)**

***Siddha Swami's Commentary:***

To understand this verse, one must first research into one's connection with the material energy. One can then see how such energy is divested into three general categories with three general types of effect in terms of giving perception of it, causing one to become involved with itself, and causing the reduction of one's sensual status in relation to itself. This is studied in *samādhi* practice. When in *brahma yoga*, the yogi realizes this, he goes further to find the Supreme Being Who, unlike him, is not affected by the subtle material energy. Then he checks into the categorical difference between himself and the Lord. He understands the effects of the Supreme Being upon material nature and its subsequent influence upon himself.

A limited being by himself could not have energized material nature, no more than a small battery could move the very large turbines in a megawatt generator; nor could a set of limited entities combine together to electrify material nature. It was the Supreme Being and He alone Who did this. This is discovered by the *brahma yogi* in higher meditations. *Śrī Patañjali Mahārṣi* gave many hints in Chapter Three of his *Sūtras*. These realizations only occur in *samādhi* practice.

त्रिभिर्गुणमयैर्भावैर्
एभिः सर्वमिदं जगत् ।
मोहितं नाभिजानाति
मामेभ्यः परमव्ययम् ॥७.१३॥
tribhirguṇamayairbhāvair
ebhiḥ sarvamidaṁ jagat
mohitaṁ nābhijānāti
māmebhyaḥ paramavyayam (7.13)

*tribhir = tribhiḥ — by three; guṇamayair = guṇamayaiḥ — by mundane influence produced; bhāvair = bhāvaiḥ — by states of being; ebhiḥ — by these; sarvam — all; idam — this; jagat — world; mohitam — stupified; nābhijānāti = na — not + abhijānāti — recognizes; mām — Me; ebhyaḥ — than these; param — higher; avyayam — unaffected*

**All this world is stupefied by the three states of being, which are produced by the mundane influence. The world does not recognize Me, Who is higher than these energies and Who is unaffected. (7.13)**

***Siddha Swami's Commentary:***

Trapped in the subtle mundane psychology, a limited being is forced to accept conclusions shown to him within his mental and emotional energy *(cittavritti, Yoga Sūtra 1.2)*. Thus he is usually stupefied and moves about in the material world as pushed and pulled by the energies, forming affiliations and causing disintegrations as he moves about randomly. He cannot recognize divine beings because he is not usually under the influence of the *sāttvikā* perceptive force, and when he is under that influence, it reveals to him only what promotes his involvement with that energy. Thus it is very rare to find an individual who could recognize *Śrī* Krishna or His parallel divinities when They choose to act through a gross or subtle material body.

*Śrī* Krishna as He described is higher than the energies, but knowing and perceiving that directly is a feat for the limited beings in this world. Their vision is processed through the mental and emotional energies and thus they are unable to truly see.

दैवी ह्येषा गुणमयी
मम माया दुरत्यया ।
मामेव ये प्रपद्यन्ते
मायामेतां तरन्ति ते ॥७.१४॥

*daivī — supernatural; hy = hi — indeed; eṣā — this; guṇamayī — quality-controlled; mama — of Me; māyā — magical display; duratyayā — difficult to transcend; mām — Me; eva — indeed; ye — who; prapadyante — they rely on;*

daivī hyeṣā guṇamayī
mama māyā duratyayā
māmeva ye prapadyante
māyāmetāṁ taranti te (7.14)

*māyām – bewitching energy; etām — this; taranti — they can see beyond; te — they*

**Indeed this quality controlled illusion of Mine is supernatural and difficult to transcend. Only those who rely on Me, can see beyond this bewitching energy. (7.14)**

***Siddha Swami's Commentary:***

Just as I stated that a limited entity or even a group of limited beings could not energize this world, so the limited spirits cannot transcend this existence all by themselves. They would require the help of the Supreme Person. For one, since the energy of the Supreme Person is mixed into the material energy, it is supernatural *(daivī)*. It is not ordinary. By His mere proximity, the mundane potency has magnetically picked up a portion of His powers. Unless one gets in proximity to Him, keeping one's focus on Him, one cannot effectively transcend the mundane potency.

न मां दुष्कृतिनो मूढाः
प्रपद्यन्ते नराधमाः ।
माययापहृतज्ञाना
आसुरं भावमाश्रिताः ॥७.१५॥
na māṁ duṣkṛtino mūḍhāḥ
prapadyante narādhamāḥ
māyayāpahṛtajñānā
āsuraṁ bhāvamāśritāḥ (7.15)

*na — not; mām — Me; duṣkṛtino = duṣkṛtinaḥ — evil-doers; mūḍhāḥ — confused; prapadyante — they take shelter; narādhamāḥ — lowest of human beings; māyayāpahṛtajñānā = māyayā — by misconception + apahṛta — erased + jñānā — discrimination; āsuram — corrupted; bhāvam — existence; āśritāḥ — attached*

**The confused evildoers, the lowest of human beings, those whose discrimination is erased by misconceptions, do not take shelter of Me. They are attached to a corrupted existence. (7.15)**

***Siddha Swami's Commentary:***

The *māyayā*, the misconceptions which erase *(apahṛta)* the discrimination *(jñānā)* of the living entity were defined previously by *Śrī* Krishna:

*śrībhagavānuvāca kāma eṣa krodha eṣa rajoguṇasamudbhavaḥ*
*mahāśano mahāpāpmā viddhyenamiha vairiṇam (3.37)*
*dhūmenāvriyate vahnir yathādarśo malena ca*
*yatholbenāvṛto garbhas tathā tenedamāvṛtam (3.38)*
*āvṛtaṁ jñānametena jñānino nityavairiṇā*
*kāmarūpeṇa kaunteya duṣpūreṇānalena ca (3.39)*

***The Blessed Lord said: This force is craving. This power is anger. The passionate emotion is the source. It has a great consuming power and does much damage. Recognize it as the enemy in this case.***

***As the sacrificial fire is obscured by smoke, and similarly as a mirror is shrouded by dust or as an embryo is covered by a skin, so a man's insight is blocked by the passionate energy.***

***The discernment of educated people is adjusted by their eternal enemy which is the sense of yearning for various things. O son of Kuntī, the lusty power, is as hard to satisfy as it is to keep a fire burning. (3.37-39)***

The limited entities become attached to a corrupted existence in material nature. The conceptions they form about existence are usually derived from the impressions their subtle senses gave them. Thus there is no clear idea about the origin of the world, and there is doubt about the existence of a Supreme Being.

Without realizing it, one becomes condemned in this existence, merely by taking shelter of material existence alone, and by believing whatever one's mind presents as firm conclusions in the psyche. The only way to break away from this is to realize the various components of consciousness and become detached from them one by one, so that one becomes free to accept higher influences.

चतुर्विधा भजन्ते मां
जनाः सुकृतिनोऽर्जुन ।
आर्तो जिज्ञासुरर्थार्थी
ज्ञानी च भरतर्षभ ॥७.१६॥
caturvidhā bhajante māṁ
janāḥ sukṛtino'rjuna
ārto jijñāsurarthārthī
jñānī ca bharatarṣabha (7.16)

*caturvidhā — four kinds; bhajante — worship; mām — Me; janāḥ — people; sukṛtino = sukṛtinaḥ — good people; 'rjuna = arjuna — Arjuna; ārto = ārtaḥ — distressed person; jijñāsur = jijñāsuḥ — inquisitive person; arthārthī — needy person; jñānī — informed person; ca — and; bharatarṣabha — O bullish man of the Bharata family*

**Four kinds of good people worship Me, O Arjuna: the distressed one, the inquisitive one, the needy one, and the informed one, O bullish man of the Bharata family. (7.16)**

***Siddha Swami's Commentary:***

These four kinds of devotees are categorized according to their relative positions in relationship to material nature. One is progressively freed from nature's influence, as one submits oneself to the Supreme Being. But such submission is only complete when one exerts oneself to change the extroverted habits of the psyche.

Those who are **distressed** *(ārto)* are persons who have faith in the Supreme Being but who are harassed by time and circumstances anyway. This proves that mere faith in God will not protect a person from hassles. The hassles will go on regardless but the person may take shelter in the idea that God is in the background, and that God certainly has the power to remove the botherations. This is a very basic form of religious belief. It is materialistic because it does not take into account the eternal soul. It does not even accommodate the idea that there is a subtle body which will survive the gross one. A devotee in this category actually feels that he or she is the material body. Even though God recognizes such a devotee, that same God may do little to influence that devotee,s advancement. This is because that person is unable to delve deeply into things of a mystic and spiritual nature. Thus God is patient in His dealings with such persons. The *Bhagavad Gītā* is heard by such devotees, but they do not take it seriously. And they hear it mostly from speakers who cheapen the texts and offer promises which *Śrī* Krishna did not endorse in the conversation with Arjuna. Thus many such devotees are fooled into thinking that God will do whatever is necessary to transfer them to a heaven at the death of their material bodies. Somehow they feel, because they are God's devotees, He will see to it that they do not die but will be translated into spiritual beings at the time of their bodies' deaths. Such an attitude however, is condemned by *Śrī* Krishna Himself in a previous verse:

*na kartṛtvaṁ na karmāṇi lokasya sṛjati prabhuḥ*
*na karmaphalasaṁyogaṁ svabhāvastu pravartate (5.14)*
*nādatte kasyacitpāpaṁ na caiva sukṛtaṁ vibhuḥ*
*ajñānenāvṛtaṁ jñānaṁ tena muhyanti jantavaḥ (5.15)*

***The Lord does not create the means of action, nor the actions of the creatures, nor the action-consequence cycle. But the inherent nature causes this.***

***The Almighty God does not receive from anyone, an evil consequence or a good reaction. The knowledge of this is shrouded by ignorance through which the people are deluded. (5.14-15)***

Even those distressed devotees are devotees in fact, because of their faith that there is a Supreme Being. Still, their approach to Him is flawed, because they feel that He will do things which cannot or would not be done by Him. And their very faith holds within it a cause for frustration. Gradually they may begin to realize the defect. This happens if they get some higher association.

Such devotees do benefit from the mission of the Supreme Lord, when He takes on a material body or sends an agent to establish righteousness and stamp out causes of irreligious activity. Because they are focused down into the material world, such persons think that God's existence only concerns righteousness in this world, and they under-rate the glory of God, trying to restrict Him as being a Regulator of human behavior in creature existence. This, however, is their flaw.

Those who are **inquisitive** *(jijñāsuh)*, eager to ask questions, do inquire of a guru about *Śrī* Krishna. Such persons, who are also devoted to *Śrī* Krishna, strike a bargain to get the association of Krishna or His agent, intending to ask questions while associating with a divine being. Some of these persons lose interest over time. Some develop a sincere regard for the Lord and a lively concern for their spiritual development. A few rare individuals develop an interest in yoga for the sake of experiencing divine reality, so as to confirm or deny in their consciousness, the things they were told either by *Śrī* Krishna or by His agent. These persons graduate to become very advanced devotees.

The **needy** devotee *(arthārthī)* is the one who strives for something but who regards *Śrī* Krishna as the person who would award that item, whatever it may be. Some of these persons have *Śrī* Krishna as their cherished wish. Others want something or someone else but feel that *Śrī* Krishna should arrange for them to have it. They subscribe that *Śrī* Krishna is the provider of everything. Some of these devotees develop an intense attraction to *Śrī* Krishna and by that force, they make the necessary sacrifice for purification. Thus they attain Him.

The last of the devotees mentioned is the **informed** person *(jñānī)*. This is someone who has definite information about *Śrī* Krishna and who has enough mystic and spiritual perception or intuition, to sense the reality of *Śrī* Krishna as the Supreme Being. This person does not waver in austerities. He is determined to attain purity of consciousness, so that he may relate to the divine persons face to face. He does not try to exploit the mercy of the Lord and works for divine grace through honest endeavor.

तेषां ज्ञानी नित्ययुक्त
एकभक्तिर्विशिष्यते ।
प्रियो हि ज्ञानिनोऽत्यर्थम्
अहं स च मम प्रियः ॥७.१७॥

*teṣām — of these; jñānī — the informed man; nityayukta — constantly disciplined in yoga; ekabhaktir = ekabhaktiḥ — one who is singularly devoted; viśiṣyate — is distinguished; priyo = priyaḥ — fond; hi — indeed; jñānino = jñāninaḥ — of the informed person; 'tyartham = atyartham — very;*

teṣāṁ jñānī nityayukta
ekabhaktirviśiṣyate
priyo hi jñānino'tyartham
ahaṁ sa ca mama priyaḥ (7.17)

*aham — I; sa = sah — he; ca — and; mama — of Me; priyaḥ — fond*

**Of these, the informed man who is constantly disciplined in yoga, being singularly devoted, is distinguished indeed. I am fond of this person and he is fond of Me. (7.17)**

***Siddha Swami's Commentary:***

*Ekabhaktih* is being singularly devoted to *Śrī* Krishna and no one else. This is the reason for stating *eka* which means one or singular. Such devotees must also be ***nityayuktah*** or constantly disciplined in yoga as *Śrī* Krishna explained so far in the *Bhagavad Gītā*, especially proficiency of *buddhi yoga*. Such a person is distinguished, certainly. He is or she is *vaśiṣyate*. *Śrī* Krishna is fond of this person and that one holds the Lord to be dear.

If devotion to *Śrī* Krishna *(bhakti)* was itself the one and only qualification, *Śrī* Krishna would not have added *nityayukta* in terms of His teachings and the practices of *buddhi yoga* as He originally taught it.

उदाराः सर्व एवैते
ज्ञानी त्वात्मैव मे मतम् ।
आस्थितः स हि युक्तात्मा
मामेवानुत्तमां गतिम् ॥७.१८॥
udārāḥ sarva evaite
jñānī tvātmaiva me matam
āsthitaḥ sa hi yuktātmā
māmevānuttamāṁ gatim (7.18)

*udārāḥ — exalted; sarva — all; evaite = eva — indeed + ete — these; jñānī — informed person; tv = tu — but; ātmaiva = ātmā — personal self + eva — indeed; me — of Me; matam — is considered; āsthitaḥ — situated with; sa = saḥ — he; hi — truly; yuktātmā — one who is disciplined in yoga practice; mām — Me; evānuttamām = eva — indeed + anuttamām — supreme; gatim — objective*

**All these are exalted people. But the informed one is considered to be my personal representative. Indeed, he who is disciplined in yoga practice, is situated with Me as the Supreme Objective. (7.18)**

***Siddha Swami's Commentary:***

The value of yoga practice as it is coordinated with devotion *(bhaktih)* to *Śrī* Krishna is hereby declared. That yogi who is devoted to *Śrī* Krishna, gains the focus on *Śrī* Krishna as the Supreme Objective *(anuttamām gatim),* so that he does not waver and does not have many objectives. Due to mastership of *buddhi yoga*, he is not distracted like the other three classes of devotees described in verse 16.

बहूनां जन्मनामन्ते
ज्ञानवान्मां प्रपद्यते ।
वासुदेवः सर्वमिति
स महात्मा सुदुर्लभः ॥७.१९॥
bahūnāṁ janmanāmante
jñānavānmāṁ prapadyate
vāsudevaḥ sarvamiti
sa mahātmā sudurlabhaḥ (7.19)

*bahūnām — of many; janmanām — of births; ante — at the end; jñānavān — the informed devotee; mām — Me; prapadyate — surrenders to; vāsudevaḥ — son of Vasudeva; sarvam — everything; iti — thus; sa = saḥ — he; mahātmā — great soul; sudurlabhaḥ — hard to locate*

**At the end of many births, the informed devotee surrenders to Me, thinking that the son of Vasudeva is essential to everything. Such a great soul is hard to locate. (7.19)**

***Siddha Swami's Commentary:***

The fact is that it takes many births, as *Śrī* Krishna clarified in this verse. This is because the *buddhi* yogi devotee needs time to master the psyche which he was awarded by providence. It does not happen overnight. Due to the complexity of the subtle machinery, such a devotee must first control it before he can be liberated. He or she must personally control the psyche. No one else does it. When one conquers over the psychic nature, then one can attain freedom from material existence.

A devotee gives in totally to *Śrī* Krishna, only after all the psychic mechanisms are purified, perfectly restrained and then abandoned. This is achieved by mastership of the *buddhi yoga* process. It does not matter if that system of psychic control is called *kriyā yoga*, *brahma yoga*, *ātma* yoga or whatever. It may be called *rāja* yoga or *aṣṭanga* yoga. That is not the argument. It is the proficiency which must be gained. Many surrender to *Śrī* Krishna but they cannot do so fully until the psychic energies are purified. Then and only then is the surrender complete.

कामैस्तैस्तैर्हृतज्ञानाः
प्रपद्यन्तेऽन्यदेवताः ।
तं तं नियममास्थाय
प्रकृत्या नियताः स्वया ॥७.२०॥
kāmaistaistairhṛtajñānāḥ
prapadyante'nyadevatāḥ
taṁ taṁ niyamamāsthāya
prakṛtyā niyatāḥ svayā (7.20)

*kāmaiḥ — by desires; taistair = taihtaiḥ — by whose, by these, contrary; hṛtajñānāḥ — persons whose experience is overshadowed; prapadyante — they plead with; 'nyadevatāḥ = anyadevatāḥ = anya — other + devatāḥ — supernatural rulers; taṁtam — this or that; niyamam — religious procedures; āsthāya — following; prakṛtyā — by material nature; niyatāḥ — restricted; svayā — by their own*

**Persons whose experience was overshadowed by contrary desires, plead with other supernatural rulers, following this or that religious procedure, being restricted by their own material nature. (7.20)**

***Siddha Swami's Commentary:***

This applied locally at *Kurukṣetra* and to other situations as well. So long as *Śrī* Krishna is not particular about any situation, another person might win out; someone's desire might prevail. But when the Supreme Person is determined, no one else may predominate.

Material nature itself, *prakṛtyā*, adheres to and cooperates more with the Supreme Being. Thus in any contest of wills, the Supreme Will prevails. In as much as a limited being has an affiliation to material nature, in as much as providence seems to favor a limited being on occasion, so also does fate side with the Supreme Being more than often. Thus anyone at *Kurukṣetra* who worshipped other supernatural rulers besides *Śrī* Krishna, and who expected that their desires would be fulfilled in opposition to *Śrī* Krishna, were frustrated for sure.

In the previous verse, *Śrī* Krishna acknowledged that even devotees may go to other supernatural rulers *(anya devatāh)* for assistance to fulfill desires, which *Śrī* Krishna does not respond to or is slow in regarding. But even so, one does this on the basis of contrary desires and an attraction to popular gods who promise this or that but who may not always fulfill their guarantees.

यो यो यां यां तनुं भक्तः
श्रद्धयार्चितुमिच्छति ।
तस्य तस्याचलां श्रद्धां
तामेव विदधाम्यहम् ॥६.२१॥
yo yo yāṁ yāṁ tanuṁ bhaktaḥ
śraddhayārcitumicchati
tasya tasyācalāṁ śraddhāṁ
tāmeva vidadhāmyaham (7.21)

*yo yo = yaḥ yaḥ — whoever; yāṁ yām — whatever; tanum — deity form; bhaktaḥ — devotedly worship; śraddhayārcitum = śraddhayā — with belief + arcitum — to worship; icchati — desires; tasya — of him; tasyācalām = tasya — of him + acalām — unwavering; śraddhām — confidence; tām — it; eva — indeed; vidadhāmy = vidadhāmi — allow; aham — I*

**I grant unwavering faith to anyone, who with belief, wants to worship any worshipable deity form. (7.21)**

***Siddha Swami's Commentary:***

The Supreme Person, *Śrī* Krishna, is not biased towards any other living being. All the living beings may exhibit some autonomy from time to time, in terms of having inalienable rights and in terms of discovering this or that gross or subtle aspect. The Supreme Being usually does not infringe on anyone's claims. His mission of establishing righteousness serves to sort conflicting claims of various entities. For Himself, the Supreme Person is not much interested in the subtle or gross commodities which are to be found in this existence.

Thus He grants unwavering faith, best wishes and all good intentions to anyone, who with belief, wants to worship any worshipable deity form of any other authority besides Himself. Everyone has a right to learn through personal experience but the Supreme Being may limit the harm one may inflict on others while doing so.

स तया श्रद्धया युक्तस्
तस्या राधनमीहते ।
लभते च ततः कामान्
मयैव विहितान्हि तान् ॥७.२२॥
sa tayā śraddhayā yuktas
tasyā rādhanamīhate
labhate ca tataḥ kāmān
mayaiva vihitānhi tān (7.22)

*sa = saḥ — he; tayā — with this; śraddhayā — by faith; yuktaḥ — endowed; tasyārādhanam = tasya — of this + ārādhanam — worshipfully petitioning a deity; īhate — thinks of; labhate — gets; ca — and; tataḥ — from that; kāmān — desires; mayaiva = maya — by Me + eva — indeed; vihitān — permitted; hi — truly; tān — them*

**Being endowed with this confidence, he thinks of worshipfully petitioning the deity and gets from that source, his desires, as those fulfillments are permitted by Me. (7.22)**

***Siddha Swami's Commentary:***

All the powerful entities have circumscription or limits about them, even the Supreme Being has a limit for His activity in this world. He too must respect others, even the most limited of the limited souls. According to the layout of this existence, according to how it was formulated originally, according to the amount of divine energy invested into it by the Supreme Person, each entity is allotted certain powers and controls. Thus when one worships another supernatural person besides *Śrī* Krishna, that person has limitations which must be recognized. He or she cannot reward one unlimitedly nor support one inordinately.

A very powerful person, a god, a spiritual master or any other authority does not become more powerful or more capable of awarding boons to followers, merely by the increase in affection of the worshipper. Those authorities who become conceited by having many worshippers and receiving the affections of such dependents, do frustrate both themselves and their followers, because they over-reach their capability and are frustrated.

अन्तवत्तु फलं तेषां
तद्भवत्यल्पमेधसाम् ।
देवान्देवयजो यान्ति
मद्भक्ता यान्ति मामपि ॥७.२३॥
antavattu phalaṁ teṣāṁ
tadbhavatyalpamedhasām
devāndevayajo yānti
madbhaktā yānti māmapi (7.23)

*antavat — something with an end, short-lived; tu — but; phalam — results; teṣām — of them; tad — this; bhavaty = bhavati — it is; alpamedhasām — of those with little intelligence; devān — supernatural rulers; devayajo = devayajaḥ — those who worship the supernatural rulers; yānti — go; madbhaktā — those who worship Me; yānti — go; mām — to Me; api — surely*

**But for those with little intelligence, the result is short-lived. The worshippers of the supernatural rulers go to those gods. Those who worship Me, surely go to Me. (7.23)**

***Siddha Swami's Commentary:***

The revelation about the Supreme Person, about *Śrī* Krishna, came about gradually in India. For instance, in the *Vedas* the stress is on various supernatural rulers like Indra and *Varuṇa*. In the *Rāmāyaṇa*, we find focus on *Brahmā*, on *Agni devata* and on *Vāyu*, the wind deity, the supposed father of *Hanumān*. But in the Upanishads, it is more of a focus on *brahman*. The rishis of the Upanishads did mystic research on and argued about the position and importance of *brahman*.

The worship of the supernatural rulers was established by Lord *Brahmā*, the *Prajāpati*, or at least this is what *Śrī* Krishna told us in Chapter Three. *Śrī* Krishna condemned such worship and in his speech with His foster father, Nanda, just prior to the lifting of Govardhana Hill, Lord Krishna berated the worship of the *devatas*, especially the Indra *yajña*. Here He stated that His devotees *(madbhaktā)* go to Him and those who worship the other supernatural rulers, find those gods as a result. This is a condemnation of the worship of any other powerful person besides *Śrī* Krishna.

अव्यक्तं व्यक्तिमापन्नं
मन्यन्ते मामबुद्धयः ।
परं भावमजानन्तो
ममाव्ययमनुत्तमम् ॥७.२४॥
avyaktaṁ vyaktimāpannaṁ
manyante māmabuddhayaḥ
paraṁ bhāvamajānanto
mamāvyayamanuttamam (7.24)

*avyaktam — that which is beyond the sensual range; vyaktim — that which is grossly perceived; āpannam — within range, limited; manyante — they think; mām — Me; abuddhayaḥ — unintelligent ones; param — higher; bhāvam — being; ajānanto = ajānantaḥ — not realizing; mamāvyayam = mama — of Me + avyayam — imperishable; anuttamam — supermost*

**Though I am beyond their sensual range, the unintelligent think of Me as being limited to their gross perception. They do not realize My higher existence which is imperishable and supermost. (7.24)**

***Siddha Swami's Commentary:***

In ordinary dealings, everything is regulated by convention. This means that normally we see things in terms of gross sense perception. This is alright for social dealings in this world. To find the subtle existence, one has to leave aside convention and enter the mystic terrains.

One should not feel that *Śrī* Krishna or anyone else is merely the material appearance of that person or thing. We should check the subtle counterpart if we want to understand the actual basis and significance of anyone or anything.

Although *Śrī* Krishna manifested a material body, a *vyaktim*, still He has an unmanifested existence, an *avyaktam*. We should seek to know His unmanifested existence, as well as our subtle selves. This is the purpose of *brahma yoga* practice, to find out about the unmanifested personal selves of all beings.

नाहं प्रकाशः सर्वस्य
योगमायासमावृतः ।
मूढोऽयं नाभिजानाति
लोको मामजमव्ययम् ॥७.२५॥
nāhaṁ prakāśaḥ sarvasya
yogamāyāsamāvṛtaḥ
mūḍho'yaṁ nābhijānāti
loko māmajamavyayam (7.25)

*nāham = na — not + aham — I; prakāśaḥ — visible; sarvasya — of everyone; yoga – yogically self-controlled + māyā — mystic power + samāvṛtaḥ — shielded; mūḍho = mūḍhaḥ — stupified; 'yam = ayam — this; nābhijānāti = na — not + abhijānāti — recognizes; loko = lokaḥ — population; mām — Me; ajam — not subjected to birth shocks; avyayam — not liable to existential pressures of change*

**I am not visible to everyone, because I am shielded by My yogicly, self-controlled mystic powers. This stupefied population does not recognize Me as not being subjected to shocks of birth and not being liable to existential pressures of change. (7.25)**

***Siddha Swami's Commentary:***

Even though this may be accepted and understood mentally, this can only be realized in fact by the perfection of *brahma yoga* practice in higher meditation, where one sees into the spiritual atmosphere and can judge the relative powers of the limited spirits and the Supreme Person.

What is visible by convention, by virtue of this physical body, is only part of the whole existence. In fact it is a minor part. A material body shows us only the indication of a spirit. And the acts of *Śrī* Krishna show us a small portion of His powers. The physical body of *Śrī* Krishna was visible to all those on the battlefield who were within physical visionary range, but the complete *Śrī* Krishna who manifested that body, was hardly seen by anyone, except for persons like Bhishma who were versed in *brahma yoga* practice.

Unless one develops the mystic and spiritual insight, one cannot see anything beyond what is physical. And so one is apt to physical ratings only. On the other hand, one has to know that the shocks of birth and the existential pressures of change which a limited person endures in the transmigrations are not to be experienced in the same way by the Supreme Soul. This is due to God's infallibility. Even though God is a spirit and the limited persons too are spirits, still, God is a special type of spirit Who is exempt from being overpowered by subtle mundane energy. If God were of the same quality as the limited spirits, then there would be no reason to distinguish Him from others.

वेदाहं समतीतानि
वर्तमानानि चार्जुन ।
भविष्याणि च भूतानि
मां तु वेद न कश्चन ॥७.२६॥

*vedāham = veda — know + aham — I; samatītāni — the departed souls; vartamānāni — the living creatures; cārjuna = ca — and + arjuna — Arjuna; bhaviṣyāni — those who are to be born; ca — and; bhūtāni — creatures; mām*

vedāhaṁ samatītāni
vartamānāni cārjuna
bhaviṣyāṇi ca bhūtāni
māṁ tu veda na kaścana (7.26)

*— Me; tu — but; veda — recognizes; na — not; kaścana — anyone*

**I know the departed souls and the living creatures, O Arjuna, as well as those beings who are to be born. But no one recognizes Me. (7.26)**

***Siddha Swami's Commentary:***

Some special features of the Supreme Person are explained. Others might have these capacities periodically and fragmentally but not fully. These are eternal denotations of the Supreme Being.

One should not be embarrassed because one does not have these capacities. And one should not aspire to have these in full either. It is not a requirement for anyone else but the Supreme Being. Knowing all the persons who are alive in this physical world, either as humans, animals, or vegetations, and knowing those who have departed forms here, as well as those who are in transit to take bodies and who are now in embryonic forms, is a responsibility for the Supreme Being and no one else. One should aspire, if anything, to cooperate with the Supreme Person as He fulfills His responsibilities. One should not desire to replace or compete with Him.

इच्छाद्वेषसमुत्थेन
द्वंद्वमोहेन भारत ।
सर्वभूतानि संमोहं
सर्गे यान्ति परंतप ॥७.२७॥
icchādveṣasamutthena
dvaṁdvamohena bhārata
sarvabhūtāni saṁmohaṁ
sarge yānti paraṁtapa (7.27)

*icchādveṣasamutthena = icchā — liking + dveṣa — disliking + samutthena — through the urge; dvandvamohena = dvandva — two-fold sensuality + mohena — by the delusive influence; bhārata — O man of the Bharata family; sarvabhūtāni — all beings; saṁmoham — delusion; sarge — at the beginning of the creation; yānti — they are influenced by; paraṁtapa — O scorcher of the enemy*

**O man of the Bharata family, at the beginning of any creation, all beings are influenced by delusion through the urge of liking or disliking and by the delusive influence of the two-fold sensuality. So it is, O scorcher of the enemy. (7.27)**

***Siddha Swami's Commentary:***

The limited entities in this world are stymied by the liking and disliking urges within their minds and emotions. These feelings exert delusive influences which entertain and entangle the living being, keeping him or her enthralled with social affairs. This has taken place since the very onset of the creation. This is primeval. This bewilderment is ancient.

येषां त्वन्तगतं पापं
जनानां पुण्यकर्मणाम् ।
ते द्वंद्वमोहनिर्मुक्ता
भजन्ते मां दृढव्रताः ॥७.२८॥
yeṣāṁ tvantagataṁ pāpaṁ
janānāṁ puṇyakarmaṇām
te dvaṁdvamohanirmuktā
bhajante māṁ dṛḍhavratāḥ (7.28)

*yeṣām — of whom; tv = tu — but; antagatam = anta — terminated + gatam — gone; pāpam — sinful propensity; janānām — of people; puṇyakarmaṇām — of persons of righteous actions; te — they; dvandvamohanirmukta = dvandva — two-fold + moha — delusion + nirmuktā — free from; bhajante — worship; mām — Me; dṛḍhavratāḥ — those who maintain firm vows of austerity*

**But those people whose sinful propensities are terminated, whose actions are righteous, who are free from the two-fold delusion, who are maintaining firm vows of austerity, do worship Me. (7.28)**

***Siddha Swami's Commentary:***

Even a detached person, a *sannyāsi*, should perform pious actions *(puṅyakarmaṇām)* whenever he is socially-involved. Renunciation is no excuse to act whimsically, to be out of one's mind or to perform actions supportive of crimes in the material world. One should always remember that the Supreme Being took it upon Himself to cut down anyone who performed or supported irreligious activities. Thus one should not, in the name of renunciation, take to irreligious actions.

When one becomes freed from the duality which *Śrī* Krishna condemned *(dvandvamohena*, Bg. 7.27), one sees clearly what to do to support the supreme will and one no longer works to contravene it. This does not mean that every *yogin* should remain tied to social affairs. Those who have advanced into higher yoga, should if possible, be isolated from such dharmic life so that they can take up the higher duty of becoming eligible for transfer into the spiritual atmosphere.

Firms vows of austerity for purifications of the psyche, should remain through a devotee's life, so that he can advance progressively on and on, from this world into the transcendental environment.

जरामरणमोक्षाय
मामाश्रित्य यतन्ति ये ।
ते ब्रह्म तद्विदुः कृत्स्नम्
अध्यात्मं कर्म चाखिलम् ॥७.२९॥
jarāmaraṇamokṣāya
māmāśritya yatanti ye
te brahma tadviduḥ kṛtsnam
adhyātmaṁ karma cākhilam (7.29)

*jarāmaraṇamokṣāya = jarā — bodily deterioration + maraṇa — bodily death + mokṣāya — to permanent release; mām — Me; āśritya — being dependent; yatanti — strive; ye — who; te — they; brahma — spiritual existence; tad — this; viduḥ — they know; kṛtsnam — complete; adhyātmam — Supreme Self; karma — cultural activity; cākhilam = ca — and + akhilam — entirely*

**Those who, being dependent on Me, strive for permanent release from bodily deterioration and death, know this spiritual existence completely, as well as the Supreme Spirit and the value of cultural activity. (7.29)**

***Siddha Swami's Commentary:***

One who is dependent on *Śrī* Krishna, must also strive with all his psychological strength for permanent release from bodily deterioration and death. This means that a devotee should strive for liberation so that he can shed the need for material bodies. That is a requirement. It is not sufficient to be a devotee of *Śrī* Krishna.

One must also exert oneself in higher yoga, in the mystic terrain, to overcome the need for gross existence. This is the highest duty one has towards the Supreme Being, for unless one achieves that, one must continue in the material world transmigrating and enduring the inherently haphazard life, something which the Supreme Being must regulate and pay attention to even in the smallest way.

Cultural activity *(karma)* holds value in giving an opportunity to free oneself from the needs for a social life. But one must endeavor and not be lazy and hazy about liberation. It is improper and an injustice to the Supreme Being for one to continue on and on in worldly cultural life, since the only Supreme Being can effectively maintain that and give us the opportunity to convert our cultural activities into the realization that we should not be in the material world in the first place.

साधिभूताधिदैवं मां
साधियज्ञं च ये विदुः ।
प्रयाणकालेऽपि च मां
ते विदुर्युक्तचेतसः ॥७.३०॥
sādhibhūtādhidaivaṁ māṁ
sādhiyajñaṁ ca ye viduḥ
prayāṇakāle'pi ca māṁ
te viduryuktacetasaḥ (7.30)

*sādhibhūtādhidaivam = sa — with + adhibhūta — Lord of mundane beings + adhidaivam — Lord of the supernatural rulers and powers; mām — Me; sādhiyajñam = sa — with + adhiyajñam — Supreme Master of religious discipline; ca — and; ye — who; viduḥ — they know; prayāṇakāle — at the time of final departure from the body; 'pi = api — even; ca — and; mām — Me; te — they; vidur = viduḥ — know; yuktacetasaḥ — those with concentrated mental focus*

**Those who know Me as the Lord of mundane beings, Lord of the supernatural rulers and powers, and Supreme Master of religious disciplines, and who know Me even at the time of the final departure from the body, are the ones who know Me with concentrated mental focus. (7.30)**

***Siddha Swami's Commentary:***

The complete spiritual realization of a *mahāyogin* is described in this verse. All yogi students should take note of it and strive to achieve it step by step. One should be patient, since these realizations will come on gradually. One will see the spiritual evidence little by little as one practices higher yoga, not otherwise.

*Yuktacetasah* means those who have concentrated mental and emotional focus, so that all their interest and concerns, all their affections become streamlined into their quest for spiritual realization. When one is completely given over to that, one will, in time, come to see all this on the spiritual plane.

# CHAPTER 8

## Paramam Puruṣam Divyam

## The Divine Supreme Person*

*abhyāsayogayuktena cetasā nānyagāminā*
*paramaṁ puruṣaṁ divyaṁ yāti pārthānucintayan (8.8)*
*kaviṁ purāṇamanuśāsitāram aṇoraṇīyāṁsamanusmaredyaḥ*
*sarvasya dhātāram acintyarūpam ādityavarṇaṁ tamasaḥ parastāt (8.9)*

***With a mind that does not venture outwards, which is disciplined by yoga practice, a person goes to the divine Supreme Person, while deeply meditating, O son of Pṛthā.***

***He who meditates on the Person Who knows everything, the most ancient of people, the Supreme Supervisor, the most minute factor, the one with unimaginable form, with a radiant body, free of grossness, (8.8-9)***

**Siddha Swami assigned this chapter title on the basis of verses 8 and 9 of this chapter.*

अर्जुन उवाच
किं तद्ब्रह्म किमध्यात्मं
किं कर्म पुरुषोत्तम ।
अधिभूतं च किं प्रोक्तम्
अधिदैवं किमुच्यते ॥८.१॥
arjuna uvāca
kiṁ tadbrahma kimadhyātmaṁ
kiṁ karma puruṣottama
adhibhūtaṁ ca kiṁ proktam
adhidaivaṁ kimucyate (8.1)

*arjuna — Arjuna; uvāca — said; kim — what; tad — this; brahma — spiritual reality; kim — what; adhyātmam — Supreme Soul; kim — what; karma — cultural activity; puruṣottama — Supermost Personality; adhibhūtam — sum total gross reality; ca — and; kim — what; proktam — authoritatively described as; adhidaivam — Supreme Supernatural Person and Power; kim — what; ucyate — is described*

**Arjuna said: What is this spiritual reality? What is the Supreme Soul? What is cultural activity, O Supermost Personality? Concerning the sum total gross reality, how is that described authoritatively? And speaking of the Supreme Supernatural Person and Power, what is that described to be? (8.1)**

***Siddha Swami's Commentary:***

Even though Śrī Krishna stated in the beginning of the last chapter, that He would give Arjuna both the knowledge and experience (*jñānam te'ham savijñānam* Bg. 7.2), still so far, Arjuna got knowledge only. In reality, from the beginning of the discourse, Śrī Krishna imparted both knowledge and experience, since as the Supreme Being, He perceives on the spiritual plane at all times. Unfortunately, Arjuna could not make contact with that spiritual level. Thus all of Śrī Krishna's explanations and experiences were not being sensed and realized by Arjuna, who was focused on the material side of existence only.

This proves that a limited being must become purified before he can have transcendental experience, or he has to be energized by his guru or by the God Himself. In either case, that of personal purification through yoga austerity or that of instant but temporary purification through inducement of power from a divine being *(śaktipāt)*, the devotee can only experience the transcendence in one of those ways. Personal purification by yoga austerities is the sure way, because it brings a permanent purification, while the inducement of a guru or of *Śrī* Krishna produces temporary ability to see into the transcendental reality. Arjuna was infused but it did not last, because he again tried to get *Śrī* Krishna to infuse him after the battle of *Kurukṣetra*. At the time *Śrī* Krishna told Arjuna the *Anu Gītā*.

Arjuna asked some very important questions in this chapter, but unfortunately the complete answer to these queries can only be given by personal vision into the spiritual reality. No amount of explanation can give the devotee complete understanding of these inquiries.

His first question was about *brahma*, spiritual reality. This is an age-old question, one answered extensively in the Upanishads, since many students inquired of it from gurus like *Yajñavalka* and *Gautama Rishi*. Whatever lies beyond this material world and is the ultimate basis of existence, used to be called *brahma* or *brahman*. Thus during the time of the Upanishads, that subject was hotly debated in the courts of many *karma* yogi rulers. They would invite ascetic brahmins to give contesting statements based on mystic researches into the Absolute Truth. In the time of Arjuna, *brahma* remained a mystery and enigma, and thus Arjuna took the opportunity to get clarification from Krishna.

The second inquiry was about the Supreme Soul, *adhyātmam*, the primal *(adhi)* spirit *(ātmam)*. Is there such a person? Some ascetics deny that there is such a person and others assert that person with great conviction. *Śrī* Krishna was not the first person in the history of India who claimed to be that Godhead. Elsewhere in other parts of the world, others proclaimed themselves as such.

*Adhi* means over and above. Thus a*dhi ātmam* or a*dhyātmam* means the Over-soul, the Soul above the other souls. Who is that person? What are the implications of His existence? Is that person male or female? Or is that Person sexless or dual-sexed?

The third question is regarding cultural activity *(karma)*. What is that? What are its implications? Can cultural activity be a means of release from this troublesome existence? Or is it only a means of continuing in this miserable life, always uncertain about the outcome?

The fourth question is about the Supermost Personality *(puruṣottama)*. In Indian philosophy the *Adhyātmam* or Oversoul is discussed in a different way to that of the Supermost Personality, for it is explained that the Oversoul is distant from this world, while the Supermost Personality exhibits involvement through cultural activities (*līlās)*. But some say that there is no distinction between the Oversoul and the Supermost Personality, that He is one and the same. Others feel that the Oversoul throws off parallel forms of Himself who function in this world or that world, as Supermost Personalities by taking *avatār* or incarnation status among embodied creatures.

The fifth question addresses the sumtotal gross reality *(adhibhūtam)*. This is a gigantic configuration of all the planets in any given universe. This consists of tons and tons of matter and many species of life, both potential and actual. This concerns the material elements which our scientists are enamored by. Even though this is matter, still it has potency. In fact the limited entities are seen to be more attached to that gross material than to their very selves.

The sixth question concerns the Supreme Supernatural Person and Power *(adhidaivam)*. This has relevance because it is somewhere between the Oversoul and the material existence. Supernatural or *daivam* means that which is supervisory over the material world but which is supervised by the spiritual world. Whatever is supernatural, is in the transitional levels between the gross material and the ultimate spiritual worlds.

Each of these inquiries can only be understood completely by revelation, either by divine grace through infusement of power, as happened to Arjuna, or by divine grace through performance of austerity to purify the psyche where it becomes capable of bearing the supernatural and spiritual insights.

अधियज्ञः कथं कोऽत्र
देहेऽस्मिन्मधुसूदन ।
प्रयाणकाले च कथं
ज्ञेयोऽसि नियतात्मभिः ॥८.२॥
adhiyajñaḥ kathaṁ ko'tra
dehe'sminmadhusūdana
prayāṇakāle ca kathaṁ
jñeyo'si niyatātmabhiḥ (8.2)

*adhiyajñaḥ — Supreme Regulator of religious ceremonies and disciplines; katham — how; ko = kaḥ — who; 'tra = atra — here; dehe — in the body; 'smin = asmin — in this; madhusūdana — O slayer of Madhu; prayāṇakāle — at the time of departure from the body; ca — and; katham — how; jñeyo = jñeyaḥ — to be known; 'si = asi — you are; niyatātmabhiḥ = niyata — subdued + ātmabhiḥ — by persons*

**Who is the Supreme Regulator of religious ceremonies and disciplines? How is He located here in this body, O killer of Madhu? And how, at the time of departure from the body, are You to be known by those persons who are subdued? (8.2)**

***Siddha Swami's Commentary:***

*Adhiyajñah* could mean the supreme religious ceremony and discipline. But since Arjuna asked about who *(kah),* he meant the supreme regulator of the religious ceremonies and disciplines. He wanted to know where such a person was located in the human body, in what dimension was that person located, because if that person were isolated to the physical body, he would be misplaced at the time of the body's death. He had to be in some imperishable location. That was the seventh inquiry.

The eighth question regards how persons would know and find *Śrī* Krishna at the time of departure from their material bodies. But Arjuna asked only about the spiritually-subdued persons, the *niyatātmabhih*, because others would have no chance of finding someone who used a transcendental form and lived in a transcendental dimension, even if such a place was interspaced into their bodies.

श्रीभगवानुवाच
अक्षरं ब्रह्म परमं
स्वभावोऽध्यात्ममुच्यते ।
भूतभावोद्भवकरो
विसर्गः कर्मसंज्ञितः ॥८.३॥
śrībhagavānuvāca
akṣaraṁ brahma paramaṁ
svabhāvo'dhyātmamucyate
bhūtabhāvodbhavakaro
visargaḥ karmasaṁjñitaḥ (8.3)

*śrībhagavān — the Blessed Lord; uvāca — said; akṣaram — unaffected; brahma — spiritual reality; paramam — supreme; svabhāvo = svabhāvaḥ — personal nature; 'dhyātmam = adhyātmam — supreme soul; ucyate — it is said; bhūtabhāvodbhavakaro = bhūtabhāva — existence of mundane forms + udbhava — production + karo (karaḥ) — causing; visargah — creative power; karmasaṁjñitaḥ = karma — cultural activity + saṁjñitaḥ — is known*

**The Blessed Lord said: The spiritual reality is unaffected and supreme. The Supreme Soul is described as a personal existence Who causes the production of the mundane world. Cultural action is known as creative power. (8.3)**

***Siddha Swami's Commentary:***

If one searches carefully though the Upanishads, he will conclude that the great sages mentioned therein, believed mostly that the *brahma* or *brahman* spiritual reality was a power which was unaffected and supreme, while the material energy is affected and relative to that *brahman*. This was verified by many ascetics through higher yoga practice.

In contrast the Oversoul is said to be a personal existence, who has *sva* or sense of ownership. In the histories in the *Purāṇas*, there is dispute regarding who that Oversoul might be. There is even dispute as to the Oversoul's gender. Is the Oversoul male or female? Is the Oversoul Shiva or *Durgā*? Is the Oversoul *Brahmā*, Vishnu or Shiva? Is the Oversoul *Rāma* of the *Rāmāyaṇa* fame or *Śrī* Krishna of the *Bhagavad Gītā* fame? Some have simplified this issue by stating that the Oversoul is one, Who divested or manifested as Shiva, as *Durgā*, as *Rāma*, as Krishna, as Vishnu and as *Brahmā Prajāpatih*. In other countries, some say that the Oversoul is Yahweh or Jehovah and that His only begotten son is Lord Jesus Christ. Others say that Mohammed is His last prophet.

According to *Śrī* Krishna, that Oversoul causes the production of the mundane world. In this respect, many agree that God must be the one who created the sun, the moon, the other planets and any of the creatures who existed, exist and will exist in the future.

*Śrī* Krishna, without going into many details, stated that cultural activity is a form of creative power. It is denoted *(samjñitah)* by the expression of creative power in this world. It is based on the force of desire which stimulates the psyche of the limited entities.

अधिभूतं क्षरो भावः
पुरुषश्चाधिदैवतम् ।
अधियज्ञोऽहमेवात्र
देहे देहभृतां वर ॥८.४॥
adhibhūtaṁ kṣaro bhāvaḥ
puruṣaścādhidaivatam
adhiyajño'hamevātra
dehe dehabhṛtāṁ vara (8.4)

*adhibhūtam — sum total gross reality; kṣaro = kṣaraḥ — ever-changing; bhāvaḥ — nature; puruṣaścādhidaivatam = puruṣa — master of the world + ca — and + adhidaivatam — Lord of the Supernatural rulers and powers; adhiyajño = adhiyajñaḥ — the Supreme Regulator of religious ceremonies and disciplines; 'ham = aham — I; evātra = eva — indeed + atra — here; dehe — in the body; dehabhṛtām vara — O best of the embodied souls*

**The sum total gross reality is ever-changing nature. The master of the world is the Lord of the supernatural rulers and powers. O best of the embodied souls, I, Who exist here in the body, am the Supreme Regulator of religious ceremonies and disciplines. (8.4)**

***Siddha Swami's Commentary:***

The sumtotal gross reality, *adhibhūtam*, is ever-changing. That is its feature, as contrasted to the stable, non-changing *brahman*. The chief person in this world must be the one who is most superior among the supernatural rulers. As in all cases, anyone with the most capacity is regarded as the greatest. *Śrī* Krishna presented Himself as the *adhiyajna*, the Supreme Regulator of religious ceremonies and disciplines. He gave His location as being in the material body and gave more details of this elsewhere in the *Gītā*.

अन्तकाले च मामेव
स्मरन्मुक्त्वा कलेवरम् ।
यः प्रयाति स मद्भावं
याति नास्त्यत्र संशयः ॥८.५॥
antakāle ca māmeva
smaranmuktvā kalevaram
yaḥ prayāti sa madbhāvaṁ
yāti nāstyatra saṁśayaḥ (8.5)

*antakāle — at the end of life; ca — and; mām — Me; eva — in particular; smaran — remembering; muktvā — giving up; kalevaram — body; yaḥ — who; prayāti — departs the body; sa = saḥ — he; madbhāvam — My condition of existence; yāti — is elevated; nāsty (nasti) = na — not + asti — is; atra — here; saṁśayaḥ — doubt*

**If at the end of one's life, one recalls Me in particular, as one gives up the body, one is elevated to My condition of existence. There is no doubt about this. (8.5)**

***Siddha Swami's Commentary:***

Usually a person who departs from a physical body, adheres to whatever person, things and location that he is most habituated. A person follows his normal attachments and adheres to these in the subtle body even if forced to abandon them in the gross existence. Hence if someone is attached to *Śrī* Krishna's spiritual existence, that person will, by the force of such attachment, go to *Śrī* Krishna at the time of death of the body. One has to recall *Śrī* Krishna in particular on the basis of a lifelong attachment to *Śrī* Krishna's spiritual self, just as normally one adheres to relatives and loved ones, and stays with them as a subtle being after being forced out of the premises which we know as the material body.

यं यं वापि स्मरन्भावं
त्यजत्यन्ते कलेवरम् ।
तं तमेवैति कौन्तेय
सदा तद्भावभावितः ॥८.६॥
yaṁ yaṁ vāpi smaranbhāvaṁ
tyajatyante kalevaram
taṁ tamevaiti kaunteya
sadā tadbhāvabhāvitaḥ (8.6)

*yaṁ yam — whatever; vāpi = va — or + api — also, moreover; smaran — recalling; bhāvam — texture of existence; tyajaty = tyajati — abandons; ante — in the end; kalevaram — the body; taṁtam — that that; evaiti = eva — indeed + eti — is projected; kaunteya — O son of Kuntī; sadā — always; tad — that; bhāva — status of life; bhāvitaḥ — being transformed*

**Moreover, whatever texture of existence is recalled when a person abandons his body in the end, to that same type of life, he is projected, O son of Kuntī, always being transformed into that status of life. (8.6)**

***Siddha Swami's Commentary:***

A living being attains a gross existence in the next life on the basis of his subtle interest in his former life. The subtle interest, if it was focused on the gross world, will cause the person to gravitate towards another gross existence. This is how a living being transmigrates from one gross body to another. Thus by that law of shifting existence, if one generates an interest in the subtle world or in the supernatural or spiritual world during one's gross life, then one might gravitate towards such places after leaving the gross body. It is the *bhāva* of the person, the normal texture of his consciousness, which determines where he will be drawn to in the next life. By instinct, one goes to the next existence, not by determination. Whatever instincts one develops in this life, will dictate the kind of place one will emerge from in the next existence.

तस्मात्सर्वेषु कालेषु
मामनुस्मर युध्य च ।
मय्यर्पितमनोबुद्धिर्
मामेवैष्यस्यसंशयः ॥८.७॥
tasmātsarveṣu kāleṣu
māmanusmara yudhya ca
mayyarpitamanobuddhir
māmevaiṣyasyasaṁśayaḥ (8.7)

*tasmāt — therefore; sarveṣu — at all; kāleṣu — at times; mām — Me; anusmara — remember; yudhya — fight; ca — and; mayy = mayi — on Me; arpitamanobuddhir (arpitamanobuddhiḥ) = arpita — anchor + manobuddhiḥ — mind and intelligence; mām — to Me; evaiṣyasy (evaiṣyasi) = eva — indeed + eṣyasi — will be with; asaṁśayaḥ — without doubt*

**Therefore, at all times, remember Me and fight. Anchor your mind and intelligence on Me. You will be with Me without doubt. (8.7)**

***Siddha Swami's Commentary:***

*Śrī* Krishna encouraged Arjuna to make use of their relationship by anchoring the mind and intelligence upon *Śrī* Krishna alone and to forego other relationships, such as Arjuna's fondness for Bhishma and *Droṇa* and other elders of the Kuru family. *Śrī* Krishna assured Arjuna that wherever *Śrī* Krishna would go after departing from this world, Arjuna too would follow along, provided Arjuna was able to recall Krishna in particular *(mām eva smaran*, 8.5). Through service to Krishna, by helping Krishna in the mission of protecting righteousness and righteous people and eliminating irreligion and irreligious people, Arjuna would earn his keep to remain with *Śrī* Krishna, by such performance of *karma yoga*, which is *Śrī* Krishna's self-appointed work.

On that basis alone, *Śrī* Krishna assured Arjuna of elevation to *Śrī* Krishna's existence *(madbhāvam*, Bg 8.5) after Arjuna left his body. This explains the path of *bhakti yoga*, comprised of *buddhi yoga* mastership with *karma yoga*, resulting in *bhakti yoga* advancement. This operates mainly on the basis of an attachment to *Śrī* Krishna, just as Arjuna had. One would have to be devoted to *Śrī* Krishna and friendly to the divinity as well *(bhakto'si me sakhā* Bg 4.3).

Amazingly, teachers who do not know *Śrī* Krishna, as Arjuna did personally, offer this guarantee to others. It is sufficient in the course of *brahma yoga*, for the student yogi to observe in great admiration of both Arjuna and Lord Krishna, this relationship which afforded Arjuna such a privilege. Arjuna is to be greatly admired and praised, and even worshiped. All student *brahma yogis* are to acknowledge Arjuna in great admiration and without any envy whatsoever.

अभ्यासयोगयुक्तेन
चेतसा नान्यगामिना ।
परमं पुरुषं दिव्यं
याति पार्थानुचिन्तयन् ॥८.८॥
abhyāsayogayuktena
cetasā nānyagāminā
paramaṁ puruṣaṁ divyaṁ
yāti pārthānucintayan (8.8)

*abhyāsa — practice;. yoga — yoga; yuktena — by discipline; cetasā — by the mind; nānyagāminā = na — not + anya — other + gāminā — by venturing outward; paramam — supreme; puruṣam — person; divyam — divine; yāti — one goes; pārthānucintayan = pārtha — son of Pṛthā + anucintayan — deeply meditating*

**With a mind that does not venture outwards, which is disciplined by yoga practice, a person goes to the divine Supreme Person, while deeply meditating, O son of Pṛthā. (8.8)**

***Siddha Swami's Commentary:***

Now this is the statement which the *brahma yoga* teachers may advertise to others. This does not hinge on a relationship such as Arjuna had, because others who do not have such a relationship will not get it, merely by impinging or by hoping for it. One either has it or he or she does not. In which case, then, *Śrī* Krishna gave this statement in verse 8.

By the perfection of *buddhi yoga* practice, in the stage of *aṣṭanga* yoga known as *pratyāhār*, where the mind does not venture outwards *(cetasā nānyagāminā)* and being disciplined in yoga practice, one does while deeply meditating *(anucintayan)* go to the divine Supreme person. One's spiritual vision opens up and one sees into the spiritual atmosphere and can develop the relationship to the divine beings who reside there.

Arjuna's situation was quite different, for he was one of those divine beings, who came with the Supreme Person, *Śrī* Krishna, from that divine place, and who was assured of going back there, just on the basis of his devoted and friendly relationship with the Lord.

Those who do not have the relationship which Arjuna had, should pay close attention to this verse, which gives them the key to how they would go to *Śrī* Krishna after leaving their material bodies at death.

कविं पुराणमनुशासितारम्
अणोरणीयांसमनुस्मरेद्यः ।
सर्वस्य धातारमचिन्त्यरूपम्
आदित्यवर्णं तमसः परस्तात् ॥८.९॥

*kavim — the person who knows everything; purāṇam — the most ancient; anuśāsitāram — the supreme supervisor; aṇor (aṇoḥ) — than the atom; aṇīyāṁsam — more minute; anusmared (anusmaret) — should meditate on; yaḥ —*

kaviṁ purāṇamanuśāsitāram
aṇoraṇīyāṁsamanusmaredyaḥ
sarvasya dhātāram acintyarūpam
ādityavarṇaṁ tamasaḥ parastāt
(8.9)

*who; sarvasya — of all; dhātāram — supporter; acintya — unimaginable; rūpam — form; ādityavarṇam = āditya — radiance + varṇam — category; tamasaḥ — grossness; parastāt — distinct form*

**He who meditates on the Person Who knows everything, the most ancient of people, the Supreme Supervisor, the most minute factor, the one with unimaginable form, with a radiant body, free of grossness, (8.9)**

***Siddha Swami's Commentary:***

This verse and the previous one consists of *brahma yoga technique*. This is given by *Patañjali* under the terms of *īśvarapraṇidhānāni (Yoga Sūtra* 2.32). Though elementary in the *Patañjali* system of yoga, this is very advanced. This is difficult to achieve for modern yogis, due to the multiple distractions in the modern civilization.

One not situated in a relationship like Arjuna, must start meditating on the Supreme Person as described in these verses. Student yogis should note every detail of these descriptions and work hard in higher yoga and spiritual perception to come face to face with these truths using the spiritual senses which develop after stunting or snubbing out the normal ways of using the psychic equipments.

Of particular notice is *Śrī* Krishna's definition of the unimaginable form, with a radiant body free of grossness. Such a form cannot be perceived in the usual way with the usual psychic equipments. Thus the student *yogin* should endeavor to develop spiritual senses. Once those senses are developed, whatever is in the spiritual environment may be automatically seen. *Śrī* Krishna particularly used the word *rūpam*, which means a form with limbs and senses. These are the divine forms of the Personalities of Godhead and Their associates.

प्रयाणकाले मनसाचलेन
भक्त्या युक्तो योगबलेन चैव ।
भ्रुवोर्मध्ये प्राणमावेश्य सम्यक्
स तं परं पुरुषमुपैति दिव्यम् ॥८.१०॥
prayāṇakāle manasācalena
bhaktyā yukto yogabalena
caiva
bhruvormadhye prāṇam
āveśya samyak
sa taṁ paraṁ puruṣamupaiti
divyam (8.10)

*prayāṇakāle — at the time of death; manasācalena = manasā — by the mind + acalena — by unwavering; bhaktyā — with devotion; yukto = yuktaḥ — connected; yogabalena — with psychological power developed through yoga practice; caiva = ca — and + eva — indeed; bhruvor = bhruvoḥ — of the two eyebrows; madhye — in the middle; prāṇam — energizing breath; āveśya — having caused to enter; samyak — precisely; sa = saḥ — he; tam — this; param — supreme; puruṣam — person; upaiti — he goes; divyam — divine*

**...and that meditator who even at the time of death, with an unwavering mind, being connected devotedly, with psychological power developed through yoga practice, and having caused the energizing breath to enter between the eyebrows with precision, goes to the Divine Supreme Person. (8.10)**

***Siddha Swami's Commentary:***

This is possible through *yogabalena*, the psychological strength developed through yoga practice, but it is possible also through devotedness and friendliness to *Śrī* Krishna and adherence to the mission of the Lord, as in the case of Arjuna. However, persons like Arjuna did practice yoga and in the case of others, such as the gopi women-friends of *Śrī* Krishna, their adherence to *Śrī* Krishna which was based on an existential connection with Him, did cause their attainment of Him by the psychological strength developed, not through yoga but through their eternal relationship with the Lord. Here I mean a spiritual family relationship, not a love relationship, even though love is included in that spiritual family connection.

The details in this verse should be adhered to by all aspiring *brahma yogis*. These details are:

- Meditation with unwavering mind at the time of death, through perfecting the *buddhi yoga* practice.
- Being devotedly connected to *Śrī* Krishna by developing devotedness and friendliness to the teacher who is the agent of *Śrī* Krishna and to *Śrī* Krishna Himself.
- Having psychological power developed through yoga practice, mastering the same *buddhi yoga* process.
- Causing the energizing breath to enter between the eyebrows, by virtue of mastering kundalini yoga, having a cleaned-out, cleared *suśumnā* central passage in the subtle spine, having kundalini shakti come into the brain through abandonment of sexual practices.

One who masters this, certainly goes to the Supreme Divine Person after leaving aside the gross body at its death.

यदक्षरं वेदविदो वदन्ति
विशन्ति यद्यतयो वीतरागाः ।
यदिच्छन्तो ब्रह्मचर्यं चरन्ति
तत्ते पदं संग्रहेण प्रवक्ष्ये ॥८.११॥
yadakṣaraṁ vedavido vadanti
viśanti yadyatayo vītarāgāḥ
yadicchanto brahmacaryaṁ caranti
tatte padaṁ saṁgraheṇa pravakṣye
(8.11)

*yad — which; akṣaram — imperishable; vedavido = vedavidaḥ — knowers of the Veda; vadanti — they described; viśanti — they enter; yad — which; yatayo = yatayaḥ — ascetics; vītarāgāḥ — free from cravings; yad — which; icchanto = icchantaḥ — desiring; brahmacaryam — life of celibacy; caranti — they follow; tat = tad — this; te — to you; padam — process; saṁgraheṇa — in brief; pravakṣye — I will explain*

**I will briefly explain the process to you, which the knowers of the Veda describe as imperishable, which the ascetics who are free from cravings enter and who desiring to be transferred there, they follow a life of celibacy. (8.11)**

***Siddha Swami's Commentary:***

Before Arjuna would ask any questions about the yoga process described, *Śrī* Krishna decided to elaborate on it, for the benefit of all concerned. To qualify for this teaching of *brahma yoga* practice, one is required to be free from cravings, to have a desire to be transferred out of material existence completely, and must follow a life of yogically-regulated celibacy. This is a time-tested process, which worked for many ancient ascetics and which would work today for anyone who wants to painstakingly practice. It is a definite process.

सर्वद्वाराणि संयम्य
मनो हृदि निरुध्य च ।
मूर्ध्न्याधायात्मनः प्राणम्
आस्थितो योगधारणाम् ॥८.१२॥
sarvadvārāṇi saṁyamya
mano hṛdi nirudhya ca
mūrdhnyādhāyātmanaḥ prāṇam
āsthito yogadhāraṇām (8.12)

*sarvadvārāṇi = sarva – all + dvārāṇi — entrances; saṁyamya — controlling; mano = manaḥ — mind; hṛdi — in the core of consciousness; nirudhya — confining; ca — and; mūrdhny = mūrdhni — in the brain; ādhāyātmanaḥ = ādhāya — situating + ātmanaḥ — of the soul; prāṇam — energizing breath; āsthito = āsthitaḥ — remain fixed; yogadhāraṇām — yoga concentration*

**Controlling all openings of the body, and restricting the mind in the core of consciousness, situating the energizing energy of the soul in the brain, remaining fixed in yoga concentration, (8.12)**

***Siddha Swami's Commentary:***

This technique was stressed by *Mahāyogin* Gorakshnatha. This was propagated by Rishi Gorakshnatha, that flawless *yogin*. Even in the time of *Śrī* Krishna, thousands of years before Gorakshnatha, this procedure was known. Usually this is done in isolation after practicing the austerities of *haṭha* yoga. One must raise kundalini consistently. One must master *buddhi yoga* to restrict the mind in the core of the consciousness in the head of the subtle body. One must relocate kundalini energy into the head. One must enter into *samādhi* by *yogadhāraṇām*, which is linking the attention of the self into higher concentration forces. This graduates into yoga *dhyāna* which is the effortless linkage of the same, and then it progresses into yoga *samādhi* which is the continuous effortless linkage of the same. These were pooled together as *samyama* by *Śrī Patañjali*.

*deśa bandhaḥ cittasya dhāraṇā*
*tatra pratyaya ekatānatā dhyānam*
*tadeva arthamātranirbhāsaṁ svarūpaśūnyam iva samādhiḥ*
*trayam ekatra saṁyamaḥ*

***Linking of the attention to a concentration force or person, involves a restricted location in the mento-emotional energy.***

***When in that location, there is one continuous threadlike flow of one's instinctive interest, that is the effortless linking of the attention to a higher concentration force or person.***

***That same effortless linkage of the attention when experienced as illumination of the higher concentration force or person, while the yogi feels as if devoid of himself, is samādhi or continuous effortless linkage of his attention to the special person, object, or force.***

***The three as one practice is the complete restraint. (Yoga Sūtra 3.1-4)***

ओमित्येकाक्षरं ब्रह्म
व्याहरन्मामनुस्मरन् ।
यः प्रयाति त्यजन्देहं
स याति परमां गतिम् ॥८.१३॥
omityekākṣaraṁ brahma
vyāharanmāmanusmaran
yaḥ prayāti tyajandehaṁ
sa yāti paramāṁ gatim (8.13)

*om — the uttered sound om; ity = iti — thus saying; ekākṣaram — one syllable; brahma — spiritual reality; vyāharan — chanting; mām — Me; anusmaran — meditating on; yaḥ — who; prayāti — passes on; tyajan — renouncing; deham — body; sa = saḥ — he; yāti — attains; paramām — supreme; gatim — objective*

**...uttering *Om,* the one-syllable sound which represents the spiritual reality, meditating on Me, the yogi who passes on, renouncing the body, attains the highest objective. (8.13)**

***Siddha Swami's Commentary:***

Uttering *Om* is a standard procedure in yoga practice. It leads to the discovery in the psyche of the naad *praṇava* sound. A yogi reaching this, does indeed go to the Supreme. A student *yogin* should utter *Om* audibly at first. Then it should be uttered mentally only. That should be done only for as long as he does not hear the natural un-uttered *Om*, the naad sound, which is a continuous sound resonating in the psyche of all beings. From there, from that sound, one will develop supernatural vision to see into the spiritual atmosphere. These practices take time. Much practice must be done by the student *yogin*.

अनन्यचेताः सततं
यो मां स्मरति नित्यशः ।
तस्याहं सुलभः पार्थ
नित्ययुक्तस्य योगिनः ॥८.१४॥
ananyacetāḥ satataṁ
yo māṁ smarati nityaśaḥ
tasyāhaṁ sulabhaḥ pārtha
nityayuktasya yoginaḥ (8.14)

*ananyacetāḥ — one whose mind does not go to another focus; satatam — perpetually; yo = yaḥ — who; mām — Me; smarati — he remembers; nityaśaḥ — constantly; tasyāham = tasya — to him + aham — I; sulabhaḥ — easy to reach; pārtha — O son of Pṛthā; nityayuktasya — of one who is constantly disciplined in yoga; yoginaḥ — of the devotee*

**He whose mind does not go to another focus at any time, who thinks of Me constantly, for that yogi who is constantly disciplined in yoga, I am easy to reach, O son of Pṛthā. (8.14)**

***Siddha Swami's Commentary:***

*Śrī* Krishna stressed the memory of Himself, *yo mām smarati nityaśah*. This means that the *yogin* must keep in mind what he has to do to please *Śrī* Krishna and reach the Lord's location after leaving the physical body. It is not just remembering *Śrī* Krishna and *Śrī* Krishna's cultural activities *(līlā)* on earth, but rather more about remembering what one must do to please *Śrī* Krishna in karma yoga activities and become purified with a nature similar to *Śrī* Krishna's. Such attainment is accomplished through purity of the psyche attained through buddhi yoga practice, as stated many times in previous verses. For such a *yogin*, *Śrī* Krishna is easy to reach.

मामुपेत्य पुनर्जन्म
दुःखालयमशाश्वतम् ।
नाप्नुवन्ति महात्मानः
संसिद्धिं परमां गताः ॥८.१५॥
māmupetya punarjanma
duḥkhālayamaśāśvatam
nāpnuvanti mahātmānaḥ
saṁsiddhiṁ paramāṁ gatāḥ (8.15)

*mām — Me; upetya — approaching; punarjanma — rebirth; duḥkhālayam = duḥkha — misery + ālayam — location; aśāśvatam — shifty; nāpnuvanti = na — not + apnuvanti — subjected to; mahātmānaḥ — great souls; saṁsiddhim — perfect; paramām — supreme; gatāḥ — gone*

**Approaching me in this way, those great souls who went to supreme perfection are not subjected to rebirth in this shifty, miserable location. (8.15)**

***Siddha Swami's Commentary:***

The completion of *brahma yoga* brings on a result such as this, whereby the *yogin* is not again subjected to taking a physical body. One does not have to stay in the material world to please *Śrī* Krishna or any other of His parallel divinities. In fact, if one develops so that one attains a spiritual body, then as one progresses, others move up the evolutionary system, and they will take up whatever duties one performed previously in *karma yoga*. One cannot progress without causing others to progress. As a *yogin* moves up, others come up after him. There is no fear that such a *yogin* would not be replaced if he left the material universe for good. Others will surely advance by his progression, and they would in turn take his place and complete whatever *karma yoga* duties he performed.

आ ब्रह्मभुवनाल्लोकाः
पुनरावर्तिनोऽर्जुन ।
मामुपेत्य तु कौन्तेय
पुनर्जन्म न विद्यते ॥८.१६॥
ā brahmabhuvanāllokāḥ
punarāvartino'rjuna
māmupetya tu kaunteya
punarjanma na vidyate (8.16)

*ā – up to; brahmabhuvanāl = brahmabhuvanāt — to Brahmā's world; lokāḥ — populations; punarāvartino = punarāvartinaḥ — subjected to repeated birth and death; 'rjuna = arjuna — Arjuna; mām — Me; upetya — approaching; tu — but; kaunteya — O son of Kuntī; punarjanma — impulsion of rebirth; na — not; vidyate — is experienced*

**Up to Brahmā's world, the populations are subjected to repeated births and deaths, O Arjuna. But in approaching Me, rebirth is not experienced, O son of Kuntī. (8.16)**

***Siddha Swami's Commentary:***

This is a very famous verse used by many Vaishnava preachers to encourage people to take up the Krishna *Bhakti* religion and to forsake all other systems of worship in India. However this verse is very technical. Indeed, only a few ascetics, only a few devotees even, will get up as far as *Brahmā*'s world. Even though all populations are subjected to repeated births and deaths, still there are different durations for each location or dimension. As such, a person who hailed from a place with 100 years as a life span, would naturally consider a place with 10,000 years life span to be fabulous. In *Brahmā*'s world, the life span is many, many thousands of years. To a human being, that is an eternity. Thus the human being cannot imagine anything as fabulous as life in the spiritual atmosphere.

There is another technicality. Even though *Śrī* Krishna stated that in approaching Him, rebirth is not experienced, this also means that in approaching Him, one might well have to take limited bodies like the earthly one, but one would retain divine consciousness throughout those births. It does not necessarily mean that in all cases, the perfected *yogin*, the devotee of Krishna, will not have to take a temporary body. For indeed that would contradict the very physical presence of Krishna and Arjuna on the *Kurukṣetra* battlefield.

सहस्रयुगपर्यन्तम्
अहर्यद्ब्रह्मणो विदुः ।
रात्रिं युगसहस्रान्तां
तेऽहोरात्रविदो जनाः ॥८.१७॥

*sahasra — one thousand; yuga — time cycle; paryantam — limit; ahar — day; yad — which; brahmaṇo = brahmaṇaḥ — of Brahmā; viduḥ — they know; rātrim — night; yugasahasrāntāṁ = yuga — time cycle +*

sahasrayugaparyantam
aharyadbrahmaṇo viduḥ
rātriṁ yugasahasrāntāṁ
te'horātravido janāḥ (8.17)

*sahasra – one thousand + antam — end; te — they; 'horātravido (ahoratravidaḥ) = ahoratra — day and night + vidaḥ — knowers; janāḥ — people*

**Those who know the day of Brahmā, which has a limit of one thousand time cycles, and the night of Brahmā, which ends in a thousand time cycles, are the people who know day and night. (8.17)**

***Siddha Swami's Commentary:***

The day of *Prajāpati Brahmā*, as well as his night, lasts for many thousands of years by earthly calculation. To the earthly mind, that would be like an eternity, because a human intellect cannot comprehend it. In *brahma yoga*, we get some idea of it when in timelessness we enter *samādhi*; otherwise it cannot be understood by a human mind, either by a devotee or anyone else.

An ordinary devotee, even one on the level of Arjuna at the time he heard this *Gītā*, cannot understand this type of day and night which pertains to *Brahmā*. But if the ordinary person were to master the *buddhi yoga* process, he could get a glimpse of this through *samādhi* practice, where he could translate himself into higher existences and experience the life there in other dimensions.

Vedic authorities from figures given in the *Purāṇas* and the *Mahābhārata*, give one day of *Brahmā* as 432 million earthly years. Even if that figure were to be contested, still the time for one day of the Creator Lord, *Brahmā*, is beyond the imagination of a human being. We can only understand these time spans by entering other dimensions in *samādhi* practice.

अव्यक्ताद्व्यक्तयः सर्वाः
प्रभवन्त्यहरागमे ।
रात्र्यागमे प्रलीयन्ते
तत्रैवाव्यक्तसंज्ञके ॥८.१८॥
avyaktādvyaktayaḥ sarvāḥ
prabhavantyaharāgame
rātryāgame pralīyante
tatraivāvyaktasaṁjñake (8.18)

*avyaktād = avyaktāt — from the invisible world; vyaktayaḥ — the visible world; sarvāḥ — all; prabhavanty = prabhavanti — they are produced; aharāgame — at the beginning of Brahmā's day; rātryāgame — at the beginning of Brahmā's night; pralīyante — they are reverted back; tatraivāvyaktasaṁjñake = tatra — at the time + eva — indeed + avyakta — invisible world + saṁjñake — is understood as*

**When the day of Creator Brahmā begins, all this visible world is produced from the invisible world. When his night comes, the manifested energies are reverted back into the invisible world. (8.18)**

***Siddha Swami's Commentary:***

How invisible matter converts into visible materials, is a mystery which our material scientists are still troubled with. As soon as they can figure that out, they will be like magicians, just like the ancient *asuras* who are mentioned in the Vedic texts. *Prajāpati Brahmā* is the one who converts the invisible matter into visible objects. Therefore what is invisible has potential for manifestation under certain conditions.

भूतग्रामः स एवायं
भूत्वा भूत्वा प्रलीयते ।
रात्र्यागमेऽवशः पार्थ
प्रभवत्यहरागमे ॥८.१९॥

*bhūtagrāmaḥ — multitude of beings; sa = saḥ — this; evāyam = eva — indeed + ayam — this; bhūtvā bhūtvā — repeatedly manifesting; pralīyate — is shifted out of visibility; rātryāgame — at the arrival of Brahmā's night; 'vaśaḥ = avaśaḥ — happening*

bhūtagrāmaḥ sa evāyaṁ
bhūtvā bhūtvā pralīyate
rātryāgame'vaśaḥ pārtha
prabhavatyaharāgame (8.19)

*naturally; pārtha — O son of Pṛthā; prabhavaty = prabhavati — it comes into existence; aharāgame — on the onset of Brahmā's day*

**O son of Pṛthā, this multitude of beings which is repeatedly manifested, is naturally shifted out of visibility at the arrival of each of Brahmā's nights. It again comes into existence at the onset of Brahmā's day. (8.19)**

***Siddha Swami's Commentary:***

We may conclude that this manifested world is dependent on the mental energy of *Śrī Brahmāji*, the Procreator Lord. Such a thing is not impossible, for even materially some large enterprises are dependent on the great mind or minds which conceive of it and are instrumental in manifesting it. It is seen that sometimes when an entrepreneur leaves his body, his projects collapse because his managers are unable to maintain the business. This is because it depended mostly on the founder's mind. Smaller minds, even if they work together, are usually unable to continue a great enterprise which a great person initiated and maintained.

But when again that entrepreneur takes a new body, he again creates large enterprises which work by the infusion of his energies, and again when he leaves that body, those concerns perish.

There are many aborigines in a forest, but rarely are any of them able to create an alphabet to expand their language and as a result their civilization remains primitive. Thus we know that certain persons are more capable than others. We can therefore accept that such a person as *Prajāpati Brahmā* is a superior entity, whose mind might sustain this creation.

In *brahma yoga* practice, in advanced *buddhi yoga* practice, one makes mystic research into this, to see who is behind the creation. Great yogins like Markandeya did this and understood the foundation of this manifested world.

परस्तस्मात्तु भावोऽन्यो
ऽव्यक्तोऽव्यक्तात्सनातनः ।
यः स सर्वेषु भूतेषु
नश्यत्सु न विनश्यति ॥८.२०॥
parastasmāttu bhāvo'nyo
'vyakto'vyaktātsanātanaḥ
yaḥ sa sarveṣu bhūteṣu
naśyatsu na vinaśyati (8.20)

*paraḥ — high; tasmāt — than this; tu — but; bhāvo = bhāvaḥ — existence; 'nyo = anyaḥ — another; 'vyakto = avyaktaḥ — invisible; 'vyaktāt = avyaktāt — than the unmanifest state of the dissolvable creation; sanātanaḥ — primeval; yaḥ = which; sa = saḥ — it; sarveṣu — in all; bhūteṣu — in creation; naśyatsu — in the disintegration; na — not; vinaśyati — is disintegrated*

**But higher than this, there is another invisible existence, which is higher than the primeval unmanifested states of this dissolvable creation. When all these creatures are disintegrated, that is not affected. (8.20)**

***Siddha Swami's Commentary:***

There are two invisible existences. One is the mundane potency in its unmanifested form, and beyond that, there is the spiritual dimension. This place cannot be reached except by the spirit. None of the subtle or gross material equipments used by a spirit can enter into that place, since they all become dissolved in their respective levels of manifestation. Thus to see into the spiritual place, one must develop the spiritual interest without using the psychic equipments. This means the practice of *brahma yoga*.

Both invisible existences, the primal material energy as well as the spiritual world, are not to be destroyed or changed at anytime, even though in the primal mundane energy, some of that force appears to click into manifestation in certain time pockets which are created by the Supreme Lord and developed further by a person like *Prajāpati Brahmā*.

अव्यक्तोऽक्षर इत्युक्तस्
तमाहुः परमां गतिम् ।
यं प्राप्य न निवर्तन्ते
तद्धाम परमं मम ॥८.२१॥
avyakto'kṣara ityuktas
tamāhuḥ paramāṁ gatim
yaṁ prāpya na nivartante
taddhāma paramaṁ mama (8.21)

*avyakto = avyaktaḥ — invisible world; 'kṣara = akṣara — unalterable; ity = iti — thus; uktaḥ — is declared; tam — it; āhuḥ — authorities say; paramām — supreme; gatim — objective; yam — which; prāpya — attaining; na — not; nivartante — return here; tad — that; dhāma — residence; paramam — supreme; mama — My*

**That invisible world is unalterable, so it is declared. The authorities say that it is the supreme objective. Attaining that, they do not return here. That place is My supreme residence. (8.21)**

***Siddha Swami's Commentary:***

The spiritual places, known in the language of the Upanishads as *brahman*, came to be described as being unalterable *(akṣara),* as invisible *(avyaktah)* and as supreme *(paramam).* Other adjectival terms are used as well. This place is fabled and became known as *akṣar dhāma, vaikuntha*, the kingdom of God and other such names like Krishna *loka*. Some say it is Shiva *loka*. Some say heaven.

*Śrī* Krishna identified the place as His supreme abode, *dhāma paramam mama*, and he attested that persons who attain that place do not return to this material world. That is doubtful, however, if it means that they never actually come back here, since *Śrī* Krishna and Arjuna as well, were indicated by *Śrī* Krishna Himself as having taken repeated births in this very same material world. He must therefore mean that a person situated in the spiritual world, does not lose contact with that locale even when in this world and is never completely given over to this place when visiting here. *Śrī* Krishna said previously:

*śrībhagavānuvāca*
*bahūni me vyatītāni janmāni tava cārjuna*
*tānyahaṁ veda sarvāṇi na tvaṁ vettha paraṁtapa (4.5)*

***The Blessed Lord said: Many of My births transpired, and yours, Arjuna. I recall them all. You do not remember, O scorcher of the enemies. (4.5)***

The indication is, therefore, that once a finite entity develops a spiritual body with limbs and senses, those spiritual utilities remain permanently for him, and as such he does not have to endeavor to develop them again. Thus if he enters the material world, then still, because his spirituality is permanently developed, he will again gravitate to the spiritual world regardless, while others who have not developed their spiritual selves, who are mere specks of spiritual light, are baffled and confused in the material existences, and do rely on gross existence for objective life.

पुरुषः स परः पार्थ
भक्त्या लभ्यस्त्वनन्यया ।
यस्यान्तःस्थानि भूतानि
येन सर्वमिदं ततम् ॥८.२२॥
puruṣaḥ sa paraḥ pārtha
bhaktyā labhyastvananyayā
yasyāntaḥsthāni bhūtāni
yena sarvamidaṁ tatam (8.22)

*puruṣaḥ — person; sa = saḥ — this; paraḥ — supreme; pārtha — O son of Pṛthā; bhaktyā — by a devotional relationship; labhyaḥ — attainable; tv = tu — but; ananyayā — not by any other; yasyāntaḥsthāni = yasya — of which + antaḥsthāni — existing within; bhūtāni — beings; yena — by which; sarvam — all; idam — this; tatam — energized*

**That Supreme Person, O son of Pṛthā, is attainable through a devotional relationship and not by any other means. Within His influence, all beings exist. By Him, all the universe is energized. (8.22)**

***Siddha Swami's Commentary:***

It appears that the spiritual place which was identified merely as *brahman* in the Upanishads, is attainable without specific devotion to this Supreme Person, *puruṣah parah*, which is mentioned by *Śrī* Krishna in this verse. But the Supreme Person Himself, the resident of that place, is only attainable through specific devotion, *bhaktyā*.

*Śrī* Krishna attests to the fact that all these beings in this material world exist within His influence and that by Him all this universe is energized. His influence is all-pervasive and is all-causative. Thus He cannot be avoided. But to attain His association in particular, one has to have a devotional relationship with Him, *bhaktyā*.

It does not mean, however, that one will not have to become expert at *buddhi yoga*. After all, Arjuna will have to develop that expertise in order to serve *Śrī* Krishna efficiently as a *karma* yogi. It is appropriate that this devotion be such as to inspire the devotee to take up the austerities which would bring the purity required for translation of his interest into the spiritual atmosphere. The devotion should not be a weak type which discourages the devotee from the austerities of *buddhi* yoga, which *Śrī* Krishna Himself inaugurated.

यत्र काले त्वनावृत्तिम्
आवृत्तिं चैव योगिनः ।
प्रयाता यान्ति तं कालं
वक्ष्यामि भरतर्षभ ॥८.२३॥
yatra kāle tvanāvṛttim
āvṛttiṁ caiva yoginaḥ
prayātā yānti taṁ kālaṁ
vakṣyāmi bharatarṣabha (8.23)

*yatra — where; kāle — in time; tv = tu — but; anāvṛttim — not return; āvṛttim — return; caiva = ca — and + eva — indeed; yoginaḥ — yogis; prayātā — departing; yānti — go; tam — this; kālam — time; vakṣyāmi — I will tell; bharatarṣabha — O bullish man of the Bharata family*

**O bullish man of the Bharata family, I will tell you of the departure for the yogis who do or do not return. (8.23)**

***Siddha Swami's Commentary:***

*Śrī* Krishna explained to Arjuna, how the yogis venture away from a material body, how they are either successful or frustrated in the attempt to reach the spiritual places or to reach *Śrī* Krishna, the Supreme Person, in particular.

अग्निर्ज्योतिरहः शुक्लः
षण्मासा उत्तरायणम् ।
तत्र प्रयाता गच्छन्ति
ब्रह्म ब्रह्मविदो जनाः ॥८.२४॥
agnirjyotirahaḥ śuklaḥ
ṣaṇmāsā uttarāyaṇam
tatra prayātā gacchanti
brahma brahmavido janāḥ (8.24)

*agnir = agniḥ — summer season; jyotir = jyotiḥ — bright atmosphere; ahaḥ — daytime; śuklaḥ — bright moonlight; saṇmāsā — six months; uttarāyaṇam — the time when the sun appears to move north; tatra — at that time; prayātā — departing; gacchanti — they go; brahma — to the spiritual location; brahmavido = brahmavidaḥ — knowers of the spiritual dimension; janāḥ — people*

**The summer season, the bright atmosphere, the daytime, the bright moonlight, the six months when the sun appears to move north; if at that time, they depart the body, those people who know the spiritual dimension, go to the spiritual location. (8.24)**

***Siddha Swami's Commentary:***

These descriptions of passing to other dimensions, pertain specifically to yogis (*yoginah*, 8.23). This verse applies to practiced mystics who learned the psychic geography of the dimensions in the hereafter. This is why *Śrī* Krishna used the term *brahmavido*, which means the knowers *(vido)* of brahman spiritual locations *(brahma)*.

These descriptions deal with the pure, impure or partially-pure status of the subtle body of the person, particularly of the yogi. If the yogi has not mastered kundalini shakti, then for certain, he cannot take advantage of the subtle benefits which accrue in the subtle atmosphere during the summer season in either the northern or southern hemisphere. The sun and moon do have effects on the living being, both materially and psychically affecting the subtle body of the finite souls.

A yogi has no fantasies about salvation, since during his life, he experiences the hereafter night after night when his subtle body separates from the gross one. Thus he knows what will happen. He knows the possibilities depend on the status of his purity alone. Others who have hopes and promises, make up all sorts of fantastic projections about salvation at the time of death, and they neglect the pure or impure status of the subtle body which they experience night after night in dreams.

धूमो रात्रिस्तथा कृष्णः
षण्मासा दक्षिणायनम् ।
तत्र चान्द्रमसं ज्योतिर्
योगी प्राप्य निवर्तते ॥८.२५॥
dhūmo rātristathā kṛṣṇaḥ
ṣaṇmāsā dakṣiṇāyanam
tatra cāndramasaṁ jyotir
yogī prāpya nivartate (8.25)

*dhūmo = dhūmaḥ — smoky, misty or hazy season; rātris — night time; tathā — as well as; kṛṣṇaḥ — the dark moon time; saṇmāsā — six months; dakṣiṇāyanam — the time when the sun appears to move south; tatra — at that time; cāndramasam — moon; jyotir = jyotiḥ — light; yogī — yogi; prāpya — attaining; nivartate — is born again*

**The smoky, misty or hazy season, as well as in the night-time, the dark-moon time, the six months when the sun appears to move south; if the yogi departs at that time, he attains moonlight, after which he is born again. (8.25)**

***Siddha Swami's Commentary:***

*Śrī* Krishna applies these statements to the yogins and to no one else, but somehow others feel that these verses apply to them or that these verses may be adjusted to accommodate them. In verse 23, Lord Krishna said that He would tell Arjuna of the departure for the yogis who do or do not return to the gross material existence, as we endure it in material bodies. These descriptions apply to such persons.

One who departs from the body under the influence of energy from the moon, will have to return to the earthly planet, because that is how that energy operates; while those yogins who leave under the influence of the solar planet, get stimulus and impetus to go higher or at least to live in a yoga siddha body which is made of sunlight. Living in such a body for a time, and associating with higher yogins, such an ascetic may complete his austerities and not have to return again to a gross body to do penances.

शुक्लकृष्णे गती ह्येते
जगतः शाश्वते मते ।
एकया यात्यनावृत्तिम्
अन्ययावर्तते पुनः ॥८.२६॥
śuklakṛṣṇe gatī hyete
jagataḥ śāśvate mate
ekayā yātyanāvṛttim
anyayāvartate punaḥ (8.26)

*śuklakṛṣṇe — light and dark; gatī — two paths; hyete = hy (hi) — indeed + ete — these two; jagataḥ — of the universe; śāśvate — perpetual; mate — is considered; ekayā — by one; yāty = yāti — goes away; anāvṛttim — not return; anyayāvartate = anyayā — by other + āvartate — comes back; punaḥ = punar — again*

**The light and the dark times are two paths which are considered to be perpetually available for the universe. It is considered so by the authorities. By one, a person goes away not to return; by the other he comes back again. (8.26)**

***Siddha Swami's Commentary:***

The two courses are perpetually available, because no matter on which material planet one may take a gross body, still one will fall under the influence of a solar planet and also of a moon or moons. These spheres have subtle counterparts which express influences on the inhabitants. As people from a certain part of this planet have similar characteristics, which were developed under geographic and atmospheric circumstances, so in each part of the universe, inhabitants have to accept certain conditions. This is unavoidable. A yogi gets into a position to study the positive and negative influences and then he may select which of these he desires to utilize for his benefit. That is the advantage of yoga practice. It gives one more insight into how to select one influence or another for spiritual benefit.

In the *Mahābhārata* history, Bhishma, the aged Kuru leader, was such a yogi that he selected which influences prevailed when he departed from his body. Thus he left aside his material body and took recourse to the influence of the solar planet.

नैते सृती पार्थ जानन्
योगी मुह्यति कश्चन ।
तस्मात्सर्वेषु कालेषु
योगयुक्तो भवार्जुन ॥८.२७॥
naite sṛtī pārtha jānan
yogī muhyati kaścana
tasmātsarveṣu kāleṣu
yogayukto bhavārjuna (8.27)

*naite = na — not + ete — these two; sṛtī — two paths; pārtha — O son of Pṛthā; jānan — knowing; yogī — yogi; muhyati — is confused; kaścana — at all; tasmāt — therefore; sarveṣu — in all; kāleṣu — in times; yogayukto = yogayuktaḥ — disciplined in yoga practice; bhavārjuna = bhava — be + arjuna — Arjuna*

**Knowing these two paths, O son of Pṛthā, the yogi is not confused at all. Therefore at all times, be disciplined in yoga practice, O Arjuna. (8.27)**

***Siddha Swami's Commentary:***

A *yogin* should study his local planetary situation and gage his position in the hereafter before he leaves the body. He should not leave the opportunity to chance. He should not live in hope that God will save him at the end merely because he is God's devotee or because he is a disciple of a prominent, reputed spiritual master. One should work step by step in *buddhi yoga* for a definite goal at the time of leaving the body. At least one should have a clear idea of one's progression and thus be able to honestly gage where one will end up after leaving the body.

वेदेषु यज्ञेषु तपःसु चैव
दानेषु यत्पुण्यफलं प्रदिष्टम् ।
अत्येति तत्सर्वमिदं विदित्वा
योगी परं स्थानमुपैति चाद्यम् ॥८.२८॥
vedeṣu yajñeṣu tapaḥsu caiva
dāneṣu yatpuṇyaphalaṁ pradiṣṭam
atyeti tatsarvamidaṁ viditvā
yogī paraṁ sthānamupaiti
cādyam (8.28)

*vedeṣu — from study of the Vedas; yajñeṣu — from religious ceremonies and disciplines; tapaḥsu — from austerities; caiva — and indeed; dāneṣu — from scripturally-recommended acts of charity; yat = yad — which; puṇyaphalam — good result; pradiṣṭam — described; atyeti — goes beyond; tat — this; sarvam — all; idam — this; viditvā — having known; yogī — yogi; param — supreme; sthānam — state; upaiti — goes; cādyam = cā — and + adyam — primal*

**The yogi, having known all this, goes beyond the good results which are derived from study of the Veda, beyond religious ceremonies and disciplines, beyond austerities and beyond offering scripturally-recommended gifts in charity. He goes to the Supreme Primal State.**

***Siddha Swami's Commentary:***

The masterful, successful *buddhi* yogi, or a *brahma yogi*, tests the various means of salvation. Thus he knows what will pay dividends and what is just fantasy. *Śrī* Krishna praised and accredited the perfected yogi: *param sthānam upaiti cādyam.*

# CHAPTER 9

# Bhaktyā

# The Devotional Attitude*

*patraṁ puṣpaṁ phalaṁ toyaṁ yo me bhaktyā prayacchati*
*tadahaṁ bhaktyupahṛtam aśnāmi prayatātmanaḥ (9.26)*

***I do accept that given devotion from a disciplined, purified person who offers Me a leaf, flower, fruit or water with a devotional attitude. (9.26)***

**Siddha Swami assigned this chapter title on the basis of verse 26 of this chapter.*

श्रीभगवानुवाच
इदं तु ते गुह्यतमं
प्रवक्ष्याम्यनसूयवे ।
ज्ञानं विज्ञानसहितं
यज्ज्ञात्वा मोक्ष्यसेऽशुभात् ॥९.१॥
śrībhagavānuvāca
idaṁ tu te guhyatamaṁ
pravakṣyāmyanasūyave
jñānaṁ vijñānasahitaṁ
yajjñātvā mokṣyase'śubhāt (9.1)

*śrībhagavān — the Blessed Lord; uvāca — said; idam — this; tu — but; te — to you; guhyatamam — most secret; pravakṣyāmy = pravakṣyāmi — I will explain; anasūyave — to one who is not cynical; jñānam — knowledge; vijñānasahitaṁ = vijñāna — experienced + sahitam — with; yaj = yad — which; jñātvā — having known; mokṣyase — you will be freed; 'śubhāt = aśubhāt — from impurity*

**The Blessed Lord said: But I will explain to you who are not cynical, the most secret truths, the knowledge with the experience, which having known, you will be freed from impurities. (9.1)**

***Siddha Swami's Commentary:***

Previously, Śrī Krishna said he would give Arjuna the knowledge and experience *(jñānam te'ham savijñānam 7.2)* but that was in reference to being absorbed in Krishna, practicing yoga, being dependent on Him and knowing Him fully without a doubt:

*śrībhagavānuvāca*
*mayyāsaktamanāḥ pārtha yogaṁ yuñjanmadāśrayaḥ*
*asaṁśayaṁ samagraṁ māṁ yathā jñāsyasi tacchṛṇu (7.1)*

> ***The Blessed Lord said: With attention absorbed in Me, O son of Pṛthā, practising yoga, being dependent on Me, you will know of Me fully without a doubt. Hear of this. (7.1)***

*Śrī* Krishna wanted to give Arjuna more confidential information and experience, regarding the transcendental world and how to attain it. Arjuna's special qualification to receive this information is his lack of cynicism while hearing *Śrī* Krishna. The Lord claimed that hearing and experiencing this, one becomes freed from impurities. Thus hearing itself is not sufficient. The experience must be gained.

Arjuna had certain qualifications. He was devoted and friendly to *Śrī* Krishna (*bhakto'si me sakhā*, 4.3). He was not cynical. This means that for one to hear this information properly, one should have these qualities. And certainly to experience all this in fact on the spiritual plane, one has to be purified.

राजविद्या राजगुह्यं
पवित्रमिदमुत्तमम् ।
प्रत्यक्षावगमं धर्म्यं
सुसुखं कर्तुमव्ययम् ॥९.२॥
rājavidyā rājaguhyaṁ
pavitramidamuttamam
pratyakṣāvagamaṁ dharmyaṁ
susukhaṁ kartumavyayam (9.2)

*rājavidyā — ultimate information; rājaguhyam — greatest secret; pavitram — purifier of consciousness; idam — this; uttamam — transcendental; pratyakṣa — by direct experience; avagamam — understood; dharmyam — the principle of religion; susukham — very happy; kartum — to execute; avyayam — everlasting.*

**This is the ultimate information, the greatest secret, the purifier of consciousness. It is plain to see, righteous, easy to practice and thoroughly consistent. (9.2)**

***Siddha Swami's Commentary:***

*Rājavidyā* means the royal knowledge or ultimate information. *Rājaguhyam* means the royal secret or greatest of the secrets. But *Śrī* Krishna acclaimed this as being the purifier of consciousness and something that was plain to see or obvious to perception, as well as being righteous, easy to practice and thoroughly consistent.

A question arises as to why people do not perceive this normally. The answer is that this is easy for *Śrī* Krishna and others like Himself, not others. It is easy to practice if one is in the association with *Śrī* Krishna in the way that Arjuna was, otherwise it is impossible to do this.

अश्रद्दधानाः पुरुषा
धर्मस्यास्य परंतप ।
अप्राप्य मां निवर्तन्ते
मृत्युसंसारवर्त्मनि ॥९.३॥
aśraddadhānāḥ puruṣā
dharmasyāsya paraṁtapa
aprāpya māṁ nivartante
mṛtyusaṁsāravartmani (9.3)

*aśraddadhānāḥ — having no faith; puruṣā — people; dharmasyāsya = dharmasya — of the righteous behavior + asya — of this; paraṁtapa — stern subduer of the enemy; aprāpya — not attaining; mām — to Me; nivartante — they are born again; mṛtyusaṁsāravartmani = mṛtyu — death + saṁsāra — cyclic rebirth + vartmani — in the course*

**People who have no faith in this righteous behavior, who have not attained Me, are born again in the cyclic course of death and rebirth, O stern subduer of the enemy. (9.3)**

***Siddha Swami's Commentary:***

*Mṛtyu samsāra vartmani* is the course of material existence, consisting of a circular route of taking a body, using it, being forced to part with it, taking another similar body and doing the same thing repeatedly without any objective idea that one is repeatedly doing this. Liberation means to stop this process.

*Śrī* Krishna again stressed the necessity to accept His process of *karma yoga*, so that one may engage in a righteous lifestyle personally as well as support such a life for the entire human society, under His direction.

This verse is an ultimatum to one and all, that if one does not fall under the influence of *Śrī* Krishna and His way of doing things as explained in the *Gītā and* is not attracted to Him at all, then one will be condemned to a cyclic course of death and rebirth.

For progression out of the material world, one take lessons from *Śrī* Krishna, first in *buddhi yoga*, then in its application to cultural activities. That application is called *karma yoga*. From there one may advance to the transcendence in one way or the other, according to the rate of progression and one's existential relationship to *Śrī* Krishna.

मया ततमिदं सर्वं
जगदव्यक्तमूर्तिना ।
मत्स्थानि सर्वभूतानि
न चाहं तेष्ववस्थितः ॥९.४॥
mayā tatamidaṁ sarvaṁ
jagadavyaktamūrtinā
matsthāni sarvabhūtāni
na cāhaṁ teṣvavasthitaḥ (9.4)

*mayā — by Me; tatam — pervaded; idam — this; sarvam — all; jagad = jagat — world; avyaktamūrtinā = avyakta — invisible + mūrtinā — by form; matsthāni — standing on Me, surviving on Me; sarvabhūtāni — all beings; na — not; cāham = ca — and + aham — I; teṣv = teṣu — in them; avasthitaḥ — standing on, surviving on*

**This world is pervaded by My invisible form. All beings survive on My energy but I am not surviving on theirs. (9.4)**

***Siddha Swami's Commentary:***

*Mūrtinā* means a form. It is not just an all-pervasive influence. That is an actual invisible form which passes through everything in the material world. This means every gross, subtle or super-subtle aspect.

For this to be realized or contested, a *yogin* would have to enter superconscious *samādhi* to check for such a spiritually, all-pervasive influence coming from a universal form. This form must be all-encompassing.

न च मत्स्थानि भूतानि
पश्य मे योगमैश्वरम् ।
भूतभृन्न च भूतस्थो
ममात्मा भूतभावनः ॥९.५॥
na ca matsthāni bhūtāni
paśya me yogamaiśvaram
bhūtabhṛnna ca bhūtastho
mamātmā bhūtabhāvanaḥ (9.5)

*na — not; ca — and; matsthāni — standing on Me, surviving on Me; bhūtāni — beings; paśya — behold; me — My; yogam = yoga — psychological power; aiśvaram — supremacy; bhūtabhṛn = bhūtabhṛt — sustaining beings; na — not; ca — and; bhūtastho = bhūtasthaḥ — existing on the beings; mamātmā = mama — My + ātmā — self; bhūtabhāvanaḥ — causing beings to be*

**And the created beings are not existing on Me. Behold My psychological supremacy. While sustaining the beings and not existing on them, I Myself cause them to be. (9.5)**

***Siddha Swami's Commentary:***

This is part of the previous verse. Research for verification of this takes place only in the *samādhi* practice of *brahma yoga*. No one can confirm or deny this otherwise. Mostly, the created beings are a hodge-podge, rag-tag combination of spiritual, psychological and physical components.

Despite the disordered and haphazard way in which most of the forms operate, they are functional in terms of creature survival in one material location or another. The God of the world stands apart and allows the world to function for better or worse, but He is still the all-pervading influence in which births, continued existences and deaths take place.

यथाकाशस्थितो नित्यं
वायुः सर्वत्रगो महान् ।
तथा सर्वाणि भूतानि
मत्स्थानीत्युपधारय ॥९.६॥
yathākāśasthito nityaṁ
vāyuḥ sarvatrago mahān
tathā sarvāṇi bhūtāni
matsthānītyupadhāraya (9.6)

*yathākāśasthito = yathākāśasthitaḥ = yathā — as + ākāśa — space + sthitaḥ — situated; nityam — always; vāyuḥ — wind; sarvatrago = sarvatragaḥ — everywhere going, pervasive; mahān — powerful; tathā — so; sarvāṇi — all; bhūtāni — beings; matsthānīty (matsthānīti) = matsthānī — exist under Me + iti — thus; upadhāraya — consider thoroughly*

**As the powerful wind is always situated in space and is pervasive, so all beings exist under My influence. Consider this thoroughly. (9.6)**

***Siddha Swami's Commentary:***

The analogy of the mighty wind, which is always situated in space, is quite apt to understand the force of the all-pervasive influence of the Supreme. In fact, a human being or animal may resist the Supreme for some time but not for all occasions. Whatever body one assumed may have within it the potential for circumventing the supreme will but such a body can only last for some years. Big trees may resist the throwing force of the wind but eventually they succumb to it and fall to the ground.

सर्वभूतानि कौन्तेय
प्रकृतिं यान्ति मामिकाम् ।
कल्पक्षये पुनस्तानि
कल्पादौ विसृजाम्यहम् ॥९.७॥
sarvabhūtāni kaunteya
prakṛtiṁ yānti māmikām
kalpakṣaye punastāni
kalpādau visṛjāmyaham (9.7)

*sarvabhūtāni — all beings; kaunteya — son of Kuntī; prakṛtim — material nature; yānti — retrogress into; māmikām — my own; kalpakṣaye — at the end of a day of Brahmā; punas = punar — again; tāni — they; kalpādau — at the beginning of a day of Brahmā; visṛjāmy = visṛjāmi — I produce; aham — I*

**O son of Kuntī, all beings retrogress into My own material nature at the end of Brahmā's day. I produce them again at the beginning of Brahmā's next day. (9.7)**

***Siddha Swami's Commentary:***

*Śrī* Krishna was specific in claiming the material nature as His energy, as He did elsewhere in the *Gītā*:

*bhūmirāpo'nalo vāyuḥ khaṁ mano buddhireva ca*
*ahaṁkāra itīyaṁ me bhinnā prakṛtiraṣṭadhā (7.4)*

***Solid substance, liquid substance, flame, gas, space, mindal energy, intelligence, and initiative are My apportioned, eight-sectioned mundane energy. (7.4)***

It may be said that it would be impossible for the spiritual selves, the finite souls, to go into material nature at the dissolution. But we should observe that right now those spiritual selves are involved with material nature all the same. In fact, most of the souls in this creation have forgotten all about their spiritual category and carry on existence as if they were the material nature which is fused with them. Thus in the dissolution, that fusion will remain with them but without any objective consciousness of either themselves or material nature. The fusion or unity of the spiritual selves and material nature, is an illusion in fact, since the spiritual selves cannot be unified with the material energy. However, to them, in their unliberated state, it seems that they are the bodies. And so even if the creation subsides, the limited selves remain allied to or existing alongside the unmanifested subtle material nature.

प्रकृतिं स्वामवष्टभ्य
विसृजामि पुनः पुनः ।
भूतग्राममिमं कृत्स्नम्
अवशं प्रकृतेर्वशात् ॥९.८॥
prakṛtiṁ svāmavaṣṭabhya
visṛjāmi punaḥ punaḥ
bhūtagrāmamimaṁ kṛtsnam
avaśaṁ prakṛtervaśāt (9.8)

*prakṛtim — material nature; svām — own; avaṣṭabhya — supported on, founded on; visṛjāmi — I produce; punaḥ punaḥ — repeated, again and again; bhūtagrāmam — the multitude of beings; imam — this; kṛtsnam — whole; avaśam — powerless; prakṛter = prakṛteḥ — of material nature; vaśāt — in respect to the potency*

**On the foundation of material nature, I repeatedly produce this whole multitude of beings, which is powerless in respect to the potency of material nature. (9.8)**

***Siddha Swami's Commentary:***

This statement of *Śrī* Krishna should be noted by one and all, by those seeking liberation from the material potency and those who wish to remain fused into it. Those who do not accept these statements of *Śrī* Krishna about Himself, may consider, however, that whosoever that Supreme Being may be, He or She or It, would have the power to produce this whole multitude of beings and they would be, in turn, powerless in respect to the mundane potency to which they are bound.

For a *brahma yogin*, this information is vital, to inform him that he must get help from the Supreme Being, if he is to attain freedom from fusion into the mundane energy. By himself or herself, a finite soul cannot possibly break the spell of the energy, even though he or she may periodically experience a transcendental state. For a full exemption from the material energy, one has to take shelter with the Supreme Being.

In *brahma yoga* practice, the efforts are made to put the self in a position, where it can continuously be in the mercy energy of the Supreme, so as to consistently and permanently avoid the influence of the mundane potency.

न च मां तानि कर्माणि
निबध्नन्ति धनंजय ।
उदासीनवदासीनम्
असक्तं तेषु कर्मसु ॥९.९॥
na ca māṁ tāni karmāṇi
nibadhnanti dhanaṁjaya
udāsīnavadāsīnam
asaktaṁ teṣu karmasu (9.9)

*na — not; ca — and; mām — Me; tāni — these; karmāṇi — cultural acts; nibadhnanti — they bind; dhanaṁjaya — conqueror of rich countries; udāsīnavad = udāsīnavat — indifferently; āsīnam — sitting, being situated; asaktam — unattached; teṣu — in these; karmasu — in cultural actions*

**And these cultural activities do not bind Me, O conqueror of rich countries. Since I am situated indifferently, I remain unattached to the activities. (9.9)**

***Siddha Swami's Commentary:***

This is one of the reasons for taking shelter of *Śrī* Krishna or a great soul whose nature is similar to the Lord. One has to develop this indifference to cultural activities to be successful as a *karma yogin*, but one must also be detached from laziness and procrastination such that if one is requested to perform some cultural act, one does it promptly without wanting a benefit in return. One must be indifferent and also free to act if requested by the Supreme Personality.

*Śrī* Krishna stated that even though He is so involved in the production of the manifested material world, still He is detached. It does not cast a spell on Him or create a reaction for Him.

मयाध्यक्षेण प्रकृतिः
सूयते सचराचरम् ।
हेतुनानेन कौन्तेय
जगद्विपरिवर्तते ॥९.१०॥

*mayādhyakṣeṇa = mayā — with Me + adhyakṣeṇa — as supervisor; prakṛtiḥ — material nature; sūyate — produces; sacarācaram — moving and non-moving*

mayādhyakṣeṇa prakṛtiḥ
sūyate sacarācaram
hetunānena kaunteya
jagadviparivartate (9.10)

*things; hetunānena = hetunā — by cause of + anena — by this; kaunteya — son of Kuntī; jagad = jagat — world; viparivartate — operates*

**With Me as the supervisor, material nature produces moving and nonmoving things. By this cause, O son of Kuntī, the universe operates. (9.10)**

***Siddha Swami's Commentary:***

The *adhyakṣena (adhi akṣena)* is the supreme overseer of an operation. There may be more than one person overseeing and supervising a project, since various parts of the work might be commissioned out to different engineers. The one who has the final say is the *adhyakṣena*. Even though there are many supervisors in the material world and many supernatural controllers as well, still the person who oversees everything is regarded as special, because His approval or disapproval supersedes all others.

अवजानन्ति मां मूढा
मानुषीं तनुमाश्रितम् ।
परं भावमजानन्तो
मम भूतमहेश्वरम् ॥९.११॥
avajānanti māṁ mūḍhā
mānuṣīṁ tanumāśritam
paraṁ bhāvamajānanto
mama bhūtamaheśvaram (9.11)

*avajānanti — they hold a low opinion; mām — Me; mūḍhā — the foolish people; mānuṣīm — human; tanum — body; āśritam — having assumed; param — higher; bhāvam — being; ajānanto = ajānantaḥ — not knowing; mama — of Me; bhūtamaheśvaram = bhūta — being + maheśvaram — Almighty God*

**The foolish people, not knowing My higher existence as the Almighty God of the beings, hold a low opinion of Me as having a human body. (9.11)**

***Siddha Swami's Commentary:***

Before one can understand the transcendental position of the Supreme Being, of *Śrī* Krishna, one needs some perception about the transcendence of one's own finite soul. Some spiritual experience of the subtlety of the spirit soul causes one to have an inkling into the nature of the Almighty God; otherwise one may hold a low opinion not only of God but of oneself as well.

If we regard ourselves as human bodies only, then we will regard all others in the same way, and no matter our religious faith or belief, we will remain glued to a materialistic temperament and will not form a proper assessment of the spirits and the Supreme Spirit.

मोघाशा मोघकर्माणो
मोघज्ञाना विचेतसः ।
राक्षसीमासुरीं चैव
प्रकृतिं मोहिनीं श्रिताः ॥९.१२॥
moghāśā moghakarmāṇo
moghajñānā vicetasaḥ
rākṣasīmāsurīṁ caiva
prakṛtiṁ mohinīṁ śritāḥ (9.12)

*moghāśā — people with vain hopes; moghakarmāṇo = moghakarmāṇaḥ — people with purposeless actions; moghajñānā — people with incorrect information; vicetasaḥ — without discrimination; rākṣasīm — wicked; āsurīm — devilish; caiva — and indeed; prakṛtim — mode of material nature; mohinīm — deluding feature; śritāḥ — relying on*

**Persons with vain hopes, purposeless actions, and incorrect information, who lack discrimination, being wicked and devilish, rely on the deluding feature of material nature. (9.12)**

***Siddha Swami's Commentary:***

The more one lacks discrimination *(vicetasah)*, the more one is prone to being influenced by the deluding feature of material nature *(prakṛtim mohinīm)*. Thus it pays for each of the limited souls to take the time to develop insight.

महात्मानस्तु मां पार्थ
दैवीं प्रकृतिमाश्रिताः ।
भजन्त्यनन्यमनसो
ज्ञात्वा भूतादिमव्ययम् ॥९.१३॥
mahātmānastu māṁ pārtha
daivīṁ prakṛtimāśritāḥ
bhajantyananyamanaso
jñātvā bhūtādimavyayam (9.13)

*mahātmānaḥ — great souls; tu — but; mām — Me; pārtha — son of Pṛthā; daivīm — supernatural; prakṛtim — material energy; āśritāḥ — being reliant; bhajanty = bhajanti — they worship; ananyamanaso = ananyamanasaḥ — persons whose minds do not deviate; jñātvā — knowing; bhūtādim — originator of beings; avyayam — constant factor*

**But great souls, being reliant on the supernatural level of material nature, worship Me, without deviation, knowing Me as the originator of beings, the constant factor. (9.13)**

***Siddha Swami's Commentary:***

One should contrast between the deluding feature of material nature and the enlightening aspect of it, which gives the supernatural people in the celestial world, their higher perceptions. The deluding feature is sponsored by the *tamo guṇa* or dulling aspect, while the enlightening force is sponsored by the *sattva guṇa* or clarifying feature.

*Daivīm prakṛtim* is not *brahman,* nor is it the *akṣara brahma paramam*, unaffected supreme spiritual reality. If it were, *Śrī* Krishna would have named it in this verse. *Prakṛtim* in His vocabulary does not mean anything about the unadulterated spiritual existence. *Śrī* Krishna used terms like *akṣara brahman paramam* (8.3), *avyaktah* (8.20), and *avyaktah akṣara* (8.21) to describe the divine places.

The great souls, *mahātmānas*, described in this verse are the accomplished yogins who successfully shifted their reliance from the lower modes of material nature, *tamo guṇa* and *rajo guṇa*, to the highest level of it which is *sattva guṇa*. These persons will graduate further to the divine reliance in full when they progress completely out of the material world.

सततं कीर्तयन्तो मां
यतन्तश्च दृढव्रताः ।
नमस्यन्तश्च मां भक्त्या
नित्ययुक्ता उपासते ॥९.१४॥
satataṁ kīrtayanto māṁ
yatantaśca dṛḍhavratāḥ
namasyantaśca māṁ bhaktyā
nityayuktā upāsate (9.14)

*satatam — always; kīrtayanto = kīrtayantaḥ — glorifying; mām — Me; yatantaśca = yatantaḥ — endeavoring + ca — and; dṛḍhavratāḥ = dṛḍha — firm + vratāḥ — vows; namasyantaśca = namasyantaḥ — paying respects to + ca — and; mām — Me; bhaktyā — with devotion; nityayuktā = nitya — always + yuktā — disciplined; upāsate — worship*

**Always glorifying Me, endeavoring with firm vows, paying respect to Me with devotion, being always disciplined, they worship Me. (9.14)**

***Siddha Swami's Commentary:***

One has to do this for quite some time before one can attain perfection. It is not an easy course. This was explained in a previous verse as follows:

*bahūnāṁ janmanāmante jñānavānmāṁ prapadyate*
*vāsudevaḥ sarvamiti sa mahātmā sudurlabhaḥ (7.19)*

***At the end of many births, the informed devotee surrenders to Me, thinking that the son of Vasudeva is essential to everything. Such a great soul is hard to locate. (7.19)***

Some feel that this statement does not apply to great devotees but only to foolish yogins who take a long time to realize who *Śrī* Krishna is in fact. However, *Śrī* Krishna Himself did not give that opinion. The mental realization of *Śrī* Krishna's position as He explained is one thing, the emotional attachment to *Śrī* Krishna despite one's impure nature is another thing, and the actual transcendental experience which gives one first-hand insight into what the spiritual reality is, is a separate accomplishment for the devotee or for any sincere seeker.

There are many different features to the worship of *Śrī* Krishna. Temple worship of the Deity is only one feature of it. Service to the popular devotee of *Śrī* Krishna, who has earned a name for himself as Krishna's foremost servant, is another feature. Much more is required before the devotee reaches perfection. And even though in some speeches *Śrī* Krishna stressed or listed a certain aspect, especially the devotion to Him as paramount, still that does not mean that the other features may be neglected. All the features must be practiced for a well-rounded achievement in reaching *Śrī* Krishna. This is why in verse after verse, so many different disciplines are mentioned.

One devotee may be always glorifying *Śrī* Krishna as best as that devotee can, but he or she may not be endeavoring with firm vows. Another may be paying respect in whatever ways he or she was shown by an authority but that person may not be disciplined internally in terms of mind and sense control. One other devotee may engage in Deity Worship as an expert *pujārī*, in terms of mastership of ceremonial routines, but that devotee may forget to always glorify the Lord, due to his seniority and managerial position in the community of devotees. Thus due to their respective short-comings, each of those devotees will progress slowly. This is why it takes many, many births *(bahūnām janmanām ante*, Bg. 7.19)

ज्ञानयज्ञेन चाप्यन्ये
यजन्तो मामुपासते ।
एकत्वेन पृथक्त्वेन
बहुधा विश्वतोमुखम् ॥९.१५॥
jñānayajñena cāpyanye
yajanto māmupāsate
ekatvena pṛthaktvena
bahudhā viśvatomukham (9.15)

*jñānayajñena = jñāna — concept + yajñena — by discipline; cāpy (capi) = ca — and + api — also; anye — others; yajanto = yajantaḥ — performing regulated worship; mām — Me; upāsate — they worship; ekatvena — with the singular basis; pṛthaktvena — as variety; bahudhā — variously shown; viśvatomukham — facing all levels*

**By the discipline of concepts, others do perform regulated worship of Me as the Singular Basis and as the Variety, facing all levels of reality simultaneously. (9.15)**

***Siddha Swami's Commentary:***

In the animal kingdom, the living entity does not bother with many ideas. There, a simple life is normal and one hardly aspires for anything except food and shelter. Philosophy is not important to the animals. However, with many human beings also, philosophical ideas are a source of boredom. The few human beings who relish philosophy grapple with many concepts presented to them by teachers and sprung into their own minds.

By the discipline of these concepts, weaning out the useless and irrational ones, and the ones which are not explanatory of existence, a person begins to approach the truth. One such person might do regulated worship of *Śrī* Krishna after considering that He is or might be the Singular Basis of this world and that He is or might be the Cause of all this variety. Then in visions one might see the God facing all levels of reality simultaneously, as Arjuna saw when the Universal Form was revealed to him.

अहं क्रतुरहं यज्ञः
स्वधाहमहमौषधम् ।
मन्त्रोऽहमहमेवाज्यम्
अहमग्निरहं हुतम् ॥९.१६॥
ahaṁ kraturahaṁ yajñaḥ
svadhāhamahamauṣadham
mantro'hamahamevājyam
ahamagnirahaṁ hutam (9.16)

*aham — I; kratur — Vedic ritual; aham — I; yajñaḥ — sacrificial ceremony; svadhāham = svadhā — sanctified offering + aham — I; auṣadham — medicinal herb; mantro = mantraḥ — sacred sound; 'ham = aham — I; evājyam = eva — indeed + ājyam — ghee; aham — I; agnir = agniḥ — fire; aham — I; hutam — oblation*

**I am represented as the Vedic ritual. I may also be seen as the sacrificial ceremony or as the sanctified offering. I may be regarded as the medicinal herb. I may be seen as the ghee, fire or oblation given. (9.16)**

***Siddha Swami's Commentary:***

These instructions have to do with the discipline of concepts which was mentioned in the previous verse. A devotee who submits to this may not get a revelation of *Śrī* Krishna as the Singular Basis or as the Variety, facing all levels of reality simultaneously. A vision of this sort was given to the residents of *Vṛndāvana* when *Śrī* Krishna instructed them to perform the Annakuta ceremony on Govardhana Hill. Arjuna received the vision of the Universal Form as related to the battle of *Kurukṣetra*, showing how *Śrī* Krishna's supremacy over the supernatural controllers who reside in the heavenly worlds.

If, however, one does not get this revelation, then one should endeavor to understand the Supreme Being's position by considering *Śrī* Krishna in the way described in this verse, and the next three verses (9.17-19). *Śrī* Krishna should be regarded as being represented by the Vedic ritual, sacrificial ceremony, sacrificial offering, medicinal herb, sacred sound used, ghee, fire and oblations which concern the Vedic fire sacrifice *(kratuh).*

If one complies with this instruction of *Śrī* Krishna, which is a theoretical way of understanding how He pervades the world, then over time, one will get the revelations which show how *Śrī* Krishna empowers and enthuses all.

पिताहमस्य जगतो
माता धाता पितामहः ।
वेद्यं पवित्रमोंकार
ऋक्साम यजुरेव च ॥९.१७॥

*pitāham = pitā — father + aham — I; asya — of this; jagato = jagataḥ — of the universe; mātā — mother; dhātā — creator; pitāmahaḥ — grandfather; vedyam — subject to be known;*

pitāhamasya jagato
mātā dhātā pitāmahaḥ
vedyaṁ pavitramoṁkāra
ṛksāma yajureva ca (9.17)

*pavitram — purifier; oṁkāra — sacred syllable Om; ṛk — Rig Veda; sāma — Sāma Veda; yajur — Yajur Veda; eva — indeed; ca — and*

**I am the father of this universe, the mother, the creator, the grandfather, the subject of education, the purifier, the sacred syllable *Om*, the *Rig*, *Sama*, and *Yajur Vedas*. (9.17)**

***Siddha Swami's Commentary:***

In terms of family relationship, one may consider *Śrī* Krishna as the father, mother, creator, and grandfather of the universe. In terms of production of this world, He should be considered as the creator. Since everything is rooted in Him as explained, He should be considered as the subject of education, or knowledge about everything. He is, in fact, the purifier of everything. He is represented by the sacred syllable *Om*, and the three primary *Vedas*, the Rig, *Sama* and *Yajur*.

गतिर्भर्ता प्रभुः साक्षी
निवासः शरणं सुहृत् ।
प्रभवः प्रलयः स्थानं
निधानं बीजमव्ययम् ॥९.१८॥
gatirbhartā prabhuḥ sākṣī
nivāsaḥ śaraṇaṁ suhṛt
prabhavaḥ pralayaḥ sthānaṁ
nidhānaṁ bījamavyayam (9.18)

*gatir = gatiḥ — objective; bhartā — supporter; prabhuḥ — master; sākṣī — observer; nivāsaḥ — existential residence; śaraṇaṁ — shelter; suhṛt — friend; prabhavaḥ — origin; pralayaḥ — cause of universal disintegration; sthānam — foundation; nidhānam — reservoir of energies; bījam — case; avyayam — non-deteriorating*

**I am the objective, the supporter, the master, the observer, the existential residence, the shelter, the friend, the origin, the cause of universal disintegration, the foundation, the reservoir of energies, and the non-deteriorating cause. (9.18)**

***Siddha Swami's Commentary:***

This is a course for developing faith in *Śrī* Krishna as the Supreme Person. This course was given by *Śrī* Krishna Himself. Thus it is valid. It concerns items and qualities which we encounter in day-to-day earthly existence. If one takes this course and faithfully practices it, training oneself in regarding things in this prescribed way, one will get the grace of *Śrī* Krishna, which will result in a revelation.

One does not need mystic yoga or *buddhi yoga* to learn this course. This course may be taken up by anyone, even by persons who have little or no mystic insight. Those who have the higher yoga expertise may research into these truths which *Śrī* Krishna declared, to verify these by personal experience on the mystic plane.

Ultimately, the Supreme Person is the objective because all other aims will in the end, terminate in Him as the Supreme Cause. If for instance one requires wealth to please one's family or to improve the status, one will have to exploit the earth for materials to sell to others. But once the wealth is achieved, one has to please the relatives by buying commodities and by exhibiting aristocratic ways. Once the relatives are satisfied, they will require more wealth to improve themselves further. At that point or at some other time in that life or the next, one will think about the means of acquiring money and the actual reason for such endeavor. Thus, ultimately, one will consider that there must be a Supreme Person, someone Who is most superior to everyone else. And in consultation with that Person one will realize that He is the ultimate objective. Relatives and friends partially represent that Supreme Person. The responsibilities one faces in life, are to a degree, representative of the mission of that Person, as explained to Arjuna in this *Gītā* about *karma yoga* and the way the ancient yogi kings like Janak were trained to serve the divine interests.

Generally people consider the father of the family as the supporter or bread-winner, the wage-earner. If the father passes away, then the eldest son takes that position. A big industrialist who opens a factory to give employment to many fathers, is considered as a city father, because he provides a means of supporting many families in the district or province. Thus, ultimately, the Supreme Person is the supporter, because through His cosmic energy, this universe was generated and is being maintained.

He is the master of this situation in real terms. He is the observer of it universally. The whole creation rests on His energy and thus He is ultimately the existential residence of this place, as the most subtle basis of this existence. He is the shelter, friend, origin, the cause of universal disintegration, foundation, reservoir of energies and non-deteriorating cause.

One should consider all this little by little and then after mastering *buddhi yoga* as taught by *Śrī* Krishna, one should enter into *samādhi* practice to realize this step by step on the supernatural plane.

तपाम्यहमहं वर्षं
निगृह्णाम्युत्सृजामि च ।
अमृतं चैव मृत्युश्च
सदसच्चाहमर्जुन ॥९.१९॥
tapāmyahamahaṁ varṣaṁ
nigṛhṇāmyutsṛjāmi ca
amṛtaṁ caiva mṛtyuśca
sadasaccāhamarjuna (9.19)

*tapāmy (tapāmi) — I produce heat; aham — I; aham — I; varṣam — rainfall; nigṛhṇāmy = nigṛhṇāmi — I withhold; utsṛjāmi — I release; ca — and; amṛtam — relatively-long life span of the celestial bodies; caiva — and indeed; mṛtyus — quick death of earthly bodies; ca — and; sad = sat — eternal life; asac = asat — short-term existence; cāham = ca — and + aham — I; arjuna — Arjuna*

**I produce heat. I withhold and release rainfall. I arrange the relatively-long life span of celestial bodies and the quick death of the earthly ones, as well as the short-term existence and eternal life. (9.19)**

***Siddha Swami's Commentary:***

These are subjects for mystic research in yoga to know if heat and atmospheric moisture are controlled by any living being. Are they haphazardly occurring? If so, under what sort of law of nature do they function? Does anyone personally supervise the weather conditions?

Are the various existences in the many dimensions regulated by anyone? What determines if one living entity will have celestial life and another a short earthly one plagued with miseries? Is this haphazardly occurring by chance factors, or is this planned by a super-entity? What is eternal life? What is short-termed existence? Why does one soul use ant bodies for centuries, while another is in a heavenly form for thousands of years? What or who determines this?

त्रैविद्या मां सोमपाः पूतपापा
यज्ञैरिष्ट्वा स्वर्गतिं प्रार्थयन्ते।
ते पुण्यमासाद्य सुरेन्द्रलोकम्
अश्नन्ति दिव्यान्दिवि देवभोगान् ॥९.२०॥

*traividyā — knowers of the three Vedas; mām — Me; somapāḥ — soma drinkers; pūta — reformed; pāpā — bad tendencies; yajñaiḥ — with sacrificial procedures; iṣṭvā — worshiping; svargatim — path of heaven; prārthayante — they desire; te —*

traividyā māṁ somapāḥ pūtapāpā
yajñairiṣṭvā svargatiṁ prārthayante
te puṇyamāsādya surendralokam
aśnanti divyāndivi devabhogān
(9.20)

*they; puṇyam — merit based; āsādya — attaining; surendra — king of the angelic people; lokam — world; aśnanti — they enjoy; divyān — angelic; divi — in the astral region; devabhogān — celestial delights*

**The knowers of the three *Vedas*, the soma drinkers, and those who are reformed of bad tendencies, worship Me with sacrificial procedures. They desire to be transferred to heaven. Attaining the merit-based world of Surendra, the king of the angelic people, they enjoy celestial delights in the astral region. (9.20)**

***Siddha Swami's Commentary:***

These three types of worshippers of *Śrī* Krishna, who use sacrificial procedures, are not the *brahma yogins*. These are persons who are educated in Sanskrit, so as to be versed in reciting the three *Vedas* and adhering to the Vedic procedures recommended in those texts. Usually these people are caste brahmins who took birth in families which by tradition repeated the Sanskrit hymns in the three *Vedas*. Some sacrificers are the soma drinkers. There were the Vedic ritualists who specialized in offering and partaking of the remnants of the Soma beverage, a drink which gave them subtle perception to perceive and communicate with the supernatural persons in the celestial world. Because of maintaining that connection during their lives, the soma drinkers went to the celestial regions temporarily, after the death of their physical forms. Some others are those who are reformed of bad tendencies, either by strict adherence to moral principles and by pious association or by the performance of austerities, which cause their bad habits to disappear. These, because of their transformed nature and character, qualify for entry into the heavenly planets at the time of death of their earthly forms, but they too, go there temporarily and then return to the earthly places.

O, how it is to be regretted, that persons take to such processes which lead them to the heavenly planets for a short or long stay, after which they must again come back to the miseries of their earthly location. One's time and energy would be better spent, remaining on earth and practicing the yoga austerities or staying in the astral regions of siddha loka where one may associate with more advanced yogins after one's material body dies. By yoga austerities one may by-pass the world of *Surendra*, overlook the petty celestial delights, and try to acquire some spiritual qualities through which one's spirit would shed off the need for the earthly incarnations. Those who stick to yoga practice should remain on the earthly planets and then go to the siddha loka place or come back to earthly place again, and then after qualifying sufficiently go on to Maharloka, Janaloka, Tapaloka and Satyaloka. Only a fool will aspire for the place of *Surendra*, that king of mundane delight.

*Devabhogān* indicated that on the *Surendra* planet, the men are playboys and the women are like movie stars and sophisticated prostitutes. What use is such a life? One can never become liberated in such an environment. It is a merit-based world, a *puṇyam lokam*, but all the same it is a supernatural place with all sorts of magical happenings *(divyān divi)*. It is similar to religious people going on a tour of sense gratificatory places on this planet. Sometimes persons who are very religious, go with their priest to a night club or cinema and embarrass themselves by dancing in vulgar ways and indulging in sensuousness and explicit sexuality. Similarly, religious people, after carefully accumulating their pious activity and being deserved of a better than earthly life, go to the heavenly planets to successfully petition for all sorts of sensual and sexual indulgences. These activities do use up their accumulated merits, just as a man's hard earned salary is used up at a luxury resort.

ते तं भुक्त्वा स्वर्गलोकं विशालं
क्षीणे पुण्ये मर्त्यलोकं विशन्ति ।
एवं त्रयीधर्ममनुप्रपन्ना
गतागतं कामकामा लभन्ते ॥९.२१॥
te taṁ bhuktvā svargalokaṁ viśālaṁ
kṣīṇe puṇye martyalokaṁ viśanti
evaṁ trayīdharmam anuprapannā
gatāgataṁ kāmakāmā labhante (9.21)

*te — they; tam — it; bhuktvā — having enjoyed; svarga – angelic paradise; lokam — world; viśālam — multi-dimensional; kṣīṇe — in being exhausted; puṇye — in pious merit; martyalokam — world of short life-duration; viśanti — they enter; evam — thus; trayī — three Vedas; dharmam — injunctions for righteous life style; anuprapannā — adhering to; gatāgatam — going away and coming back; kāmakāmā — those who aspire for pleasures and luxuries; labhante — they get the opportunity*

**Having enjoyed the multi-dimensional, angelic paradise world, exhausting their pious merits, they enter the world of short-life duration. Thus adhering to the tri-part Vedic injunctions for righteous lifestyle, those who aspire for pleasures and luxuries get the opportunity to go to heaven and come back to the earth again. (9.21)**

***Siddha Swami's Commentary:***

Many ministers, gurus and priests feel that this *svargalokam* angelic paradise world is God's kingdom. Many of them direct their followers to this place. And the followers cannot distinguish between this and the actual kingdom of God. Thus many living entities strive for this sort of heaven in the hereafter, without realizing that such a place is denoted by only one thing, frustration of one's plans and objectives. This is because after one's merits are exhausted by enjoyment there, one feels a great resentment and must turn away from that place, like a drunken gambler whose money was used out in a casino or like an aristocratic female dancer or prostitute whose body has turned too old to be enjoyed by others.

But hardly a soul wants to stay in this *martyalokam* short life-duration world, even though this place is the gateway to the real kingdom of God. The temptation to use up one's pious credits, which are based on moral behavior and righteous lifestyle, is very great and few people can tolerate it. Thus many are fooled again and again by having to behave well in the religious way on earth and then go to the heavenly world of *Surendra*, only to find out that their stay there was clocked and their celestial body deteriorated as soon as their pious merits were spent out.

अनन्याश्चिन्तयन्तो मां
ये जनाः पर्युपासते ।
तेषां नित्याभियुक्तानां
योगक्षेमं वहाम्यहम् ॥९.२२॥
ananyāścintayanto māṁ
ye janāḥ paryupāsate
teṣāṁ nityābhiyuktānāṁ
yogakṣemaṁ vahāmyaham (9.22)

*ananyāś — to no other person; cintayanto = cintayantaḥ — keeping the mind attuned to; mām — Me; ye — who; janāḥ — people; paryupāsate — they worship; teṣām — concerning them; nityābhiyuktānāṁ = nitya — always + abhiyuktānām — of those who cultivate yoga disciplines; yogakṣemam — welfare; vahāmy = vahāmi — I tend to; aham — I*

**I tend to the welfare of the persons who worship Me and no other person, who keep their minds attuned to Me, and who always cultivate the yoga disciplines. (9.22)**

***Siddha Swami's Commentary:***

This is a most reasonable declaration by *Śrī* Krishna, a promise that we can safely believe in but it does not mean that *Śrī* Krishna will live up to every expectation of His devotees. For protection under this promise, the devotee should keep his mental and emotional energy attuned to *Śrī* Krishna and to no other person. He or she must worship *Śrī* Krishna and should always cultivate the yoga disciplines which *Śrī* Krishna inaugurated in this *Bhagavad Gītā*, the most basic system of which is the *buddhi yoga* process described herein.

*Śrī* Krishna's tending to their welfare does not mean that they will dictate to Him what that welfare is. In fact *Śrī* Krishna decides for Himself as to what is their benefit, even if they do not agree with Him. As it is in every case of a guardian and dependent, the dependent may disagree with the decisions of the guardian.

येऽप्यन्यदेवता भक्ता
यजन्ते श्रद्धयान्विताः ।
तेऽपि मामेव कौन्तेय
यजन्त्यविधिपूर्वकम् ॥९.२३॥
ye'pyanyadevatā bhaktā
yajante śraddhayānvitāḥ
te'pi māmeva kaunteya
yajantyavidhipūrvakam (9.23)

*ye — who; 'py = api — even; anyadevatābhaktā = anya — other + devatā — supernatural rulers + bhaktā — worshipping; yajante — they do prescribed ceremonies and disciplines; śraddhayānvitāḥ = śraddhayā — with faith + anvitāḥ — with; te — they; 'pi = api — also; mām — Me; eva — indeed; kaunteya — son of Kuntī; yajanty = yajanti — they do prescribed ceremonies and disciplines; avidhipūrvakam — not by the recommendation*

**Those who, with religious ceremonies, disciplines and faith, devotedly worship other supernatural rulers, indirectly petition Me, O son of Kuntī, although they do not perform the ceremonies and disciplines by My recommendation. (9.23)**

***Siddha Swami's Commentary:***

There are many persons in India and elsewhere, who are devoted to other real or imagined supernatural beings besides *Śrī* Krishna. All of these do indirectly worship *Śrī* Krishna, because after all, if we are to accept His claims, it would imply that all powerful persons derive power from Him and are ultimately accountable to Him alone. All responsibility is ultimately traceable to Him.

अहं हि सर्वयज्ञानां
भोक्ता च प्रभुरेव च ।
न तु मामभिजानन्ति
तत्त्वेनातश्च्यवन्ति ते ॥९.२४॥
ahaṁ hi sarvayajñānāṁ
bhoktā ca prabhureva ca
na tu māmabhijānanti
tattvenātaścyavanti te (9.24)

*aham — I; hi — truly; sarvayajñānām = sarva — all + yajñānām — of religious ceremonies and disciplines; bhoktā — the person who appreciates; ca — and; prabhur = prabhuḥ — master; eva — indeed; ca — and; na — not; tu — but; mām — Me; abhijānanti — they recognize; tattvenātaś = tattvena — by reality + ataḥ — hence; cyavanti — they deviate from the path of virtue; te — they*

**Indeed I am the Master of all religious ceremonies and disciplines and I am the person Who should appreciate such procedures. But they do not recognize Me; hence they deviate from the path of virtue. (9.24)**

***Siddha Swami's Commentary:***

There are many priests, spiritual masters and religious figureheads the world over. Some of these persons are self-made authorities, while others hail under the auspices of some age-old or established religious tradition. Many of these, in fact most of these make no allegiance to *Śrī* Krishna. Some deny Him outright. But according to *Śrī* Krishna, He is the master of all such religious ceremonies and disciplines. He is the person who should appreciate such procedures. They require His approval to be actually authorized.

If we accept that the standards for religion, should be given by *Śrī* Krishna and by no one else, then those who issue religious ideals and methods, and who do not tally with *Śrī* Krishna and what *He* stated in the *Bhagavad Gītā*, are deviant to the path of virtue as defined by *Śrī* Krishna.

यान्ति देवव्रता देवान्
पितृन्यान्ति पितृव्रताः ।
भूतानि यान्ति भूतेज्या
यान्ति मद्याजिनोऽपि माम् ॥९.२५॥
yānti devavratā devān
pitṝnyānti pitṛvratāḥ
bhūtāni yānti bhūtejyā
yānti madyājino'pi mām (9.25)

*yānti — they go; devavratā — those who satisfy the supernatural rulers; devān — supernatural rulers; pitṝn — pious ancestors who exist as departed spirits; yānti — go; pitṛvratāḥ — those who satisfy the pious ancestors; bhūtāni — the ghostly spirits; yānti — go; bhūtejyā — those who satisfy the ghosts; yānti — they go; madyājino = madyājinaḥ — those who satisfy Me; 'pi = api — surely; mām — Me*

**Those who satisfy the supernatural rulers, go to those authorities. Those who satisfy the pious ancestors, associate with such departed spirits. Those who try to satisfy the ghosts, go to those beings. Those who try to satisfy Me, surely approach Me. (9.25)**

***Siddha Swami gave this translation:***

**Those who are avowed to the supernatural rulers, go to those authorities. Those who are committed to the pious ancestors, associate with such departed spirits. Those who are attached to the departed entities who assumed ghostly status, go to those beings. Those who practice the religious and disciplinary procedures which I introduced, surely approach Me.**

***Siddha Swami's Commentary:***

Much of what we do in this existence is based on association and upon those from whom we seek approval and or disapproval for our activities. A person's way of life, has much to do with the persons to whom he is held accountable. The Supreme Person hardly enforces Himself upon any other entity. Thus human beings have a choice to follow either other human beings, supernatural beings, ghostly beings or even inanimate objects. Whosoever and whatsoever a man or woman respects, that person or force exerts a counter-influence.

पत्रं पुष्पं फलं तोयं
यो मे भक्त्या प्रयच्छति ।
तदहं भक्त्युपहृतम्
अश्नामि प्रयतात्मनः ॥९.२६॥
patraṁ puṣpaṁ phalaṁ toyaṁ
yo me bhaktyā prayacchati
tadahaṁ bhaktyupahṛtam
aśnāmi prayatātmanaḥ (9.26)

*patram — leaf; puṣpam — flowers; phalam — fruit; toyam — water; yo = yaḥ — who; me — Me; bhaktyā — with devotion; prayacchati — he offers; tad — that; aham — I; bhaktyupahṛtam = bhakty (bhakti) –devotional + upahṛtam — given; aśnāmi — I accept; prayatātmanaḥ = prayata – disciplined, purified + ātmanaḥ — from the person*

**I do accept that given devotion from a disciplined, purified person who offers Me a leaf, flower, fruit or water with a devotional attitude. (9.26)**

***Siddha Swami's Commentary:***

Many commentators stress the word *bhaktyā* which means with devotion, with love, with affection for *Śrī* Krishna. The word is very significant but it is not the only requirement. The quality of love is important. If *Śrī* Krishna meant just love and affection, He would not have stated *prayatātmanah* as well. The person must be of a pure and disciplined nature. And what sort of discipline would that be? It would be the sort of discipline which comes from the practice of *Śrī* Krishna's *buddhi yoga* which was explained in so much detail to Arjuna. And what sort of purity would that be? It would be purity concerning the *ātma* which *Śrī* Krishna addressed in Chapters 5 and 6, concerning the use of the body, mind and intelligence, or even the senses alone, to perform cultural acts without attachment, for self purification, and having to do with sitting in a posture, having the mind focused, controlling the thinking and sensual energy, practicing the yoga discipline for self purification (5.11, 6.12).

For the student *yogin*, *bhaktyā* affection and devotion for *Śrī* Krishna begins with being devoted and friendly to the yoga teacher who teaches a system thoroughly consistent with what *Śrī* Krishna originally taught to persons like *Vivasvat, Manu* and *Ikṣvāku*. In this *Gītā*, He explained the *karma yoga* teachings and when He spoke to Uddhava in Canto 11 of *Śrīmad Bhāgavatam*, He discussed in detail the *jñāna yoga* system and the *bhakti yoga* system, as well as *bhakti* by itself without yoga expertise. Students who know a little Sanskrit should take the time to find out the meaning of the word *prayatātmanah* by dissecting it into its root parts as *pra yata ātmanah*. *Yata* is an expansion of the root word *yam*.

Persons who, on the basis of hearing of this verse, take up the process of offering a leaf, flower, fruit or water to *Śrī* Krishna with devotion but who are not disciplined and purified by the *buddhi yoga* process explained in the *Gītā*, are admired and are to be encouraged. But such persons should be doubtful as to whether their offerings are accepted by *Śrī* Krishna, because this verse does not state that their efforts are approved by *Śrī* Krishna. They are not purified and they did not have the purification gained through the *buddhi yoga* process explained by Him to those ancient rulers and to others like Uddhava.

यत्करोषि यदश्नासि
यज्जुहोषि ददासि यत् ।
यत्तपस्यसि कौन्तेय
तत्कुरुष्व मदर्पणम् ॥९.२७॥
yatkaroṣi yadaśnāsi
yajjuhoṣi dadāsi yat
yattapasyasi kaunteya
tatkuruṣva madarpaṇam (9.27)

*yat = yad — what; karoṣi — you do; yad — what; aśnāsi — you eat; yaj = yad — what; juhoṣi — you present ceremonially; dadāsi — you gave away; yat = yad — what; yat = yad — what; tapasyasi — you perform as a discipline; kaunteya — son of Kuntī; tat = tad — that; kuruṣva — do; madarpaṇam — offering to Me*

**Whatever you do, whatever you eat, whatever you present ceremonially, whatever you give away, whatever you perform as a discipline, O son of Kuntī, do that as an offering to Me. (9.27)**

***Siddha Swami's Commentary:***

This is another verse exploited by those who are not purified as mentioned in the commentary to the previous verse. This was specifically addressed to Arjuna, as *kaunteya*, the son of *Kuntī Mātā*. Arjuna was practiced at *buddhi yoga*, but he did not apply the detachment gained in it to his cultural life. That was something which *Śrī* Krishna directed him to do while speaking *Bhagavad Gītā*. We must never forget that Arjuna was an accomplished *yogin* before the battle of *Kurukṣetra* was laid out. Arjuna was a devotee of *Śrī* Krishna who was familiar with advanced yoga practice, but he was not oriented to applying yoga expertise to cultural worldly life. He had no idea of how he could apply yoga proficiency in cultural affairs. He was taught that by *Śrī* Krishna as *karma yoga*.

*Śrī* Krishna instructed him in that verse to begin something new, which was to do anything, eat anything, present anything ceremonially, give away anything and perform anything as a discipline only as an offering to *Śrī* Krishna. This was a new teaching to Arjuna, because it meant that Arjuna would have to consider all his life actions in an entirely new and very restrictive way in terms of always gaining the approval of *Śrī* Krishna before acting.

From then onwards, if something could not be done for *Śrī* Krishna, it could not be done. If something could not be eaten by *Śrī* Krishna, it could not be eaten. If something could not be presented ceremonially to *Śrī* Krishna, it could not be presented to anyone. If something could not be given away to *Śrī* Krishna, Arjuna could not deal with the item at all, and if a discipline would not be performed with *Śrī* Krishna's approval, it could not be taken up as a practice by Arjuna.

Arjuna's life would be completely Krishna-approved in every detail of every consideration and act. Others may pretend to themselves and to their followers that they can live in this very restricted way and they may glamorize this as being very sublime, but this is a limited lifestyle given to Arjuna by *Śrī* Krishna.

शुभाशुभफलैरेवं
मोक्ष्यसे कर्मबन्धनैः ।
संन्यासयोगयुक्तात्मा
विमुक्तो मामुपैष्यसि ॥९.२८॥
śubhāśubhaphalairevaṁ
mokṣyase karmabandhanaiḥ
saṁnyāsayogayuktātmā
vimukto māmupaiṣyasi (9.28)

*śubhāśubha — good and bad; phalair (phalaiḥ) — with consequences; evam — thus; mokṣyase — you will be liberated; karmabandhanaiḥ — from the implications of action; saṁnyāsa — renunciation; yoga — yoga; yukta – disciplined; ātmā — self; vimukto = vimuktaḥ — liberated; mām — Me; upaiṣyasi — you will attain*

**Thus you will be liberated from good and bad consequences and from the implications that come from action. Being liberated by the discipline of yoga as it was applied to renunciation, you will come to Me. (9.28)**

***Siddha Swami's Commentary:***

Instead of avoiding yoga practice, specifically *buddhi yoga* practice, one should instead try to take it up, in order to comply with *Śrī* Krishna. Here again even though *Śrī* Krishna mentioned *bhaktyā* or devotion and affection for Him in the previous verse and in some other verses, still yoga is mentioned much more frequently in the *Bhagavad Gītā*. This cannot be denied. Everyone has *bhaktyā* or affection and devotional energy, to be sure, but everyone does not have that in purity. It is mostly impure. *Śrī* Krishna will not accept it in that form. He will be disinclined from taking it. Thus He recommended purity of the psyche and gave methods for doing this before. He did not say anywhere in the *Gītā* that one gets purity of the psyche by giving Him devotion or affection. This is because He would not accept affections from an impure psyche in the first place.

*Samnyāsa yoga yuktātmā* means the discipline of yoga as applied to renunciation of cultural opportunities by perfect mastery of the psyche as it is presided over by the spirit self or *ātma*. Arjuna was told that if he lived in that restricted way of getting *Śrī* Krishna's approval for his every act, then as described in the last verse, he would be liberated from good results, bad consequences and implications. This is because his destiny would be altered in such a way that his initiatives would be used up by *Śrī* Krishna and Arjuna would be doing nothing on his own, and he would not act as prompted or desired by any other person but *Śrī* Krishna.

A guru cannot be substituted here for *Śrī* Krishna, since the Lord does not in any verse substitute any person for Himself. And if Arjuna were to act in this way, then being liberated in the process of time by the discipline of yoga as it was applied to renunciation in the cultural field, he would go to *Śrī* Krishna for certain. But this cannot happen without the application of yoga expertise. It cannot happen with *bhaktyā* or affection and devotion alone. The purity must be there. And such purity must come in the way *Śrī* Krishna Himself recommended in these verses of the *Gītā*. Otherwise we are not discussing the *Bhagavad Gītā* but something else. And we are putting forward someone else's standard and falsely thinking that it is Krishna's.

समोऽहं सर्वभूतेषु
न मे द्वेष्योऽस्ति न प्रियः ।
ये भजन्ति तु मां भक्त्या
मयि ते तेषु चाप्यहम् ॥९.२९॥
samo'haṁ sarvabhūteṣu
na me dveṣyo'sti na priyaḥ
ye bhajanti tu māṁ bhaktyā
mayi te teṣu cāpyaham (9.29)

*samo = samaḥ — equally disposed; 'ham = aham — I; sarvabhūteṣu — to all beings; na — not; me — of Me; dveṣyo = dveṣyaḥ — shunned; 'sti = asti — is; na — not; priyaḥ — especially dear; ye — who; bhajanti — they worship; tu — but; mām — Me; bhaktyā — with devotion; mayi — in Me; te — they; teṣu — in them; cāpy = cāpi — and too; aham — I*

**I am equally disposed to all beings. No one is shunned by Me nor is anyone especially dear to Me. But those who worship Me with devotion are My favorite and I am special to them too. (9.29)**

***Siddha Swami's Commentary:***

Now here is a verse where *Śrī* Krishna mentioned only devotion, *bhaktyā*, and nothing else. Yoga is not mentioned. But still to say that yoga is not relevant is a distortion and is a rejection of all else that *Śrī* Krishna stressed throughout the *Bhagavad Gītā*. *Bhaktyā* in this verse means the kind of *bhaktyā* which entails what was discussed before. One should not haphazardly quote verses like this one, lifting them out of the *Gītā* and presenting them to mislead others.

It is through His equal disposition to everyone that *Śrī* Krishna regards devotees as being His favorites. It is a reciprocal relationship, like any other connection between ordinary persons in the material world. We find this kind of treatment even among the animals. An animal becomes very affectionate to anyone who treats it kindly. This is a common experience.

Krishna reciprocates but that does not mean that the quality of devotion does not figure in. It does. One who has pure devotion gets more special treatment from *Śrī* Krishna. A person with impure affection will not get the same treatment. In fact, a person who follows the purity discipline of *buddhi yoga* given in the *Gītā*, will get the most affectionate and special treatment from the Lord.

However, spiritual masters and religious leaders who hail in Krishna's name should not prostitute or misuse these statements of *Śrī* Krishna, in order to increase their following in the name of *Śrī* Krishna. That is improper and it will bear unfavorable consequences for such leading devotes. *Śrī* Krishna never instructed anyone to make cheap devotees by watering down and distorting His statements in the *Gītā*. In fact it is very disrespectful to *Śrī* Krishna to do this. It is also a dishonor to Arjuna.

अपि चेत्सुदुराचारो
भजते मामनन्यभाक् ।
साधुरेव स मन्तव्यः
सम्यग्व्यवसितो हि सः ॥९.३०॥
api cetsudurācāro
bhajate māmananyabhāk
sādhureva sa mantavyaḥ
samyagvyavasito hi saḥ (9.30)

*api — also; cet = ced — if; sudurācāro = sudurācāraḥ — wicked person; bhajate — worships; mām — Me; ananyabhāk — without being devoted to another; sādhur = sādhuḥ — saintly; eva — indeed; sa = sah — he; mantavyaḥ — should be considered; samyag = samyac — correctly; vyavasito = vyavasitaḥ — decided; hi — indeed; saḥ — he*

**If a wicked person worships Me without being devoted to any other authority, he is considered saintly, for he decided correctly. (9.30)**

***Siddha Swami's Commentary:***

*Śrī* Krishna stressed only His worship in this verse. This has religious connotation in acceptance of *Śrī* Krishna as the Supreme God. *Bhajate* is from the Sanskrit root word *bhaj* which means worshiping, honoring, venerating and religiously respecting. This same root is the source of *bhaktyā* which means devotion and affectionate love or attachment. *Ananyabhāk* means that the person religiously worships *Śrī* Krishna as the Supreme God, forgetting all other supernatural and natural authorities. If even a wicked person does this, then he is considered to be saintly, a *sadhu* in fact, just because he decided correctly that Krishna is the Supreme Person and Krishna's counsel is the best advisory.

The stress here and credit given, is based on the decision to religiously worship *Śrī* Krishna and no other person, going to *Śrī* Krishna alone for shelter. Usually a wicked person will do this, thinking that others misled Him into doing acts for which he suffered greatly, giving him false assurances and encouraging him in vices which led to his downfall. The stress here is on Krishna Himself, not on other persons, not even on priests and teachers who advocate *Śrī* Krishna, since they do, from time to time, give advice which Krishna disapproves.

क्षिप्रं भवति धर्मात्मा
शश्वच्छान्तिं निगच्छति ।
कौन्तेय प्रतिजानीहि
न मे भक्तः प्रणश्यति ॥९.३१॥
kṣipraṁ bhavati dharmātmā
śaśvacchāntiṁ nigacchati
kaunteya pratijānīhi
na me bhaktaḥ praṇaśyati (9.31)

*kṣipram — quickly; bhavati — he becomes; dharmātmā — a person whose character is virtuous; śaśvacchāntim = śaśvac (śaśvat) — eternal + chāntim (śāntim) — spiritual peace; nigacchati — he experiences; kaunteya — son of Kuntī; pratijānīhi — take note!; na — not; me — of Mine; bhaktaḥ — devotees; praṇaśyati — is ruined permanently*

**He quickly becomes a person whose character is virtuous. He experiences the eternal spiritual peace. O son of Kuntī, take note of it! No devotee of Mine is ruined permanently. (9.31)**

***Siddha Swami's Commentary:***

A wicked person who takes to religiously worshiping *Śrī* Krishna and who sticks to that, because he decided correctly that *Śrī* Krishna is the Supreme God, will, by taking the divine association, become virtuous in character. If we find that one becomes such a devotee of *Śrī*

Krishna, and the person's character remains the same, then it means that he is not really in touch with *Śrī* Krishna, even though he may be worshiping the Krishna Murti and chanting the names of *Śrī* Krishna or doing any other services or vows which are usually identified as Krishna-related acts.

Character reformation is an important sign of a person who advances in Krishna association. If one claims to be a devotee and has not become a *dharmātma*, a person whose character is consistent with morality and righteous lifestyle, then it is understood that one has not really made contact with divine association.

All the same, *Śrī* Krishna declared that no devotee of His is ruined permanently, *pratijānīhi na me bhaktah praṇaśyati*. This means any devotees of His, even the bad devotee who has a record of irreligious activities, the *sudurācāro*. When we break apart the root word formations of *sudurācāro*, we get *su-* very, *dur-* bad, wicked, *ācār-* to act, practice. But we must establish caution in applying this to all persons who appear to be devotees and who have bad character, because we must be sure that such persons are religiously-worshiping *(bhajate) Śrī* Krishna and no other natural or supernatural being.

It is important also to understand the protection guaranteed to such a person as contrasted to what *Śrī* Krishna assured before about the undisciplined person with faith who deviated from yoga practice (*ayatih śraddhyopeto yogāccalitamānasah*, 6.37). For the fallen yogi, that is the fallen *buddhi* yogi, that person, if promoted to the heavenly planets, will come back again to the earth, taking birth in a well-do-do pious family or in a family of advanced yogis and will complete the *buddhi yoga* practice.

मां हि पार्थ व्यपाश्रित्य
येऽपि स्युः पापयोनयः ।
स्त्रियो वैश्यास्तथा शूद्रास्
तेऽपि यान्ति परां गतिम् ॥९.३२॥
māṁ hi pārtha vyapāśritya
ye'pi syuḥ pāpayonayaḥ
striyo vaiśyāstathā śūdrās
te'pi yānti parāṁ gatim (9.32)

*mām — Me; hi — indeed; pārtha — son of Pṛthā; vyapāśritya — by relying on; ye — who; 'pi = api — also; syuḥ — they should be; pāpayonayaḥ — persons from sinful parentage; striyo = striyaḥ — women; vaiśyāḥ — businessmen; tathā — even; śūdrās — laborers; te – they; 'pi = api — also; yānti — they move towards; parām — supreme; gatim — goal*

**O son of Pṛthā, by relying on Me, even persons from sinful parentage, even women, businessmen, even laborers, do move towards the supreme goal. (9.32)**

***Siddha Swami's Commentary:***

The rate of progression of each type of devotee would depend on the degree of reliance on *Śrī* Krishna *(mām vyapāśritya)*, but all such devotees would move towards the supreme goal *(yānti parām gatim)*. After discussing the progression of the yogis who take up *Śrī* Krishna's *buddhi yoga* course, the Lord explained the protection offered to others who rely on Him.

किं पुनर्ब्राह्मणाः पुण्या
भक्ता राजर्षयस्तथा ।
अनित्यमसुखं लोकम्
इमं प्राप्य भजस्व माम् ॥९.३३॥

*kim — how; punar — more again, more accessible; brāhmaṇāḥ — brahmins; puṇyā — piously-inclined; bhaktā — devoted; rājarṣayaḥ — yogi kings; tathā — also; anityam — temporary; asukham —*

kiṁ punarbrāhmaṇāḥ puṇyā
bhaktā rājarṣayastathā
anityamasukhaṁ lokam
imaṁ prāpya bhajasva mām (9.33)

*miserable; lokam — world; imam — this; prāpya — having acquired; bhajasva — devote yourself; mām — Me*

**How much more accessible then, is it for the piously-inclined brahmins and yogi kings? Having acquired an opportunity in this temporary, miserable world, you should devote yourself to Me. (9.33)**

***Siddha Swami's Commentary:***

The piously-inclined and devoted brahmins and yogi-kings are those who take up *buddhi yoga* either to apply it to *jñāna yoga* or to *karma yoga* respectively, as explained in the *Gītā* before. The brahmins should avoid *karma yoga*, except for their advisories to the yogi-kings and their performance of religious ceremonies for public usage. But the yogi-king should practice the *karma yoga* to proficiency as was advised for Arjuna. These have special coverage from *Śrī* Krishna, even though all other devotees are regarded on the basis of their reliance on Him.

मन्मना भव मद्भक्तो
मद्याजी मां नमस्कुरु ।
मामेवैष्यसि युक्त्वैवम्
आत्मानं मत्परायणः ॥९.३४॥
manmanā bhava madbhakto
madyājī māṁ namaskuru
māmevaiṣyasi yuktvaivam
ātmānaṁ matparāyaṇaḥ (9.34)

*manmanā — one whose mind is fixed on Me; bhava — be; madbhakto = madbhaktaḥ — being devoted to Me; madyājī — performing ceremonial worship of Me; mām — to Me; namaskuru — make obeisance; mām — Me; evaiṣyasi = eva — indeed + esyasi — you will come; yuktvaivam = yuktva — disciplined + evam — thus; ātmānam — self; matparāyaṇaḥ — with Me as the Supreme Objective*

**With the mind fixed on Me, being devoted to me, performing ceremonial worship to Me, make obeisance to Me. Being thus disciplined, with Me as the Supreme Objective, you will come to Me. (9.34)**

***Siddha Swami's Commentary:***

As Arjuna was on the course of *karma yoga*, he was given the requirements for that system:

*manmanā —fixation of the mind on Sri Krishna*
*bhava madbhakto — being completely devoted or given over to Sri Krishna*
*madyājī mām — performing ceremonial worship of Sri Krishna*
*namaskuru — making obeisances to Sri Krishna*
*yuktvaivam ātmānam — being self disciplined by buddhi yoga practice*
*matparāyaṇam — living as if Sri Krishna were the Supreme Objective*

# CHAPTER 10

## Tejah Amśa Sambhavam

## A Fraction of Krishna's Splendor*

*yadyadvibhūtimatsattvaṁ śrīmadūrjitameva vā*
*tattadevāvagaccha tvaṁ mama tejoṁśasaṁbhavam (10.41)*

***You should realize that whatever fantastic existence, whatever prosperous or powerful object there is, in any case, it originates from a fraction of My splendor. (10.41)***

***Siddha Swami assigned this chapter title on the basis of verse 41 of this chapter.**

श्रीभगवानुवाच
भूय एव महाबाहो
श्रृणु मे परमं वचः ।
यत्तेऽहं प्रीयमाणाय
वक्ष्यामि हितकाम्यया ॥ १०.१ ॥
śrībhagavānuvāca
bhūya eva mahābāho
śṛṇu me paramaṁ vacaḥ
yatte'haṁ prīyamāṇāya
vakṣyāmi hitakāmyayā (10.1)

*śrī bhagavān — the Blessed Lord: uvāca — said; bhūya — again; eva — indeed; mahābāho — O powerful man; śṛṇu — hear; me — from Me; paramam — supreme; vacaḥ — information; yat = yad — which; te — to you; 'ham = aham — I; prīyamāṇāya — to one who is beloved; vakṣyāmi — I will explain; hitakāmyayā — desiring your welfare*

**The Blessed Lord said: Again, O powerful man, hear from Me of the supreme information. Desiring your welfare, I will explain it, O beloved one. (10.1)**

***Siddha Swami's Commentary:***

In giving the supreme information *(paramam vacah),* one verse is not sufficient for understanding and for motivating the student to pursue the inquiry to the point of real experience. Thus *Śrī* Krishna said more to Arjuna, a devotee who was beloved to *Śrī* Krishna *(priyamāṇāya).*

न मे विदुः सुरगणाः
प्रभवं न महर्षयः ।
अहमादिर्हि देवानां
महर्षीणां च सर्वशः ॥ १०.२ ॥
na me viduḥ suragaṇāḥ
prabhavaṁ na maharṣayaḥ
ahamādirhi devānāṁ
maharṣīṇāṁ ca sarvaśaḥ (10.2)

*na — not; me — of Me; viduḥ — they know; suragaṇāḥ — the supernatural rulers; prabhavam — the origin; na — nor; mahārṣayaḥ — great yogi sages; aham — I; ādir = ādiḥ — source; hi — in fact; devānām — of the supernatural rulers; mahārṣīnām — of the great yogi sages; ca — and; sarvaśaḥ — in all respects*

**The supernatural rulers do not know My origin, nor do the great yogi sages. In all respects, I am the source of the supernatural rulers and the great yogi sages. (10.2)**

***Siddha Swami's Commentary:***

*Śrī* Krishna wanted Arjuna to know that the Supreme Soul, Krishna Himself, was unknown to some extent even to the supernatural rulers and even to the great yogi sages who had a reputation for penetrating all supernatural and spiritual reality.

The *rājarṣis* (4.2) are the yogi kings like Janak. They were proficient in *buddhi yoga* and knew its application to cultural life, a skill which was known as *karma yoga*. But the *mahārṣis* are higher than the *rājarṣis*. The *mahārṣis* are the yogi sages, who were expert in *jñāna yoga*, the application of *buddhi yoga* to supernatural and spiritual affairs.

The *devas* are the supernatural rulers who were appointed to rule over human beings. They do so without manifesting themselves physically. *Śrī* Krishna claimed to be the source of such persons, indicating that there was no way for any of them to realize His existence fully. This is obvious since anything produced cannot fully transcend its origination.

यो मामजमनादिं च
वेत्ति लोकमहेश्वरम् ।
असंमूढः स मर्त्येषु
सर्वपापैः प्रमुच्यते ॥ १०.३ ॥

*yo = yaḥ — who; mām — Me; ajam — birthless; anādim — beginningless; ca — and; vetti — knows; lokamaheśvaram — Almighty God of the world; asaṁmūḍhaḥ — unconfused,*

yo māmajamanādiṁ ca
vetti lokamaheśvaram
asaṁmūḍhaḥ sa martyeṣu
sarvapāpaiḥ pramucyate (10.3)

*perceptive; sa = saḥ — he; martyeṣu — of those who use perishable bodies; sarvapāpaiḥ — from all faults; pramucyate — is freed*

**Of those who use perishable bodies, the one who regards Me as birthless and beginningless and who knows that I am the Almighty God of the world, is the perceptive person. He is freed from all faults. (10.3)**

***Siddha Swami's Commentary:***

This person is freed from faults because of mastership of *buddhi yoga* and because of its application to spiritual insight into the spiritual world. Knowledge alone about *Śrī* Krishna's birthless and beginningless condition, as well as His identify as the Almighty God of the world, is not sufficient for freedom from faults. The knowledge of this may or may not spur sufficient purification to gain the insight. Some have the knowledge but not the purity from which they would get the spiritual insight into these statements of *Śrī* Krishna.

बुद्धिर्ज्ञानमसंमोहः
क्षमा सत्यं दमः शमः ।
सुखं दुःखं भवोऽभावो
भयं चाभयमेव च ॥१०.४॥
buddhirjñānamasaṁmohaḥ
kṣamā satyaṁ damaḥ śamaḥ
sukhaṁ duḥkhaṁ bhavo'bhāvo
bhayaṁ cābhayameva ca (10.4)

*buddhir = buddhiḥ — intelligence; jñānam — knowledge; asaṁmohaḥ — non-confusion, sanity; kṣamā — patience; satyam — truthfulness; damaḥ — self-control; śamaḥ — tranquility; sukham — pleasure; duḥkham — pain; bhavo = bhavaḥ — existence; 'bhāvo = abhāvaḥ — non-existence; bhayam — fear; cābhayam = ca — and + abhayam — fearlessness; eva — indeed; ca — and*

अहिंसा समता तुष्टिस्
तपो दानं यशोऽयशः ।
भवन्ति भावा भूतानां
मत्त एव पृथग्विधाः ॥१०.५॥
ahiṁsā samatā tuṣṭis
tapo dānaṁ yaśo'yaśaḥ
bhavanti bhāvā bhūtānāṁ
matta eva pṛthagvidhāḥ (10..5)

*ahiṁsā — non-violence; samatā — impartiality; tuṣṭiḥ — contentment; tapo = tapaḥ — austerity; dānam — charity; yaśo = yaśaḥ — fame; 'yaśaḥ = ayaśaḥ — infamy; bhavanti — are; bhāvā — existential conditions; bhūtānām — of the beings; matta — from Me; eva — alone; pṛthagvidhāḥ — multiple*

**Intelligence, knowledge, sanity, patience, truthfulness, self-control, tranquility, pleasure, pain, existence, non-existence, fear, fearlessness, (10.4)**

**...non-violence, impartiality, contentment, austerity, charity, fame and infamy, are multiple existential conditions, which are derived from Me alone. (10.5)**

***Siddha Swami's Commentary:***

These qualities come on in material nature through its contact with the power of the God. Limited entities assume these qualities according to their relationship with material nature and their alignment with the God. *Śrī* Krishna explained already that for the most part, the limited beings are stupefied by material nature. This is because material nature is supernatural. It is enthused by the power of the God.

*tribhirguṇamayairbhāvair ebhiḥ sarvamidaṁ jagat*
*mohitaṁ nābhijānāti māmebhyaḥ paramavyayam (7.13)*
*daivī hyeṣā guṇamayī mama māyā duratyayā*
*māmeva ye prapadyante māyāmetāṁ taranti te (7.14)*

***All this world is stupefied by the three states of being, which are produced by the mundane influence. The world does not recognize Me, Who is higher than these energies and Who is unaffected.***

***Indeed this quality controlled illusion of Mine is supernatural and difficult to transcend. Only those who rely on Me, can see beyond this bewitching energy. (7.13-14)***

When *Śrī* Krishna stated that the multiple existential conditions are derived from Him alone, He meant Himself in conjunction with material nature. Initially, only the Supreme Being is aware of the possibility of life in material nature. By the expansion of His energy into material nature, various aspects manifest. All of these aspects form later as tendencies of the limited beings, causing them to identify in terms of the various qualities. The finite souls latch onto those combinations of these qualities and they are usually unaware of the Supreme Lord.

What is described here as *bhāvā* or existential conditions, is the effect seen in material nature by the presence of the Supreme Being. These are manifested effects of His proximity to subtle matter. These qualities, in turn, appear to be idiosyncrasies or special habits of the various limited entities.

महर्षयः सप्त पूर्वे
चत्वारो मनवस्तथा ।
मद्भावा मानसा जाता
येषां लोक इमाः प्रजाः ॥१०.६॥
maharṣayaḥ sapta pūrve
catvāro manavastathā
madbhāvā mānasā jātā
yeṣāṁ loka imāḥ prajāḥ (10.6)

*mahārṣayaḥ — great yogi sages; sapta — seven; pūrve — in ancient times, of old; catvāro = catvāraḥ — four celibate boys; manavaḥ — primal sexually-disciplined procreators; tathā — also; madbhāvā — coming from Me; mānasā — mentally; jātā — produced; yeṣāṁ — of whom; loka — universe; imāḥ — these; prajāḥ — creatures*

**The seven great yogi sages of old, the four celibate boys, and also the primal sexually-disciplined procreators come from Me, being produced mentally. From them, the creatures of this universe evolved. (10.6)**

***Siddha Swami's Commentary:***

One should not hereby assume that *Śrī* Krishna created or will create in the future, the individual limited spirits, or material nature, or any combination in which we find spiritual and material energy. The material energy is eternal and so are the individual finite persons, the spirits. The Supreme Being is also eternal. The God, however, is responsible for the productions which come about by the combinations of the spirits and material nature. He is also responsible for the spread of all influences.

As a grandfather is regarded as the head of a family, so the Supreme Lord, *Śrī* Krishna, may be regarded as the head of all families. And the seven great yogi sages, the four celibate boys who are reputed sons of Procreator *Brahmā*, as well as the primal, sexually-disciplined sub-creators are the parents of everyone else.

The material energy remains there eternally. But the Supreme Lord, through His proximity to it, stimulates it into activity. As such He is the efficient remote cause.

एतां विभूतिं योगं च
मम यो वेत्ति तत्त्वतः ।
सोऽविकम्पेन योगेन
युज्यते नात्र संशयः ॥१०.७॥
etāṁ vibhūtiṁ yogaṁ ca
mama yo vetti tattvataḥ
so'vikampena yogena
yujyate nātra saṁśayaḥ (10.7)

*etām — this; vibhūtim — divine glory; yogam — yoga, extensive mystic discipline; ca — and; mama — of My; yo = yaḥ — who; vetti — experience; tattvataḥ — in reality; so = saḥ — he; 'vikampena = avikampena — by consistent; yogena — by yoga practice; yujyate — is harmonized with; nātra = na — not + atra — here; saṁśayaḥ — doubt*

**Whosoever experiences in reality, this divine glory and extensive mystic discipline of Mine, becomes harmonized with Me by consistent yoga practice. There is no doubt about this. (10.7)**

***Siddha Swami's Commentary:***

Higher yoga and higher yoga alone, namely *buddhi yoga* and *jñāna yoga* which is the advanced form of *buddhi yoga*, gives a limited being the required insight into the divine glory and extensive mystic discipline of *Śrī* Krishna. *Buddhi yoga* was described in detail in the latter part of Chapter Two and elsewhere. *Karma yoga* is the application of *buddhi yoga* to cultural affairs, but *jñāna yoga* begins when one abandons cultural concerns and takes to spiritual insight alone. This is why *Śrī* Krishna accredited the *jñānī* or practitioner of *jñāna yoga*.

*teṣāṁ jñānī nityayukta ekabhaktirviśiṣyate*
*priyo hi jñānino'tyartham ahaṁ sa ca mama priyaḥ (7.17)*

***Of these, the informed man who is constantly disciplined in yoga, being singularly devoted, is distinguished indeed. I am fond of this person and he is fond of Me. (7.17)***

When all is said and done about devotion to Krishna, about *bhakti*, the purity of it is the main concern. If one can attain that purity by higher yoga practice, one would be a fool not to practice. In the name of laziness, people do not learn yoga, but they dismiss their inertia by criticizing the possibility of yoga in this era. Yoga is possible now but one must be serious about the objective.

अहं सर्वस्य प्रभवो
मत्तः सर्वं प्रवर्तते ।
इति मत्वा भजन्ते मां
बुधा भावसमन्विताः ॥१०.८॥
ahaṁ sarvasya prabhavo
mattaḥ sarvaṁ pravartate
iti matvā bhajante māṁ
budhā bhāvasamanvitāḥ (10.8)

*aham — I; sarvasya — of all; prabhavo = prabhavaḥ — originator; mattaḥ — from Me; sarvam — everything; pravartate — proceeds; iti — thus, in this way; matvā — having thought; bhajante — they worship; mām — Me; budhā — intelligent person; bhāvasamanvitāḥ = bhāva — states of being, meditative ability + samanvitāḥ — endowed with*

**I am the originator of all. From Me, everything proceeds. Thinking of Me in this way, the intelligent persons, who are endowed with meditative ability, worship Me. (10.8)**

***Siddha Swami's Commentary:***

The worship of *Śrī* Krishna is wonderful; that is the Deity Worship in the temples. The worship of *Śrī* Krishna in localized ways in the home, by devotees who heard about *Śrī* Krishna and who have a natural liking to Him, is also distinguished, for how many people are able to do it? How many persons hear of Krishna and are attracted to His *līlā* pastimes?

But greater in wonderment is the worship by intelligent persons who are endowed with meditative ability and who reach *Śrī* Krishna in the spiritual world. One must perfect the *brahma yoga* practice, to find the Cause of all causes, the originator of all. Then with that firsthand experience, one would worship the Supreme Person sincerely and with infallible faith.

मच्चित्ता मद्गतप्राणा
बोधयन्तः परस्परम् ।
कथयन्तश्च मां नित्यं
तुष्यन्ति च रमन्ति च ॥१०.९॥
maccittā madgataprāṇā
bodhayantaḥ parasparam
kathayantaśca māṁ nityaṁ
tuṣyanti ca ramanti ca (10.9)

*maccittā — those who think of Me; madgataprāṇā — those who concentrate the life energy onto Me; bodhayantaḥ — enlighten; parasparam — one another; kathayantasca = kathayantaḥ — speaking of + ca — and; mām — of Me; nityam — constantly; tuṣyanti — they are content; ca — and; ramanti — they are happy; ca — and*

**Those who think of Me, who concentrate the life energy on Me, who enlighten one another and speak of Me constantly, are content and happy. (10.9)**

***Siddha Swami's Commentary:***

The value of higher yoga practice, the proficiency of *buddhi yoga*, should not be underestimated in this service and worship to *Śrī* Krishna. Arjuna himself, who was beloved and friendly to *Śrī* Krishna, was advised by the Lord to apply yoga proficiency in *karma yoga* and work at *Kurukṣetra* in the disagreeable war concerns of the Kurus. *Śrī* Krishna did not tell Arjuna that all he needed was love and devotion to *Śrī* Krishna. In verse after verse, the Lord stressed yoga, and He impressed also the great and irreplaceable value of *bhakti* to Him and no other person, not even any of the supernatural rulers, the *devas* who were worshipped all over India in the time of *Śrī* Krishna.

*Maccittā* is the thorough application of one's mental and emotional energies to *Śrī* Krishna. To do this, however, one has to master *buddhi yoga*, otherwise the attempt will be thwarted by an unruly intellect, memory and sensual energy. This concerns the organization and supervision of the organs in the head of the subtle body.

*Madgataprāṇā* is the concentration and dedication of the life energy, *prāṇa*, on *Śrī* Krishna. This can be done thoroughly only through kundalini yoga practice. This concerns the energy in the spine of the subtle body. The other aspects of enlightening one another and speaking of *Śrī* Krishna constantly cannot be done fully without a purified psyche, since otherwise, the impure psychology will minimize such efforts and cause them to be inefficiently done.

Real contentment and happiness comes only to those advanced yogi devotees who do this to completion. But others also find happiness in their endeavors to please *Śrī* Krishna, as much as they are allowed by their unruly psyches.

तेषां सततयुक्तानां
भजतां प्रीतिपूर्वकम् ।
ददामि बुद्धियोगं तं
येन मामुपयान्ति ते ॥१०.१०॥

*teṣām — of these; satatayuktānām = satata – constantly + yuktānām — of the disciplined; bhajatām — of the worshippers; prītipūrvakam — with affection; dadāmi — I give; buddhiyogam — technique of insight yoga, application of yoga to*

teṣāṁ satatayuktānāṁ
bhajatāṁ prītipūrvakam
dadāmi buddhiyogaṁ taṁ
yena māmupayānti te (10.10)

*the use of intelligence; tam — it; yena — by which; mām — Me; upayānti — they draw near; te — they*

**Of those who are constantly disciplined, who worship with affection, I give the technique by which they draw near to Me. (10.10)**

***Siddha Swami's Commentary:***

*Bhajatām prītipūrvakam* definitely means those who worship with affection (*prīti*). But again there must be the purity which comes from the practice of higher yoga, *buddhi yoga*. *Śrī* Krishna said herein that to those persons He gives the *buddhi yogam* techniques. This means they must practice it. *Śrī* Krishna does not and cannot bestow it without the devotee's practice. Through the practice described before, which is bestowed by Him, the devotee draws near to *Śrī* Krishna.

The whole of the *Bhagavad Gītā* gets a fresh, new and very practical meaning for the student devotee, if it is understood in this way. This stands over the idea that by worshiping the Krishna Murti, chanting *Śrī* Krishna's holy name, and eating foods offered to *Śrī* Krishna with an impure psyche, one will derive the benefits of *buddhi yoga* without practice. One will achieve nothing of the sort in that way.

तेषामेवानुकम्पार्थम्
अहमज्ञानजं तमः ।
नाशयाम्यात्मभावस्थो
ज्ञानदीपेन भास्वता ॥१०.११॥
teṣāmevānukampārtham
ahamajñānajaṁ tamaḥ
nāśayāmyātmabhāvastho
jñānadīpena bhāsvatā (10.11)

*teṣām — of them; evānukampārtham = eva — indeed + anukampā — assistance + artham — interest; aham — I; ajñānajam — ignorance produced; tamaḥ — stupifying influence of material nature; nāśayāmy = nāśayāmi — I caused to be banished; ātmabhāvastho = ātmabhāvasthaḥ — situated in the self; jñānadīpena = jñāna — knowledge, realized + dīpena — with light, with insight (jñānadīpena – with realized insight); bhāsvatā — clear, shining, clarity of consciousness*

**In the interest of assisting them, I who am situated within their beings, cause the ignorance, produced by the stupefying influence of material nature to be banished by their clear realized insight. (10.11)**

***Siddha Swami's Commentary:***

*Teṣām* or them in this verse means the devotees of *Śrī* Krishna who endeavor in *buddhi yoga* practice and who by practice make some headway in purifying the subtle equipments, like the *buddhi* intellect, memory, sensual energies and life survival powers. When a devotee endeavors with *Śrī* Krishna's *buddhi yoga* practice, then in the interest of assisting that student *yogin*, *Śrī* Krishna, Who is already situated in the psyche, helps to replace the ignorance of spiritual perception, produced by the stupefying influence of material nature, with the student's assumption of clear, realized insight, supernatural and spiritual perception.

*Ātmabhāvasthah* is *sthah* or situated, *bhāva* or in the being or existential environment of, and *ātma* or spirit self. *Śrī* Krishna claimed to be situated in the existential environment of every spirit self. He claimed to be already there, even when the person lacks spiritual insight. He does act to remove that ignorance, when the person takes up and ardently practices *buddhi yoga* as He taught it to the ancient rulers like *Vivasvat, Manu* and *Ikṣvāku*. He did not say that He banished the ignorance by mystic power but rather that it is banished when He assists the devotee in acquiring clear, realized insight.

The darkness in the mind of the student yogi disappears when he masters the buddhi yoga practice. Then his intellect, which is termed in this verse *jñānadīpa*, becomes *bhāsvatā* or clear and shining, so that it is no longer something dark in his subtle head (*jñānavimūḍhām* 3.32).

अर्जुन उवाच
परं ब्रह्म परं धाम
पवित्रं परमं भवान् ।
पुरुषं शाश्वतं दिव्यम्
आदिदेवमजं विभुम् ॥१०.१२॥
arjuna uvāca
paraṁ brahma paraṁ dhāma
pavitraṁ paramaṁ bhavān
puruṣaṁ śāśvataṁ divyam
ādidevamajaṁ vibhum (10.12)

*arjuna — Arjuna; uvāca — said; param — supreme; brahma — spiritual reality; param — supreme; dhāma — refuge; pavitram — reformer; paramam — supreme; bhavān — You, O Lord; puruṣam — person; śāśvatam — eternal; divyam — divine; ādidevam — Primal God; ajam — birthless; vibhum — one whose influence spreads everywhere*

**Arjuna said: Hail to You Who are the Supreme Reality, the Supreme Refuge, the Supreme Reformer, O Lord. You are the eternal divine Person, the Primal God Who is birthless, and Whose influence spreads everywhere. (10.12)**

***Siddha Swami's Commentary:***

This is Arjuna's appraisal of *Śrī* Krishna on the basis of *Śrī* Krishna's assertions, and also on the basis of what Arjuna heard from others.

आहुस्त्वामृषयः सर्वे
देवर्षिर्नारदस्तथा ।
असितो देवलो व्यासः
स्वयं चैव ब्रवीषि मे ॥१०.१३॥
āhustvāmṛṣayaḥ sarve
devarṣirnāradastathā
asito devalo vyāsaḥ
svayaṁ caiva bravīṣi me (10.13)

*āhuḥ — they declare; tvām — You; ṛṣayaḥ — yogi sage; sarve — all; devarṣir = devarṣiḥ — supernatural yogi sage; nāradaḥ — Narada; tatha — as well as; asito devalo —Asita Devala; vyāsaḥ — Vyāsa; svayam — your own self; caiva = ca — and + eva — indeed; bravīṣī — You state; me — to Me*

**All the yogi sages, as well as the supernatural yogi sage Narada, Asita Devala, and Vyasa declare this of You. And You Yourself state this to me. (10.13)**

***Siddha Swami's Commentary:***

Of these, *Nārada* stands out as the yogi sage recognized in the assembly of the *devas* or supernatural rulers. *Vyāsa* is the teacher of Arjuna's eldest brother, Yudhishthira. *Vyāsa* instructed him in the techniques of *buddhi yoga*. And he, Yudhishthira, in turn was said to instruct Arjuna. This is related in the *Mahābhārata*.

Since *Nārada* is an authority on the heavenly planets, Arjuna could authoritatively refer to him. Arjuna, after mastering some higher yoga, had journeyed to the celestial realms even before this sacred discourse with *Śrī* Krishna.

सर्वमेतदृतं मन्ये
यन्मां वदसि केशव ।
न हि ते भगवन्व्यक्तिं
विदुर्देवा न दानवाः ॥१०.१४॥
sarvametadṛtaṁ manye
yanmāṁ vadasi keśava
na hi te bhagavānvyaktiṁ
vidurdevā na dānavāḥ (10.14)

*sarvam — all; etad — this; ṛtam — true; manye — I believe; yan = yad — which; mām — me; vadasi — you say; keśava — O Keśava; na — not; hi — indeed; te — to you; bhagavan — O Blessed Lord; vyaktim — form; vidur = viduḥ — they know; devā — the supernatural rulers; na — nor; dānavāḥ — descendants of Danu, enemies of the supernatural rulers*

**All that You say to me is true. I believe it, O Keśava. Indeed it is not possible to understand You, O Bhagavan, Blessed Lord. Neither the supernatural rulers nor their enemies, the descendants of Danu, can know Your form. (10.14)**

***Siddha Swami's Commentary:***

*Śrī* Krishna's form, *vyaktim*, which cannot be known by these authorities, is His transcendental form, which was mentioned before as *param bhāvam*:

*avyaktaṁ vyaktimāpannaṁ manyante māmabuddhayaḥ*
*paraṁ bhāvamajānanto mamāvyayamanuttamam (7.24)*

***Though I am beyond their sensual range, the unintelligent think of Me as being limited to their gross perception. They do not realize My higher existence which is imperishable and supermost. (7.24)***

If such a form cannot be seen or known by the supernatural rulers, then it cannot be apprehended by the impure senses even of a devotee here on earth. First one must purify the psyche through the practice of *buddhi yoga* and then one may perceive the transcendental form of *Śrī* Krishna, as *Nārada* and others like *Asita Devala* and *Vyāsa* did.

स्वयमेवात्मनात्मानं
वेत्थ त्वं पुरुषोत्तम ।
भूतभावन भूतेश
देवदेव जगत्पते ॥१०.१५॥
svayamevātmanātmānaṁ
vettha tvaṁ puruṣottama
bhūtabhāvana bhūteśa
devadeva jagatpate (10.15)

*svayam — yourself; evātmanā = eva — indeed + ātmanā — by yourself; 'tmānam = ātmānam — yourself; vettha — you know; tvam — you; puruṣottama — Supreme Person; bhūtabhāvana — one who sustains the existence of all others; bhūteśa — Lord of created beings; devadeva — God of the gods; jagatpate — Lord of the universe*

**You alone know Yourself, O Supreme Person, O maintainer of the creatures, O Lord of the created beings, O God of gods, O Lord of the universe. (10.15)**

***Siddha Swami's Commentary:***

*Śrī* Krishna explained this before in different words, from another angle of perception as follows:

*vedāhaṁ samatītāni vartamānāni cārjuna*
*bhaviṣyāṇi ca bhūtāni māṁ tu veda na kaścana (7.26)*

***I know the departed souls and the living creatures, O Arjuna, as well as those beings who are to be born. But no one recognizes Me. (7.26)***

वक्तुमर्हस्यशेषेण
दिव्या ह्यात्मविभूतयः ।
याभिर्विभूतिभिर्लोकान्
इमांस्त्वं व्याप्य तिष्ठसि ॥१०.१६॥
vaktumarhasyaśeṣeṇa
divyā hyātmavibhūtayaḥ
yābhirvibhūtibhirlokān
imāṁstvaṁ vyāpya tiṣṭhasi (10.16)

*vaktum — to describe; arhasy = arhasi — you can; aśeṣeṇa — without deleting anything, thoroughly; divyā — supernatural; hy = hi — in truth; ātmavibhūtayaḥ — wondrous manifestations of Yourself; yābhir = yābhiḥ — by which; vibhūtibhir = vibhūtibhiḥ — wondrous manifestations; lokān — worlds; imāṁs — these; tvam — you; vyāpya — pervading; tiṣṭhasi — you are situated*

**Please describe thoroughly, Your supernatural wondrous manifestations by which You pervade these worlds and are situated in them. (10.16)**

***Siddha Swami's Commentary:***

Arjuna asked here not for a revelation but only for a more detailed description. Such a description may be verified in the *brahma yoga* practice during periods of *samādhi* insight.

कथं विद्यामहं योगिंस्
त्वां सदा परिचिन्तयन् ।
केषु केषु च भावेषु
चिन्त्योऽसि भगवन्मया ॥१०.१७॥
kathaṁ vidyāmahaṁ yogiṁs
tvāṁ sadā paricintayan
keṣu keṣu ca bhāveṣu
cintyo'si bhagavānmayā (10.17)

*katham — how; vidyām I will know; aham — I; yogin — O mystic master; tvām — You; sadā — constantly; paricintayan — meditating; keṣukeṣu — in what, in what; ca — and; bhāveṣu — in aspects of existence; cintyo = cintyah — to be considered; 'si = asi — You are; bhagavan — Blessed Lord; mayā — by me*

**How will I know You, Mystic Master, O Yogi? Is it by constantly meditating? In what aspects of existence are You to be considered by Me, O Blessed Lord? (10.17)**

***Siddha Swami's Commentary:***

This is a very good question posted to *Śrī* Krishna by Arjuna on everyone's behalf. Whatever *Śrī* Krishna said is to be proven to anyone who is interested. But how would it be proven? Can one research this in meditation by constant *samādhi* practice? And what aspects are to be focused on and in what order? It is interesting because *Śrī Patañjali Mahārṣi* has related a sequence of *samādhis* in his yoga sutras.

It is interesting because Arjuna's position is unique. He had the revelation merely by asking for it as related in the next chapter. Does that apply to everyone? Arjuna was just granted divine vision by *Śrī* Krishna as we heard.

One should note, however, that Arjuna asked about higher meditation to see into these aspects of existence (*bhāveṣu*). This is because *Nārada*, *Asita Devala* and *Vyāsa* got their information from actual experiences of the supernatural and divine worlds in meditation.

विस्तरेणात्मनो योगं
विभूतिं च जनार्दन ।
भूयः कथय तृप्तिर्हि
शृण्वतो नास्ति मेऽमृतम् ॥१०.१८॥

*vistareṇātmano (vistareṇātmanaḥ) = vistareṇa — with detail + ātmanaḥ — of Yourself; yogam — yoga, self-disciplinary methods and the resultant mystic power; vibhūtim — splendrous form; ca — and; janārdana — O motivator of the people; bhūyaḥ*

vistareṇātmano yogaṁ
vibhūtiṁ ca janārdana
bhūyaḥ kathaya tṛptirhi
śṛṇvato nāsti me'mṛtam (10.18)

*— more; kathaya — explain; tṛptir = tṛptiḥ — final satisfaction; hi — indeed; śṛṇvato = śṛṇvataḥ — of hearing; nāsti = na — not + asti — is; me — of me; 'mṛtam = amrtam — sweetness*

**Explain in more detail about Your self-disciplinary methods and the resultant mystic power and of Your splendorous form, O motivator of the people. There is no final satisfaction for me in hearing Your sweet words. (10.18)**

***Siddha Swami's Commentary:***

Arjuna is overjoyed by this conversation with *Śrī* Krishna. He wants insight into the mystery of *Śrī* Krishna's supremacy over the world. And he also requests more explanation about *Śrī* Krishna's self disciplinary methods and the resultant mystic control, as well as *Śrī* Krishna's splendid form through which He powerfully regulates what happens in the material world *(vibhūtim)*.

श्रीभगवानुवाच
हन्त ते कथयिष्यामि
दिव्या ह्यात्मविभूतयः ।
प्राधान्यतः कुरुश्रेष्ठ
नास्त्यन्तो विस्तरस्य मे ॥१०.१९॥
śrībhagavānuvāca
hanta te kathayiṣyāmi
divyā hyātmavibhūtayaḥ
prādhānyataḥ kuruśreṣṭha
nāstyanto vistarasya me (10.19)

*śrībhagavān — the Blessed Lord; uvāca — said; hanta — listen; te — to you; kathayiṣyāmi — I will talk of; divyā — supernaturally; hy = hi — truly; ātmavibhūtayaḥ — own wondrous forms; prādhānyataḥ — most prominent; kuruśreṣṭha — O best of the Kuru clan; nāsty (nasti) = na — not + asti — is; anto = antaḥ — limit; vistarasya — to the influence; me — My*

**The Blessed Lord said: Listen, I will talk to you of the most prominent of my supernatural manifestations, O best of the Kuru clan, for there is no limit to My influence. (10.19)**

***Siddha Swami's Commentary:***

*Śrī* Krishna briefly spoke of this in Chapter Nine when He discussed the worship of Himself as the Singular Basis and as the Variety, facing all levels of reality simultaneously (*ekatvena pṛthaktvena bahudhā viśatomukham*, 9.15). He claims that there is no limit to His influence.

अहमात्मा गुडाकेश
सर्वभूताशयस्थितः ।
अहमादिश्च मध्यं च
भूतानामन्त एव च ॥१०.२०॥
ahamātmā guḍākeśa
sarvabhūtāśayasthitaḥ
ahamādiśca madhyaṁ ca
bhūtānāmanta eva ca (10.20)

*aham — I; ātmā — self; guḍākeśa — sleep-regulator; sarvabhūtāśayasthitaḥ = sarva — all + bhūta — beings + āśaya — mystic resting place + sthitaḥ — situated in; aham — I; ādiśca = ādiḥ — beginning + ca — and; madhyam — middle; ca — and; bhūtānām — of the beings; anta — end; eva — indeed; ca — and*

**O sleep regulator, I am the person Who is situated in the mystic resting place of all beings. I am responsible for the beginning, middle, and end of all beings. (10.20)**

***Siddha Swami's Commentary:***

Whatever *Śrī* Krishna would describe about Himself and about anything else or anyone else, also about His relation to all else, could be researched by the interested *yogin*. By carefully hearing what *Śrī* Krishna told Arjuna, a *yogin* could decide for himself what holds his interest. Then he could develop insight into those supernatural and spiritual matters in higher yoga practice. For Arjuna it is different, since *Śrī* Krishna gave Arjuna the revelation of the Universal Form and of the four-handed, divine form. Such visions may not be bestowed upon others, and even for Arjuna it was not a permanent vision, for it subsided when Arjuna requested that *Śrī* Krishna remove the vision of the Universal Form and just after *Śrī* Krishna granted the divine vision to see the four-handed Form.

*Śrī* Krishna will give more details about His presence as the one Who is situated in the mystic resting place of all beings. To realize Him, one should do *samādhi* practice. One must first master perception of one's spiritual self. Then one may see that super-person, *Śrī* Krishna, existing in the psyche as well.

आदित्यानामहं विष्णुर्
ज्योतिषां रविरंशुमान् ।
मरीचिर्मरुतामस्मि
नक्षत्राणामहं शशी ॥ १०.२१ ॥
ādityānāmahaṁ viṣṇur
jyotiṣāṁ raviraṁśumān
marīcirmarutāmasmi
nakṣatrāṇāmahaṁ śaśī (10.21)

*ādityānām — of the Adityas; aham — I; viṣṇur = viṣṇuḥ — Vishnu; jyotiṣām — of lights; ravir = raviḥ — the sun; aṁśumān — radiant; marīcir = marīciḥ — Marici; marutām — of the thunderstormers; asmi — I am; nakṣatrāṇām — of the stars; aham — I; śaśī — the moon*

**Of the Ādityas, I am Vishnu. Of lights, I am represented by the radiant sun. Of the thunderstorms, I am represented by Marīci. Of the stars, I am signified by the moon. (10.21)**

***Siddha Swami's Commentary:***

One begins spiritual disciplines by hearing of the wonders of the world. But one should strive to realize these in fact. One should not be satisfied to remain as a person who only perceives things grossly and who may know of supernatural and spiritual aspects through hearing alone. For indeed, what is the value of such a belief, if one cannot at any rate, realize it by direct perception? And why should one have to wait until the time of death to see beyond this physical world. If there is something beyond this physical appearance, why can it not be experienced while using a material body?

Initially spiritual life begins with faith in the scripture and the spiritual master, the religious teacher. *Śrī* Krishna related many details which can be accepted merely on the basis of faith in Him and in the person who teaches one about Him.

These descriptions of *Śrī* Krishna relate mostly to the religious belief in India at the time of this discourse with Arjuna. In other countries, people might be unable to follow these explanations because of unfamiliarity with the Indian religions. The comparison of the moon with the stars, indicating that the moon is the most prominent of the stars, is based on ordinary vision, whereby the moon appears to be white just as the stars do, while the sun appears to be brilliant whitish-yellow. Modern astronomy does not regard the moon as a star. They regard the sun as a small star. However, *Śrī* Krishna's comparisons may be taken at face value, and one can appreciate His main point in showing how one may relate Him to all phenomena and even to prevailing religious ideas.

वेदानां सामवेदोऽस्मि
देवानामस्मि वासवः ।
इन्द्रियाणां मनश्चास्मि
भूतानामस्मि चेतना ॥ १०.२२ ॥
vedānāṁ sāmavedo'smi
devānāmasmi vāsavaḥ
indriyāṇāṁ manaścāsmi
bhūtānāmasmi cetanā (10.22)

*vedānām — of the Vedas; sāmavedo = sāmavedaḥ — Sāma Veda; 'smi = asmi — I am; devānām — of the supernatural rulers; asmi — I am; vāsavaḥ — Vāsava Indra; indriyāṇām — of the senses; manaścāsmi = manas — mind + ca — and + asmi — I am; bhūtānām — of the creature forms; asmi — I am; cetanā — consciousness*

**Of the *Vedas*, I am represented by the Sāma Veda. Of the supernatural rulers, I am represented as Vāsava Indra. Of the senses, I am represented as the mind. In creature forms, I am represented as consciousness. (10.22)**

***Siddha Swami's Commentary:***

Each of the comparisons should be carefully studied by the student *yogin*, so that He understands how he is to regard *Śrī* Krishna and how he should be Krishna conscious, even in relation to the natural and supernatural material world.

*Cetanā* means the mental, emotional and life impulse force which is in creature forms. Usually we feel that this power represents life. When a body no longer exhibits that life, we discard it as a dead form. The overall living force in the body comprises several aspects of natural, supernatural and spiritual forces. Together these are representative of the Supreme Being.

रुद्राणां शंकरश्चास्मि
वित्तेशो यक्षरक्षसाम् ।
वसूनां पावकश्चास्मि
मेरुः शिखरिणामहम् ॥ १०.२३ ॥
rudrāṇāṁ śaṁkaraścāsmi
vitteśo yakṣarakṣasām
vasūnāṁ pāvakaścāsmi
meruḥ śikhariṇāmaham (10.23)

*rudrāṇām — of the cosmic destroyers; śaṁkaraścāsmi = śaṁkaraḥ — Shankara Shiva + ca — and + asmi — I am; vitteśo = vitteśaḥ — Kubera; yakṣarakṣasām — of the Yakshas and Rakshas; vasūnām — of the Vasus; pāvakaścāsmi = pāvakaḥ — Pavāka + ca — and + asmi — I am; meruḥ — Meru; śikhariṇām — of the mountains; aham — I*

**Of the cosmic destroyers, I am represented by the Shankara Shiva. Of the Yakshas and Rakshas, I am best represented as Vittesha Kubera. Of the Vasus, I am represented by Pāvaka Agni. Of the mountains, I am represented as Mount Meru. (10.23)**

***Siddha Swami's Commentary:***

Persons unfamiliar with the gods of the Vedic religions in India, cannot make good use of this analogy, but *Śrī* Krishna gave sufficient descriptions of ordinary phenomena like the moon and the stars. In that way, each person, even from varied backgrounds with varied religious upbringings, will be able to grasp the lessons of this Krishna-conscious way of viewing the world.

Those of Indian religious orientation should take the time to study this chapter since the most elementary way of meeting with *Śrī* Krishna is given herein. This basic training does not require yoga expertise but it serves as a motivation for one to take up higher yoga in order to verify what *Śrī* Krishna said. One should not be lazy in the acceptance and subsequent verification in what *Śrī* Krishna taught to Arjuna.

पुरोधसां च मुख्यं मां
विद्धि पार्थ बृहस्पतिम् ।
सेनानीनामहं स्कन्दः
सरसामस्मि सागरः ॥१०.२४॥
purodhasāṁ ca mukhyaṁ māṁ
viddhi pārtha bṛhaspatim
senānīnāmahaṁ skandaḥ
sarasāmasmi sāgaraḥ (10.24)

*purodhasām — of the family priest; ca — and; mukhyam — chief; mām — me; viddhi — know; pārtha — son of Pṛthā; bṛhaspatim — Bṛhaspati; senānīnām — of the commanders; aham — I; skandaḥ — Skanda; sarasām — of the seas; asmi — I am; sāgaraḥ — the ocean*

**O son of Pṛthā, know Me as being represented by Brihaspati, the chief of the family priests. Of military commanders, I am represented by Skanda. Of the seas, I am symbolized by the ocean. (10.24)**

***Siddha Swami's Commentary:***

For the purpose of *brahma yoga*, the advanced level of *buddhi yoga* when it is converted into *jñāna yoga*, the yogi loses interest both in this world and in its controllers. Thus most of the description of how to relate gross and subtle objects to the Supreme Person is not used in that practice. However, a student should have learned this relational course and should know how to apply it whenever he or she interacts with the subtle or gross material energy. One must also know this for the purpose of teaching persons who are not advanced. Thus this course of elementary Krishna consciousness should be studied in detail by everyone.

The construction, maintenance and demolition of things in the material world are really of no interest to an advanced *brahma yogi*. He searches out the spiritual self of himself and then tries to penetrate into the spiritual environment which has no subtle or super-subtle material energy. These are his primary concerns.

महर्षीणां भृगुरहं
गिरामस्म्येकमक्षरम् ।
यज्ञानां जपयज्ञोऽस्मि
स्थावराणां हिमालयः ॥१०.२५॥
maharṣīṇāṁ bhṛguraham
girāmasmyekamakṣaram
yajñānāṁ japayajño'smi
sthāvarāṇāṁ himālayaḥ (10.25)

*maharṣīṇām — of the great yogi sages; bhṛgur = bhṛguḥ — Brigu; aham — I; girām — of spoken words; asmy = asmi — I; ekamakṣaram — one-syllable sound; yajñānām — of the religiously-motivated disciplines; japayajño = japayajñaḥ — the discipline of uttering prayers; 'smi = asmi — I am; sthāvarāṇām — of the stationary objects; himālayaḥ — Himalaya*

**Of the great yogi sages, Bhrigu is one who I am best represented by. Of the spoken words, I am represented by the one-syllable sound. Of the religiously-motivated disciplines, I am represented best by the discipline of uttering prayers. Of stationary objects, I am best represented by the Himalayas. (10.25)**

***Siddha Swami's Commentary:***

Names like *Bhṛgu*, *Nārada*, *Indra* and *Brahmā* are used as status names in the Vedic scriptures. This means that one person who has that post or position is awarded that title, just as the president of a country is called Mr. President, rather than by his personal name. *Bhṛgu* is the chief great yogi sage on the Maharloka planets situated above the Svargaloka heavenly worlds. Or rather, whosoever is the greatest of those yogi sages is called *Bhṛgu*.

In the religious and spiritual life, one has to start where he or she is. If the student is materialistic, he should start there by taking this course of how to relate gross objects to the

Supreme Person. Then gradually, as one advances, one may become introspective to pursue what is supernatural and spiritual.

अश्वत्थः सर्ववृक्षाणां
देवर्षीणां च नारदः ।
गन्धर्वाणां चित्ररथः
सिद्धानां कपिलो मुनिः ॥१०.२६॥
aśvatthaḥ sarvavṛkṣāṇāṁ
devarṣīṇāṁ ca nāradaḥ
gandharvāṇāṁ citrarathaḥ
siddhānāṁ kapilo muniḥ (10.26)

*aśvatthaḥ — sacred fig tree; sarvavṛkṣāṇāṁ = sarva — all + vṛksāṇām — of trees; devarṣīṇām — of the celestial supernatural yogi sages; ca — and; nāradaḥ — Narada; gandharvāṇām — of the supernatural singers; citrarathaḥ — Citraratha; siddhānām — of the perfected souls; kapilo = kapilaḥ — Kapila; muniḥ — yogi philosopher*

**Of all trees, I am best represented by the Ashvattha sacred fig tree. Of the supernatural yogi sages, I am represented by Narada. Of the supernatural singers, it is Chitraratha; of the perfected souls, the yogi philosopher Kapila. (10.26)**

***Siddha Swami's Commentary:***

*Nārada* is another status name. *Nārada* is the person who does errands for *Prajāpatih Brahmā*. By qualification, this person is a devotee of the Lord and is also a *mahāyogin*. The word *devarṣīṇām* indicates that such a person is regarded as a yogi philosopher in the assembly of the *deva* supernatural rulers. The siddhas or perfected souls are those who left aside *karma yoga* and pursue *jñāna yoga* for the highest perfection. Among them Kapila Rishi *Mahāyogin* is the greatest. He is rated as an incarnation of Godhead.

The siddhas are persons who gained an exemption from cultural activities, and thus they are only pursuing the course of spiritual perfection.

उच्चैःश्रवसमश्वानां
विद्धि माममृतोद्भवम् ।
ऐरावतं गजेन्द्राणां
नराणां च नराधिपम् ॥१०.२७॥
uccaiḥśravasamaśvānāṁ
viddhi māmamṛtodbhavam
airāvataṁ gajendrāṇāṁ
narāṇāṁ ca narādhipam (10.27)

*uccaihśravasam — the supernatural horse Uccaihśrava; aśvānām — of the horses; viddhi — know; mām — me; amṛtodbhavam = amṛta — a sweet celestial sea + udbhavam — born from; airāvatam — Airāvata; gajendrāṇām — of kingly elephants; narāṇām — of men; ca — and; narādhipam — King of men*

**Of horses, know Me as represented by the supernatural horse Uccaihśrava, which was born of the sweet celestial sea. Of the kingly elephants, know Me as represented by Airāvata, and know Me as the King of men. (10.27)**

***Siddha Swami's Commentary:***

A ruler, even a bad one, represents the supreme authority, even though the unprincipled leader deviates from righteousness.

आयुधानामहं वज्रं
धेनूनामस्मि कामधुक् ।
प्रजनश्चास्मि कन्दर्पः
सर्पाणामस्मि वासुकिः ॥१०.२८॥

*āyudhānām — of weapons; aham — I; vajram — supernatural thunderbolt; dhenūnām — of cows; asmi — I am; kāmadhuk — supernatural Kamadhuk cow;*

āyudhānāmahaṁ vajraṁ
dhenūnāmasmi kāmadhuk
prajanaścāsmi kandarpaḥ
sarpāṇāmasmi vāsukiḥ (10.28)

*prajanaścāsmi = prajanas — begetting + ca — and + asmi — I am; kandarpaḥ — Kandarpa, the god of romance; sarpāṇām — of serpents; asmi — I am; vāsukiḥ — Vāsuki*

**Of weapons, I am compared to the Vajra supernatural thunderbolt. Of cows, I am represented as the supernatural Kāmadhuk. And in the case of begetting, I am represented by Kandarpa, the god of romance. Of serpents, I am represented by Vāsuki. (10.28)**

***Siddha Swami's Commentary:***

Whatever is the greatest principle or the greatest object is representative of the Supreme. But in higher yoga, one leaves aside things of mundane origin and focuses on finding the Supreme in the supernatural and spiritual realities.

अनन्तश्चास्मि नागानां
वरुणो यादसामहम् ।
पितृणामर्यमा चास्मि
यमः संयमतामहम् ॥ १०.२९॥
anantaścāsmi nāgānāṁ
varuṇo yādasāmaham
pitṝṇāmaryamā cāsmi
yamaḥ saṁyamatāmaham (10.29)

*anantaścāsmi = anantaḥ — Ananta + ca — and + asmi — I am; nāgānām — of supernatural snakes; varuṇo = varuṇaḥ — Varuṇa; yādasām — of the aquatics; aham — I; pitṝṇām — of the piously-departed ancestors; aryamā — Aryamā; cāsmi = ca — and + asmi — I am; yamaḥ — Yama; saṁyamatām — of the subduers; aham — I*

**I am represented by Ananta among the supernatural snakes. I am represented by Varuṇa, among the aquatics. Among the piously-departed spirits, I am represented by Aryamā. Of the subduers, I am represented by Yama. (10.29)**

***Siddha Swami's Commentary:***

In the creation, we are always confronted with comparisons, even competitions between various entities in the same species or in the same family. Whatever seems to be the greatest should be regarded as representative of the Supreme.

Regardless of whether we like it or not, we have to respect whatever is greater than ourselves. If confronted, we give in to whatever is superior.

प्रह्लादश्चास्मि दैत्यानां
कालः कलयतामहम् ।
मृगाणां च मृगेन्द्रोऽहं
वैनतेयश्च पक्षिणाम् ॥ १०.३०॥
prahlādaścāsmi daityānāṁ
kālaḥ kalayatāmaham
mṛgāṇāṁ ca mṛgendro'haṁ
vainateyaśca pakṣiṇām (10.30)

*prahlādaścāsmi = prahlādaḥ — Prahlāda + ca — and + asmi — I am; daityānām — of the titan descendants of Diti; kālaḥ — time; kalayatām — of the monitors; aham — I; mṛgāṇām — of the animals; ca — and; mṛgendro = mṛgendraḥ — king of the beasts; 'ham = aham — I; vainateyaśca = vainateyaḥ — son of Vinata + ca — and; pakṣiṇām — of the birds*

**And I am represented as Prahlāda among the titan descendants of Diti, as time of the monitors, as the king of beasts among the animals, as the son of Vinata among the birds. (10.30)**

***Siddha Swami's Commentary:***

God is easily understood by studying the regulation of time. A human being, however great he may be, cannot supersede time. During the life of one's body, one learns how to make use of time, but ultimately time continues and pushes one's body aside. One should learn how to respect time as being superior over all limited souls.

As living beings come and go, live and die, and live again and die, time supervises them, allowing them to appear in one place, flourish and then perish. Time is to be respected as being representative of the Supreme.

पवनः पवतामस्मि
रामः शस्त्रभृतामहम्।
झषाणां मकरश्चास्मि
स्रोतसामस्मि जाह्नवी ॥१०.३१॥
pavanaḥ pavatāmasmi
rāmaḥ śastrabhṛtāmaham
jhaṣāṇāṁ makaraścāsmi
srotasāmasmi jāhnavī (10.31)

*pavanaḥ — the wind; pavatām — of the cleansers; asmi — I am; rāmaḥ — Rāma; śastrabhṛtām — of the weapon carriers; aham — I; jhaṣāṇām — of sea monsters; makaraścāsmi = makaraḥ — shark + ca — and + asmi — I am; srotasām — of rivers; asmi — I am; jāhnavī — daughter of Jahnu*

**Among the cleansers, I am best represented by the wind. Of the weapon carriers, I am best represented by Rāma. Of the sea monsters, I am represented by the shark. Of the rivers, I am represented by Jahnu's daughter. (10.31)**

***Siddha Swami's Commentary:***

The power of God cannot be known fully by any of the limited spirits. Still one should endeavor to know God and one should know God in so far as one is capable of assessing His power and glory. Thus whatever is great, whatever is beyond comparison, whatever is the most beautiful and most charming, and whatever is the most dangerous gives some idea about God. When one appreciates whatever is before one's eyes, as being representative of God, one practices humility, and from that one makes progress and gets the grace of the Almighty. This is how one progresses in the religious way.

सर्गाणामादिरन्तश्च
मध्यं चैवाहमर्जुन ।
अध्यात्मविद्या विद्यानां
वादः प्रवदतामहम् ॥१०.३२॥
sargāṇāmādirantaśca
madhyaṁ caivāhamarjuna
adhyātmavidyā vidyānāṁ
vādaḥ pravadatāmaham (10.32)

*sargāṇām — of creations; ādir = ādiḥ — formation; antaśca = antaḥ — ending + ca — and; madhyam — continuation; caivāham = ca — and + eva — indeed + aham — I; arjuna — Arjuna; adhyātmavidyā — knowledge of the Supreme Soul; vidyānām — of sciences; vādaḥ — conclusion; pravadatām — of the logicians; aham — I*

**Of creations, I am represented by the formation, continuation and ending. O Arjuna, of the sciences, I am knowledge of the Supreme Soul. I am represented by the conclusion of the logicians. (10.32)**

***Siddha Swami's Commentary:***

By a careful study of how objects appear, we get some view about the formation, continuation and ending of things which are manifested. But by what force do the formations occur in the first place? How did this material energy manifest? What is its basic state? What will it disappear into in the end?

There is *ātmavidyā* and *adhyātmavidyā*, knowledge and experience of the soul and of the Supreme Soul. One should strive for this. It is only possible to understand the Supreme Soul after assessing oneself. The Supreme Soul is subtler than the limited spirit.

अक्षराणामकारोऽस्मि
द्वंद्वः सामासिकस्य च ।
अहमेवाक्षयः कालो
धाताहं विश्वतोमुखः ॥ १०.३३ ॥
akṣarāṇāmakāro'smi
dvaṁdvaḥ sāmāsikasya ca
ahamevākṣayaḥ kālo
dhātāhaṁ viśvatomukhaḥ (10.33)

*akṣarāṇām — of letters; akāro = akāraḥ — the letter A; 'smi = asmi — I am; dvandvaḥ — two-word compound; sāmāsikasya — of the word combinations; ca — and; aham — I; evākṣayaḥ = eva — indeed + akṣayaḥ — infinite; kālo = kālaḥ — time; dhātāham = dhātā — Dhātā Brahmā + aham — I; viśvatomukhaḥ — one who faces all directions, four-faced*

**Of letters, I am represented by the letter A. Of the word combinations, I am represented by the two-word compound. I am comparable to infinite time. I am represented by Dhātā, the four-faced Brahmā. (10.33)**

***Siddha Swami's Commentary:***

Whatever took place, takes place, and will take place, does so within the span of time. Time itself is considered to be infinite. Whatever exists must occur within the space of time. Thus time is all comprehensive. It directly represents the Supreme Being.

मृत्युः सर्वहरश्चाहम्
उद्भवश्च भविष्यताम् ।
कीर्तिः श्रीर्वाक्च नारीणां
स्मृतिर्मेधा धृतिः क्षमा ॥ १०.३४
mṛtyuḥ sarvaharaścāham
udbhavaśca bhaviṣyatām
kīrtiḥ śrīrvākca nārīṇāṁ
smṛtirmedhā dhṛtiḥ kṣamā (10.34)

*mṛtyuḥ — death; sarvaharaścāham = sarvaharaḥ — all-devouring + ca — and + aham — I; udbhavaśca = udbhavaḥ — origin + ca — and; bhaviṣyatām — of things which are to be produced; kīrtiḥ — Kīrti, goddess of fame; śrīr = śrīḥ — Shri, goddess of fortune; vāk — Vāk, goddess of speech; ca — and; nārīṇām — of women; smṛtir = smṛtiḥ — Smṛti, goddess of recollection; medhā — Medhā, goddess of counsel; dhṛtiḥ — Dhṛti, goddess of faithfulness; kṣamā — Kṣamā, goddess of patience*

**I am represented as all-devouring death. I am the foundation of things that are to be produced. And among women, I am represented by Kīrti, the goddess of fame, Śrī, the goddess of fortune, Vāk, the goddess of speech, Smṛti, the goddess of recollection, Medhā, the goddess of counsel, Dhṛti, the goddess of faithfulness and Kṣama, the goddess of patience. (10.34)**

***Siddha Swami's Commentary:***

God is also represented by death, something that hardly anyone can appreciate. Death is serviceable in expediting the disintegration of the formations in the subtle and gross material world. Death is a utility for transforming one form into another. And whatever is to be produced already exists in potential form. That potentiality represents the Supreme Being.

बृहत्साम तथा साम्नां
गायत्री छन्दसामहम् ।
मासानां मार्गशीर्षोऽहम्
ऋतूनां कुसुमाकरः ॥ १०.३५ ॥

*bṛhatsāma — Brihat Sāma melody; tathā — also; sāmnām — of the Sāma Veda chants; gāyatrī — Gayatri; chandasām — of the poetic hymns; aham — I; māsānām — of*

bṛhatsāma tathā sāmnāṁ
gāyatrī chandasāmaham
māsānāṁ mārgaśīrṣo'ham
ṛtūnāṁ kusumākaraḥ (10.35)

*months; mārgaśīrṣo = mārgaśīrṣaḥ — November-December lunar month; 'ham = aham — I; ṛtūnām — of seasons; kusumākaraḥ — spring*

**Of the Sāma Veda chants, the Brihat Sāma melody represents Me. Of the poetic hymns, I am the Gāyatrī. Of months, I am best represented by the November-December lunar month. Of the seasons, I am best compared to Spring. (10.35)**

***Siddha Swami's Commentary:***

The *Gāyatrī* hymn like the *Om* sound was used by many ascetics in the quest for perfection. Thus these two sounds represent the Supreme Person. There are many *Gāyatrī* mantras but the chief is:

*om bhūr bhuvah svah tat savitur vareṇyam*
*bhargo devasya dhīmahi dhi yo yo na prachodayāt*

द्यूतं छलयतामस्मि
तेजस्तेजस्विनामहम् ।
जयोऽस्मि व्यवसायोऽस्मि
सत्त्वं सत्त्ववतामहम् ॥ १०.३६ ॥
dyūtaṁ chalayatāmasmi
tejastejasvināmaham
jayo'smi vyavasāyo'smi
sattvaṁ sattvavatāmaham (10.36)

*dyūtam — gambling skill; chalayatām — of the swindlers; asmi — I am; tejaḥ — splendor; tejasvinām — of the splendid things; aham — I; jayo = jayaḥ — victory; 'ham = asmi — I am; vyavasāyo = vyavasāyaḥ — endeavor; 'smi = asmi — I am; sattvam — reality; sattvavatām — of the real things; aham — I*

**I am represented as the gambling skill of the swindlers. I am compared to the splendor of the splendid things. I am compared to victory and endeavor. I am the reality of the realistic things. (10.36)**

***Siddha Swami's Commentary:***

Elementary religion is concerned with appreciating what is good for human beings. It includes what is pleasant, desirable and what gives security to human beings. Thus one should appreciate the splendor of the splendid thing *(tejah tejasvinām)*. And God should be regarded as the reality in real things.

वृष्णीनां वासुदेवोऽस्मि
पाण्डवानां धनंजयः ।
मुनीनामप्यहं व्यासः
कवीनामुशना कविः ॥ १०.३७ ॥
vṛṣṇīnāṁ vāsudevo'smi
pāṇḍavānāṁ dhanaṁjayaḥ
munīnāmapyahaṁ vyāsaḥ
kavīnāmuśanā kaviḥ (10.37)

*vṛṣṇīnām — of the Vrishnis; vāsudevo = vāsudevaḥ — the son of Vasudeva; 'smi = asmi — I am; pāṇḍavānām — of the Pandavas; dhanaṁjayaḥ — Arjuna; munīnām — of the yogi philosophers; apy = api — also; aham — I; vyāsaḥ — Vyasa; kavīnām — of poets; uśanā — Ushana; kaviḥ — respected poet*

**Of the Vṛṣṇis, I am the son of Vasudeva. Of the Pāṇḍavas, I am represented by Arjuna. Of the yogi philosophers, I am compared to Vyāsa. Of the poets, I am represented by the respected poet Uśanā. (10.37)**

***Siddha Swami's Commentary:***

Since *Śrī* Krishna was known as the son of *Vasudeva* and was called *Vāsudeva*, He is acclaimed as that cultural identity. He is not factually the son of *Vasudeva*, but for social purposes He is regarded in that way. Krishna wanted to be regarded as being Arjuna among the Pandavas. Arjuna was His foremost devotee among the sons of Pandu. And of the yogi philosophers, he is identified with Krishna *Dvaipāyaṇa*, *Vyāsa*, the son of *Satyavatī* and *Parāśar Muni*. Of the great Sanskrit poets, Krishna is represented in the seer named *Uśanā*.

दण्डो दमयतामस्मि
नीतिरस्मि जिगीषताम् ।
मौनं चैवास्मि गुह्यानां
ज्ञानं ज्ञानवतामहम् ॥ १०.३८ ॥
daṇḍo damayatāmasmi
nītirasmi jigīṣatām
maunaṁ caivāsmi guhyānāṁ
jñānaṁ jñānavatāmaham (10.38)

*daṇdo = daṇdaḥ — authority to punish; damayatām — of the rulers; asmi — I am; nītir = nītiḥ — morality; asmi — I am; jigīṣatām — of those seeking victory; maunam — silence; caivāsmi = ca — and + eva — indeed + asmi — I am; guhyānām — of secrets; jñānam — knowledge; jñānavatām — of those who know; aham — I*

**Of rulers, I am the authority to punish. For those seeking victory, I may be compared to the means of morality; of secrets, I am represented by silence. In wise men, I am represented as knowledge. (10.38)**

***Siddha Swami's Commentary:***

The authority to punish shifts from one ruler or judge to another. That authority itself is representative of *Śrī* Krishna. For those seeking victory over others, there is no better means than the righteous way of living. *Śrī* Krishna Himself establishes righteous lifestyle. The battle of *Kurukṣetra* was fought by King Yudhishthira for establishing and upholding righteousness. *Śrī* Krishna represents silence. It is in silence, that yogins master the higher yoga.

यच्चापि सर्वभूतानां
बीजं तदहमर्जुन ।
न तदस्ति विना यत्स्यान्
मया भूतं चराचरम् ॥ १०.३९ ॥
yaccāpi sarvabhūtānāṁ
bījaṁ tadahamarjuna
na tadasti vinā yatsyān
mayā bhūtaṁ carācaram (10.39)

*yac = yad — which; cāpi = ca — and + api — also; sarvabhūtānām — of all created beings; bījam — origin point; tad — that; aham — I; arjuna — Arjuna; na — not; tad — that; asti — is; vinā — without; yat = yad — which; syān = syāt — should be; mayā — through My influence; bhūtam — existing; carācaram — active or stationary*

**And O Arjuna, I am the origin of all created beings. There is nothing active or stationary which could exist without My influence. (10.39)**

***Siddha Swami's Commentary:***

The Supreme Being is Himself the origin point or *bījam* of all created beings. There is in fact, nothing active or stationary which could exist without His influence. He permeates all.

नान्तोऽस्ति मम दिव्यानां
विभूतीनां परंतप ।
एष तूद्देशतः प्रोक्तो
विभूतेर्विस्तरो मया ॥ १०.४० ॥

*nānto (nāntaḥ) = na — no + antaḥ — end; 'sti = asti — is; mama — of My; divyānām — of the supernatural; vibhūtīnām — manifestations; paraṁtapa — burner of enemy forces; eṣa — this; tūddeśataḥ = tu —*

nānto'sti mama divyānāṁ
vibhūtīnāṁ paraṁtapa
eṣa tūddeśataḥ prokto
vibhūtervistaro mayā (10.40)

*but + uddeśataḥ — for a sample; prokto = proktaḥ — explained; vibhūter = vibhūteḥ — of the opulences; vistaro = vistaraḥ — of the spreading, extensive; mayā — by Me*

**There is no end to My supernatural manifestations, O burner of the enemy forces. This was explained by Me as a sampling of My extensive opulence. (10.40)**

***Siddha Swami's Commentary:***

The power of God cannot be sufficiently rated by any limited being. Still, all persons should endeavor for understanding His glories to whatever extent their minds could hold. That is our duty to the Supreme Being.

यद्यद्विभूतिमत्सत्त्वं
श्रीमदूर्जितमेव वा ।
तत्तदेवावगच्छ त्वं
मम तेजोंऽशसंभवम् ॥ १०.४१ ॥
yadyadvibhūtimatsattvaṁ
śrīmadūrjitameva vā
tattadevāvagaccha tvaṁ
mama tejoṁśasaṁbhavam (10.41)

*yad yad — what, whatever; vibhūtimat — fantastic; sattvam — real object; Śrīmad = śrīmat — prosperous; ūrjitam — powerful; eva — indeed; vā — or; tat tad = tad tat — this, that, any case; evāvagaccha = eva — indeed + avagaccha — realize; tvam — you; mama — of Me; tejo = tejaḥ — splendor; 'mśasaṁbhavam (aṁśasaṁbhavam) = aṁśa — fraction + saṁbhavam — origin*

**You should realize that whatever fantastic existence, whatever prosperous or powerful object there is, in any case, it originates from a fraction of My splendor. (10.41)**

***Siddha Swami's Commentary:***

This realization about the supreme is more or less a mental assessment in wonderment. But one must go further to experience some of this on the supernatural and spiritual planes.

अथ वा बहुनैतेन
किं ज्ञातेन तवार्जुन ।
विष्टभ्याहमिदं कृत्स्नम्
एकांशेन स्थितो जगत् ॥ १०.४२ ॥
atha vā bahunaitena
kiṁ jñātena tavārjuna
viṣṭabhyāhamidaṁ kṛtsnam
ekāṁśena sthito jagat (10.42)

*athavā — but; bahunaitena = bahunā — with extensive + etena — with this; kim — what is the value?; jñātena — with information; tavārjuna = tava — of you + arjuna — Arjuna; viṣṭabhyāham = viṣṭabhya — supporting + aham — I; idam — this; kṛtsnam — entire; ekāṁśena = eka — one + aṁśena — by a fraction; sthito = sthitaḥ — based, standing; jagat — world*

**But Arjuna, what is the value of this extensive information? As the foundation, I support this entire universe with a fraction of Myself. (10.42)**

***Siddha Swami's Commentary:***

Each devotee must research into the origin of himself or herself, as well as the origin of this material world. Each needs to understand this to a greater or lesser degree. Thus it is up to the particular student, as to how far he will inquire and pry into this.

*Śrī* Krishna opined that since with a fraction of Himself He supported this universe, there was really no need for an extensive explanation in cataloging the items of this world and His relationship to these. In other words, it would be better to leave aside the wonders of this world and go to their source, which is the Supreme Spirit Himself. And that is the quest of *brahma yoga* practice.

# CHAPTER 11

# Paramam Rūpam Aiśvaram

## The Supreme Form

## The Supernatural Glory*

*saṁjaya uvāca*
*evamuktvā tato rājan mahāyogeśvaro hariḥ*
*darśayāmāsa pārthāya paramaṁ rūpamaiśvaram (11.9)*

***Sanjaya said: O King, having said that, the great Master of yoga, Hari, the God Vishnu, revealed to the son of Pṛthā, the Supreme Form, the supernatural glory. (11.9)***

****Siddha Swami assigned this chapter title on the basis of verse 9 of this chapter.***

अर्जुन उवाच
मदनुग्रहाय परमं
गुह्यमध्यात्मसंज्ञितम् ।
यत्त्वयोक्तं वचस्तेन
मोहोऽयं विगतो मम ॥ ११.१ ॥
arjuna uvāca
madanugrahāya paramaṁ
guhyamadhyātmasaṁjñitam
yattvayoktaṁ vacastena
moho'yaṁ vigato mama (11.1)

*arjuna — Arjuna: uvāca — said; madanugrahāya — kindness to me, as a matter of mercy to me; paramaṁ — highest; guhyam — private; adhyātmasaṁjñitam = adhyātma — Supersoul + samjñitam — known as; yad — which; tvayoktaṁ = tvaya — by you + uktam — explained; vacaḥ — lecture; tena — by this; moho = mohaḥ — delusion; 'yam = ayam — this; vigato = vigataḥ — departed; mama — of me (11.1)*

**Arjuna said: As a matter of mercy to me, the highest, most private information of the Supreme Soul was explained by You in this lecture. Subsequently, the delusion departed from me. (11.1)**

***Siddha Swami's Commentary:***

Merely by hearing of the Supreme Soul *(adhyātmasamjñitam),* without even the experience to verify the information, Arjuna's delusion departed from his psyche. Thus he praised *Śrī* Krishna for having, as a matter of mercy *(madanugrahāya),* given the highest, most private information. However, one's doubts are not removed merely by hearing. Through Arjuna's faith in *Śrī* Krishna, his trust of the Lord, he was able to loosen himself from the delusion. Still Arjuna would require the experience to personally verify the truths which *Śrī* Krishna explained.

The lack of delusion does not indicate that Arjuna or anyone else received an experience merely by hearing. The delusion overcame the devotee at some other time and bog him down in the mire of indecision, sabotaging his ability to follow the instructions of *Śrī* Krishna.

भवाप्ययौ हि भूतानां
श्रुतौ विस्तरशो मया ।
त्वत्तः कमलपत्राक्ष
माहात्म्यमपि चाव्ययम् ॥ ११.२ ॥
bhavāpyayau hi bhūtānāṁ
śrutau vistaraśo mayā
tvattaḥ kamalapatrākṣa
māhātmyamapi cāvyayam (11.2)

*bhavāpyayau = bhava — origin + apy (api) — also + ayau — ruination; hi — indeed; bhūtānām — of the beings; śrutau — both were heard; vistaraśo = vistaraśaḥ — in detail; mayā — by me; tvattaḥ — from you; kamalapatrākṣa = kamala — lotus + patra — petal + akṣa — eyed; māhātmyam — majestic glory; api — also; cāvyayam = ca — and + avyayam — eternally*

**The description of the origin and ruination of the beings was heard in detail by me, O Person Whose eyes are shaped like lotus petals. You also described Your eternal majestic glory. (11.2)**

***Siddha Swami's Commentary:***

This eternal majestic glory *(māhātmyam api cāvyayam)* is mostly a description of how the Supreme Being relates to and regulates His relationship with this material world. This is not so much an interest in the higher yoga practice. Higher yoga really concerns only what is spiritual in itself and not how the spiritual interacts with the material. But still one needs to understand this eternal majestic glory, otherwise one's quest in higher yoga will he forestalled. Unless one understands the relationship between the spiritual reality and the material energy, one will not transcend one's connection with subtle material nature, and hence one's progression will be nil.

Arjuna admired the material form which was used by *Śrī* Krishna. Arjuna heard descriptions of *Śrī* Krishna's divine form from persons like *Nārada*, *Asita Devala* and *Vyāsa*. Thus he wondered about the spiritual beauty of *Śrī* Krishna, Who even materially had incomparable beauty.

एवमेतद्यथात्थ त्वम्
आत्मानं परमेश्वर ।
द्रष्टुमिच्छामि ते रूपम्
ऐश्वरं पुरुषोत्तम ॥११.३॥
evametadyathāttha tvam
ātmānaṁ parameśvara
draṣṭumicchāmi te rūpam
aiśvaraṁ puruṣottama (11.3)

*evam — thus; etad — this; yathāttha = yathā — as + attha — you explain; tvam — you; ātmānam — yourself; parameśvara — O Supreme Lord; draṣṭum — to see; icchāmi — I wish; te — your; rūpam — form; aiśvaram — majesty; puruṣottama — O Supreme Person*

**This is as You explained about Yourself, O Supreme Lord. I wish to see Your Majestic Form, O Supreme Person. (11.3)**

***Siddha Swami's Commentary:***

Even though Arjuna felt a relief from the delusive energy which invaded his psyche after seeing the Kuru armies before him, still he remained unconvinced by *Śrī* Krishna's explanation about the origin and ruination of the beings (*bhavāpyayau hi bhutānām*, 11.2). Arjuna wanted to see that directly with firsthand supernatural vision. Thus he frankly told *Śrī* Krishna that he wanted to see the majestic form *(rūpam aiśvaram puruṣottama).*

मन्यसे यदि तच्छक्यं
मया द्रष्टुमिति प्रभो ।
योगेश्वर ततो मे त्वं
दर्शयात्मानमव्ययम् ॥११.४॥
manyase yadi tacchakyaṁ
mayā draṣṭumiti prabho
yogeśvara tato me tvaṁ
darśayātmānamavyayam (11.4)

*manyase — you think; yadi — if; tac = tad — that; chakyam = sakyam — possible; mayā — by me; draṣṭum — to see; iti — thus; prabho — O Lord; yogeśvara — Master of yoga technique; tato = tataḥ — then; me — to me; tvam — you; darśayātmānam = darśayā — make it be seen + ātmānam — self; avyayam — eternal*

**If You think that it is possible for me to see this, O Lord, Master of the yoga technique, then make me see You in that Eternal Form. (11.4)**

***Siddha Swami's Commentary:***

Arjuna asked to see the *ātmanam avyayam* which is the eternal self-form of *Śrī* Krishna, but the matter is not that simple, for *Śrī* Krishna will reveal His Universal Form which regulated the incidence at *Kurukṣetra*, an immediate concern for Arjuna. Such a form, though supernatural, is not perpetual. Such a form may be regarded as enduring only in reference to the material world but not in reference to the pure spiritual environment.

This Universal Form was required for Arjuna because he, like every other devotee, must progress from where he stands. Everyone must start with his own concerns and gradually work his way up and out of the material world. Arjuna rightly addressed *Śrī* Krishna as Master of the yoga technique, *Yogeśvara*, and he requested humbly that if possible, he should be made to see the Form which was behind all action in the material world and which was effective in approving or disapproving any activity.

**श्रीभगवानुवाच**
**पश्य मे पार्थ रूपाणि**
**शतशोऽथ सहस्रशः ।**
**नानाविधानि दिव्यानि**
**नानावर्णाकृतीनि च ॥ ११.५ ॥**
śrībhagavānuvāca
paśya me pārtha rūpāṇi
śataśo'tha sahasraśaḥ
nānāvidhāni divyāni
nānāvarṇākṛtīni ca (11.5)

*śrībhagavān – the Blessed Lord; uvāca — said; paśya — see; me — My; pārtha — son of Pṛthā; rūpāṇi — forms; śataśo = śataśaḥ — hundred; 'tha = atha — or; sahasraśaḥ — thousand; nānāvidhāni — variously manifested; divyāni — supernatural; nānāvarṇākṛtīni = nānā — various + varṇa — color + ākṛtīni — shapes + ca — and*

**The Blessed Lord said: O son of Pṛthā, see My forms in the hundreds or rather in the thousands, variously manifested, supernatural and of the various colors and shapes. (11.5)**

***Siddha Swami's Commentary:***

The vision of a supernatural or divine form has two distinct parts to it. First, the form must be revealed. Second, the person to whom the revelation is given must have supernatural vision. We must realize that these supernatural forms are existing right now alongside this world. In that sense, they are already revealed, but we must develop the vision to perceive them.

*Śrī* Krishna opened a gap between this level of existence and the dimension in which the Universal Form was manifested, but Arjuna did not yet have the vision to see through the gap. Sometimes in higher yoga, a *yogin* perceives such a gap. Looking through it, he sees the supernatural personalities and their environment. In that case, the *yogin* developed *jñāna-dīpah* (10.11) vision to see into the supernatural worlds. However in the case of Arjuna, even though *Śrī* Krishna created a link or opening between this level and that supernatural plane, still Arjuna could not see through it.

The fact that *Śrī* Krishna had to reveal this on special request, indicates that those dimensions are naturally sealed off from us in this world. We have to develop or be awarded special vision to verify the existence of that level.

**पश्यादित्यान्वसून्रुद्रान्**
**अश्विनौ मरुतस्तथा ।**
**बहून्यदृष्टपूर्वाणि**
**पश्याश्चर्याणि भारत ॥ ११.६ ॥**
paśyādityānvasūnrudrān
aśvinau marutastathā
bahūnyadṛṣṭapūrvāṇi
paśyāścaryāṇi bhārata (11.6)

*paśyādityān = paśya — look at + ādityān — supernatural rulers; vasūn — Vasus; rudrān — supernatural destroyers; aśvinau — two supernatural doctors; marutaḥ — supernatural stormers; tathā — also; bahūny = bahūni — many; adṛṣṭapūrvāṇi = adṛṣṭa — unseen + pūrvāṇi — before; paśyāścaryāṇi = paśya — view + āścaryāṇi — wonders; bhārata — O relation of the Bharata family*

**Look at the supernatural rulers, the supernatural destroyers, the two supernatural doctors and the supernatural stormers. View many wonders which were unseen before, O relation of the Bharata family. (11.6)**

***Siddha Swami's Commentary:***

These wonders have to do with the material existence, especially in relation to control by higher personalities whose existences are manifested in other worlds or dimensions.

इहैकस्थं जगत्कृत्स्नं
पश्याद्य सचराचरम् ।
मम देहे गुडाकेश
यच्चान्यद्द्रष्टुमिच्छसि ॥ ११.७॥

ihaikasthaṁ jagatkṛtsnaṁ
paśyādya sacarācaram
mama dehe guḍākeśa
yaccānyaddraṣṭumicchasi (11.7)

*ihaikastham = iha — here + ekastham — situated in one reality; jagat — universe; kṛtsnam — entire; paśyādya = pasya — see + adya — now; sacarācaram — with active and inactive; mama — of Me; dehe — in the body; guḍākeśa — O conqueror of sleep; yac = yad — what; cānyad = cānyat = ca — and + anyat — other; draṣṭum — to see; icchasi — you desire*

**Here, O conqueror of sleep, you see the entire universe with all active and inactive manifestations, situated as one reality, in My body. And observe any other manifestations which you desire to see. (11.7)**

***Siddha Swami's Commentary:***

Just as the limited entity has a physical, subtle and causal body, so the Supreme Person, *Śrī* Krishna, has more than one body. This body being revealed is the Universal Form with specific reference to the affairs of this gross world. As a pregnant body and psyche has more than one entity in it, so this form of the Supreme Lord has many powerful entities within it, functioning in various roles, for controlling the material manifestation.

*Śrī* Krishna invited Arjuna to look carefully and to observe what was revealed and to also take the opportunity to observe any other manifestation which he desired to see specifically. In that way, all doubts about *Śrī* Krishna would be removed. Thus when Arjuna would lose this vision, the memory of it would be sufficient to cause Arjuna to trust *Śrī* Krishna completely.

न तु मां शक्यसे द्रष्टुम्
अनेनैव स्वचक्षुषा ।
दिव्यं ददामि ते चक्षुः
पश्य मे योगमैश्वरम् ॥ ११.८॥ ॥

na tu māṁ śakyase draṣṭum
anenaiva svacakṣuṣā
divyaṁ dadāmi te cakṣuḥ
paśya me yogamaiśvaram (11.8)

*na — not; tu — but; mām — Me; śakyase — you can; draṣṭum — to see; anenaiva = anena — by this + iva (eva) — indeed; svacakṣuṣā — with your vision; divyam — supernatural; dadāmi — I give; te — to you; cakṣuḥ — sight; paśya — look at; me — Me; yogam — mystic power; aiśvaram — majesty*

**But you cannot see with your vision. I give you supernatural sight to look at My mystic majesty. (11.8)**

***Siddha Swami's Commentary:***

*Śrī* Krishna revealed the Universal Form by creating a gap between this dimension and the supernatural one, but at first Arjuna could not take advantage of the vision, for he had no supernatural insight. This means that there may be a gap or a parting of the separation energies between this place and others, and still one would not be able to see into the other places, if one does not have the vision to penetrate and perceive supernaturally.

During daylight hours everything in this world is very plain to see, but still a person with defective eyes cannot perceive any of it. During higher yoga, gaps may open up between this world and others but the *yogin* cannot use these if he has not developed sufficient supernatural insight and if the opened gaps occur only momentarily.

With natural vision, *svacakṣuṣā*, Arjuna would only see what was revealed by sunlight or by firelight. Thus *Śrī* Krishna, as a matter of mercy and to convince Arjuna, gave supernatural vision, *divyam cakṣuh*. This means that Arjuna was so important as an agent for *Śrī* Krishna at *Kurukṣetra*, that Krishna gave the vision; it is not merely because Arjuna was a dear devotee of *Śrī* Krishna. Many other dear devotees have longed for this vision, and still to this day have not been graced to either develop it or have it bestowed on them.

संजय उवाच
एवमुक्त्वा ततो राजन्
महायोगेश्वरो हरिः ।
दर्शयामास पार्थाय
परमं रूपमैश्वरम् ॥११.९॥
saṁjaya uvāca
evamuktvā tato rājan
mahāyogeśvaro hariḥ
darśayāmāsa pārthāya
paramaṁ rūpamaiśvaram (11.9)

*saṁjaya — Sanjaya; uvāca — said; evam — thus; uktvā — having said; tato = tataḥ — then; rājan — O King; mahāyogeśvaro = mahāyogeśvaraḥ — the great master of yoga; hariḥ — Hari, the God Vishnu; darśayāmāsa — reveals; pārthāya — to the son of Pṛthā; paramam — supreme; rūpam — form; aiśvaram — supernatural glory*

**Sanjaya said: O King, having said that, the great Master of yoga, Hari, the God Vishnu, revealed to the son of Pṛthā, the Supreme Form, the supernatural glory. (11.9)**

***Siddha Swami's Commentary:***

Sanjaya, a student of *brahma yoga* as it was taught by *Śrīla Vyāsaji*, rightfully and respectfully addressed *Śrī* Krishna as the great Master of yoga, *mahāyogeśvarah*. Sanjaya was using supernatural vision to see these events as he described them to King *Dhṛtarāṣṭra*. Thus he was qualified to address *Śrī* Krishna fittingly without flattery. Sanjaya took the opportunity to alert *Dhṛtarāṣṭra* that *Śrī* Krishna was none other than the God Vishnu, *Harih*, and that the Supreme Form, the supernatural glory, *paramam rūpam aiśvaram*, was seen clearly by Arjuna.

अनेकवक्त्रनयनम्
अनेकाद्भुतदर्शनम् ।
अनेकदिव्याभरणं
दिव्यानेकोद्यतायुधम् ॥११.१०॥
anekavaktranayanam
anekādbhutadarśanam
anekadivyābharaṇaṁ
divyānekodyatāyudham (11.10)

*anekavaktranayanam = aneka — countless + vaktra — mouth + nayanam — eye; anekādbhutadarśanam = aneka — countless + adbhuta — wonders + darśanam — vision; anekadivyābharaṇaṁ = aneka — countless + divya — supernatural + ābharaṇam — ornament; divyānekodyatāyudham = divya — supernatural + aneka — countless + udyata — uplifted + āyudham — weapon*

**Countless mouths, eyes, wondrous visions, countless supernatural ornaments, supernatural uplifted weapons, (11.10)**

***Siddha Swami's Commentary:***

These are supernatural formations, not the gross material existences that we know. To see these one has to develop or be graced with supernatural vision to see into the particular dimension in which these forms are manifested.

दिव्यमाल्याम्बरधरं
दिव्यगन्धानुलेपनम् ।
सर्वाश्चर्यमयं देवम्
अनन्तं विश्वतोमुखम् ॥११.११॥
divyamālyāmbaradharaṁ
divyagandhānulepanam
sarvāścaryamayaṁ devam
anantaṁ viśvatomukham (11.11)

*divyamālyāmbaradharam = divya — supernatural + mālya — garland + ambara — garment + dharam — wearing; divyagandhānulepanam = divya — supernatural + gandha — perfume + anulepanam — ointment; sarvāścaryamayam = sarvaścarya – all wonder + mayam — made of; devam — God; anantam — infinite; viśvatomukham — facing all directions*

**...wearing supernatural garlands and garments, with supernatural perfumes and ointments, appearing all wonderful, the God appeared infinite as He faced all directions. (11.11)**

***Siddha Swami's Commentary:***

Even though the God appeared infinite, this universal form was infinite only in comparison to what it controlled in the material world. It was the face of the Absolute which pointed in the direction of this specific sector of the material energies. He and His assistant male beings wore supernatural garlands and garments, with supernatural perfumes and ointments, appearing all wonderfully on that supernatural plane. Everything, their bodies, their ornaments and whatever they used, was made of light. Nothing on that supernatural plane was heavy like earth or water. Everything was made of light rays.

दिवि सूर्यसहस्रस्य
भवेद्युगपदुत्थिता ।
यदि भाः सदृशी सा स्याद्
भासस्तस्य महात्मनः ॥११.१२॥
divi sūryasahasrasya
bhavedyugapadutthitā
yadi bhāḥ sadṛśī sā syād
bhāsastasya mahātmanaḥ(11.12)

*divi — in the sky; sūryasahasrasya = sūrya — sun + sahasrasya — of one thousand; bhaved = bhavet — should be; yugapad — at once; utthitā — risen; yadi — if; bhāḥ — brilliance; sadṛśi — such; sā — it; syād — it might be; bhāsaḥ — of brightness; tasya — of it; mahātmanaḥ — of the great personality*

**Imagine in the sky, a thousand suns, being at once risen together. If such a brilliance were to be, it might be compared to that Great Personality. (11.12)**

***Siddha Swami's Commentary:***

To give us some idea of the power and glory of that Supreme Person's Universal Form, Sanjaya made comparison to a thousand suns *(sūryasahasrasya)*. If we could imagine seeing such brilliance *(bhāh)*, then we would have some idea of the wonder and glory of those personalities who comprise the Universal Form of *Śrī* Krishna. But the power was being shown on the supernatural level. And we must ponder as to how it is administered and felt on this physical plane.

तत्रैकस्थं जगत्कृत्स्नं
प्रविभक्तमनेकधा ।
अपश्यद्देवदेवस्य
शरीरे पाण्डवस्तदा ॥११.१३॥

*tatraikastham = tatra there + ekastham — one position; jagat — universe; kṛtsnam — entire; pravibhaktam — divided; anekadhā — in many ways; apaśyad = apaśyat — he saw;*

tatraikasthaṁ jagatkṛtsnaṁ
pravibhaktamanekadhā
apaśyaddevadevasya
śarīre pāṇḍavastadā (11.13)

*devadevasya — of the God of gods; śarīre — in the body; pāṇḍavas — Arjuna Pandava; tadā — then*

**There the entire universe existed as one reality divided in many ways. Arjuna Pandava then saw the God of gods in that body. (11.13)**

***Siddha Swami's Commentary:***

Existentially that location of the Universal Form was the centralized place from which these manifestations originated. From there, these manifestations spiral outward, and to that place, these worlds are linked. Arjuna was focused on the Supreme Person of that Universal Form, the God of gods, *devadeva*. Since Arjuna saw that supernatural form and appears to have lost contact with physical vision, we may assume that his attention is a spiritual force which may be applied either to supernatural or physical perception. In this case, by the yogic power of *Śrī* Krishna, Arjuna's attention was focused through supernatural sight and it disconnected with his physical visionary apparatus.

ततः स विस्मयाविष्टो
हृष्टरोमा धनंजयः ।
प्रणम्य शिरसा देवं
कृताञ्जलिरभाषत ॥११.१४॥
tataḥ sa vismayāviṣṭo
hṛṣṭaromā dhanaṁjayaḥ
praṇamya śirasā devaṁ
kṛtāñjalirabhāṣata (11.14)

*tataḥ — then; sa = saḥ — he; vismayāviṣṭo = vismayāviṣṭaḥ — one who is amazed; hṛṣṭaromā — one whose hair is bristled; dhanamjayaḥ — Arjuna, conqueror of rich countries; praṇamya — bowing; śirasā — with the head; devam — God; kṛtāñjalir = kṛtāñjaliḥ — making reverence with palms pressed for prayers; abhāsata — he spoke*

**Then he, who was amazed, whose hair bristled, Arjuna, the conqueror of rich countries, bowing his head to the God, with palms pressed for prayers, spoke. (11.14)**

***Siddha Swami's Commentary:***

To offer respect to *Śrī* Krishna, after hearing His glories, either directly from Him as Arjuna did, or through some other person like *Nārada*, *Asita Devala* or *Vyāsa*, is not equivalent to seeing glories with supernatural vision and then offering all due respects. The solemnity of Arjuna is many, many degrees higher than the respects offered to *Śrī* Krishna before seeing the Universal Form directly. Nothing compares to personal experience by direct perception of reality.

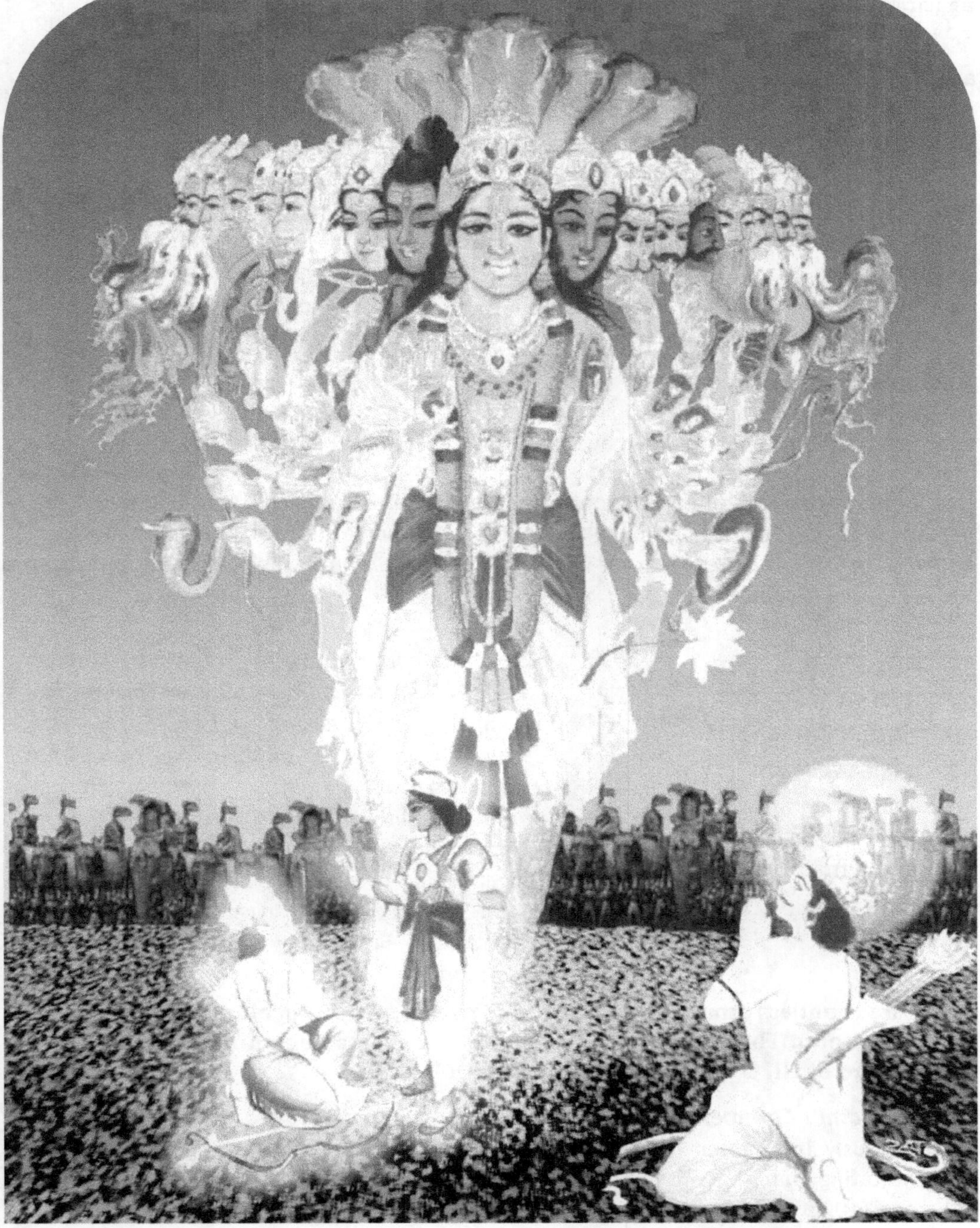

*Terri Stokes-Pineda Art*

अर्जुन उवाच
पश्यामि देवांस्तव देव देहे
सर्वांस्तथा भूतविशेषसंघान् ।
ब्रह्माणमीशं कमलासनस्थम्
ऋषींश्च सर्वानुरगांश्च दिव्यान् ॥ ११.१५॥
arjuna uvāca
paśyāmi devāṁstava deva dehe
sarvāṁstathā bhūtaviśeṣasaṁghān
brahmāṇamīśaṁ kamalāsanastham
ṛṣīṁśca sarvānuragāṁśca divyān
(11.15)

*arjuna — Arjuna; uvāca — said; paśyāmi — I see; devāṁs — spiritual rulers; tava — your; deva — O God; dehe — in the body; sarvāṁs — all; tathā — as well as; bhūtaviśeṣasaṁghān = bhūta — being + viśeṣa — variety + saṁghān — assembled; brahmāṇam — Lord Brahmā; īśam — Lord; kamalāsanasthaṁ = kamala — lotus + āsana — seat + stham — situated; ṛṣīṁśca = ṛṣīn — yogi sages + ca — and; sarvān — all; uragāṁśca = uragān — serpents + ca — and; divyān — supernatural*

**Arjuna said: I see the supernatural rulers in Your body, O God, as well as all varieties of beings assembled there, Lord Brahmā, who is lotus-seated, all the yogi sages and the supernatural serpents. (11.15)**

***Siddha Swami's Commentary:***

All beings which became visible in the material world, even those which are extinct or which were not yet manifested, have supernatural forms. The physical form is emblematic of a supernatural configuration.

There was sexual differentiation in that Universal Form, since Arjuna saw the major personalities as male beings only and not as the powerful female deities like *Durgā*, *Chandikā* or even the great warrior woman, *Kālī*. Lord *Brahmā* was prominent and so were the yogi sages of repute.

अनेकबाहूदरवक्त्रनेत्रं
पश्यामि त्वां सर्वतोऽनन्तरूपम् ।
नान्तं न मध्यं न पुनस्तवादिं
पश्यामि विश्वेश्वर विश्वरूप ॥ ११.१६॥
anekabāhūdaravaktranetraṁ
paśyāmi tvām sarvato'nantarūpam
nāntaṁ na madhyaṁ na
punastavādiṁ
paśyāmi viśveśvara viśvarūpa
(11.16)

*anekabāhūdaravaktranetram = aneka — countless + bāhu — arm + udara — belly + vaktra — face + netram — eye; paśyāmi — I see; tvām — you; sarvato = sarvataḥ — all directions; 'nantarūpam = anantarūpam = ananta — infinite + rūpam — form; nāntam = na — not + antam — end; na — not; madhyam — middle; na — no; punas = punar — again even; tavādim = tava — of you + ādim — beginning; paśyāmi — I observe; viśveśvara — O Lord of all; viśvarūpa — form of everything*

**There are countless arms, bellies, faces, and eyes. I see You in all directions, O person of infinite form. There is no end, no middle, nor even a beginning of You. I observe You, O Lord of all, O Form of everything. (11.16)**

***Siddha Swami's Commentary:***

Previously in Chapter Ten, *Śrī* Krishna declared Himself as the origin of all created beings, stating that there is nothing active or stationary which could exist without His influence (10.39). Arjuna got proof of that statement. Wherever Arjuna looked into the supernatural plane, he could see only *Śrī* Krishna in all directions, infinite, without end, middle or beginning. Thus like *Nārada*, *Asita Devala* and *Vyāsa*, Arjuna declared *Śrī* Krishna to be the Form of everything, the Lord of all *(viśveśvara viśvarūpa).*

किरीटिनं गदिनं चक्रिणं च
तेजोराशिं सर्वतो दीप्तिमन्तम् ।
पश्यामि त्वां दुर्निरीक्ष्यं समन्ताद्
दीप्तानलार्कद्युतिमप्रमेयम् ॥११.१७॥
kirīṭinaṁ gadinaṁ cakriṇaṁ ca
tejorāśiṁ sarvato dīptimantam
paśyāmi tvāṁ durnirīkṣyaṁ samantād
dīptānalārkadyutim aprameyam
(11.17)

*kirīṭinam — crowned; gadinam — armed with a club; cakriṇam — bearing a discus; ca — and; tejo — splendor + rāśim — a mass; sarvato = sarvataḥ — on all sides; dīptimantam — shining wondrously; paśyāmi — I see; tvām — you; durnirīkṣyam — difficult to behold; samantāt — in entirety; dīptānalārkadyutim = dīpta — blazing + anala — fire + arka — sun + dyutim — effulgence; aprameyam — immeasurable*

**This Form is crowned, armed with a club, bearing a discus, a mass of splendor on all sides, shining wondrously with immeasurable radiance of the sun and blazing fire. I see You in entirety, You Who are difficult to behold. (11.17)**

***Siddha Swami's Commentary:***

As Arjuna testified, the Universal Form and specifically the Central Figure of it, was formally crowned. He was armed with a club and discus. He appeared to be a mass of splendor on all sides. He shone wondrously with immeasurable radiance of the sun and with blazing fire. He was difficult for a limited person like Arjuna to behold but Arjuna saw the apparition in entirety as he looked through the opening from this world to that one.

त्वमक्षरं परमं वेदितव्यं
त्वमस्य विश्वस्य परं निधानम् ।
त्वमव्ययः शाश्वतधर्मगोप्ता
सनातनस्त्वं पुरुषो मतो मे ॥११.१८॥
tvamakṣaraṁ paramaṁ veditavyaṁ
tvamasya viśvasya paraṁ nidhānam
tvamavyayaḥ śāśvatadharmagoptā
sanātanastvaṁ puruṣo mato me
(11.18)

*tvam — you; akṣaram — imperishable; paramam — supreme; veditavyam — to be revealed; tvam — you; asya — of it; viśvasya — of all; param — ultimate; nidhānam — shelter; tvam — you; avyayaḥ — imperishable; śāśvatadharmagoptā = śāśvata — eternal + dharma — law + goptā — guardian; sanātanaḥ — most ancient; tvam — you; puruṣo = puruṣaḥ — person; mato = mataḥ — thought; me — of me*

**You are the indestructible Supreme Reality to be realized. You are the ultimate shelter of all. You are the imperishable, eternal guardian of law. It seems to me that You are the most ancient person. (11.18)**

***Siddha Swami's Commentary:***

We emphatically agree with Arjuna that the Supreme Person is the indestructible Supreme Reality Who is to be realized. He should be everyone's aim and objective. As the ultimate objective, He should be thought of continuously by everyone. As the eternal guardian of law *(dharmagoptā),* He should be respected by everyone. Each human being should strive to gain His approval. He is everyone's superior as the most ancient person.

अनादिमध्यान्तमनन्तवीर्यम्
अनन्तबाहुं शशिसूर्यनेत्रम्
पश्यामि त्वां दीप्तहुताशवक्त्रं
स्वतेजसा विश्वमिदं तपन्तम् ॥११.१९॥

*anādimadhyāntam = an — without + ādi — beginning + madhya — middle + antam — end; anantavīryam = ananta — unlimited + vīryam — manly power; anantabāhuṁ = ananta — unlimited + bāhum — arm; śaśisūryanetram =*

anādimadhyāntam anantavīryam
anantabāhuṁ śaśisūryanetram
paśyāmi tvāṁ dīptahutāśavaktraṁ
svatejasā viśvamidaṁ tapantam
(11.19)

*śaśi — moon + sūrya — sun + netram — eye; paśyāmi — I see; tvām — you; dīptahutāśavaktraṁ = dīpta — blazing + hutāśa — oblation-eating + vaktram — mouth; svatejasā — with Your splendor; viśvam — universe; idam — this; tapantam — heating*

**You who are without beginning, middle, or ending, Who has infinite manly power, Who has unlimited arms, Who has the sun and moon as Your eyes, I see You, with the blazing oblation-eating mouth, heating this universe with Your Own splendor. (11.19)**

***Siddha Swami's Commentary:***

As he requested, Arjuna got evidence of *Śrī* Krishna's supernatural, wondrous manifestations by which Krishna pervades these worlds and is situated in them ( Bg. 10.16). He got evidence of how *Śrī* Krishna sustains these worlds even on the physical level, even how *Śrī* Krishna takes oblations through ceremonial rites which are approved by Him.

द्यावापृथिव्योरिदमन्तरं हि
व्याप्तं त्वयैकेन दिशश्च सर्वाः ।
दृष्ट्वाद्भुतं रूपम् उग्रं तवेदं
लोकत्रयं प्रव्यथितं महात्मन् ॥११.२०॥

dyāvāpṛthivyoridam antaraṁ hi
vyāptaṁ tvayaikena diśaścasarvāḥ
dṛṣṭvādbhutaṁ rūpam ugraṁ tavedaṁ
lokatrayaṁ pravyathitaṁ mahātman (11.20)

*dyāvāpṛthivyor = dyāvāpṛthivyoḥ — of heaven and earth; idam — this; antaram — space between; hi — indeed; vyāptam — pervaded; tvayaikena = tvaya — by you + ekena — alone; diśaḥ — directions; ca — and; sarvāḥ — all; dṛṣtvā — having seen; adbhutam — marvelous; rūpam — form; ugram — terrible; tavedam = tava — your + idam — this; lokatrayam = loka — world + trayam — three; pravyathitam — trembling; mahātman — O great personality*

**In all directions, the space between heaven and earth is pervaded by You alone. Seeing Your marvelous Form, of a terrible feature, the three worlds tremble, O great Personality. (11.20)**

***Siddha Swami's Commentary:***

This apparition of the Universal Form of *Śrī* Krishna occurred on a supernatural plane and not on this physical level. The Form was not projected into this physical world, except through the agency of *Śrī* Krishna's physical body, Arjuna's physical body and the physical body of any other person who served at any time as Its agent. The directions mentioned *(diśah)*, the space between heaven and earth, are all supernatural locations and not physical ones. It is not that this apparition of the Universal Form was seen by physical eyes. Sanjaya saw the Form through supernatural vision which he developed through yoga practice and by the grace of *Śrīla Vyāsaji*, his spiritual teacher.

That marvelous Form, of a terrible feature, and Its effects upon the three worlds as Arjuna perceived, occurred only on the supernatural plane. The distribution of those effects into other subtle and gross dimensions occurred through particular channels which caused the inhabitants of those locales not to track those disciplinary energies to *Śrī* Krishna. This is why Arjuna asked *Śrī* Krishna previously about His self disciplinary methods and mystic powers, in order to see exactly how that energy moves from the supernatural level to the subtle and gross dimensions. Arjuna inquired previously:

*vistareṇātmano yogaṁ vibhūtiṁ ca janārdana*
*bhūyaḥ kathaya tṛptirhi śṛṇvato nāsti me'mṛtam (10.18)*

***Explain in more detail about Your self-disciplinary methods and the resultant mystic power and of Your splendrous form, O motivator of the people. There is no final satisfaction for me in hearing Your sweet words. (10.18)***

Arjuna was burdened with a sense of responsibility for influencing the Kurus to avert that family quarrel which led to war. He hoped to show Krishna's supremacy, feeling that if they saw it, they would be convinced to live in a way which pleased *Śrī* Krishna. But Arjuna will be unable to show them this reality of the Universal Form, and how such a form, which existed in another dimension isolated from this one, would affect anything in this physical world.

Arjuna got the proof he wanted but was unable to show that to others. He did not have the mystic power to do such a thing. Even for him it was a great feat to trace out the connection between *Śrī* Krishna's Universal Form and what took place in this world.

अमी हि त्वा सुरसंघा विशन्ति
केचिद्भीताः प्राञ्जलयो गृणन्ति ।
स्वस्तीत्युक्त्वा महर्षिसिद्धसंघाः
स्तुवन्ति त्वां स्तुतिभिः पुष्कलाभिः ॥
११.२१॥

amī hi tvā surasaṁghā viśanti
kecidbhītāḥ prāñjalayo gṛṇanti
svastītyuktvā
maharṣisiddhasaṁghāḥ
stuvanti tvāṁ stutibhiḥ
puṣkalābhiḥ (11.21)

*amī — those; hi — truly; tvām — you; surasaṁghā = sura — supernatural ruler + saṁghā — groups; viśanti — they enter; kecid — some; bhītāḥ — terrified; prāñjalayo = prāñjalayaḥ — bowing with palms pressed together; gṛṇanti — they offer praise; svastīty = svastīti = sv (su) — suitable + asti — there be + iti — thus; uktvā — saying; maharṣisiddhasaṁghāḥ = mahārṣi — great yogi sages + siddha — perfected yogis + saṁghāḥ — groups; stuvanti — they praise; tvām — you; stutibhiḥ — with glorification; puṣkalābhiḥ — with lavish*

**Those groups of supernatural rulers enter You. Some being terrified, bowing with palms pressed together, offer praise. "May everything be suitable," they say. The groups of great yogi sages and perfected yogis praise You with lavish glorification. (11.21)**

***Siddha Swami's Commentary:***

*Dhṛtarāṣṭra* was the only one who heard of this from Sanjaya at the time of the discourse but *Dhṛtarāṣṭra* did not have the supernatural vision as did Arjuna and Sanjaya. *Dhṛtarāṣṭra* depended on hearing of this from a reliable witness who was Sanjaya. Such hearing, though impressive on the mind of the hearer, does not have the full convincing effect of direct perception; hence the need existsfor higher yoga practice to develop the required insight.

The *mahārṣi* great yogi sages and the siddha perfected or near-to-being-perfected yogins do not have duties for establishing, maintaining and enforcing dharmic righteous living in the material creation. As such they simply offer praise to the Universal Form with lavish glorification. However, the *surasaṅghā* groups of supernatural rulers who supervise moral behavior are accountable to the Central Figure in the Universal Form, *Śrī* Krishna, for completion of duties. Thus some of them were terrified for having lapsed in responsibility. All of them were bowing as Arjuna and Sanjaya reported, with palms pressed together, offering praise saying: *'May everything be suitable. Whatever is to happen should be such that it is approved by You.'*

रुद्रादित्या वसवो ये च साध्या
विश्वेऽश्विनौ मरुतश्चोष्मपाश्च ।
गन्धर्वयक्षासुरसिद्धसंघा
वीक्षन्ते त्वां विस्मिताश्चैव सर्वे ॥
११.२२॥

rudrādityā vasavo
ye ca sādhyā
viśve'śvinau
marutaścoṣmapāśca
gandharvayakṣā
surasiddhasaṁghā
vīkṣante tvām vismitāś
caiva sarve (11.22)

*rudrādityā = rudra — supernatural destroyers + ādityāḥ — supernatural rulers; vasavo = vasavaḥ — Vasus, assistants to supernatural rulers; ye — who; ca — and; sādhyā — Sādhya, guardian angels; viśve — Vishvadevas supernatural priests; 'śvinau = aśvinau — two primal supernatural doctors; marutaścoṣmapāś = marutaḥ — supernatural stormers + ca — and + uṣmapāḥ — spirits who take vapor bodies; ca — and; gandharvayakṣāsurasiddhasaṁghā = gandharva — celestial musicians + yakṣa — spirits guarding natural resources + asura — supernatural rebels + siddha — perfected souls + saṁghā — groups; vīkṣante — they behold; tvām — you; vismitāścaiva = vismitāḥ — amazed + ca — and + iva (eva) — indeed; sarve — all*

**The supernatural destroyers, the supernatural rulers, the assistants to those rulers, these and the Sādhya guardian angels, the Vishvadeva supernatural priests, the two primal supernatural doctors, the supernatural stormers, the spirits who take vapor bodies, the groups of celestial musicians, the spirits guarding natural resources, the supernatural rebels and the perfected souls, behold You. And they are all amazed. (11.22)**

### *Siddha Swami's Commentary:*

The very fact that these supernatural personalities were all amazed at the apparition of the Universal Form, indicated that the manifestation or phase of the Form which was revealed to Arjuna, is not normally seen even by the elevated beings in higher dimensions. Even some of the persons who comprise the Form do not usually see the whole configuration of it, but they became aware of the entire Form, when *Śrī* Krishna revealed that to Arjuna. It was remarkable that Arjuna and Sanjaya, along with many of the elevated beings in this and other dimensions, saw that Universal Form in fullness.

रूपं महत्ते बहुवक्त्रनेत्रं
महाबाहो बहुबाहूरुपादम् ।
बहूदरं बहुदंष्ट्राकरालं
दृष्ट्वा लोकाः प्रव्यथितास्तथाहम्॥ ११.२३॥
rūpaṁ mahatte bahuvaktranetraṁ
mahābāho bahubāhūrupādam
bahūdaraṁ bahudaṁṣṭrākarālaṁ
dṛṣṭvā lokāḥ pravyathitās tathāham
(11.23)

*rūpam — form; mahat — great; te — your; bahuvaktranetram = bahu — many + vaktra — mouth + netram — eye; mahābāho — O mighty-armed Person; bahubāhūrupādam = bahu — many + bāhu — arm + ūru — thigh + pādam — foot; bahūdaram = bahu – many + udaram — belly; bahudaṁṣṭrākarālam = bahu – many + daṁṣṭrā — teeth + karālam — terrible; dṛṣṭvā — having seen; lokāḥ — the world; pravyathitāḥ — trembling; tathā — as well as; 'ham = aham — I*

**O mighty-armed Person, having seen Your great Form with many mouths, and many arms, thighs, and feet, many bellies and many terrible teeth, the worlds tremble as well as I. (11.23)**

### *Siddha Swami's Commentary:*

The apparition of the Universal Form was nothing but disciplinary and terrifying in aspect to all limited beings like Arjuna and Sanjaya. Arjuna realized that the Form was a living threat to the three worlds and that it could bring on widespread disasters for ordinary living beings who were unaware of the Form's presence but who would nevertheless be affected if the Form acted in a hostile way.

Arjuna lost his interest in proving that *Śrī* Krishna was God to the Kurus, and now Arjuna will become concerned only with complying with the request of *Śrī* Krishna, for enforcing a righteous lifestyle among the officials of the Kuru clan.

नभःस्पृशं दीप्तमनेकवर्णं
व्यात्ताननं दीप्तविशालनेत्रम् ।
दृष्ट्वा हि त्वां प्रव्यथितान्तरात्मा
धृतिं न विन्दामि शमं च विष्णो ॥ ११.२४॥
nabhaḥspṛśaṁ dīptamanekavarṇaṁ
vyāttānanaṁ dīptaviśālanetram
dṛṣṭvā hi tvāṁ pravyathitāntarātmā
dhṛtiṁ na vindāmi śamaṁ ca viṣṇo
(11.24)

*nabhaḥspṛśaṁ = nabhaḥ — sky + spṛśaṁ — touching, extending; dīptam — glowing; aneka — many; varṇam — colors; vyātta — open; ānanam — mouths; dīpta — glowing; viśāla — very great; netram — eyes; dṛṣṭvā — seeing; hi — certainly; tvām — You; pravyathita — perturbed; antaḥ — within; ātmā — soul; dhṛtim — steadiness; na — not; vindāmi — I have; śamam — mental tranquillity; ca — also; viṣṇo — O Lord Viṣṇu*

**Having seen You, sky extending, blazing, multi-colored, with gaping mouths and blazing vast eyes, there is a shivering in my soul. I find no courage, nor stability, O God Vishnu. (11.24)**

***Siddha Swami's Commentary:***

As a finite and very limited being, even though devoted to *Śrī* Krishna and on friendly terms with the Lord, Arjuna felt isolated and his spirit shivered seeing the extensive influence, blazing powers, multicolored forms, gaping mouths and vast, light-flashing eyes of the Form. Arjuna found no courage to resist *Śrī* Krishna as he did in Chapter One of this discourse when he argued for allowing the Kurus to carry on their government in peace. He felt very insecure by the disapproving looks of the Form.

दंष्ट्राकरालानि च ते मुखानि
दृष्ट्वैव कालानलसंनिभानि ।
दिशो न जाने न लभे च शर्म
प्रसीद देवेश जगन्निवास ॥ ११.२५॥
daṁṣṭrākarālāni ca te mukhāni
dṛṣṭvaiva kālānalasaṁnibhāni
diśo na jāne na labhe ca śarma
prasīda deveśa jagannivāsa (11.25)

*daṁṣṭrā — teeth; karālāni — terrible; ca — also; te — Your; mukhāni — faces; dṛṣṭvā — seeing; eva — thus; kāla-anala — the fire of death; sannibhāni — as if; diśaḥ — the directions; na — not; jāne — I know; na — not; labhe — I obtain; ca — and; śarma — grace; prasīda — be pleased; deva-īśa — O Lord of all lords; jagat-nivāsa — O refuge of the worlds*

**And seeing Your Form with many mouths, having terrible teeth, glowing like the fire of universal destruction, I cannot determine the cardinal points. I do not find any peace of mind. Have mercy, O Lord of the gods, Abode of the universe. (11.25)**

***Siddha Swami's Commentary:***

Arjuna lost his footing or existential reference point in relationship to this earth. He could not find security anywhere else in that vast supernatural terrain which was perceived as reality by him. Thus he appealed to *Śrī* Krishna for mercy, crying out to the Lord of the gods, to the Abode of the universe.

अमी च त्वां धृतराष्ट्रस्य पुत्राः
सर्वे सहैवावनिपालसंघैः ।
भीष्मो द्रोणः सूतपुत्रस्तथासौ
सहास्मदीयैरपि योधमुख्यैः ॥११.२६॥
amī ca tvāṁ dhṛtarāṣṭrasya putrāḥ
sarve sahaivāvanipālasaṁghaiḥ
bhīṣmo droṇaḥ sūtaputrastathāsau
sahāsmadīyairapi odhamukhyaiḥ
(11.26)

*amī — those; ca — and; tvāṁ — you; dhṛtarāṣṭrasya — of Dhṛtarāṣṭra; putrāḥ — sons; sarve — all; sahaivāvanipālasaṁghaiḥ = saha — with + eva — indeed + avāvanipāla — rulers of the earth + saṁghaiḥ — with groups; bhīṣmo = bhīṣmaḥ — Bhishma; droṇaḥ — Droṇa; sūtaputraḥ — Karna, son of the charioteer; tathāsau = tathā — as well as + asau — that; saha — along with + asmadīyaiḥ — with ours; api — also; yodhamukhyaiḥ — with chief warriors*

**And those, all the sons of Dhṛtarāṣṭra, along with the groups of rulers, Bhishma, Droṇa, as well as that son of the charioteer, along with our men and also our chief warriors, are in contrast to You. (11.26)**

***Siddha Swami's Commentary:***

The limited beings in this world, are usually in contrast to the Supreme Being, because those limited souls are not aware of the will of the Personality of Godhead. They do not usually understand that their views are in conflict with the Supreme. Arjuna and Sanjaya saw firsthand how even those chief warriors on Arjuna's side were thinking in an isolated way. They had feelings about the battle of *Kurukṣetra* without any consideration of *Śrī* Krishna's views in the Universal Form.

The pressures of the supreme will which were vividly expressed on that supernatural plane were not so obvious on the material level and some persons felt that their duty was to resist it. They did not understand the repercussions which could follow in the wake of defiance. Arjuna also, before the discussion of the *Gītā*, felt that *Śrī* Krishna was just another person in the world, a person who could be contested. But seeing that vision of the Universal Form, Arjuna came to a different conclusion.

वक्त्राणि ते त्वरमाणा विशन्ति
दंष्ट्राकरालानि भयानकानि ।
केचिद्विलग्ना दशनान्तरेषु
संदृश्यन्ते चूर्णितैरुत्तमाङ्गैः ॥११.२७॥
vaktrāṇi te tvaramāṇā viśanti
daṁṣṭrākarālāni bhayānakāni
kecidvilagnā daśanāntareṣu
saṁdṛśyante cūrṇitair uttamāṅgaiḥ
(11.27)

*vaktrāṇi — mouths; te — your; tvaramāṇā — speedily; viśanti — they enter; daṁṣṭrākarālāni = daṁṣṭrā — teeth + karālāni — dreadful; bhayānakāni — fearful; kecid (kecit) — some: vilagnā — clinging: daśanāntareṣu = daśana — tooth + antareṣu — in between; saṁdṛśyante — they are seen'; cūrṇitaiḥ — with crushed; uttamāṅgaiḥ — with heads*

**They speedily enter Your fearful mouths, which have dreadful teeth. Some cling between the teeth. They are seen with crushed heads. (11.27)**

***Siddha Swami's Commentary:***

The arguments between *Śrī* Krishna and others was seen quite differently on the supernatural level, where Arjuna looked and perceived the opponents speedily entering *Śrī* Krishna's fearful mouths which had dreadful teeth. Some of them clinged between the teeth of that Universal form. Arjuna saw some with crushed heads. This happened to the subtle forms of the persons who opposed *Śrī* Krishna's views.

यथा नदीनां बहवोऽम्बुवेगाः
समुद्रमेवाभिमुखा द्रवन्ति ।
तथा तवामी नरलोकवीरा
विशन्ति वक्राण्यभिविज्वलन्ति ॥११.२८॥
yathā nadīnāṁ bahavo'mbuvegāḥ
samudramevābhimukhā dravanti
tathā tavāmī naralokavīrā
viśanti vaktrāṇyabhivijvalanti (11.28)

*yathā — as; nadīnāṁ — of the rivers; bahavo – bahavaḥ — many; 'mbuvegāḥ = ambuvegāḥ — water currents; samudram — sea; evābhimukhā = eva — indeed + abhimukhā — facing towards; dravanti — they flow; tathā—so; tavāmī = tava — of you + ami — those; naralokavīrā = nara — man + loka — world + vīrā — heroes; viśanti — they enter; vaktràni — mouths; abhivijvalanti — they are flaming*

**As the water currents of many rivers flow to the sea, so the earthly heroes enter Your mouths, which are flaming. (11.28)**

***Siddha Swami's Commentary:***

Due to the power of the Supreme Person, all others must be attracted to Him even if they do not like Him, even if they disagree with Him. Thus Arjuna saw even the opponents rushing into Krishna's supernatural mouths, being helplessly drawn into the body of that Form. On the physical level this was experienced as an attraction in opposition and defiance to *Śrī* Krishna. Duryodhana, the chief opponent of the Pandavas, as well as his uncle Shakuni, were being pulled by a strong force into *Śrī* Krishna's Universal Body. Even though they disliked *Śrī* Krishna because He did not submit to their views, still they always thought of Him and worried about His disapproval. That is how the supernatural level was ushered over into physical existence.

यथा प्रदीप्तं ज्वलनं पतंगा
विशन्ति नाशाय समृद्धवेगाः ।
तथैव नाशाय विशन्ति लोकास्
तवापि वक्राणि समृद्धवेगाः ॥११.२९॥
yathā pradīptaṁ jvalanaṁ pataṁgā
viśanti nāśāya samṛddhavegāḥ
tathaiva nāśāya viśanti lokās
tavāpi vaktrāṇi samṛddhavegāḥ (11.29)

*yathā — as; pradīptaṁ — blazing; jvalanaṁ — fire; pataṁgā — moths; viśanti — enter; nāśāya — to destruction; samṛddhavegāḥ — with great speed; tathaiva = tathā — so + iva (eva) — indeed; nāśāya — to ruination; viśanti —enter; lokāh — worlds; tavāpi = tava — you + api — also; vaktrāṇi — mouths; samṛddhavegāḥ — with great speed*

**As moths speedily enter a blazing fire to destruction, so to ruination, the worlds enter Your mouths with great speed. (11.29)**

***Siddha Swami's Commentary:***

Arjuna perceived even other existences, which are separate but parallel, and which flowed into *Śrī* Krishna's Universal Body. Many of these were doing that in defiance, in disagreement to *Śrī* Krishna as their time for particular manifestations had come to an end and He, the Central Person in that Form, pulled those existences into that Universal Body, which He tightly controlled.

लेलिह्यसे ग्रसमानः समन्ताल्
लोकान्समग्रान्वदनैर्ज्वलद्भिः ।
तेजोभिरापूर्य जगत्समग्रं
भासस्तवोग्राः प्रतपन्ति विष्णो ॥११.३०॥

*lelihyase — you lick; grasamānaḥ — swallow; samantāt — from all sides; lokān — the worlds; samagrān — all; vadanaiḥ — with mouths; jvaladbhiḥ — with flaming; tejobhiḥ — with splendor; āpūrya*

lelihyase grasamānaḥ samantāl
lokānsamagrānvadanair jvaladbhiḥ
tejobhirāpūrya jagatsamagraṁ
bhāsastavogrāḥ pratapanti viṣṇo (11.30)

*— filling; jagat — universe; samagraṁ — all; bhāsaḥ — rays; tavogrāḥ = tava — your + ugrāh — horrible; pratapanti — burns; viṣṇo — O Lord Vishnu*

**You lick, swallowing from all sides, all the worlds with Your flaming mouths, filling the universes with splendor, Your horrible blazing rays burn it, O Lord Vishnu. (11.30)**

***Siddha Swami's Commentary:***

Even though there is an impersonal and mere physical side to existence, there is also interwoven with it, the personal and subtle psychic existence. In the atmosphere, for instance, we may see clouds, rainfall, lightning, mists, sunlight and rainbows but that does not mean that any of these mere physical phenomena do not have personal counterparts to them. Unless we can see into the subtle world, we should not form conclusions that such physical aspects are not the gross result of psychic actions of personalities.

The licking, swallowing, flaming and horrible blazing was seen by Arjuna to be personally conducted by Persons in that Universal Form, but on the physical level, such actions may translate into something that appears to be natural disasters to human beings. People sometimes say that events like earthquakes, lightning strikes, hailstorms and other disasters are acts of God, even though no person has seen a physical body producing such dreadful features. But from what Arjuna observed, we can assume that actions on the supernatural level would translate into natural disasters and even holocausts and warfare on the earthly plane. It is definitely a clash of wills.

आख्याहि मे को भवानुग्ररूपो
नमोऽस्तु ते देववर प्रसीद ।
विज्ञातुमिच्छामि भवन्तमाद्यं
न हि प्रजानामि तव प्रवृत्तिम् ॥ ११.३१ ॥
ākhyāhi me ko bhavānugrarūpo
namo'stu te devavara prasīda
vijñātumicchāmi bhavantamādyaṁ
na hi prajānāmi tava pravṛttim (11.31)

*ākhyāhi — explain; me — to me; ko = kaḥ — who; bhavān — respected person; ugrarūpo — ugrarūpaḥ — of terrible form; namo = namaḥ — homage; 'stu — astu — may it be; te — to you; devavara — best of the gods; prasīda — have mercy; vijñātum — to understand; icchāmi — I want; bhavantam — Your lordship; ādyaṁ — primal person; na — not: hi — indeed; prajānāmi — I know; tava — your; pravṛttim — intention*

**Explain to me who You are, O respected Person of terrible form. I gave my homage to You, O best of gods. Have mercy! I want to understand You, O Primal Person. I do not know Your intentions. (11.31)**

***Siddha Swami's Commentary:***

While before, Arjuna related to *Śrī* Krishna as dear friend and cousin, as someone who was very fond of Him and of Whom he was endearing, after the vision of the Universal Form, Arjuna inquired afresh about the identity of *Śrī* Krishna. Arjuna spoke to Krishna as the Central Person in the Form. Arjuna lost touch with his cousin and friend *Śrī* Krishna, the human being to whom he expressed views in the first chapter of the discourse.

Arjuna lost interest in his own views about the *Kurukṣetra* conflict. Now he wanted to know of the intentions, the desires of that Supreme Person, because he felt obligated to assist that supreme will, rather than to bargain with it or to try to change and influence it as before. Arjuna gave homage to *Śrī* Krishna as the best of the gods: *namo'stu te devavara prasīda*.

श्रीभगवानुवाच
कालोऽस्मि लोकक्षयकृत्प्रवृद्धो
लोकान्समाहर्तुमिह प्रवृत्तः ।
ऋतेऽपि त्वा न भविष्यन्ति सर्वे
येऽवस्थिताः प्रत्यनीकेषु योधाः ॥ ११.३२ ॥
śrībhagavānuvāca
kālo'smi lokakṣayakṛt pravṛddho
lokānsamāhartumiha pravṛttaḥ
ṛte'pi tvāṁ na bhaviṣyanti sarve
ye'vasthitāḥ pratyanīkeṣu yodhāḥ
(11.32)

*śrī bhagavān — the Blessed Lord; uvāca — said; kālo = kālah — time-limit; 'smi = asmi — I am; lokaksayakṛt = loka — world + ksaya — destruction + kṛt — causing; pravṛddho = pravṛddhaḥ — mighty; lokān — worlds; samāhartum — to annihilate; iha — here; pravṛttaḥ — appeared; ṛte — without; 'pi = api — also; tvāṁ — you na — not, cease; bhaviṣyanti — they will live; sarve — all; ye — who; 'vasthitāḥ = avasthitāḥ — armored; pratyanikeṣu — on both armies; yodhāḥ — warriors*

**The Blessed Lord said: I am the time limit, the mighty world-destroying Cause, appearing here to annihilate the worlds. Even without you, all the armored warriors in both armies will cease to live. (11.32)**

***Siddha Swami's Commentary:***

It is a fact that on occasion one individual entity carries with him the life or death of many. Take for example, generals of armies, or militant presidents of countries. These fellows do on occasion exercise national power to kill off much of the population. Hence we can easily believe what *Śrī* Krishna had to say about His identity as the time-limit, the mighty world-destroying Cause.

A person does not have to act physically to cause destruction to others on the physical plane. Some great men, particularly great industrialists and bankers, have caused wars which reaped great destruction for many families. And still such wealthy individuals remained hidden from physical view, since others functioned on their behalf to do the actual killing of many common people.

*Śrī* Krishna's claim is that even without the assistance of Arjuna, all the armored warriors in both armies would face destruction, because that was the supreme will which would, in one way or the other, manifest itself physically. Arjuna was not an essential element, unless he was willing to cooperate as an agent of Krishna; otherwise, the supreme will would find other ways to do what it desired. This was in answer to Arjuna's question regarding *Śrī* Krishna's intention:

*ākhyāhi me ko bhavānugrarūpo namo'stu te devavara prasīda*
*vijñātumicchāmi bhavantamādyaṁ na hi prajānāmi tava pravṛttim (11.31)*

***Explain to me who You are, O respected Person of terrible form. I gave my homage to You, O best of gods. Have mercy! I want to understand You, O Primal Person. I do not know Your intentions. (11.31)***

तस्मात्त्वमुत्तिष्ठ यशो लभस्व
जित्वा शत्रून्भुङ्क्ष्व राज्यं समृद्धम् ।
मयैवैते निहताः पूर्वमेव
निमित्तमात्रं भव सव्यसाचिन् ॥ ११.३३ ॥

*tasmāt — therefore; tvam — you; uttiṣṭha — stand; yaśaḥ — glory; labhasva — get; jitvā — having conquered; śatrūn — enemies; bhuṅkṣva — enjoy; rājyaṁ — country; samṛddham — prosperous; mayaivaite =*

tasmāttvamuttiṣṭha yaśo labhasva
jitvā śatrūnbhuṅkṣva rājyaṁ samṛddham
mayaivaite nihatāḥ pūrvameva
nimittamātraṁ bhava savyasācin (11.33)

*mayā — by me + eva — indeed + ete — these; nihatāḥ — supernaturally-destroyed; pūrvam — already; eva — indeed; nimitta— agent; mātraṁ — only; bhava — be; savyasācin — O ambidextrous archer*

**Therefore you should stand up! Get the glory! Having conquered the enemies, enjoy a prosperous country. These fellows are supernaturally disposed by Me. Be only the agent, O ambidextrous archer. (11.33)**

***Siddha Swami's Commentary:***

*Śrī* Krishna encouraged Arjuna to participate on behalf of the Universal Form. Since on the supernatural level, Arjuna saw that the opponents to *Śrī* Krishna's views were wiped out already, there was no point in Arjuna's hesitation to assist the Universal Form. Arjuna was asked to be an agent only, not to take the responsibility. Krishna Himself would carry all liabilities.

द्रोणं च भीष्मं च जयद्रथं च
कर्णं तथान्यानपि योधवीरान् ।
मया हतांस्त्वं जहि मा व्यथिष्ठा
युध्यस्व जेतासि रणे सपत्नान् ॥ ११.३४॥
droṇaṁ ca bhīṣmaṁ ca jayadrathaṁ ca
karṇaṁ tathānyānapi yodhavīrān
mayā hatāṁstvaṁ jahi mā vyathiṣṭhā
yudhyasva jetāsi raṇe sapatnān (11.34)

*droṇaḥ — Droṇa; ca — and; bhīṣmaṁ — Bhishma; ca — and; jayadrathaṁ — Jayadratha; ca — and; karṇaṁ — Karṇa; tathānyān = tathā — as well as; anyān— others; api — also; yodhavīrān — battle heroes; mayā — by me; hatāṁ — supernaturally hurt; tvaṁ — you; jahi — physically kill; mā — not; vyathiṣṭhā — hesitate; yudhyasva — fight; jetāsi — you will conquer; raṇe — in battle; sapatnān — enemies*

**Droṇa, Bhishma, Jayadratha, and Karṇa, as well as other battle heroes, were supernaturally hurt by Me. You may physically kill them. Do not hesitate. Fight! You will conquer the enemies in battle. (11.34)**

***Siddha Swami's Commentary:***

The student learns in higher yoga of the various influences under which human beings function. No one is independent. It is a matter of selecting which influence one may be subordinate to. In fact, in most cases, the human beings, even if they realize the various influences and the resultant consequences, still impulsively act as puppets for a particular force under which they function.

Arjuna, for instance, was under the influence of the family expansion of the Kurus. Thus he used every argument he could muster, even quoting from the Vedic scriptures of his time, regarding what was right or wrong in social affairs. Those arguments were designed to justify the continued corruption of the Kurus on the basis of saying that it was better to tolerate what they did, than to stop them through the use of violence. Thus Arjuna was under that influence. *Śrī* Krishna wanted Arjuna to side-step those concerns and take up the cause of the Universal Form, which fought for righteous lifestyle at all costs.

संजय उवाच
एतच्छ्रुत्वा वचनं केशवस्य
कृताञ्जलिर्वेपमानः किरीटी ।
नमस्कृत्वा भूय एवाह कृष्णं
सगद्गदं भीतभीतः प्रणम्य ॥ ११.३५॥

*saṁjaya — Sanjaya; uvāca — said; etat — this; śrutvā — having heard; vacanaṁ — speech; keśavasya — of the handsome-haired Krishna; kṛtāñjalil— offering respects with joined palms; vepamānah — trembling; kirīṭī — Arjuna, the crowned one; namaskṛtvā = namaḥ —*

saṁjaya uvāca
etacchrutvā vacanaṁ keśavasya
kṛtāñjalirvepamānaḥ kirīṭī
namaskṛtvā bhūya evāha kṛṣṇaṁ
sagadgadaṁ bhītabhītaḥ praṇamya
(11.35)

*obeisances + krtvā — having made; bhūya — again; evāha = eva— indeed + aha — said; kṛṣṇaṁ — Kṛṣṇaṁ; sagadgadaṁ — stutteringly; bhītabhītaḥ — very frightened; praṇamya — prostrations*

**Sanjaya said: Having heard the speech of the handsome-haired Krishna, Arjuna, the crowned one, who was trembling, offered respect with joined palms. Bowing again, he stutteringly, with much fright and prostrations, spoke to Krishna. (11.35)**

***Siddha Swami's Commentary:***

Arjuna was not shifted back to the material plane. Hence he did not immediately respond to *Śrī* Krishna's request that he fight as an instrument of the Form. Arjuna remained in the supernatural vision and therefore he stutteringly, with much fright and prostrations, spoke to *Śrī* Krishna, the Central Person in the Form. This was told to King *Dhṛtarāṣṭra* to explain why Arjuna did not respond, saying that he would fight on *Śrī* Krishna's behalf.

अर्जुन उवाच
स्थाने हृषीकेश तव प्रकीर्त्या
जगत्प्रहृष्यत्यनुरज्यते च ।
रक्षांसि भीतानि दिशो द्रवन्ति
सर्वे नमस्यन्ति च सिद्धसंघाः ॥११.३६॥
arjuna uvāca
sthāne hṛṣīkeśa tava prakīrtyā
jagatprahṛṣyatyanurajyate ca
rakṣāṁsi bhītāni diśo dravanti
sarve namasyanti ca siddhasaṁghāḥ
(11.36)

*arjuna — Arjuna; uvāca — said; sthāne — in position; hṛṣīkeśa — masterful controller of the senses; tava — your; prakīrtyā — by fame; jagat — universe; prahṛṣyati — rejoices; anurajyate — is delighted; ca — and; rakṣāṁsi — demons; bhītāni — terrified; diśo = diśaḥ — directions; dravanti — they flee; sarve—all; namasyanti — they will reverentially bow; ca — and; siddhasaṁghāḥ — groups of perfected souls*

**Arjuna said: Everything is in position, O Hṛṣīkeśa, masterful controller of the senses. The universe rejoices and is delighted by Your fame. The demons being terrified, flee in all directions. All the groups of perfected souls will reverentially bow to You. (11.36)**

***Siddha Swami's Commentary:***

After a little while, Arjuna adjusted to the supernatural level and he was no longer afraid of the Universal Form. He lost touch with the physical plane and its social insecurities which cause a limited being to side with other limited spirits, even against all odds in being defiant towards the supreme will.

Arjuna anticipated that the groups of perfected souls would reverentially bow down to *Śrī* Krishna. That was enough moral support for Arjuna on the physical level, so that even the irreligiously-inclined persons would be worried about Krishna and would be terrified, fleeing in all directions. Arjuna was no longer concerned about them even if they were relatives on the physical plane.

The groups of perfected souls, *siddha saṅghāh*, were of interest to Arjuna, who was an accomplished *buddhi* yogi. Arjuna wanted to be rated among them and to be with them. Thus he segregated himself from others, who are not in the mood of praising *Śrī* Krishna and bowing reverentially to the God.

कस्माच्च ते न नमेरन्महात्मन्
गरीयसे ब्रह्मणोऽप्यादिकर्त्रे ।
अनन्त देवेश जगन्निवास
त्वमक्षरं सदसत्तत्परं यत् ॥ ११.३७॥
kasmācca te na nameran mahātman
garīyase brahmaṇo'pyādikartre
ananta deveśa jagannivāsa
tvamakṣaraṁ sadasattat paraṁ yat (11.37)

*kasmāt — why; ca — and; te — to you; na—not; nameran — they should bow; mahātmān — O great soul; garīyase — greater; brahmaṇaḥ — than Brahmā; 'pi = api — also; ādikartre = ādi — original + kartre — to the creator; ananta — infinite; deveśa — lord of the gods; jagan (jagat) — universe; nivāsa — resort; tvam — you; akṣaraṁ — imperishable basis of energies; sat — sum total permanent life; asat — sum total temporary existence; tatparaṁ — that which is beyond; yat = yad — whatever*

**And why should they not bow to You, O great soul, original creator, Who is also greater than Brahmā, Who is the infinite Lord of the gods, the resort of the world? You are the imperishable basis of energies, the sum total permanent life, the sum total temporary existence, and whatever is beyond all that. (11.37)**

***Siddha Swami's Commentary:***

Arjuna's demeanor changed after he viewed the Universal Form, especially after he became integrated into the supernatural body through which he could see the Form. All of Arjuna's doubts and misgivings about the authority of *Śrī* Krishna disappeared.

Arjuna will again be reinstated into his physical body but the memory of this experience remained with him for some time during the battle of *Kurukṣetra*. Thus he consistently, for the most part, agreed with *Śrī* Krishna from then on, and he did not again gravitate towards the social world of the Kuru family.

त्वमादिदेवः पुरुषः पुराणस्
त्वमस्य विश्वस्य परं निधानम् ।
वेत्तासि वेद्यं च परं च धाम
त्वया ततं विश्वमनन्तरूप ॥ ११.३८॥
tvamādidevaḥ puruṣaḥ purāṇas
tvamasya viśvasya paraṁ nidhānam
vettāsi vedyaṁ ca paraṁ ca dhāma
tvayā tataṁ viśvamanantarūpa (11.38)

*tvam — you; ādidevaḥ — first God; puruṣaḥ — spirit; purāṇaḥ— most ancient; tvam— you; asya — of it; viśvasya — of the universe; paraṁ — supreme; nidhānam — refuge; vettāsi = vettā — knower + asi — you are; vedyaṁ — that which is to be known; ca — and; paraṁ — ultimate; ca — and; dhāma— sanctuary; tvayā — by you; tataṁ — pervaded; viśvam — universe; anantarūpa — Person of Infinite Form*

**You are the First God, the most ancient spirit. You are the knower, You are the supreme refuge of all the worlds. You are that which is to be known. You are the ultimate sanctuary. By You, the universe is pervaded, O Person of Infinite Form. (11.38)**

***Siddha Swami's Commentary:***

Arjuna's testimony is now to be added to that of *Nārada*, *Asita Devala* and *Vyāsa*. This also was proclaimed separately by Sanjaya, who narrated this to *Dhṛtarāṣṭra*. The conclusion then is that one should hear of this, ponder on it sufficiently and then take whatever steps are necessary to perceive this on the supernatural plane. This may be done through *samādhi* practice. Arjuna did indeed experience this through the grace of *Śrī* Krishna in causing Arjuna's spiritual focus of soul to move from the physical to the supernatural level. But others may enter that level through *samādhi* practice in higher yoga.

वायुर्यमोऽग्निर्वरुणः शशाङ्कः
प्रजापतिस्त्वं प्रपितामहश्च ।
नमो नमस्तेऽस्तु सहस्रकृत्वः
पुनश्च भूयोऽपि नमो नमस्ते ॥ ११.३९ ॥
vāyuryamo'gnirvaruṇaḥ
śaśāṅkaḥ
prajāpatistvaṁ prapitāmahaśca
namo namaste'stu
sahasrakṛtvaḥ
punaśca bhūyo'pi namo
namaste (11.39)

*vāyuḥ — Vāyu wind regulator; yamo — yamaḥ — Yama, Death Supervisor; 'gniḥ = agniḥ= Agni, fire controller; varuṇaḥ — Varuṇa, Master of the waters; śaśāṅkaḥ — Śaśāṅka moon lord; prajāpatiḥ — procreator Brahmā; tvaṁ — you; prapitāmahaḥ— father of Brahmā; ca — and; namo = namaḥ — obeisances: namaḥ — obeisances repeated; te — to you; 'stu = astu — let it be; sahasrakṛtvaḥ — a thousand times made; punasca = punaḥ (punar) — again + ca — and; bhūyo = bhuyaḥ— again; 'pi = api — also; namo – namaḥ — obeisances repeated; te — to you*

**You are represented by Vāyu, the wind regulator; Yama, the death supervisor; Agni, the fire controller; Varuṇa, the master of the waters; Śāśaṅka, the moon Lord; Procreator Brahmā; and you are the father of Brahmā. Obeisances unto You a thousand times repeatedly. Again and again, honor to You! (11.39)**

***Siddha Swami's Commentary:***

*Śrī* Krishna declared that the supernatural rulers and the great yogi sages did not know His origin, because in all respects He is the source of those authorities (10.2). Arjuna saw this visually on the supernatural level. He particularly saw *Vāyu*, the wind regulator, *Yama*, the death supervisor, Agni the fire controller, *Varuṇa* the master of the waters, *Śāśaṅka*, the moon lord and Procreator *Brahmā,* as being representative of *Śrī* Krishna and not as authorities in their own right. He saw that the perfected siddhas and their disciples were bowing down to *Śrī* Krishna.

Taking hints from their behavior, Arjuna offered obeisances to *Śrī* Krishna repeatedly, as if to do so a thousand times, again and again in honor.

नमः पुरस्तादथ पृष्ठतस्ते
नमोऽस्तु ते सर्वत एव सर्व ।
अनन्तवीर्यामितविक्रमस्त्वं
सर्वं समाप्नोषि ततोऽसि सर्वः ॥ ११.४० ॥
namaḥ purastādatha pṛṣṭhataste
namo'stu te sarvata eva sarva
anantavīryāmitavikramastvaṁ
sarvaṁ samāpnoṣi tato'si sarvaḥ
(11.40)

*namaḥ — reverence; purastāt — from in front; atha — and then; pṛṣṭhataḥ — from behind; te — to you; namo = namaḥ — obeisances; 'stu = astu — let there be; te — to you; sarvata — on all sides; eva — also; sarva — sum total reality; anantavīryāmitavikramaḥ = ananta — infinite + vīrya — power + amita — immeasurable + vikramaḥ — might; tvaṁ — you; sarvaṁ — everything; samāpnoṣi — you penetrate; tato = tataḥ — thus, in that sense; 'si = asi — you are; sarvaḥ — everything*

**Reverence to You from the front, from behind. Let there be obeisances to You on all sides, O sum total Reality. You are infinite power, immeasurable might. You penetrate everything. In that sense, You are Everything. (11.40)**

***Siddha Swami's Commentary:***

Since *Śrī* Krishna is the ultimate power source, as Arjuna experienced, the Person underlying everything, He may be addressed as Everything. Arjuna saw visually that *Śrī* Krishna was the location from which everything had effectively emerged.

सखेति मत्वा प्रसभं यदुक्तं
हे कृष्ण हे यादव हे सखेति.।
अजानता महिमानं तवेदं
मया प्रमादात्प्रणयेन वापि ॥ ११.४१ ॥
sakheti matvā prasabhaṁ yaduktaṁ
he kṛṣṇa he yādava he sakheti
ajānatā mahimānaṁ tavedaṁ
mayā pramādāt praṇayena vāpi (11.41)

*sakheti = sakhā — friend + iti — such as; matvā— considering; prasabhaṁ — impulsively; yat — whatever; uktaṁ — was said; he —hey; kṛṣṇa — Kṛṣṇa; he — hey; yādava — family man of the Yadus; he— hey; sakheti = sakhā — buddy + iti — thus; ajānatā — through ignorance; mahimānaṁ — majestic supernatural glory; tavedaṁ = tava — your + idam — this; mayā — by me; pramādāt — from familiarity; pranayena — with affection; vāpi = va — or + api — even*

**Whatever was said impulsively, considering You as a friend, such as, "Hey, Krishna! Hey, family man of the Yadus! Hey, buddy!" was done by me through ignorance of Your majestic supernatural glory or even by affectionate familiarity. (11.41)**

***Siddha Swami's Commentary:***

The physical view and the supernatural one may be variant. In some cases a powerful human being has much supernatural authority. But in other situations, a powerful person may have little or no supernatural impact. *Śrī* Krishna criticized those persons who did not estimate his majestic supernatural glory and who considered Him to be merely His material body. He said:

*avyaktaṁ vyaktimāpannaṁ manyante māmabuddhayaḥ*
*paraṁ bhāvamajānanto mamāvyayamanuttamam (7.24)*

***Though I am beyond their sensual range, the unintelligent think of Me as being limited to their gross perception. They do not realize My higher existence which is imperishable and supermost. (7.24)***

यच्चावहासार्थमसत्कृतोऽसि
विहारशय्यासनभोजनेषु ।
एकोऽथ वाप्यच्युत तत्समक्षं
तत्क्षामये त्वामहमप्रमेयम् ॥ ११.४२ ॥
yaccāvahāsārthamasatkṛto'si
vihāraśayyāsanabhojaneṣu
eko'tha vāpyacyut tatsamakṣaṁ
tatkṣāmaye tvām aham aprameyam (11.42)

*yat — that; cāvahāsārtham = ca — and + avahāsa — joking + artham — intention; asatkṛto — asatkṛtaḥ — disrespectfully; 'si = asi — you are; vihāraśayyāsanabhojaneṣu = vihāra — play + śayyā — couch + āsana — sitting + bhojaneṣu — in dining; eko = ekaḥ — alone, privately; 'thavāpi = athavāpi = athava — nor + api — also; acyuta — O infallible Kṛṣṇa; tatsamakṣaṁ — before the public; tat — that; kṣāmaye — I ask forgiveness; tvām — of you; aham — I; aprameyam — one who is boundless*

**And with intent to joke, You were disrespectfully treated, while playing, while on a couch, while sitting, while dining privately or even in public, O infallible Krishna. For that I ask forgiveness of You Who are boundless. (11.42)**

***Siddha Swami's Commentary:***

In the *brahma yoga* practice, one stops taking social relationships for granted. One tries by mystic and supernatural means to determine the spiritual status of each living being one encounters in any of the worlds.

A *brahma yogi* does honor the traditional social norms of any society he ventures into but he keeps track of the spiritual glory of the various individual entities he encounters.

Before Arjuna saw the Universal Form, he did not have the supernatural vision. He could not assess the value of *Śrī* Krishna in reference to everyone else. Thus he rated *Śrī* Krishna only as a relative, buddy and friend. Even though he was told by others like *Nārada*, *Asita Devala* and *Vyāsa*, that *Śrī* Krishna was in fact the Supreme Person, still Arjuna, not having any conscious experience of that, regarded *Śrī* Krishna only in the social way.

In retrospect, Arjuna regretted his former behavior. He offered apology to *Śrī* Krishna.

The two visions occur on separate planes of consciousness, but a *brahma yogin* has to be aware of both levels in order to apply himself appropriately in any given circumstance. *Nārada* had the vision. *Śrīla Vyāsa* had the vision. They knew how to honor a person in the social way and also apply spiritual ratings fittingly. In *brahma yoga* practice, one is taught how to do this.

पितासि लोकस्य चराचरस्य
त्वमस्य पूज्यश्च गुरुर्गरीयान् ।
न त्वत्समोऽस्त्यभ्यधिकः कुतोऽन्यो
लोकत्रयेऽप्यप्रतिमप्रभाव ॥११.४३॥
pitāsi lokasya carācarasya
tvamasya pūjyaśca gururgarīyān
na tvatsamo
'styabhyadhikaḥ kuto'nyo
lokatraye'pyapratim aprabhāva
(11.43)

*pitāsi = pitā — father + asi — you are; lokasya — of the world; carācarasya — of the moving and non-moving; tvam — you; asya — of this; pūjyaśca = pūjyaḥ — worshipable + ca — and; guruḥ — spiritual master; garīyān — gravest; na — not; tvatsamo = tvatsamaḥ = tyat (tvam) —you + samaḥ — similar, like; 'sti = asti — there is; abhyadhikaḥ— greater; kuto = kutaḥ — how; 'nyo = anyaḥ — other; lokatraye — in the three partitions of the universe; 'pi = api — also; apratimaprabhāva — person of incomparable splendor*

**You are the father of the world, of the moving and non-moving objects. You are the worshipable and gravest spiritual master. There is none like You in the three partitions of the universe. How could anyone be greater, O person of incomparable splendor? (11.43)**

***Siddha Swami's Commentary:***

After hearing from authorities like *Nārada*, Arjuna got his own experience of the divinity of *Śrī* Krishna. He testified by what he saw, stating that *Śrī* Krishna was the father of the world, of the animate and inanimate creations. *Śrī* Krishna is indeed the worshipable and gravest spiritual master. *Śrī* Krishna is unique. There is none like Him in the three partitions of the universe. His splendor in terms of power and influence is incomparable. He is the Supreme Being.

तस्मात्प्रणम्य प्रणिधाय कायं
प्रसादये त्वामहमीशमीड्यम् ।
पितेव पुत्रस्य सखेव सख्युः
प्रियः प्रियायार्हसि देव सोढुम् ॥११.४४॥
tasmātpraṇamya praṇidhāya kāyaṁ
prasādaye tvāmahamīśamīḍyam
piteva putrasya sakheva sakhyuḥ
priyaḥ priyāyārhasi deva soḍhum
(11.44)

*tasmāt — therefore; praṇamya — bowing with reverence; praṇidhāya — lying down; kāyaṁ— body; prasadaye — I ask mercy; tvām — you; aham — of you; īśam — Lord; īḍyam — to be praised; piteva = pitā — father + eva — as; putrasya — of a son; sakheva = sakhā — friend + eva — as; sakhyuḥ— of a chum; priyaḥ — beloved; priyāyārhasi = priyāya — to a lover + arhasi — you should; deva — O God; soḍhum — to be merciful*

**Therefore, bowing with reverence, lying my body down, I ask for mercy of You, O Lord Who is to be praised. As a father to a son, as a friend to his chum, as a beloved to a lover, You should be merciful, O God. (11.44)**

***Siddha Swami's Commentary:***

Arjuna asked for pardon because formerly he berated *Śrī* Krishna by acting with undue familiarity in almost every circumstance. He spoke to *Śrī* Krishna previously, as if *Śrī* Krishna was just another limited person like himself, and he tried to deny *Śrī* Krishna's rights to override the decision of others in the Kuru family. Arjuna considered this and asked for pardon.

अदृष्टपूर्वं हृषितोऽस्मि दृष्ट्वा
भयेन च प्रव्यथितं मनो मे ।
तदेव मे दर्शय देव रूपं
प्रसीद देवेश जगन्निवास ॥ ११.४५ ॥
adṛṣṭapūrvaṁ hṛṣito'smi dṛṣṭvā
bhayena ca pravyathitaṁ mano me
tadeva me darśaya deva rūpaṁ
prasīda deveśa jagannivāsa (11.45)

*adṛṣṭapūrvaṁ = adṛṣṭa — never seen + pūrvaṁ — previously; hṛṣito = hṛṣitaḥ — delighted; 'smi = asmi — I am; dṛṣṭvā— having seen; bhayena — with fear; ca — and, but; pravyathitaṁ — trembling; mano = manaḥ — mind; me — my; tat — that; eva — indeed: me — to me; darśaya — to see; deva — O God; rūpaṁ — God-form; prasīda — have mercy; deveśa — Lord of gods; jagannivāsa — shelter of the world*

**Seeing what was never seen before, I am delighted but my mind trembles with fear. Now, O God, cause me to see the God-form. Have mercy, O Lord of the gods, shelter of the world. (11.45)**

***Siddha Swami's Commentary:***

Arjuna had a secret desire to see the God-form. Thus we may wonder why Arjuna did not ask *Śrī* Krishna to reveal this before. The answer is that Arjuna was unsure that *Śrī* Krishna was in fact the Supreme Person. Arjuna did not know for sure that Krishna could reveal these facets of supernatural and spiritual reality.

Arjuna asked to see how *Śrī* Krishna controlled the material circumstances in the most minute details, especially in reference to the affairs of the Kurus. Thus *Śrī* Krishna showed the Universal Form in a way that was never seen before, with special application to the world at the time of Kuru conflict. But besides this, Arjuna had another deeper desire, which was to see the God-form. Arjuna took the opportunity to ask *Śrī* Krishna for the revelation of that Divine Form.

Arjuna knew for certain that he could not view that divinity without a revelation of *Śrī* Krishna. Thus he asked the Lord to please cause that vision to be.

When discussed in terms of *brahma yoga*, the student yogi is advised to take every effort in *samādhi* practice to see the God-form, but still despite all his endeavors, he might not see. He may, however, ask for special mercy from the Lord, so that the Form is revealed to Him. *Brahma yoga* is mostly a study and application of how to position oneself existentially for easy viewing of the divine forms. Since a limited being cannot see the divine forms just like that, naturally, then it is only left for him or her to position themselves in such a way as to encourage the Supreme Being to reveal divinity.

किरीटिनं गदिनं चक्रहस्तम्
इच्छामि त्वां द्रष्टुमहं तथैव ।
तेनैव रूपेण चतुर्भुजेन
सहस्रबाहो भव विश्वमूर्ते ॥ ११.४६ ॥

*kirīṭinaṁ — form which wears a crown; gadinaṁ — form which is armed with a disc; cakrahastaṁ — for with a club in hand; icchāmi — I wish; tvāṁ — you; draṣṭum — to see; aham — I;*

kirīṭinaṁ gadinaṁ cakrahastam
icchāmi tvāṁ draṣṭumahaṁ tathaiva
tenaiva rūpeṇa caturbhujena
sahasrabāho bhava viśvamūrte
(11.46)

*tathaiva = tathii — as requested + eva—indeed; tenaiva = tena — with this + eva — indeed; rūpeṇa — with the form; caturbhujena — with four arms; sahasrabāho — O thousand-armed person; bhava — become; viśvamūrte — person of universal dimensions*

**I wish to see You wearing a crown, armed with a club, and with a disc in hand, as requested. Please become that four-armed form, O thousand-armed Person, O Person of universal dimensions. (11.46)**

***Siddha Swami's Commentary:***

Even though Arjuna requested the vision of the Universal Form, the thousand-armed Person, the One of universal dimensions, *Viśvamūrte*, still that was not the form that Arjuna wanted to view dearly. We must keep in mind that Arjuna was a practicing *yogin* who wanted to see the divine forms or forms of God. He had seen the divine forms of Lord Shiva and Goddess *Durgā*. But the form which he really wanted to see was the four-armed form of God, wearing a crown and being armed with a club and disc. This four-armed form is the ultimate form of divinity which faces this world in a slightly disciplinary mood for promoting righteous lifestyle. Arjuna was much interested in seeing that form. Thus he took the opportunity to request the vision.

श्रीभगवानुवाच
मया प्रसन्नेन तवार्जुनेदं
रूपं परं दर्शितमात्मयोगात् ।
तेजोमयं विश्वमनन्तमाद्यं
यन्मे त्वदन्येन न दृष्टपूर्वम् ॥११.४७॥
śrībhagavānuvāca
mayā prasannena tavārjunedaṁ
rūpaṁ paraṁ darśitam ātmayogāt
tejomayaṁ viśvamanantam ādyaṁ
yanme tvadanyena na dṛṣṭapūrvam
(11.47)

*śrī bhagavān — the Blessed Lord; uvāca — said; mayā — by me; prasannena — by grace; tavārjunedaṁ = tava — to you + arjuna — Arjuna + idam — this; rūpaṁ — form; param — supreme; darśitaṁ — manifested; ātmayogāt — from my yoga power; tejomayaṁ — made of supernatural energy; viśvam — universal; anantam — infinite; ādyaṁ — primal; yat — which; me — my; tvadanyena = tvad — besides you + anyena — by any other; na — not; dṛṣṭapūrvam = dṛṣṭa — seen + pūrvam — before*

**The Blessed Lord said: By My grace to you Arjuna, this Supreme Form was manifested from My yoga power. This Form of Mine which is made of supernatural energy, being universal, infinite and primal, was never seen by another other person besides you. (11.47)**

***Siddha Swami's Commentary:***

*Ātmayogat* refers to *Śrī* Krishna's mystic power which is manifested even in His physical body. By that, *Śrī* Krishna revealed the Universal Form to Arjuna, in a way which was never shown to anyone before. The Universal Form was not made of gross matter like a material body. Its substance was light or *tejah*.

But Arjuna no longer wanted to view that form. He wanted *Śrī* Krishna to shift the revelation to another more sublime level, where the four-handed divinity could be seen. This would mean that Arjuna would be bestowed by *Śrī* Krishna with a higher body capable of perceiving the four-handed divine form.

Arjuna must have had information about that four-armed form, otherwise he would not have asked about it. This means that he heard of the form from persons like *Nārada, Asita, Devala* and *Vyāsa*, but they did not speak of the Universal Form in the way that *Śrī* Krishna revealed the Thousand-armed Form of Universal Dimensions. Arjuna had a burning desire to perceive that four-handed form. He took the opportunity to request the vision of it.

न वेदयज्ञाध्ययनैर्न दानैर्
न च क्रियाभिर्न तपोभिरुग्रैः ।
एवंरूपः शक्य अहं नृलोके
द्रष्टुं त्वदन्येन कुरुप्रवीर ॥ ११.४८॥
na vedayajñādhyayanairna dānair
na ca kriyābhirna tapobhirugraiḥ
evaṁrūpaḥ śakya ahaṁ nṛloke
draṣṭuṁ tvadanyena kurupravīra
(11.48)

*na — not; vedayajñādhyayanaiḥ = veda — Veda + yajñā — by sacrificial ceremonies + adyayanaiḥ — by education; na — nor; danaiḥ — by charity as recommended in the Vedic literature; na — not; ca — and; kriyābhiḥ — by special ritual acts; na — not; tapobhiḥ — by austerities; ugraiḥ — by strenuous; evam — as such; rūpaḥ — form; śakya = śakye — can; ahaṁ — I; nṛloke — in the world of human beings; drastuṁ — to see; tvadanyena = tvad — except you + anyena — by another; kurupravīra — great hero of the Kurus*

**Not by Vedic sacrificial ceremonies, nor by Vedic education, not by offering charity as recommended in the Vedic literatures and not by special ritual acts, nor by strenuous austerities, can I be seen in such a form in this world of human beings except through the method used by you, O great hero of the Kurus. (11.48)**

***Siddha Swami's Commentary:***

Arjuna was done with the *Viśvamūrti* Universal Form. He no longer wanted to view that. He was convinced that *Śrī* Krishna was in fact, the Supreme Person, Who is to be obeyed. Thus Arjuna made up his mind to comply with *Śrī* Krishna's instructions; he felt it unnecessary to see that ghastly Form any longer. And still *Śrī* Krishna spoke to clarify it fully.

मा ते व्यथा मा च विमूढभावो
दृष्ट्वा रूपं घोरमीदृङ्ममेदम् ।
व्यपेतभीः प्रीतमनाः पुनस्त्वं
तदेव मे रूपमिदं प्रपश्य ॥ ११.४९॥
mā te vyathā mā ca vimūḍhabhāvo
dṛṣṭvā rūpaṁ ghoramīdṛṅmamedam
vyapetabhīḥ prītamanāḥ punastvaṁ
tadeva me rūpamidaṁ prapaśya
(11.49)

*mā — not; te — of you; vyathā — should tremble; mā — not; ca — and; vimūḍhabhāvo = vimūḍhabhāvaḥ — confused state; dṛṣṭvā — having seen; rūpam — form; ghoram — ghastly; īdṛn = īdṛḥ — such; mamedam = mama — of my + idam — this; vyapetabhīḥ = vyapeta — freed from + bhīḥ — fear; prītamanāḥ — cheerful in mind; punaḥ — again; tvam — you; tat — you; eva — indeed; me — of me; rūpam — form; idam — this; prapaśya — look at*

**You should not tremble or be confused after seeing this, My ghastly form. Be free from fear and be cheerful of mind. Again look at this form of Mine. (11.49)**

***Siddha Swami's Commentary:***

*Śrī* Krishna first down-shifted, causing Arjuna to lose perception in a supernatural body and to go down to the earthly plane to see only the special physical form of *Śrī* Krishna. Arjuna looked at the same location but instead of seeing the Universal Form, he now only saw the special physical body of *Śrī* Krishna. *Śrī* Krishna did not just switch Arjuna over to a spiritual body to see the Divine Four-handed Form. Arjuna was first reinstated to his physical identity in a physical form, as a normal social being of this world.

संजय उवाच
इत्यर्जुनं वासुदेवस्तथोक्त्वा
स्वकं रूपं दर्शयामास भूयः ।
आश्वासयामास च भीतमेनं
भूत्वा पुनः सौम्यवपुर्महात्मा ॥ ११.५० ॥
saṁjaya uvāca
ityarjunaṁ vāsudevas tathoktvā
svakaṁ rūpaṁ darśayāmāsa bhūyaḥ
āśvāsayāmāsa ca bhītamenaṁ
bhūtvā punaḥ saumyavapur
mahātmā (11.50)

*Saṁjaya — Sanjaya; uvāca — said; iti — thus; arjunam — Arjuna; vāsudevaḥ — Kṛṣṇa, the son of Vasudeva; tathoktvā = tathā — thus + uktvā — having said; svakaṁ — his own; rūpaṁ — divine form; darśayāmāsa — he revealed; bhūyaḥ — again; āsvāsayāmāsa — he caused to be calm; ca — and; bhītam — frightened person; enam — this; bhūtvā — having assumed; punaḥ — punar — again; saumyavapuḥ = saumya — pleasing + vapuḥ — attractive appearance; mahātmā — great person*

**Sanjaya said: Krishna, the son of Vasudeva, having said this to Arjuna, revealed His own Divine Form. And once again that great person assumed the pleasing, attractive form and caused the frightened Arjuna to be calm. (11.50)**

***Siddha Swami's Commentary:***

It should be noted that *Śrī* Krishna wanted Arjuna to give up confusion and fear about the Universal Form. Arjuna was afraid of the Form because he was still in touch with his cultural identity as a junior member of the Kuru family. *Śrī* Krishna wanted Arjuna to separate from that Kuru clan idea once and for all. In viewing the Universal Form, if one is fearful, it means that one still remains attached to social relationships which run contrary to the divine will for this world. A *brahma yogin* may therefore take steps to eradicate his susceptibility to such influences which cause him to support ideas not approved by *Śrī* Krishna, the Supreme Lord.

*Śrī* Krishna revealed the four-handed divine form which Arjuna made a special request to see, but Krishna still wanted Arjuna to comply with the Universal Form which regulated the details of the outcome of the battle of *Kurukṣetra*. Arjuna was one of the main agents. Even though *Śrī* Krishna was not a combatant in the war, He expressed His influence and desire through persons like Arjuna. Thus it was important for Arjuna not to be fearful of or confused about the Form.

Student *brahma yogins* should note that even though Arjuna wanted to see and be with the four-handed divine form of *Śrī* Krishna, still he was not allowed to stay with that form, or to have that vision for very long. In fact, on a careful reading of this chapter, most of the vision which Arjuna had, was of the Thousand-armed Person of Universal Dimensions Who pertained to the politics of this world. Thus one should not expect to see what one wants to see or desires dearly, but rather what *Śrī* Krishna determines is in the interest of one's mission in the current life. When meditating to see the supernatural and divine forms, one must have a flexible and submissive mentality in regards to what might be revealed.

Arjuna had to be content finally with the same special material form manifested by *Śrī* Krishna but there was a difference, in that Arjuna was aware that the person who was his cousin, buddy and friend, was the Supreme Lord in fact.

अर्जुन उवाच
दृष्ट्वेदं मानुषं रूपं
तव सौम्यं जनार्दन ।
इदानीमस्मि संवृत्तः
सचेताः प्रकृतिं गतः ॥ ११.५१ ॥
arjuna uvāca
dṛṣṭvedaṁ mānuṣaṁ rūpaṁ
tava saumyaṁ janārdana
idānīmasmi saṁvṛttaḥ
sacetāḥ prakṛtiṁ gataḥ (11.51)

*arjuna — Arjuna; uvāca — said; dṛṣṭvedaṁ = dṛṣṭvā — having seen + idam — this; mānuṣaṁ — human: rūpaṁ — form; tava — of you; saumyam — gentle; janārdana — O motivator of human beings; idānīm — now; asmi — I am; saṁvṛttaḥ — satisfied; sacetāḥ — with mind; prakṛtiṁ — to human nature, to normal condition; gataḥ — gone back, returned*

**Arjuna said: Seeing this gentle, human-like Form of Yours, O Janardana, motivator of human beings, I am satisfied with my mind returned to the normal condition. (11.51)**

***Siddha Swami's Commentary:***

It appears that Arjuna could not bear for long either the development of his psyche into the supernatural plane of the Universal Form or that of the four-handed divine form which he so much wanted to perceive. Thus he was relieved when his normal vision resumed.

Of particular interest to the student *brahma yogi*s, this means that unless they successfully relieve themselves of the mundane psychology they will be unable to maintain a supernatural or spiritual body, even if such a form were developed for them, either through efforts in yoga practice or by the divine grace of the Supreme Being or any of His parallel divinities. One must strive conscientiously and sincerely to relieve oneself of the subtle body, since its recurring tendency is to develop a gross form and be focused into the gross plane of existence.

The fact that a person as dear to *Śrī* Krishna as Arjuna, could not shed the need for physical vision and physical reality, is a sure sign of the power of the subtle body in its dead-set determination to develop gross forms. This is a warning to one and all, not to underestimate the strength of the tendencies in the subtle body.

श्रीभगवानुवाच
सुदुर्दर्शमिदं रूपं
दृष्टवानसि यन्मम ।
देवा अप्यस्य रूपस्य
नित्यं दर्शनकाङ्क्षिणः ॥ ११.५२ ॥
śrībhagavānuvāca
sudurdarśamidaṁ rūpaṁ
dṛṣṭavānasi yanmama
devā apyasya rūpasya
nityaṁ darśanakāṅkṣiṇaḥ (11.52)

*śrī bhagavān — The Blessed Lord; uvāca — said; sudurdarsam — difficult to perceive; idam — this; rūpaṁ — form; dṛṣṭvān — having seen; asi — you are; yat — which; mamā — of mine; deva — supernatural rulers; api — also; asya — of this; rūpasya — of the form; nityam — always; darśanakāṅkṣiṇaḥ = darśana — sight + kāṅkṣiṇaḥ — wishing*

**The Blessed Lord said: This Form of Mine which you saw, is difficult to perceive. Even the supernatural rulers always wish for the sight of this Form. (11.52)**

***Siddha Swami's Commentary:***

*Śrī* Krishna as the supreme master of the yoga austerities, makes it clear to Arjuna, that no one, not even Arjuna, should brush aside the vision of the Four-handed divine form of *Śrī* Krishna. After Arjuna saw the Universal Form and was spooked out of his wits, he asked to see the Four-handed divine Form, which he heard of and wanted to experience visually. Thus *Śrī* Krishna complied with that request, but still Arjuna, just after seeing that Form, again wanted to go back quickly to physical vision, which was his main interest and the main concern of the subtle body. Thus *Śrī* Krishna admonished Arjuna in this verse, alerting him and everyone else, that the four-handed Divine Form is difficult to perceive, even for persons using supernatural bodies in the celestial world. They wish to see that Four-handed Divine Form and they cannot fulfill that desire. So how could Arjuna take such a form lightly? It appears that the physical reality was more impressionable to the psyche of Arjuna.

नाहं वेदैर्न तपसा
न दानेन न चेज्यया ।
शक्य एवंविधो द्रष्टुं
दृष्टवानसि मां यथा ॥ ११.५३॥
nāhaṁ vedairna tapasā
na dānena na cejyayā
śakya evaṁvidho draṣṭuṁ
dṛṣṭavānasi māṁ yathā (11.53)

*nāhaṁ = na — neither + aham — I; vedaiḥ — by Vedic study; na — nor; tapasā — by austerity; na — nor; dānena — by charity; na — not; cejyayā = ca — and + ijyayā — by sacrificial ceremony; śakya = śakye — I can; evaṁvidho = evaṁvidhaḥ — in that way; draṣṭuṁ — to see; dṛṣṭavān — having seen; asi — you are; mām — me; yathā — as*

**Neither by Vedic study, nor by austerity, nor by charity, and not by sacrificial ceremony, can I be seen in the way you saw Me. (11.53)**

***Siddha Swami's Commentary:***

Vedic study is important at a certain stage of one's spiritual development but it is mere theory for anyone who cannot see supernaturally and spiritually to verify it. Austerity has value since by it one may upgrade one's psychology. However, one may only upgrade as much as permitted by certain laws of physical, supernatural and spiritual nature. A person who uses austerity will upgrade himself to a degree but since he is working from an ignorant stage, his progression will of necessity be haphazard and painstaking.

Charity cannot cause divine development, because the divine bodies do not need patronizing. Charity counteracts the natural tendency for selfishness but it does not remove that survival mechanism. Sacrificial ceremony allows for pleasing the authoritarian, supernatural persons who stipulate how a human being should live to develop piety. The value of piety is its effect on the subtle body, whereby it causes that body to become compatible to the forms of the supernatural rulers, but it does not have an effect on the spiritual status. Thus by these methods, one cannot develop spiritual vision to see the divine body of *Śrī* Krishna or anyone else.

भक्त्या त्वनन्यया शक्य
अहमेवंविधोऽर्जुन ।
ज्ञातुं द्रष्टुं च तत्त्वेन
प्रवेष्टुं च परंतप ॥ ११.५४॥
bhaktyā tvananyayā śakya
ahamevaṁvidho'rjuna
jñātuṁ draṣṭuṁ ca tattvena
praveṣṭuṁ ca paraṁtapa (11.54)

*bhaktyā — by devotion; tu — only; ananyayā — not in another way, undistracted; śakya = śakye — I can; aham — 1; evaṁvidho = evaṁvidhaḥ — in that way; 'rjuna = arjuna — Arjuna; jñātuṁ — to be known; draṣṭuṁ — to see; ca — and; tattvena — by reality; praveṣṭuṁ — to communicate with; ca — and; paraṁtapa — scorcher of the enemies*

**By undistracted devotion only, O Arjuna, can I be known, seen in reality, and communicated with, O scorcher of enemies. (11.54)**

***Siddha Swami's Commentary:***

*Śrī* Krishna accredited undistracted devotion alone, as being the cause of the spiritual vision which Arjuna experienced. Thus, why is it that some who claim to have this devotion, do not see the divine form of *Śrī* Krishna but instead state that the painted murti or sculptured form in the temple is identical to that divine form or that *Śrī* Krishna is non-different from His name? And why is it that some devotees, failing to see the divine form of *Śrī* Krishna, take to meditations where they imagine such forms on the basis of descriptions given in the *Bhagavad Gītā* and elsewhere? Why is it that some feel the two-handed physically visible form of *Śrī* Krishna is the divine form in fact?

The reason is simple: *bhaktyā tu ananyayā*, undistracted devotion cannot be defined by anybody but *Śrī* Krishna. No one else really can tell us what it is. But whosoever has it, gets the divine vision which Arjuna so graciously was bestowed, to see the four-handed form as described.

मत्कर्मकृन्मत्परमो
मद्भक्तः सङ्गवर्जितः ।
निर्वैरः सर्वभूतेषु
यः स मामेति पाण्डव ॥ ११.५५॥
matkarmakṛnmatparamo
madbhaktaḥ saṅgavarjitaḥ
nirvairaḥ sarvabhūteṣu
yaḥ sa māmeti pāṇḍava (11.55)

*matkarmakṛt — doing my word; matparamo = matparamaḥ — depending on me; madbhaktaḥ — being devoted to me; saṅgavarjitaḥ= sariga — attachment + varjitaḥ — abandoned; nirvairaḥ — free from hostility; sarvabhūteṣu —to all beings; yah — who; sa = saḥ — he; mām — to me; eti — comes; pāṇḍava — son of Pāndu*

**Whosoever does My work, depending on Me, being devoted to Me, abandoning attachment, being freed from hostility towards all beings, comes to Me, O son of Pṛthā. (11.55)**

***Siddha Swami's Commentary:***

This does not mean that this devotee comes instantly. It means that according to his purity and his undistracted devotion, as noted by *Śrī* Krishna, he will go to Krishna at the rate of advancement he deserves. He must do *Śrī* Krishna's work in this material world by submitting to the duties assigned to him by the Universal Form, in terms of protecting this world from irreligious activities, just as Arjuna was destined to do at *Kurukṣetra*. He has to depend on *Śrī* Krishna, otherwise he would not be able to complete those tasks, due to his susceptibility to the influence of others who are opposed to the supreme will. This was the dilemma of Arjuna in the beginning of the *Bhagavad Gītā* discourse.

The devotee should be devoted to *Śrī* Krishna, *madbhakta*, on the basis of a cordial student-to-teacher relationship as demonstrated by Arjuna in *Bhagavad Gītā*. He should abandon attachment through his psychological strength developed by mastering *buddhi yoga* practice. He should be freed from hostility to all beings, even to those who are hostile to *Śrī* Krishna, just as *Śrī Nārada* was with persons like Kamsa who were very inimical to *Śrī* Krishna. This does not mean that he would not discipline such persons or even deprive them of their material bodies. It means that on his own he would not oppose them, even though on behalf of the Universal Form he would discipline them in any way stipulated by the Central Person in the Universal Form. Such a devotee would go to *Śrī* Krishna merely by cooperation with the God and through developed devotion to Him.

# CHAPTER 12

## Mad Yogam Āśritah

## Resorting to Krishna's Yoga Process *

*athaitadapyaśakto'si kartuṁ madyogamāśritaḥ*
*sarvakarmaphalatyāgaṁ tataḥ kuru yatātmavān (12.11)*

***If you are unable to even do this, then resorting to My yoga process, abandoning all results of action, act with self restraint. (12.11)***

**Siddha Swami assigned this chapter title on the basis of verse 11 of this chapter.*

अर्जुन उवाच
एवं सततयुक्ता ये
भक्तास्त्वां पर्युपासते ।
ये चाप्यक्षरमव्यक्तं
तेषां के योगवित्तमाः ॥१२.१॥
arjuna uvāca
evaṁ satatayuktā ye
bhaktāstvāṁ paryupāsate
ye cāpyakṣaramavyaktaṁ
teṣāṁ ke yogavittamāḥ (12.1)

*arjuna — Arjuna; uvāca — said; evaṁ — thus; satatayuktā = satata — constantly + yuktā — disciplined in yoga; ye — who; bhaktāh — devoted; tvam — you; paryupāsate — they cherish; ye — who; cāpi = ca — and + api — also; akṣaram — imperishable; avyaktaṁ — invisible existence; teṣāṁ — of them; ke — which; yogavittamāḥ — those who have the highest knowledge of yoga*

**Arjuna said: Of those who are constantly disciplined in yoga, being also devoted to You, and those who cherish the imperishable invisible existence, which of these two have the highest knowledge of the yoga techniques? (12.1)**

***Siddha Swami's Commentary:***

*Satatayuktā* are those who mastered the same *buddhi yoga* which *Śrī* Krishna explained in detail in the preceding chapters. It cannot be anything else, nor any modern system of salvation which deducts such practice from the spiritual process. What we heard is what *Śrī* Krishna explained, not what any another *avatār* said. We do not have here an adjustment for fallen entities in Kali Yuga. Whatever we hear in the *Gītā* must be coordinated with what is defined in the *Gītā* itself. Other religious books have their valid or invalid proclamations but these are not to be mixed up with the *Gītā*, just for the sake of using the *Gītā* to support other declarations of other religious teachers or *avatārs* who descend.

Arjuna wanted *Śrī* Krishna to give a clear and unbiased assessment of Krishna's system of *buddhi yoga* practice while being devoted to *Śrī* Krishna, as contrasted to the other system in the time of *Śrī* Krishna. This other process was followed by yogins who mastered the same *buddhi yoga* process either through proficient teachers or by self discovery but these yogins were not devoted to *Śrī* Krishna. They were either devoted to no one in particular or had other ideas about the identity of the Supreme Person. Most of all they cherished the imperishable invisible existence as one sum total reality which they adored. They negated any idea of a Supreme Personality like *Śrī* Krishna.

Arjuna's interest in the two groups of yogis concerned which had the highest knowledge of the yoga techniques. And the answer is obvious. Those yogis who are devoted to *Śrī* Krishna, get by that confidence in Him, very advanced techniques step by step. What the others have to discover may be taught by Krishna to the yogi-devotee step by step in an integrated and thorough way.

श्रीभगवानुवाच
मय्यावेश्य मनो ये मां
नित्ययुक्ता उपासते ।
श्रद्धया परयोपेतास्
ते.मे युक्ततमा मताः ॥१२.२॥

*śrībhagavān — the Blessed Lord; uvāca — said; mayyāveśya = mayi — on me + āveśya – focusing on: mano = manaḥ — mind; ye — who; māṁ — me; nityayuktā — those who are always disciplined in yoga; upāsate — they worship; śraddhayā — with faith; parayopetās = parayā — with the highest*

śrībhagavānuvāca
mayyāveśya mano ye māṁ
nityayuktā upāsate
śraddhayā parayopetās
te me yuktatamā matāḥ (12.2)

*degree; upetāḥ — endowed; te — they; me — to me; yuktatamā — most disciplined; matāḥ — considered*

**The Blessed Lord said: Those whose minds are focused on Me, who are always disciplined in yoga, who are always involved in worship of Me, who are endowed with the highest degree of faith, they are considered to be the most disciplined. (12.2)**

***Siddha Swami's Commentary:***

In as much as this answer of *Śrī* Krishna seems straight forward and simple at a glance, if we look in detail, we will discover that this is complicated. Let us take the parts of this requirement step by step.

First the yogi devotee's mind must be focused on *Śrī* Krishna. But how is this to be done? Does this mean to focus on the holy name of *Śrī* Krishna, as popularized by many devotees today who do not practice *buddhi yoga* as explained in the *Gītā*. How should the mind be focused? What intimacy should the yogi devotee have with *Śrī* Krishna in order to make sure that his focus is actually on *Śrī* Krishna and not on his idea of Krishna, an idea developed under the influence of others who have read of *Śrī* Krishna but who never met the Lord face to face on either on the physical, subtle or spiritual levels as Arjuna did. We know that before the vision of the Universal Form, Arjuna met *Śrī* Krishna physically many times and had a friendly relationship with the Lord. In the vision of the Universal Form, Arjuna met *Śrī* Krishna on the supernatural level and then in the vision of the four-armed Form, He met the Lord spiritually. Thus for Arjuna, focusing on the Supreme Lord would be based on those encounters with *Śrī* Krishna. Arjuna did not rely on the name of *Śrī* Krishna as many devotees do today, nor even on the artistically created murti forms of *Śrī* Krishna that are seen in temples and on altars.

Secondly, as stated in the previous verse under the term *satatayukta*, the yogi devotee must be disciplined in the *buddhi yoga* practice *(nityayuktā)* as it was explained by *Śrī* Krishna in this *Bhagavad Gītā*. Yoga cannot be deducted from these requirements if we plan to follow the *Bhagavad Gītā* as it was explained to Arjuna.

Thirdly, the devotee must always be involved in worship of *Śrī* Krishna. The elaboration of this worship is not given here but this refers to formal worship in religious ceremonies, which today is called Deity worship or *archanam*.

Fourthly, the yogi devotee must be endowed with the highest degree of faith in *Śrī* Krishna. This was a preliminary requirement which *Śrī* Krishna elaborated on before.

Such a yogi devotee is rated as being the most disciplined of the yogis, and as such his spiritual progression is definite and certain.

ये त्वक्षरमनिर्देश्यम्
अव्यक्तं पर्युपासते ।
सर्वत्रगमचिन्त्यं च
कूटस्थमचलं ध्रुवम् ॥१२.३॥
ye tvakṣaramanirdeśyam
avyaktaṁ paryupāsate
sarvatragamacintyaṁ ca
kūṭasthamacalaṁ dhruvam (12.3)

*ye — who; tu — but; akṣaram — imperishable; anirdeśyam — undefinable; avyaktaṁ — invisible; paryupāsate — they cherish; sarvatragam — all-pervading; acintyam — inconceivable; ca — and; kūṭastham — unchanging; acalaṁ — immovable; dhruvam — constant*

**But those who cherish the imperishable, undefinable, invisible, all-pervading, inconceivable, unchanging, immovable, constant reality, (12.3)**

***Siddha Swami's Commentary:***

The imperishable is that which will not deteriorate under any circumstance. The undefinable is that which transcends a yogi's intelligence. The yogi may confront this level of reality in *samādhi* but he cannot make complete analysis of it because his intelligence and sensual apparatus are unable to assess it. The invisible is that which cannot be subjected to visual analysis.

The all-pervading is whatever everything else is influenced by; that is something which permeates every detail of every existence in all the dimensions of reality. The inconceivable is that which cannot be photographed in any way by the imagination. Thus a limited being cannot have a complete conception or idea of it. The unchanging is that which remains in constancy always and does not go through alternations at any stage. The immovable is that which does not exhibit any type of external or internal mobility. It is therefore termed *dhruvam* or constant.

A question may arise as to whether a yogi devotee who is devoted to *Śrī* Krishna, may ever encounter that imperishable, undefinable, invisible, all-pervading, inconceivable, unchanging, immovable and constant reality? And if such a devotee does, what should be his relation to it? What indeed is it? How is it related to *Śrī* Krishna? What is its importance?

संनियम्येन्द्रियग्रामं
सर्वत्र समबुद्धयः ।
ते प्राप्नुवन्ति मामेव
सर्वभूतहिते रताः ॥१२.४॥
saṁniyamyendriyagrāmaṁ
sarvatra samabuddhayaḥ
te prāpnuvanti māmeva
sarvabhūtahite ratāḥ (12.4)

*saṁniyamyendriyagrāmaṁ = saṁniyamya — controlling + indriyagrāmaṁ — all sensual energies; sarvatra — in all respects; samabuddhayaḥ — even-minded; te — them; prāpnuvanti — they attain; mām — me; eva — also; sarvabhūtahite = sarvabhūta — all creatures + hite — in the welfare; ratāḥ — rejoicing*

**...by controlling all sensual energies, being even-minded in all respects, rejoicing in the welfare of all creatures, they also attain Me. (12.4)**

***Siddha Swami's Commentary:***

For those who cherish the constant reality as described, the important qualification is their complete control of sensual energies. If a person does not control the sensual energies in his psyche in total, he cannot do a thorough research into the constant reality. He will be diverted by the sensual interest which will utilize his attention to investigate and become involved with the non-constant energies.

Due to the sensual energy control, that *yogin* would be even-minded in all respects, dispassionate to everything which usually stimulates others. And he would not have resentments to others. Thus he would rejoice in the welfare of all creatures. Such a yogi would attain *Śrī* Krishna as stated in this verse, because the course of his progress necessitates an encounter with the Supreme Being, the Supreme Person, *Śrī* Krishna.

क्लेशोऽधिकतरस्तेषाम्
अव्यक्तासक्तचेतसाम् ।
अव्यक्ता हि गतिर्दुःखं
देहवद्भिरवाप्यते ॥१२.५॥

*kleśo = kleśaḥ — exertion; 'dhikataraḥ = adhikataraḥ — greater; tesam — of them; avyaktāsaktacetasām = avyakta — invisible existence + āsakta — attached + cetasām — of*

kleśo'dhikatarasteṣām
avyaktāsaktacetasām
avyaktā hi gatirduḥkhaṁ
dehavadbhiravāpyate (12.5)

*minds; avyaktā — invisible reality; hi — truly; gatiḥ — goal; duḥkhaṁ — difficult; dehavadbhiḥ — by the human beings; avāpyate — is attained*

**The mental exertion of those whose minds are attached to the invisible existence is greater. The goal of reaching that invisible reality is attained with difficulty by the human beings. (12.5)**

***Siddha Swami Maharaja translated this verse as follows:***

**The mental and emotional exertion of those whose minds are attached to the invisible existence is greater. The goal of linking into that invisible energy is attained with difficulty by the human beings. (12.5)**

***Siddha Swami's Commentary:***

It is extremely difficult to link oneself into the invisible existence. Even if one can do it for a second or so, it is nearly impossible for one to do so for a long time, say for instance for one hour, what to speak of doing that permanently once and for all. Many, many great yogis endeavored to do this in their quest to end off their affiliation with the ever-changing, bothersome material nature, but many of those great persons found it to be an impossible task, just as a man who wants to touch the horizon, approaches it but can never put his finger on it.

A *yogin* who aspires for this may begin with a mental exertion in determination to achieve his goal, but he will have to focus his emotions on it also, otherwise he will be continually drawn back into the world of sensual interplay. However, the application of the emotions to something that undefinable, invisible, inconceivable and unchanging, may be boring and frustrating. It all depends on the existential status of the particular *yogin*.

While a *yogin* who is devoted to *Śrī* Krishna may apply his emotions to his relationship with *Śrī* Krishna, others who have no such relation must struggle with the demands of their sensual energies and resist the temptations which arise in these form-alluring material worlds.

ये तु सर्वाणि कर्माणि
मयि संन्यस्य मत्पराः ।
अनन्येनैव योगेन
मां ध्यायन्त उपासते ॥१२.६॥
ye tu sarvāṇi karmāṇi
mayi saṁnyasya matparāḥ
ananyenaiva yogena
māṁ dhyāyanta upāsate (12.6)

*ye — who; tu — but; sarvāṇi — all; karmāṇi — actions; mayi — in me; saṁnyasya — deferring; matparāḥ — regarding me as the most important factor; ananyenaiva = ananyena — without another, undistracted + eva — indeed; yogena — with yoga discipline; māṁ — me; dhyayānta — meditating on; upāsate — they worship*

**But those who defer all actions to Me, regarding Me as the most important factor, who meditate on Me with undistracted yoga discipline, do worship Me. (12.6)**

***Siddha Swami's Commentary:***

In comparison to the yogis who are not devotees of *Śrī* Krishna and who do not take directions from Him, those who do, by deferring their actions to Him and regarding Him as the most important factor, meditate on Him with undistracted yoga discipline through *buddhi yoga (ananyenaiva yogena mām dhyāyanta),* worship Him *(upāsate)* in the approved way. Thus their success in spiritual life is assured and it takes place rapidly by His divine grace.

तेषामहं समुद्धर्ता
मृत्युसंसारसागरात् ।
भवामि नचिरात्पार्थ
मय्यावेशितचेतसाम् ॥ १२.७॥
teṣāmahaṁ samuddhartā
mṛtyusaṁsārasāgarāt
bhavāmi nacirātpārtha
mayyāveśitacetasām (12.7)

*teṣām — of those; aham — I; samuddhartā — delivered; mṛtyusaṁsārasāgarāt = mṛtyu — death + saṁsāra — reincarnations + sāgarāt — from the vast existence; bhavāmi — I am; nacirāt — soon; pārtha — son of Pṛthā; mayyāveśitacetasām = mayi — in me + āveśita — intently, invested in + cetasām — of thoughts*

**I am the deliverer of those devotees, rescuing them from the vast existence of death and reincarnation. O son of Pṛthā, I soon deliver those devotees whose thoughts are intently invested in Me. (12.7)**

*Siddha Swami asked that this verse be translated in this way:*

**I am the deliverer of those devotees, rescuing them from the vast existence of death and reincarnation. O son of Prtha, I soon deliver those devotees whose intellect and emotions are intently invested in Me. (12.7)**

***Siddha Swami's Commentary:***

*Śrī* Krishna is the deliverer of those devotees because they rely on Him as their teacher. Their faith in Him is strong and so they take directions from Him, and as submissive students they learn from Him rapidly. He rescues them from the vast existence of death and reincarnation *(mṛtyusamsārasāgarāt)*. He does not do this independently of their cooperation, endeavor, and assistance. He does that mostly because they endeavor under His direction in the *buddhi yoga* teaching which He described previously in the *Gītā*.

For the investing *(āveśita)* of the intellect and emotions on *Śrī* Krishna, one must master *buddhi yoga* as it was taught by *Śrī* Krishna to the *Manu* and others like King Janaka. This cannot be done except by someone who knows *Śrī* Krishna personally and who met with *Śrī* Krishna either physically, supernaturally or spiritually. Merely to hear of *Śrī* Krishna from scripture will not put one in touch with *Śrī* Krishna sufficiently for one's whole being to be intent upon the Supreme Lord.

मय्येव मन आधत्स्व
मयि बुद्धिं निवेशाय ।
निवसिष्यसि मय्येव
अत ऊर्ध्वं न संशयः ॥ १२.८॥
mayyeva mana ādhatsva
mayi buddhiṁ niveśaya
nivasiṣyasi mayyeva
ata ūrdhvaṁ na saṁśayaḥ (12.8)

*mayyeva = mayi — on me + eva — alone; mana — mind; ādhatsva — place; mayi — on me; buddhiṁ — intellect; niveśaya — cause to be absorbed; nivasiṣyasi — you will be focused; mayyeva = mayi — in me + eva — indeed; ata ūrdhvaṁ — from now onwards; na — not; saṁśayaḥ — doubt*

**Placing your mind on Me alone, causing your intellect to be absorbed in Me alone, you will be focused on Me from now onwards. There is no doubt about this. (12.8)**

***Siddha Swami's Commentary:***

This, though extolled by *Śrī* Krishna, is not possible for most devotees since to do this, one needs an intimate relationship with the Lord. It is enough for us to take note of this and to admire persons like Arjuna who were in confidence with *Śrī* Krishna, being in touch with

His higher existence which is imperishable and Supermost.

*avyaktaṁ vyaktimāpannaṁ manyante māmabuddhayaḥ*
*paraṁ bhāvamajānanto mamāvyayamanuttamam (7.24)*

***Though I am beyond their sensual range, the unintelligent think of Me as being limited to their gross perception. They do not realize My higher existence which is imperishable and supermost. (7.24)***

The ability to place one's mind on *Śrī* Krishna alone, causing the intellect to be absorbed in Him alone and being focused only on Him from then onwards, can only be attained by one who masters *buddhi yoga* and develops a confidential relationship with the person of *Śrī* Krishna directly and not merely with His name and His *līlā* narrations. A *brahma yogi* may certainly aspire for this but he cannot have this until *Śrī* Krishna allows him to develop a confidential relationship and until he can see the divine form of *Śrī* Krishna. Otherwise it is not possible. Everything stated by *Śrī* Krishna may not be attained by a particular devotee and it is foolish to rate oneself as a person who would attain all the accomplishments guaranteed within the *Gītā*. Some of these attainments are to be appreciated for the time being, at least until one may advance further.

अथ चित्तं समाधातुं
न शक्नोषि मयि स्थिरम् ।
अभ्यासयोगेन ततो
मामिच्छाप्तुं धनंजय ॥१२.९॥
atha cittaṁ samādhātuṁ
na śaknoṣi mayi sthiram
abhyāsayogena tato
māmicchāptuṁ dhanaṁjaya (12.9)

*atha — if however; cittam — thought; samādhātum — to anchor; na — not; śaknoṣi — you can; mayi — on me; sthiram — steadily; abhyāsayogena = abhyāsa — practice + yogena — by yoga; tato = tataḥ — then; mām — me; icchāptum = iccha — with + āptuṁ — to attain; dhanaṁjaya — conqueror of wealthy countries*

**If, however, you cannot steadily anchor your thoughts on Me, then by yoga practice, try to attain Me, O conqueror of wealthy countries. (12.9)**

***Siddha Swami's Commentary:***

Certainly most persons in this world, even most devotees of *Śrī* Krishna, are unable to steadily anchor their mental and emotional psyche upon *Śrī* Krishna exclusively. This verse should be translated as follows:

**If, however, you cannot steadily anchor your mental and emotional energies on Me, then by yoga practice, try to attain Me, O conqueror of wealthy countries. (12.9)**

Furthermore it is clear that unless one has a relationship with Śrī Krishna like Arjuna had or like Krishna's relatives and friends in Mathura and *Vṛndāvana* had, one must take recourse to yoga practice *(abhyāsayogena)*. This means *buddhi yoga*. It does not mean *bhakti* or *bhakti yoga*. If honestly and truly, one does not have a confidential relationship with Śrī Krishna, one will not be able to place one's mental and emotional force on Krishna alone nor will one be able to focus on Śrī Krishna from then onwards as stipulated in the previous verse. Thus one should not pretend that one can do that. One should instead take this verse nine very seriously and take up the practice of buddhi yoga.

अभ्यासेऽप्यसमर्थोऽसि
मत्कर्मपरमो भव ।
मदर्थमपि कर्माणि
कुर्वन्सिद्धिमवाप्स्यसि ॥ १२.१० ॥
abhyāse'pyasamartho'si
matkarmaparamo bhava
madarthamapi karmāṇi
kurvansiddhimavāpsyasi (12.10)

*abhyāse — in practice; 'pi = api — perchance; asamartho = asamarthaḥ — incapable; 'si = asi — you are; matkarmaparamo = matkarmaparamaḥ = matkarma — my work + paramaḥ — be absorbed; bhava — be; madartham — for my sake; api — even; karmāṇi — activities; kurvan — doing; siddhim — perfection; avāpsyasi — you will attain*

**But if perchance, you are incapable of such practice, then by being absorbed in My work, or even by doing activities for My sake, you will attain perfection. (12.10)**

***Siddha Swami's Commentary:***

Now *Śrī* Krishna digressed to a lower but necessary stage for those who do not have the confidential relationship with him and for those also who cannot practice and master the *buddhi yoga* process which He taught the ancient seers and which was reviewed in the *Gītā* with Arjuna. If one is unable to meet the standards given in the previous two verses, then one should try to work for Krishna with as much attention and sincerity as one can muster. One should support *Śrī* Krishna's efforts to maintain righteous lifestyle. In that way, in time, one will attain perfection. However, one should not take this to mean that one will not have to do yoga, or go through a slow process of cultivating a confidential relationship with *Śrī* Krishna.

*Śrī* Krishna particularly stated that such a person attains perfection. This means that his or her perfection will occur in the future definitely, but it does not mean that the only requirement is working for *Śrī* Krishna's mission of *dharma*, righteous lifestyle, as He described previously. One should not undervalue the rest of the *Gītā* or feel that whatever else was required will be cancelled for one's easy salvation.

अथैतदप्यशक्तोऽसि
कर्तुं मद्योगमाश्रितः ।
सर्वकर्मफलत्यागं
ततः कुरु यतात्मवान् ॥ १२.११ ॥
athaitadapyaśakto'si
kartuṁ madyogamāśritaḥ
sarvakarmaphalatyāgaṁ
tataḥ kuru yatātmavān (12.11)

*athaitat = atha — if + etat — this; api — even: aśakto = aśaktaḥ — unable; 'si = asi — you are; kartum — to do; madyogam — my yoga; aśritaḥ — resorting to; sarvakarmaphalatyāgaṁ = sarvakarmaphala — all results of action + tyāgam — abandoning; tataḥ — then; kuru — act; yatātmavān — with restraint*

**If you are unable to even do this, then resorting to My yoga process, abandoning all results of action, act with self restraint. (12.11)**

***Siddha Swami's Commentary:***

If, however, a person cannot take up the work of *Śrī* Krishna for whatever reason, that person is advised to begin the *buddhi yoga* process as a student. After practicing for a time, a person will master the application of *buddhi yoga* to cultural activities. This is *karma yoga*. Thus in time, the person would resort to Krishna's yoga process which He described before, the same *karma yoga* which Arjuna was being schooled in during this discourse, and which was taught to *Vivasvat* and others by *Śrī* Krishna.

There is no other digression given by *Śrī* Krishna, no other easy way to satisfy or approach Him. In retrospect, He said that one should be absorbed on Him alone, in entirety.

Then if one could not do that one should take up the practice of yoga, so that eventually by the mastership of yoga, one would absorb Him. This yoga is described in Chapter Six of the *Bhagavad Gītā*.

*Śrī* Krishna said that if one could not do that yoga, then one should try to do His work of righteous lifestyle establishment. But if one could not do that, then one should take up the *buddhi yoga* practice and apply that to cultural life or *karma yoga*. And *Śrī* Krishna did not give any other alternatives such as chanting holy names, doing worship in a temple or following a guru blindly. Let us consider this if we are serious about attaining *Śrī* Krishna.

श्रेयो हि ज्ञानमभ्यासाज्
ज्ञानाद्ध्यानं विशिष्यते ।
ध्यानात्कर्मफलत्यागस्
त्यागाच्छान्तिरनन्तरम् ॥१२.१२॥
śreyo hi jñānamabhyāsāj
jñānāddhyānaṁ viśiṣyate
dhyānātkarmaphalatyāgas
tyāgācchāntiranantaram (12.12)

*śreyo = śreyaḥ — better; hi — indeed; jñānam — derived knowledge, experience; abhyāsāt — from the practice; jñānāt — than derived knowledge; dhyānaṁ — meditation; viśiṣyate — is superior; dhyānāt — than meditation; karmaphalatyāgaḥ = karmaphala — results of action + tyāgaḥ — renunciation; tyāgāt — from renunciation; śāntiḥ — spiritual peace; anantaram — instantly*

**Indeed, derived knowledge is better than practice. Meditation is superior to derived knowledge. Renunciation of results is better than meditation. From such renunciation, spiritual peace is instantly gained. (12.12)**

***Siddha Swami's Commentary:***

To prove His points and verify what He said, *Śrī* Krishna explained that derived knowledge is better than the practice which gave it. This is because the purpose of practice is the expertise gained from it. The practice provides the means to that expertise. One develops a skill from practice, and the skill supercedes the practice. Even though the practice is instrumental in the development of the skill, the skill is superior.

Derived knowledge is known as a conclusion. But once the conclusion is gained, one should take up meditation to link the mental and emotional energies to higher concentration forces. After all, once one sees that this material existence is futile, the only alternative left is to meditate so as to find higher existences. However, once these are located on the supernatural and spiritual planes, one has to return to this world and act in a way which is conducive to a natural transfer to the said higher places. To do this one must act here with detachment so that one renounces the results of whatever good or bad forces are intermeshed into one's cultural life. This renunciation of the results, or *tyāgah*, causes the experiences gained in meditation, to be remembered firmly at first. Then by continued practice, one remains linked to those higher planes even when doing cultural work, when a tiny portion of one's attention remains invested in this world and the major part of it remains anchored to the higher plane discovered.

Spiritual peace, *śāntih*, is gained from such renunciation, because one breaks free from the rules and dictates of this cultural life and escapes the thralldom of material existence, even though one still has a material body and still has to participate culturally.

अद्वेष्टा सर्वभूतानां
मैत्रः करुण एव च ।
निर्ममो निरहंकारः
समदुःखसुखः क्षमी ॥१२.१३॥

*adveṣṭā — one who does not dislike; sarvabhūtānāṁ — all creatures; maitraḥ — friendly; karuṇa — compassionate; eva — indeed; ca — and; nirmamo = nirmamaḥ — free from*

adveṣṭā sarvabhūtānāṁ
maitraḥ karuṇa eva ca
nirmamo nirahaṁkāraḥ
samaduḥkhasukhaḥ kṣamī (12.13)

*attachment to possessions; nirahaṁkāraḥ — free from the propensity of, "I am the creator of my actions"; samaduḥkhasukhaḥ = sama — equally disposed + duḥkha — pain + sukhaḥ — pleasure; kṣamī — be patient*

**One who does not dislike any of the creatures, who is friendly and compassionate, free from attachment to possessions, free from the propensity of "I am the creator of my actions," being equally disposed towards pain and pleasure, being patient, (12.13)**

***Siddha Swami's Commentary:***

This verse and the remaining seven verses of this chapter, a total of eight verses, describe a person who became proficient in the *buddhi yoga* practice and who additionally developed the devotion to *Śrī* Krishna.

*Adveṣṭā*, the **tendency not to dislike anyone**, even persons who are wicked and irreligious, is gained by the mastery of kundalini yoga practice. This cannot be consistently attained by determination alone or by saintly association only. One has to purify the force that creates prejudices in one's nature. This force is the kundalini force in the subtle body. If one does not purify that, then one will assume an attitude of:

**'I am a devotee of *Śrī* Krishna and he is not. We are devotees and they are worldly people. We are superior. He does not believe in *Śrī* Krishna, therefore he should be shunned.'**

By taking in a higher grade of energy into the subtle body, one's nature sheds off the polluted pranic energies which sponsored prejudices and thus one becomes **friendly and compassionate** to others but one is not fooled by others, even though one may overlook their faults.

**Freedom from attachment to possessions** comes about by transferring one's attention to other levels of existence, to other more subtle energies. Arjuna, for instance, was very much in possession of his Kuru cultural identity, but after he viewed the Universal Form, he discarded that attachment and no longer considered the material plane to be the total reality. Freedom from attachment to possessions does not occur consistently by efforts to give up possession. Such efforts are a good show for making a reputation as an ascetic, but that is not what *Śrī* Krishna spoke of.

**Freedom from the propensity of 'I am the creator of my actions,'** comes about by keeping in touch with the Universal Form. Unless one keeps in contact with the instructions of that Form, one is bound to take on the **'I am the creator of my actions'** attitude, even if one is a recognized devotee. For contact with the Universal Form, one needs to have mystic perception as a permanent part of one's psyche. Usually this is attained by yoga practice, specifically *buddhi yoga*. Arjuna, as a devotee, was affected by the **'I am the creator of my actions'** attitude, and that proves that merely being a devotee of *Śrī* Krishna is insufficient for shedding that propensity.

**Being equally disposed to pleasure and pain** comes about by mastering one's emotions. An emotional person, who has not curbed his feelings by keeping his attention segregated, cannot be equally disposed to pain and pleasure. This comes about by mastership in *buddhi yoga* practice. This was Arjuna's psychological fault when he first began speaking in the *Gītā*, but gradually Arjuna was lifted from that level of existence by *Śrī* Krishna. He was lifted not because he was a devotee but rather through his importance as an agent of the Universal Form of *Śrī* Krishna. Other devotees on that battlefield, who were just as dear as Arjuna, were not lifted in the same way because they were not as important to the occasion of the battle of *Kurukṣetra*. The Supreme Person can certainly lift up a limited being merely by His glance, by His grace, but that usually does not happen. Usually one has to endeavor in yoga for the upliftment.

**Being patient** comes about by being in touch with the Universal Form and knowing that the Central Person in the Form commands this creation ultimately. One adapts an attitude of submission to providence and does not try to force the hand of the Almighty or counteract most of disturbances which one encounters in this creation.

संतुष्टः सततं योगी
यतात्मा दृढनिश्चयः ।
मय्यर्पितमनोबुद्धिर्
यो मद्भक्तः स मे प्रियः ॥१२.१४॥
saṁtuṣṭaḥ satataṁ yogī
yatātmā dṛḍhaniścayaḥ
mayyarpitamanobuddhir
yo madbhaktaḥ sa me priyaḥ (12.14)

*saṁtuṣṭaḥ — contented; satataṁ — always; yogī — yogi; yatātmā — one with a controlled self; draḍhaniścayaḥ — determined; mayi — on me; arpitamanobuddhiḥ = arpita — focused + mano = manas — mind + buddhiḥ — intellect; yo = yaḥ — who; madbhaktaḥ — devoted to me; sa = saḥ — he; me — of me; priyaḥ — dear*

**...the yogi who is always content, who has a controlled self, who is determined, whose mind and intellect are focused on Me, who is devoted to Me, is dear to Me. (12.14)**

***Siddha Swami's Commentary:***

Sincerity in yoga practice combined with the understanding that the limited living entity must participate in the achievement of his salvation, results in an attitude that makes the *yogin* compatible to *Śrī* Krishna. Such a *yogin* does not expect that the Lord should save him merely because he chants the name of Krishna or bows to the worshipable *Śrī* Krishna Murti idol form in the temple or because he feels that the requirement for salvation should be adjusted from era to era, in upgrades and downgrades to suit the elevated or degraded cultural situation of human society.

A sincere *yogin* listens to the divinity and complies with the request for austerities which will result not in beliefs about salvation that promise a glorious end after death of his body, but in actual salvation in gradual stages. In proportion to the successful execution of austerities as they are described in this *Bhagavad Gītā*, he does not accept that he cannot perform the austerities which will cause him to become a controlled spirit *(yatātmā)*.

The **dearness to *Śrī* Krishna** *(priyah)* was a status which Arjuna had throughout his lifetime on earth, before that and thereafter. But for others who do not have that sort of contact with *Śrī* Krishna, such dearness must be developed by complying with *Śrī* Krishna's request for mastership of *buddhi yoga* and its application into cultural life as *karma yoga*, and further progressions in *brahma yoga* as indicated by the Supreme Lord. This *brahma yoga* is termed as *jñāna yoga* or *samkhya yoga*. *Bhakti yoga* which is a higher stage, has its place, perhaps on the top of the list of the yogas because it cannot be practiced except with a completely purified psyche, since the application of one's affections to *Śrī* Krishna, will reach the Lord only when one's psyche is completely purified of its prejudices in the subtle material nature. Hence *bhakti yoga* is, in fact, quite distinct and different to how it is defined by most commentators.

Anyone serious about *bhakti yoga* should begin by being devoted to *Śrī* Krishna and to a teacher who sticks to the *Gītā* as it was taught to Arjuna, not to an adjusted rendition of the *Gītā* which forges into the text something modern which was introduced by empowered souls after the time of *Śrī* Krishna. One begins that devotion to *Śrī* Krishna by showing a willingness to accept the *Gītā* as taught to Arjuna and by endeavoring in the discipline of *buddhi yoga*. Then one becomes dear to the same *Śrī* Krishna who instructed Arjuna.

यस्मान्नोद्विजते लोको
लोकान्नोद्विजते च यः ।
हर्षामर्षभयोद्वेगैर्
मुक्तो यः स च मे प्रियः ॥१२.१५॥
yasmānnodvijate loko
lokānnodvijate ca yaḥ
harṣāmarṣabhayodvegair
mukto yaḥ sa ca me priyaḥ (12.15)

*yasmāt — from whom; nodvijate = na — not + udvijate — is repulsed; loko = lokaḥ — world; lokat — from the world; nodvijate = na — not + udvijate — is repulsed; ca — and; yaḥ — who; harṣāmarṣabhayodvegaiḥ = harṣa — excitement + amarṣa — impatience + bhaya — fear + udvegaiḥ — with distress; mukto = muktaḥ — freed; yaḥ — who; sa = saḥ— he; ca — and; me — of me; priyaḥ — dear*

**He from whom the world is not repulsed, and who is not repulsed from the world, who is free from excitement, impatience, fear and distress, is dear to Me. (12.15)**

***Siddha Swami's Commentary:***

There is much evidence that these requirements are everlasting, not changing from era to era. These qualities precede liberation. A spiritual teacher cannot award these qualities to a disciple but can show the disciple how to best cultivate such qualities. When the disciple has made sufficient endeavor, a change in his nature will cause the desired qualities to manifest.

The negative qualities of excitement, impatience, fear and distress may be experienced by neophyte yogins and by common people as either enjoyable or detestable but very necessary qualities. This is due to their inability to regulate their core self's relationship with the *citta* mento-emotional force. As soon as a *yogin* advances sufficiently, his close relationship with the mento-emotional energy comes to an end. It is ruptured so that he feels the distinction between his core self and the emotional power. Then a detachment comes about, such that he can sort between his emotions, his sensual energies, the subtle senses, the calculative intellect, the ever-activating memory and all other facets of psychology. Thus he is no longer repulsed or attracted to the world on the basis of prejudiced notions.

Even in an advanced *yogin*, the mento-emotional force does not give up its counterproductive stance completely, for as *Śrī Patañjali* stated, the *abhiniveśa* energy which sponsors fear and denial of impending death of one's body, is exhibited in all creatures, even in that of the advanced souls. Thus the advanced persons control their relationship to that mental-emotional power and not the power itself. The power gets its influence from its proximity to the core self. Hence if the energy it derives from that self is restricted, it is effectively curbed.

अनपेक्षः शुचिर्दक्ष
उदासीनो गतव्यथः ।
सर्वारम्भपरित्यागी
यो मद्भक्तः स मे प्रियः ॥१२.१६॥

*anapekṣaḥ — impartial; śuciḥ — hygienic; dakṣa — competent; udāsīno = udasīnāḥ — indifferent; gatavyathaḥ — one whose anxieties are gone; sarvārambhaparityāgī = sarva — all + ārambha — undertaking +*

anapekṣaḥ śucirdakṣa
udāsīno gatavyathaḥ
sarvārambhaparityāgī
yo madbhaktaḥ sa me priyaḥ (12.16)

*parityāgi — abandoning; yo = yaḥ — who; madbhaktaḥ — devoted to me; sa = saḥ — he; me — of me; priyaḥ — dear*

**He who is impartial, hygienic, competent, indifferent, whose anxieties are gone, who has abandoned all personal undertakings, and who is devoted to Me, is dear to Me. (12.16)**

***Siddha Swami's Commentary:***

Many who are impartial and indifferent to life are, in fact, mad. They are not advanced yogis who are wise to the hidden realities behind this physical existence. Usually they are unhygienic and incompetent. A *yogin*, if advanced, will not only be detached from this life, but could, in an instant, become very attached for the completion of duties. This is due to submissiveness to the Universal Form of *Śrī* Krishna. One should be detached and should endeavor daily for the supreme dispassion but one must also do the contrary when stipulated by the Central Figure in the Universal Form or by circumstantial factors which are providential.

*Sarvārambhaparityāgī* or the abandonment of all personal undertakings does not exclude the *yogin* from mandatory duties which are assigned to him by the Universal Form. These duties must be performed or one's spiritual life will be checked by divine force which manifests as stagnation and lack of progressive realization and lack of increase in mystic perception. For his own sake, a *yogin* should be impartial and indifferent but for the sake of God he should be competent and should eagerly and efficiently take up and complete assigned tasks. This falls under the term of *karma yoga*.

यो न हृष्यति न द्वेष्टि
न शोचति न काङ्क्षति ।
शुभाशुभपरित्यागी
भक्तिमान्यः स मे प्रियः ॥१२.१७॥
yo na hṛṣyati na dveṣṭi
na śocati na kāṅkṣati
śubhāśubhaparityāgī
bhaktimānyaḥ sa me priyaḥ (12.17)

*yo = yaḥ — who; na — not; hṛṣyāti — rejoice; na — not; dveṣṭi — hates; na — not; śocati — laments; na — not; kāṅkṣati — craves; śubhāśubhaparityāgī = subhasubha — agreeable and disagreeable + parityāgī — leaving aside; bhaktimān — full of devotion; yaḥ — who; sa = saḥ — he; me — of me; priyaḥ — dear*

**One who does not rejoice, or hate, or lament, or crave, who left aside what is agreeable and disagreeable, who is full of devotion, is dear to Me. (12.17)**

***Siddha Swami's Commentary:***

A *yogin* who has to discipline someone for the Universal Form, should be so advanced in the practice of *buddhi yoga*, that he should not have an urge to rejoice or lament over the matter. He should execute it indifferently, realizing that he has nothing to do with the affair. It is just like a policeman's arrest of a wanted man. The officer should not indulge in thinking that the man is guilty or innocent but should merely arrest the individual and take him to the authorities of law.

The terms *yah sa me priyah*, which mean one who is dear to *Śrī* Krishna, as well as the use of the terms *madbhaktah* and *bhaktimān* in this verse and verses 13, 14, 15, 17, 19 and 20, show the stress placed on being a devotee of *Śrī* Krishna. And such a devotee, if he masters the *buddhi yoga* process, will exceed other yogins who are not devotees and who master *buddhi yoga* either by self discovery or by instruction from others. This is assured by *Śrī* Krishna.

समः शत्रौ च मित्रे च
तथा मानावमानयोः ।
शीतोष्णसुखदुःखेषु
समः सङ्गविवर्जितः ॥१२.१८॥
samaḥ śatrau ca mitre ca
tathā mānāvamānayoḥ
śītoṣṇasukhaduḥkheṣu
samaḥ saṅgavivarjitaḥ (12.18)

*samaḥ — equally disposed; śatrau — and to an enemy; ca — and; mitre — to friend; ca — and; tathā — similar; mānāvamānayoḥ — in honor and dishonor; śītoṣṇasukhaduḥkheṣu = śīta — cold + uṣṇa — heat + sukha — happiness + duḥkheṣu — in distress; samaḥ — same; saṅgavivarjitaḥ = saṅga — attachment + vivarjitaḥ — freedom from*

**Being equally disposed to an enemy and a friend, with a similar attitude in honor and dishonor, in cold and heat, happiness and distress, being free from attachment, (12.18)**

***Siddha Swami's Commentary:***

These qualities are developed not directly but by controlling the psyche, which consists of the mental compartment, intellect, memory, sensual energy and life force. When these are purified and controlled, then the *yogin* becomes equally disposed to enemies and friends. He develops a similar attitude when honored or ridiculed, in cold or heat, in happiness and distress. He is free from attachment because he develops a lack of interest even in his material well-being. Having become anchored in higher levels of reality, the significance of these lower dimensions decreases rapidly for him.

तुल्यनिन्दास्तुतिर्मौनी
संतुष्टो येन केनचित् ।
अनिकेतः स्थिरमतिर्
भक्तिमान्मे प्रियो नरः ॥१२.१९॥
tulyanindāstutirmaunī
saṁtuṣṭo yena kenacit
aniketaḥ sthiramatir
bhaktimānme priyo naraḥ (12.19)

*tulyanindāstutiḥ = tulya — relates to + nindā — condemnation + stutiḥ — glorification; maunī — silent; saṁtuṣṭo = saṁtuṣṭaḥ — content; yena — with what; kenacit = kenacid — with anything; aniketaḥ — without a house; sthiramatiḥ = sthira —steady + matiḥ —mind; bhaktimān — full of devotion; me — of me; priyo = priyaḥ — dear; naraḥ — person*

**...one who relates equally to condemnation and glorification, who is silent, content with anything, who is unattached to home, who has a steady mind, and who is full of devotion, that person is dear to Me. (12.19)**

***Siddha Swami's Commentary:***

In these descriptions, the importance of devotion to *Śrī* Krishna is ever present. Conversely if the *yogin* has no such devotion, but remains sincere in the practice of *buddhi yoga*, he will achieve success and will as a matter of course, realize the Supreme Being. So long as he keeps advancing, the realization of the Supreme will be attained by him. And nothing is more convincing than direct experience which *Śrī* Krishna directly attested to earlier.

Devotion to *Śrī* Krishna makes the yoga process an easier and faster one, because the *yogin* does not have to discover every stage by himself painstakingly, but moves through the course academically and practically under the teaching influence of *Śrī* Krishna and yogins who represent the Lord. These verses guarantee that if a person practices *buddhi* yogi and masters it sufficiently, he becomes very dear to Lord Krishna. By mastery of *buddhi yoga*, he sets aside the troublesome energies in the psyche and is no longer inspired to oppose the will of the Central Person in the Universal Form.

ये तु धर्म्यामृतमिदं
यथोक्तं पर्युपासते ।
श्रद्दधाना मत्परमा
भक्तास्तेऽतीव मे प्रियाः ॥ १२.२० ॥
ye tu dharmyāmṛtamidaṁ
yathoktaṁ paryupāsate
śraddadhānā matparamā
bhaktāste'tīva me priyāḥ (12.20)

*ye — who; tu — but; dharmyāmṛtam = dharmya — codes of behavior + amṛtam — life-giving; idam — this; yathoktaṁ = yathā — as + uktaṁ — declared; paryupāsate — they honor; śraddhadhānā — having confidence; matparamā — absorbed in me as top priority; bhaktāḥ— be devoted; te — they; 'tīva = atīva — very very; me — to me; priyaḥ — dear*

**Those who honor these life-giving codes of behavior, who have confidence, being intent on Me as top-priority, being devoted, are very dear. (12.20)**

***Siddha Swami's Commentary:***

By the practice of *dharmyāmṛtam*, life-giving codes of behavior, the subtle body is highly energized and the *yogin* becomes eligible for higher and higher grades of existence. Because *Śrī* Krishna is the highest of the living beings, those who are intent on Him as the top priority will eventually, as fast as they can become qualified, attain His location. It would hinge on their qualification, their ability to upgrade their psychology. The proper codes of behavior (*dharmya*) enable a living being to move from a lower to a higher status, but such a person must first adopt higher intake of subtle energy, so that the subtle system of the psyche changes in an upward direction.

The more and more pure one becomes, the dearer and dearer one becomes to *Śrī* Krishna.

# CHAPTER 13

# Anādimat Param Brahma

## The Beginningless Supreme Reality *

*jñeyaṁ yattatpravakṣyāmi yajjñātvāmṛtamaśnute*
*anādimatparaṁ brahma na sattannāsaducyate (13.13)*

***I will explain that which is to be experienced, knowing which one gets in touch with eternal life. The beginningless Supreme Reality is said to be neither substantial nor insubstantial. (13.13)***

***Siddha Swami assigned this chapter title on the basis of verse 13 of this chapter.**

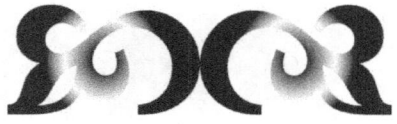

अर्जुन उवाच
प्रकृतिं पुरुषं चैव
क्षेत्रं क्षेत्रज्ञमेव च ।
एतद्वेदितुमिच्छामि
ज्ञानं ज्ञेयं च केशव ॥१३.१॥
arjuna uvāca
prakṛtiṁ puruṣaṁ caiva
kṣetraṁ kṣetrajñameva ca
etadveditumicchāmi
jñānaṁ jñeyaṁ ca keśava (13.1)

*arjuna — Arjuna; uvāca — said; prakṛtiṁ — material nature; puruṣaṁ — person; caiva — and indeed; kṣetraṁ — the living space; kṣetrajñam — the experiencer of the living space; eva — indeed; ca — and; etad — this; veditum — to know; icchāmi — I wish; jñānaṁ — conclusion; jñeyaṁ — what is to be experienced; ca — and; keśava — pretty-haired one*

**Arjuna said: What is material nature? What is the person? What is the living space? Who is the experiencer of the living space? I wish to know this. What is a conclusion? And what is experienced, O Keshava, pretty-haired One? (13.1)**

***Siddha Swami's Commentary:***

Even after seeing the glorious vision of the Universal Form, as well as the four-handed Divine Form of *Śrī* Krishna, Arjuna still had unresolved questions. This means that merely by the experience of the Universal Power and the divine forms of the Divinity, still a devotee, even one as dear as Arjuna, may need further explanations.

The idea that nothing remains to be seen after the Universal Form or even the Divine Form of *Śrī* Krishna, is true in theory. With due reason, if the Universal Form is the source of these manifestations, then Its appearance is the ultimate significance of anything that was, is, and will be. However, that still does not erase our personal need for explanations about specific features of the existences.

Arjuna needed to understand certain things in detail, and thus he persisted in questioning *Śrī* Krishna. Arjuna did not ask these questions just to query *Śrī* Krishna for our sake. Each person will need to pry into certain truths even after receiving the revelations. This verifies our individuality and its uniqueness. Each devotee has within his psychology certain things to resolve. Some of this may be resolved by supernatural visions and spiritual apparitions, but some of the questions will remain even after that and will be resolved only by in-depth mystic research by the said devotee.

Let us look at this inquiry of Arjuna. He again asked about material nature. This is certainly the most troublesome and persistent of the realities faced by a limited being. Unless one understands material nature fully, one cannot permanently transcend it. There is another facet which must be grasped, namely the relationship between the self and material nature. That relationship stymies the limited self and keeps him time bound. He must himself understand it, study it and make efforts to upgrade himself. Naturally God must help him but he must also make endeavor, or he will remain under the dominance of material nature.

Arjuna asked about the person. This is because the confusion of psychology persists. Who is the person? Is the mind the person? Is it the emotions? Is it the combination of the mind and emotions? Is it the so called ego or do these aspects make up different parts of what we call the person? What is the spirit? Arjuna witnessed much in the Universal Form and the Divine four-handed Form, but that did not help him clarify for him his own individual psychology. We should take note of this.

He asked about the living space, the psychological environment in which the ego is housed. What is that? What is it made of? As we can understand the material atmosphere and see objects floating about in the form of planets and stars, can we see the objects in the psychological space? How can this be done? Will we ever have clarity in the sky of consciousness?

He asked about the experiencer of the living space. This question is similar to the question about the *puruṣam* person. Who is the one who experiences the psychological environment? Is there more than one observer, and more than one type of such observers?

Arjuna declared that he wanted to know of that in detail. It was not sufficient to see the Universal Form and God's hold on this world nor the four-handed Divine Form of *Śrī* Krishna. In addition, he asked for a clear idea of a conclusion and of what is experienced by a living being. Is the experience merely material consisting of subtle and gross reality? Is the experience in the material world, a mixture of spiritual and material facets?

श्रीभगवानुवाच
इदं शरीरं कौन्तेय
क्षेत्रमित्यभिधीयते ।
एतद्यो वेत्ति तं प्राहुः
क्षेत्रज्ञ इति तद्विदः. ॥ १३.२ ॥
śrībhagavānuvāca
idaṁ śarīraṁ kaunteya
kṣetramityabhidhīyate
etadyo vetti taṁ prāhuḥ
kṣetrajña iti tadvidaḥ (13.2)

*śrī bhagavān — the Blessed Lord; uvāca — said; idaṁ — this; śarīraṁ — earthly body; kaunteya — O son of Kuntī; kṣetraṁ — the living space; iti — thus; abhidhīyate — it is called; etat — this; yo = yaḥ — who; vetti — knows; taṁ — him; prāhuḥ — they declare; kṣetrajña — experiencer of the living space; iti — thus; tadvidaḥ — of those knowledgeable of that*

**The Blessed Lord said: This, the earthly body, O son of Kuntī, is called the living space. Those who are knowledgeable of this, declare the person who understands this to be the experiencer of the living space. (13.2)**

***Siddha Swami's Commentary:***

*Śrī* Krishna defined each of the terms of Arjuna's query in very clear terms. He said that the living space or psychological environment is the earthly body. The term *śarīram* means the living physical body. It is interesting that *Śrī* Krishna termed that as a psychological environment. That is the teaching in *brahma yoga*. This is because the subtle body is intermeshed or interspaced into any living physical form. The subtle body itself may be termed as the psychological environment for the individual soul but higher than that body and more enduring and essential to a spirit's presence in the material world, is the causal body. Hence, the causal body, which consists of only psychic energy with identity potential, is ultimately the most basic psychological environment in this world. But so long as there is a physical body, we must accept the existence of a subtle and causal form dimensionally spaced with it. All this is to be realized and perceived directly by the yogi devotee in meditation practice. Only by psychic purity can one perceive this. So long as one's mind attaches to material objects, even sacred material objects like the Deity in the temple, one cannot have causal perception. And thus one will have to be content with information about these facets only, without the mystic perception of these.

Even though *Śrī* Krishna defined the living material body to be the living space, or the environment in which the spirit is housed, still he quoted previous authorities who stated that only those who understand this are in fact experiencers of the psyche. This means that the mere information does not qualify one as an experiencer of the psyche. The reason is this: The psyche is designed to give experiences of external phenomena in the physical environment. That is its natural capability. Hence without subtle awareness, one will not be conscious of the parts of one's own psychology, even though one will know much of the physical world outside one's body.

Let us take for example the organs within the physical body. These organs cannot be seen by the physical eyes of that body. But those eyes may easily see other objects which are outside the body. Hence unless one has mystic vision he cannot see inside his subtle body.

It is said that seeing is believing, but many teachers incorrectly speak as if believing is seeing. To be a *puruṣa* one has to see the organs in the body, specifically inside the subtle form. This is not perceived easily. That vision cannot be developed by an easy method like chanting the names and glories of *Śrī* Krishna, otherwise Arjuna would have used such a method. The subtle body becomes available for directive usage only through austerities in *buddhi yoga* practice and not otherwise, unless one is a divine being on par with or near par to *Śrī* Krishna. If one is on Arjuna's level or below, one cannot use the subtle body for subtle vision without *buddhi yoga*.

क्षेत्रज्ञं चापि मां विद्धि
सर्वक्षेत्रेषु भारत ।
क्षेत्रक्षेत्रज्ञयोर्ज्ञानं
यत्तज्ज्ञानं मतं मम ॥ १३.३
kṣetrajñaṁ cāpi māṁ viddhi
sarvakṣetreṣu bhārata
kṣetrakṣetrajñayorjñānaṁ
yattajjñānaṁ mataṁ mama (13.3)

*kṣetrajñam — the experiencer of the living space; cāpi = ca — and + api — also; māṁ — me, viddhi — know; sarvakṣetreṣu — of all living spaces; bhārata — O man of the Bhārata family; kṣetrakṣetrajñayoḥ — of the living space and the experiencer of it; jñānaṁ — information; yat — which; tat — that; jñānaṁ — knowledge; mataṁ — considered; mama — by me*

**Know also, that I am the experiencer of all living spaces, O man of the Bharata family. Information of the living space and the experiencer of it, is considered by Me to be knowledge. (13.3)**

***Siddha Swami's Commentary:***

*Śrī* Krishna accredited himself as the super-experiencer, the super-person who experiences all living spaces, all the psychological units used by the limited beings. Thus He is known as the *Mahāpuruṣa*, the Great Person, the greatest of the persons in existence, the super-perceiver.

He said that knowledge really means information about the psychology and the person who inhabits it. But conventionally, knowledge is interpreted as what is encountered in the physical world.

तत्क्षेत्रं यच्च यादृक् च
यद्विकारि यतश्च यत् ।
स च यो यत्प्रभावश्च
तत्समासेन मे शृणु ॥ १३.४॥

*tat = tad — this; kṣetraṁ — living space; yat — what; ca — and; yadṛk — what kind?; ca — and; yadvikāri = yad — what + vikāri — changes; yataśca = yataḥ— what causes?; ca — and; yat — what; sa = saḥ — he; ca — and; yo = yaḥ — who; yatprabhāvaḥ*

tatkṣetraṁ yacca yādṛk ca
yadvikāri yataśca yat
sa ca yo yatprabhāvaśca
tatsamāsena me śṛṇu (13.4)

*= yat (yad) — what + prabhāvaḥ — potential + ca — and; tat = tad — that; samāsena — with brevity, in brief; me — of me; śṛṇu — hear*

**As for this living space, as for what is, as for what kind of environment it is, as for the changes it endures, as to what causes it to change, as for he who is involved, as for his potential, hear from Me of that in brief. (13.4)**

***Siddha Swami's Commentary:***

*Śrī* Krishna decided to elaborate on the psychology, the changes within it, the pressures which affect it, the entity who is housed in it and the potential development of that individual spirit.

ऋषिभिर्बहुधा गीतं
छन्दोभिर्विविधैः पृथक् ।
ब्रह्मसूत्रपदैश्चैव
हेतुमद्भिर्विनिश्चितैः ॥१३.५॥
ṛṣibhirbahudhā gītaṁ
chandobhirvividhaiḥ pṛthak
brahmasūtrapadaiścaiva
hetumadbhirviniścitaiḥ (13.5)

*ṛṣibhiḥ — by the yogī sages; bahudhā — many times; gītaṁ — recited; chandobhiḥ — with Vedic hymns; vividhaiḥ — with various; pṛthak — distinctly; brahmasūtrapadaiścaiva = brahmasūtrapadaiḥ — with Brahma-sūtra verses + ca — and + eva — indeed; hetumadbhiḥ — with sound logic; viniścataiḥ — with definite, conclusive*

**This was distinctly recited many times with the various Vedic hymns and with the Brahma Sūtras, conclusively with sound logic, by the great yogi sages. (13.5)**

***Siddha Swami's Commentary:***

The research into these matters on the mystic plane was done before the advent of *Śrī* Krishna. But even so, to know this fully, each person must develop the *buddhi yoga* practice to get the mystic insight for personal observation of these truths. *Śrī* Krishna mentioned the recital of Vedic hymns and the *Brahma Sūtras* which explained the status of the individual person and his or her psychology.

महाभूतान्यहंकारो
बुद्धिरव्यक्तमेव च ।
इन्द्रियाणि दशैकं च
पञ्च चेन्द्रियगोचराः ॥१३.६॥
mahābhūtānyahaṁkāro
buddhiravyaktameva ca
indriyāṇi daśaikaṁ ca
pañca cendriyagocarāḥ (13.6)

*mahābhūtāni — major elements; ahaṁkāro = ahaṁkāraḥ = ahaṁ— I, person + kāraḥ — doing, initiative to act; buddhiḥ— intellect; avyaktam — unmanifested energy; eva — indeed; ca — and; indriyāṇi — senses; daśaikaṁ = dasa — ten + ekam — one; ca — and; pañca — five; cendriyagocarāḥ = ca — and + indriyagocarāḥ — attractive objects*

**The major categories of the elements, the personal initiative, the intellect, the unmanifested energy, the ten and one senses, the five attractive objects, (13.6)**

***Siddha Swami's Commentary:***

The material world, as we commonly know it and as the animals also perceive it, is based on causal forces, which are very subtle energies. Therefore in this explanation, one should not look for or expect much elaboration about physical matter. It is subtle energy which underlines the gross world. *Buddhi yoga* and *brahma yoga* concern subtle and super-subtle energy.

A human being or animal knows well the major categories of elements, for such a creature cannot avoid contact with these, which are solids, liquids, combustives, flames, gases and spaces. These have subtle counterparts. Even in the subtle body, there are substances which though subtle to a material body, are gross to an ethereal form. Thus the physical world has a subtle counterpart.

Overall the subtle energies are regarded as being light energy and radio frequencies. But besides these, there is the personal initiative which is individualized. There is an intellect or a calculating instrument which operates by light frequency. There is the unmanifested subtle material energy known as pranic psychic force. This energy operates the intellect. There are the sensual energies which divest into vision, hearing, touching, tasting and smelling. And there are the sensual utilities in the form of hands for grasping, feet for motion, vocal cord for speaking, and anus and genital for evacuating.

The gross material energy emerges as five attractive objects which are sensed as sounds, surfaces, colors, flavors and odors. This is information, but in *buddhi yoga* the information is given to motivate the student to develop psychic perception.

इच्छा द्वेषः सुखं दुःखं
संघातश्चेतना धृतिः ।
एतत्क्षेत्रं समासेन
सविकारमुदाहृतम् ॥ १३.७॥
icchā dveṣaḥ sukhaṁ duḥkhaṁ
saṁghātaścetanā dhṛtiḥ
etatkṣetraṁ samāsena
savikāramudāhṛtam (13.7)

*icchā — desire; dveṣaḥ — hatred; sukhaṁ — pleasure; duḥkhaṁ — pain; saṁghātaścetanā = saṁghātaḥ — the whole body + cetana — consciousness; dhṛtiḥ — conviction; etat = etad — this; kṣetraṁ — living space; samāsena — with brevity, briefly; savikāram — with changes; udāhṛtam — described*

**...desire, hatred, pleasure, pain, the whole body, consciousness and conviction; this is described with brevity, as the living space with its changes. (13.7)**

***Siddha Swami's Commentary:***

This verse provides evidence that the living space or psychology comprises the subtle and causal bodies in conjunction with a living physical one, since the physical body by itself is not consciousness. A dead physical body does not display the type of consciousness we observe in a living physical one.

Aspects of the psychology like desire, hatred, pleasure and pain, come from consciousness. These in turn motivate the physical body to act. But we must meditate to see that desire, hatred, pleasure, pain and conviction are parts of the subtle body and originate in the causal form.

By tradition, we feel that the whole body, the *samghātaś*, is the person. We call this the human being or animal, the man or woman, dog or cat. In reality, this whole body is an aggregate of various parts that can be studied by mystic perception in *buddhi yoga* practice.

अमानित्वमदम्भित्वम्
अहिंसा क्षान्तिरार्जवम् ।
आचार्योपासनं शौचं
स्थैर्यमात्मविनिग्रहः ॥ १३.८॥

*amānitvaṁ — a lack of pride; adambhitvam — freedom from deceit; ahiṁsā — non-violence; kṣāntiḥ — patience; ārjavam — straightforwardness; ācāryopāsanaṁ — sitting near a teacher, attendance to a teacher; śaucaṁ*

amānitvamadambhitvam
ahiṁsā kṣāntirārjavam
ācāryopāsanaṁ śaucaṁ
sthairyamātmavinigrahaḥ (13.8)

— *purity; sthairyam — stability; ātmavinigrahaḥ — ātma — self + vinigrahaḥ — restraint*

**Lack of pride, freedom from deceit, non-violence, patience, straightforwardness, attendance to a teacher, purity, stability and self-restraint, (13.8)**

***Siddha Swami's Commentary:***

*Śrī* Krishna gave definitions from the spiritual viewpoint. This is learned in the practice of *buddhi yoga*. This is different from the traditional knowledge which concerns only the gross world and how we may exploit it. Those habituated to the gross existence, even devotees who are fond of the material world, will not appreciate these definitions. However all persons may at least hear of this, since it was described by the Supreme Person. One who is materialistic, even a devotee of *Śrī* Krishna, will continue in such pursuits even after hearing and will be reluctant to take up *buddhi yoga*. Still such a person will lose nothing by considering this.

The method used to rid bad qualities and assume good ones, differs from person to person. Few are successful in trying to rid themselves permanently of bad tendencies. However, many succeed in temporarily suppressing the bad traits. By using methods which cannot possibly get to the root of the problems. In yoga practice, the two preliminary stages are *yama*, moral restraints, and *niyama*, recommended observances. These are what should be done and what should not be done. They are behavioral prohibitions and approvals. At first a person expects these to be administered and practiced only on the physical plane, because a human being gives import to the physical level, while treating the subtle ones as unsubstantial since they border on or comprise of dreams and imagination. However, when one practices yoga seriously, particularly *buddhi yoga*, one understands that the *yama* and *niyama* regulations apply to the subtle level even more than to the gross plane.

It is the subtle body which forms the bed-rock or foundation of the gross one. It is the subtle body which enjoys experiences of the gross one and which shies away from unpleasant gross experiences. Hence it is the tendencies of the subtle bodies which need to be curbed.

In higher yoga, the bad qualities are eliminated by flushing the energies in the psyche which support, sponsor and cause irregular and spiritually-destructive behaviors. That is a different approach to the one used in traditional religion, where a person struggles with bad qualities by substituting good ones. If the energy of bad qualities is removed in the subtle and causal forms, then those qualities cannot be exhibited.

This is all well and good as an explanation of the means used in higher yoga, in *buddhi yoga*, but how is this done in fact? What are the *kriyā*s or mystic and physical methods used to achieve this?

**Lack of pride**, if accomplished by a *yogin*, is achieved by regulating the energy of identity in the causal body. But a *yogin* cannot, at first, discipline the causal form. He must first take control of the subtle body, before he tries to restrict the intake of energies of the causal form. In the causal body there are two basic energies. These are the sense of *I am* and the super-subtle energy from which the sensual apparatus in the subtle form is created. This sense of, *I am,* causes pride. But pride develops in it by means of the kind of super-subtle energy it utilizes and by the kind of energy the subtle body uses. Thus in the beginning, a *yogin* has to curb his psychic energy intake to regulate this. He does this by practicing various types of *prāṇāyāma* and meditation in which he trains his psyche to reject certain subtle energies.

**Deceit** also originates from the sense of identity in the causal form. It spreads out into the subtle body and is based on the causal and subtle energy intakes. In the subtle body, deceit is sponsored by the two lower chakras, the ones which regulate excretion and sexuality. Thus a yogi has to curb that by practicing kundalini yoga to clean out the subtle system of chakras in the spine of the subtle body. In elementary religions, it is believed that by practicing honesty, one will get rid of deceit. But this is an ineffective method, since so long as the two lower chakras are impure, the psychology will have to exhibit deceitful behaviors as it is forced to do so by the nature of the impure energies. This is why in yoga, the methods of elementary religion are cast aside and the *kriyās* are adopted.

**Violence** is a basic requirement in the subtle and gross material world. But it is more of a serious problem in the gross world, since in the subtle one, the violence does not kill the body but only incapacitates it for a short period of time. Violence is sponsored by the lower four chakras in the subtle body. Its removal from the psyche is completed only if one gets rid of the subtle body. It may be decreased almost to nil by the purification of the four lower chakras that control excretion, sexuality, nutrition and affection.

In the *Bhagavad Gītā*, we learn that violence is used by the Central Person in the Universal Form, and that it exists and is exhibited even on the supernatural level, where many subtle bodies clash. Therefore violence is part and parcel of the material world and even the divinities wield it. For them it is a disciplinary tool. For others, it is a tool for survival and protection of dependents. When Arjuna saw the four-handed Divine Form, there was no exhibition of violence, even though the Form carried two tools for violence which were the disc and club.

*kirīṭinaṁ gadinaṁ cakrahastam icchāmi tvāṁ draṣṭumahaṁ tathaiva*
*tenaiva rūpeṇa caturbhujena sahasrabāho bhava viśvamūrte (11.46)*

***I wish to see You wearing a crown, armed with a club, and with a disc in hand, as requested. Please become that four-armed form, O thousand-armed Person, O Person of universal dimensions. (11.46)***

While the four-handed Form carried weapons as a formality and as insignia only, the Thousand-armed Person of Universal Dimensions carried weapons to thwart those opposed to His desires. Thus we understand that a *yogin* can only rid himself of violence if he gets an exemption from serving the Universal Form. There are many verses in the *Bhagavad Gītā* which hint at and definitely indicate such an exemption. For instance:

*adveṣṭā sarvabhūtānāṁ maitraḥ karuṇa eva ca*
*nirmamo nirahaṁkāraḥ samaduḥkhasukhaḥ kṣamī (12.13)*

***One who does not dislike any of the creatures, who is friendly and compassionate, free from attachment to possessions, free from the propensity of "I am the creator of my actions," being equally disposed towards pain and pleasure, being patient, (12.13)***

Yogis who exhibit such qualities consistently and permanently, are those who have purified their four lower chakras, or who, though having not purified those chakras in this life, did so in a relevant past life. Due to their past they carry the tendency over into this life.

**Impatience** involves the causal body, in which there is a subtle energy which converts into desire on the subtle plane. In higher yoga, one learns how to remain resistant to the penetration of that subtle energy which is converted into desire and motivation in the subtle form. Unless each yogi endeavors to curb his nature he cannot relinquish bad qualities permanently. He himself must endeavor, because his susceptibility to the subtle influences causes bad behavior. It is his own relationship to the subtle material energy which he experiences as emotional and mental force in his mind and feelings. He must develop resistance to these. God's resistance or a teacher's resistance gives one an idea of what that resistance can achieve. One may strive under their direction for mastership over lower propensities.

इन्द्रियार्थेषु वैराग्यम्
अनहंकार एव च ।
जन्ममृत्युजराव्याधि-
दुःखदोषानुदर्शनम् ॥ १३.९ ॥
indriyārtheṣu vairāgyam
anahaṁkāra eva ca
janmamṛtyujarāvyādhi-
duḥkhadoṣānudarśanam (13.9)

*indriyārtheṣu — towards the attractive objects; vairāgyam — indifference; anahaṁkāra = an — absence of + ahaṁkāra — motivated initiative; eva — indeed; ca — and; janmamṛtyujarāvyādhi = janma — birth + mṛtyu — death + jarā — old age + vyādhi — disease; duḥkhadoṣānudarśanam = duḥkha — suffering + doṣa — danger + anudarśanam — perception*

**..indifference towards the attractive objects, absence of motivated initiative, the perception of the danger of birth, death, old age, disease, and suffering, (13.9)**

***Siddha Swami's Commentary:***

Forceful and involuntary attraction to dangerous but attractive objects comes about because in the psyche resides forces which are different to the core self and which require fulfillment that runs contrary to the wellbeing of the self. Until these forces are removed from the psyche or disabled in it, one will be subjected to irresistible attractions, to dangerous and spiritually-destructive objects. These objects act in such a way as to cause one to adopt a responsibility for them and to become liable for their activities.

*Śrī Patañjali Mahārṣi* recommended the stilling of the mento-emotional energy, the *citta* force. The achievement of that is only completed by a few advanced yogins. That mental and emotional power forces the psyche, hence the core self, to chase after and to become responsible and liable for whimsical attractive objects, either animate or inanimate. Thus curbing and purifying the mental and emotional force is necessary. This is achieved in kundalini and *kriyā yoga*, which are both parts of *buddhi yoga*.

So long as there is a causal body, the sense of initiative to act cannot be removed; it is an essential and permanent part of the causal form. The motivations of that initiative are expanded in the subtle body and drive that form to seek procurements. When something is acquired by the subtle form, it is experienced either as a desirable, undesirable or non-stimulating object. These objects may be subtle. For instance, a flavor might emanate from something gross or it might occur all by itself without being borne in a gross form. The fact that flavors and other objects occur in the realm of imagination, proves that these have their own subtle form which may occur without gross embodiment.

All of the subtle body's flaws are traceable to the causal form, but in the causal situation, those flaws remain unmanifested and undisplayed. However in higher yoga, one learns to detect the causal energies and to remove oneself from their associations. If one cannot do this, one will by necessity be subjected to their exhibition in the subtle form. Since some of these exhibitions are pleasurable, one develops a reluctance to eliminate them and one becomes conditioned to them. This leads to the cultivation of vices on the material plane. These are spear-headed by the vice of sexual indulgence.

Therefore, celibacy through yoga practice is the counteracting measure for weaning the subtle body from vices and attacking the seed energies in the causal form. The subtle body specifically is subjected to the need for sexual companionship so unless that body is curbed, one cannot eliminate the need for sexual intercourse.

If one remains under the influence of desire, one cannot perceive the dangers of material existence which brings birth, suffering, disease, old age and death. This is because one's discernment is stymied by changes in the subtle body during its creation and maintenance of a gross form. Since one's attention is helplessly attached to the subtle body, its alternations become a sure distraction and so one is unable to assess material existence objectively. When at last one gets help from the Supreme Being and from His agent, one can relinquish the fascination with the subtle form, and one strives to segregate oneself from the forces which promote the predominance of the subtle form. Only then does one subjugate the causal body and get some idea of the possibility of liberation.

असक्तिरनभिष्वङ्गः
पुत्रदारगृहादिषु ।
नित्यं च समचित्तत्वम्
इष्टानिष्टोपपत्तिषु ॥१३.१०॥
asaktiranabhiṣvaṅgaḥ
putradāragṛhādiṣu
nityaṁ ca samacittatvam
iṣṭāniṣṭopapattiṣu (13.10)

*asaktiḥ — non-attachment, social detachment; anabhiṣvaṅgaḥ — absence of emotional affection; putradāragṛhādiṣu = putra — child + dāra — wife + gṛha — home + ādiṣu — beginning with, whatever is related to; nityaṁ — always; ca — and; samacittatvam — even-mindedness; iṣṭāniṣṭopapattiṣu = iṣṭa — undesired + aniṣṭa — not wanted + upapattiṣu — in matters*

**...social and emotional detachment towards child, wife, a home and whatever is related to social life, being always even-minded towards what is desired and what is not wanted, (13.10)**

***Siddha Swami's Commentary:***

Social life and the need for it is sourced in the subtle body; hence the necessity exists to bring that form under control. Whatever is problematic with the gross body is traceable to the subtle form. Therefore, to come to terms with the subtle form, one must master higher yoga in mystic actions.

No matter where one may go, one will have some type of social life. Therefore a *yogin* aspires for such life with higher entities in a superior environment. Higher association, becoming compatible with superior yogins and the divine beings, is the key to ridding oneself of the need for lower social life.

The addiction to social life in terms of children and spouse, home and whatever else that entails, is a primitive attachment, which may be overcome by mastership of kundalini yoga. So long as the kundalini system of energies is oriented downwards, it will foster the development of such social life and afflict the subtle body with such fulfillments; hence the need to perfect kundalini yoga. Women especially are victims of the need for such social life but they can overcome it by the practice of yoga combined with higher association. Many of the angelic women display a detachment from such social life and effectively avoid it by not taking birth in a situation where children are a necessary part of the generation process.

In this world, women have a tendency for expanding social life but the pains of it eventually inspire them to work for its elimination. However, unless their subtle energies are purified, no elimination can occur.

मयि चानन्ययोगेन
भक्तिरव्यभिचारिणी ।
विविक्तदेशसेवित्वम्
अरतिर्जनसंसदि ॥ १३.११ ॥
mayi cānanyayogena
bhaktiravyabhicāriṇī
viviktadeśasevitvam
aratirjanasaṁsadi (13.11)

*mayi — in me; cānanyayogena = ca — and + ananya — no other + yogena — with yoga practice; bhaktiḥ — devotion; avyabhicārinī — not wandering away, unwavering; viviktadeśasevitvam = vivikta — secluded + deśa — place + sevitvam — resorting; aratiḥ — having a dislike; janasaṁsadi — in crowds of human beings*

**...unswerving devotion to Me, with no other discipline but yoga practice, resorting to a secluded place, having a dislike for crowds of human beings, (13.11)**

***Siddha Swami's Commentary:***

Unswerving devotion to *Śrī* Krishna must include yoga practice as it is defined in Chapter Six of the *Gītā*, for without yoga practice, the psyche cannot be purified. And without such purity, one cannot in truth reach *Śrī* Krishna. One must also resort to a secluded place in order to conserve time for yoga practice and to listen on the subtle level to higher yogins and the Supreme Person.

On a close inspection of the Sanskrit for this verse, one may clarify that yoga and *bhakti* or devotion are two separate cultivations. *Yogena* means with yoga. This is why the ending of that Sanskrit word is there. *Bhaktih* means devotion, as indicated by the Sanskrit word-ending *ih*. This means both *bhakti* and yoga. Further verification is given by the terms *viviktadeśasevitvam*, resorting to a secluded place, which was a requirement listed for yoga practice in Chapter Six, verse 10.

One must have a dislike for crowds of human beings; otherwise one will never get the full purification required to complete the practice of yoga. Involvement with human beings means social occupation, which leads to lack of time for yoga practice and the remaining of oneself in environments which are hostile to yoga.

अध्यात्मज्ञाननित्यत्वं
तत्त्वज्ञानार्थदर्शनम् ।
एतज्ज्ञानमिति प्रोक्तम्
अज्ञानं यदतोऽन्यथा ॥ १३.१२ ॥
adhyātmajñānanityatvaṁ
tattvajñānārthadarśanam
etajjñānamiti proktam
ajñānaṁ yadato'nyathā (13.12)

*adhyātmajñānanityatvam = adhyātma — Supreme Spirit + jñana — information + nityatvam — constantly; tattvajñānārtha darśanam = tattva — reality + jñāna — science + artha — value + darśanam — perceiving; etat — this; jñānam — knowledge; iti — thus; proktam — declared as; ajñānaṁ — ignorance; yat — whatever; ato = ataḥ — to this; 'nyathā = anyathā — otherwise, contrary*

**...constantly considering information about the Supreme Spirit, perceiving the value of the science of reality; this is declared as knowledge. Whatever is contrary to this, is ignorance. (13.12)**

***Siddha Swami's Commentary:***

Even though existence in the material world takes up one's attention, one must resist this with all determination and take every opportunity to practice the *buddhi yoga* discipline. One should constantly consider information about the Supreme Spirit and continually shift one's mind from its preoccupation with material things. One must also shift one's emotions from attachments to pleasurable experiences. This all requires personal endeavor.

*Śrī* Krishna listed aspects in this verse, as well as in the four preceding verses. These He declared as knowledge and all else as ignorance. Thus one must fight the psyche whenever it portrays what is contrary as being knowledge. The subtle body is determined to be preoccupied with the gross world and with pleasurable experiences which lead downward into vices, but one must resist this and then study the mechanisms in the subtle form, so that one can effect their alteration.

ज्ञेयं यत्तत्प्रवक्ष्यामि
यज्ज्ञात्वामृतमश्नुते ।
अनादिमत्परं ब्रह्म
न सत्तन्नासदुच्यते ॥ १३.१३॥
jñeyaṁ yattatpravakṣyāmi
yajjñātvāmṛtamaśnute
anādimatparaṁ brahma
na sattannāsaducyate (13.13)

*jṇeyaṁ — to be known, the desired subject; yat — which; tat — that; pravakṣyāmi — I will explain; yat — which; jñātvā — knowing; 'mṛtam = amṛtam — eternal life; aśnute — he gets in touch with; anādimat — beginningless; paraṁ — supreme; brahma — reality; na — not; sat — substantial; tat — this; nāsat = na — not + asat — non-substantial; ucyate — is said*

**I will explain that which is to be experienced, knowing which one gets in touch with eternal life. The beginningless Supreme Reality is said to be neither substantial nor insubstantial. (13.13)**

***Siddha Swami's Commentary:***

A student *yogin* must observe *Śrī* Krishna's view of what is to be experienced. One must study this and compare it with the subtle body's view of what should be contacted. It is a fact that the subtle body will not always agree with *Śrī* Krishna. Hence there is a need to reform that subtle form, so that it comes into complete agreement with the Lord. Its purification must be effected.

In terms of detection by a gross body and even by the subtle one, the beginningless Supreme Reality appears to be neither substantial nor insubstantial. This is because the subtle body cannot fully detect that Supreme Reality. It cannot properly gage it. It can neither affirm nor deny it. It cannot properly assess the value of it.

सर्वतःपाणिपादं तत्
सर्वतोक्षिशिरोमुखम् ।
सर्वतःश्रुतिमल्लोके
सर्वमावृत्य तिष्ठति ॥ १३.१४॥
sarvataḥpāṇipādaṁ tat
sarvatokṣiśiromukham
sarvataḥśrutimalloke
sarvamāvṛtya tiṣṭhati (13.14)

*sarvataḥ — everywhere; pāṇi — hand; pādaṁ — foot; tat = tad — this; sarvato = sarvataḥ — everywhere; 'kṣiśiromukham = akṣiśiromukham = akṣi — eye + śiraḥ— head + mukham — face; sarvataḥśrutimat = sarvataḥ — everywhere + śrutimat — having hearing ability; loke — in the world; sarvam — all; āvṛtya — ranging over; tiṣṭhati — stands*

**Everywhere is Its hands and feet, everywhere Its eyes, head and face, everywhere is Its hearing ability in this world; It stands, ranging over all. (13.14)**

***Siddha Swami's Commentary:***

The beginningless Supreme Reality was a main subject for research in the time of the sages who spoke the Upanishads. They had many disputes and debates concerning that

Supreme Reality, as to whether it was personal or impersonal or comprising both. *Śrī* Krishna's teachings extol the personal and impersonal aspects with stress on the personal, claiming Himself as that Supreme Being, the God of gods.

सर्वेन्द्रियगुणाभासं
सर्वेन्द्रियविवर्जितम् ।
असक्तं सर्वभृच्चैव
निर्गुणं गुणभोक्तृ च ॥ १३.१५॥
sarvendriyaguṇābhāsaṁ
sarvendriyavivarjitam
asaktaṁ sarvabhṛccaiva
nirguṇaṁ guṇabhoktṛ ca (13.15)

*sarvendriyaguṇābhāsaṁ = sarva — all + indriyaḥ — sensual + guṇa — mood + ābhāsaṁ — appearance; sarvendriyavivarjitam = sarva — all + indriya — sensuousness + vivarjitam — freedom from; asaktaṁ — unattached; sarvabhṛt — maintaining everything; caiva = ca — and + eva — indeed; nirguṇaṁ — free from the influence of material nature; guṇabhoktṛ — experiencer of the modes of material nature; ca — and*

**It has the appearance of having all sensual moods, and It is freed from sensuousness. Though unattached, It maintains everything. Though free from the influence of material nature, It is the experiencer of that influence nevertheless. (13.15)**

***Siddha Swami's Commentary:***

The all-pervading nature of the Supreme Reality is explained as an unattached super-subtle presence which is transcendental to everything else, and which affects all else nevertheless. This is to be perceived in higher yoga practice of *samādhi*, the continuous linking of the attention to that Supreme Reality.

The individual spirit is sometimes described as being part of that all-pervading Supreme Reality. He or she may realize this by self focus in linking itself to the all-pervading Spirit.

बहिरन्तश्च भूतानाम्
अचरं चरमेव च ।
सूक्ष्मत्वात्तदविज्ञेयं
दूरस्थं चान्तिके च तत् ॥ १३.१६ ॥
bahirantaśca bhūtānām
acaraṁ carameva ca
sūkṣmatvāttadavijñeyaṁ
dūrasthaṁ cāntike ca tat (13.16)

*bahiḥ — outside; antaḥ — inside; ca — and; bhūtānām — of the beings; acaraṁ — non-moving; caram — moving; eva — indeed; ca — and; sūkṣmatvāt — from subtlety; tat — this; avijñeyaṁ — not to be comprehended; dūrasthaṁ — situated far off; cāntike = ca — and + antike — in the location; ca — and; tat = tad — this*

**It is outside and inside the moving and non-moving beings. Because of Its subtlety, this beginningless Supreme Reality is not comprehended. This Reality is situated far away and it is in the location as well. (13.16)**

***Siddha Swami's Commentary:***

The Ultimate is ever present but transcends all formations. To find It, one only needs to connect with the most subtle of the existences. It is not something over there, far away, for it is ever present within all realities. A human being should research into his own existence to find what is even subtler than his own spirit.

*Śrī* Krishna spoke in Chapter Twelve of the imperishable, indefinable, invisible, all-pervading, inconceivable, unchanging, immovable constant reality, which He said was difficult to reach. It is far away but it is located right here as well.

अविभक्तं च भूतेषु
विभक्तमिव च स्थितम् ।
भूतभर्तृ च तज्ज्ञेयं
ग्रसिष्णु प्रभविष्णु च ॥१३.१७॥
avibhaktaṁ ca bhūteṣu
vibhaktamiva ca sthitam
bhūtabhartṛ ca tajjñeyaṁ
grasiṣṇu prabhaviṣṇu ca (13.17)

*avibhaktam — undivided; ca — and; bhūteṣu — among the beings; vibhaktam— divided; iva — as if; ca — and; sthitam — remaining; bhūtabhartṛ = bhūta — being + bhartṛ — sustainer; ca — and; tat — this; jñeyaṁ — to be known; grasiṣṇu — absorber; prabhaviṣṇu — producer; ca — and*

**It is undivided among the beings, but It appears as if It is divided in each. It is the sustainer of the beings and this should be known. It is the absorber and producer. (13.17)**

***Siddha Swami's Commentary:***

Appearing to be split into many individual beings, the Supreme Reality was depicted by some as having assumed limitless spark-like existences in the form of the numerous *ātmas* or spirits which are centralized and which energize the psyches. But actually the Supreme Reality must be undivided, even though it is the sustainer of the beings and should be known by each. Additionally, as the absorber and the producer, it appears to be paradoxical.

ज्योतिषामपि तज्ज्योतिस्
तमसः परमुच्यते ।
ज्ञानं ज्ञेयं ज्ञानगम्यं
हृदि सर्वस्य विष्ठितम् ॥१३.१८॥
jyotiṣāmapi tajjyotis
tamasaḥ paramucyate
jñānaṁ jñeyaṁ jñānagamyaṁ
hṛdi sarvasya viṣṭhitam (13.18)

*jyotiṣām — of luminaries; api — also; tat = tad — this; jyotiḥ — light; tamasaḥ — of gross or subtle darkness; param — beyond; ucyate — declared to be; jñānaṁ — information; jñeyaṁ — education; jñānagamyaṁ = jñāna — education + gamyam — goal; hṛdi — in the psychological core; sarvasya — of all; viṣṭhitam — situated*

**This is declared as the light of the luminaries, but It is beyond gross or subtle darkness. It is the information, the education and the goal of education. It is situated in the psychological core of all beings. (13.18)**

***Siddha Swami's Commentary:***

If indeed, anything is worthy of meticulous research, it is that Supreme Reality, which is the light of the luminaries, the ultimate energy source. It is the real information and education, the supreme energizer.

इति क्षेत्रं तथा ज्ञानं
ज्ञेयं चोक्तं समासतः ।
मद्भक्त एतद्विज्ञाय
मद्भावायोपपद्यते ॥१३.१९॥
iti kṣetraṁ tathā jñānaṁ
jñeyaṁ coktaṁ samāsataḥ
madbhakta etadvijñāya
madbhāvāyopapadyate (13.19)

*iti — thus; kṣetraṁ — the living space, the psychological environment; tathā — as well as; jñanaṁ — standard knowledge; jñeyaṁ — what is to be known; coktaṁ = ca — and + uktaṁ — described; samāsataḥ — in brief; madbhakta — my devotee; etad — this; vijñāya — experiencing; madbhāvāyopapadyate = madbhāvāya — to my state of being + upapadyate — draws near*

**Thus the psychological environment as well as the standard knowledge and what is to be known, was described in brief. Experiencing this, My devotee draws near to My state of being. (13.19)**

***Siddha Swami's Commentary:***

*Brahma yoga* practice concerns the experience of this by the student *yogin*. Of course he gets the information but that is not sufficient. He is urged and encouraged to work hard in the austerities to acquire direct perception for himself or herself.

The immediate psychological environment must be studied by mystic perceptions. When that is achieved, the student may research into whatever is transcendental to his core self. Obviously, a *yogin* devotee would draw near to *Śrī* Krishna's state of being as rapidly as he could gain the spiritual perceptions.

प्रकृतिं पुरुषं चैव
विद्ध्यनादी उभावपि ।
विकारांश्च गुणांश्चैव
विद्धि प्रकृतिसंभवान्॥ १३.२० ॥
prakṛtiṁ puruṣaṁ caiva
viddhyanādī ubhāvapi
vikārāṁśca guṇāṁścaiva
viddhi prakṛtisaṁbhavān (13.20)

*prakṛtiṁ — material nature; puruṣaṁ — spiritual personality; caiva = ca — and + eva — indeed; viddhi — know; anādī — beginningless; ubhau — both; api — also; vikārān — changes of the living space (see 13.4); ca — and; guṇāṁ — moods; caiva = ca — and + eva — indeed; viddhi — know; prakṛtisaṁbhavān = prakṛti — material nature + saṁbhavān — produced*

**Know that both material nature and the spiritual personality are beginningless, and know that the changes of the living space and the moods of material nature are produced from material nature. (13.20)**

***Siddha Swami's Commentary:***

Besides the beginningless Supreme Reality, there is the limited personality, the seemingly finite self, and there is also the material nature at large, which is a colossal power, vast and seemingly endless. *Śrī* Krishna acknowledged the power of material nature which causes moods and changes even in the psychology of the spirits who are described as being eternal.

कार्यकारणकर्तृत्वे
हेतुः प्रकृतिरुच्यते ।
पुरुषः सुखदुःखानां
भोक्तृत्वे हेतुरुच्यते ॥ १३.२१ ॥
kāryakāraṇakartṛtve
hetuḥ prakṛtirucyate
puruṣaḥ sukhaduḥkhānāṁ
bhoktṛtve heturucyate (13.21)

*kāryakaraṇakartṛtve = kārya — created work + karaṇa — sensual potency as a cause + kartṛtve — agency; hetuḥ — cause; prakṛtiḥ — material nature; ucyate — is said; puruṣaḥ — the spiritual personality; sukhaduḥkhānāṁ — of pleasure and pain; bhoktṛtve — in terms of experiencing; hetuḥ — cause; ucyate — is said*

**Material nature is said to be the cause in terms of created work, sensual potency and agency. The spiritual personality is said to be the cause in terms of experiencing pleasure and pain. (13.21)**

***Siddha Swami's Commentary:***

Material nature is only the immediate cause; behind it sits the same beginningless Supreme Reality, which transcends everything that is manifested in these worlds. But still, material nature cannot be ignored because it is empowered by that Supreme Reality. It may be argued that since the spirits are part and parcel of the Supreme Reality, they should not have to play games with material nature. However, it is factual that the spirits struggle with material nature and try to either suppress it in terms of its influence upon them or reject it outright for gaining liberation. Thus that struggle bears testimony to its power. *Śrī* Krishna rightly credited it as being the cause in terms of created work, sensual potency and agency. When a student *yogin* researches, he first finds the subtle material nature as the cause. If he transcends that, he finds the Supreme Reality underneath as the ultimate cause, either directly or indirectly.

Of great interest is *Śrī* Krishna's declaration that the spiritual personality, the *puruṣah*, is the cause in terms of experiencing pleasure and pain. The energies which give occasion to pleasure and pain are subtle material potencies, but these sensations are felt by the *puruṣah*, the spiritual personality, through his attached psyche which he energized by helpless proximity.

If the spiritual personality, the core self, was not finite or locative, he could not be the subject of the pleasurable or painful feelings. Thus he is definitely a focus of feelings. He needs to develop detachment from the psyche and then the feelings would not reach to torment or excite him.

पुरुषः प्रकृतिस्थो हि
भुङ्क्ते प्रकृतिजान्गुणान् ।
कारणं गुणसङ्गोऽस्य
सदसद्योनिजन्मसु ॥ १३.२२ ॥
puruṣaḥ prakṛtistho hi
bhuṅkte prakṛtijānguṇān
kāraṇaṁ guṇasaṅgo'sya
sadasadyonijanmasu (13.22)

*puruṣaḥ — spirit; prakṛtistho = prakṛtisthaḥ — situated in material nature; hi — indeed; bhuṅkte — experiencing; prakṛtijān — produced on material nature; guṇān — the modes of material nature; kāraṇaṁ — the source; guṇasaṅgo = guṇasaṅgaḥ — attachment to the influence of material nature; 'sya = asya — of it; sadasadyonijanmasu = sad (sat) — reality + asad (asat) — unrealistic + yoni — birth situations + janmasu — birth*

**The spirit, being situated in material nature, experiences the modes which were produced by that nature. Attachment to the modes is the cause of the spirit's emergence from realistic and unrealistic situations. (13.22)**

***Siddha Swami's Commentary:***

*Prakṛtisthah* means **situated in material nature**. This is the problem: Since the spirit is presently situated in material nature, he or she cannot just ignore that reality. He must first perceive how he is connected to the subtle energies. Then there should be a consideration of the possibility of breaking off that connection. How did the spirit get to be so connected? Is such a connection eternal? Can it be adjusted to the advantage of the spirit or must he or she remain time-bound and energy-bound by that relationship?

*Guṇasaṅgo* or **attachment to the influence of material nature** is the key issue in terms of any freedom that might be gained by a spirit. But the spirit himself must invest all his determination to bring his connection with material nature to an end. It is not the Supreme Spirit, *Śrī* Krishna, nor the agents of the Supreme, who must bring about the freedom of a particular spirit. From within his psychology, the limited spirit must study his causeless and seemingly beginningless attachment to material nature. From that self-analysis, the spirit must endeavor for release. Otherwise, the spirit's attachment to such energies will continue unabated, causing him to emerge from realistic and unrealistic situations in these temporarily-manifested worlds.

उपद्रष्टानुमन्ता च
भर्ता भोक्ता महेश्वरः ।
परमात्मेति चाप्युक्तो
देहेऽस्मिन्पुरुषः परः ॥१३.२३॥
upadraṣṭānumantā ca
bhartā bhoktā maheśvaraḥ
paramātmeti cāpyukto
dehe'sminpuruṣaḥ paraḥ (13.23)

*upadraṣṭānumantā = upadraṣṭā —observer + anumantā — permitter; ca — and; bhartā — supporter; bhoktā — experiencer; maheśvaraḥ — Supreme Lord; paramātmeti = paramātmā — Supreme Soul + iti — thus; cāpi — and also; ukto = uktaḥ — is called; dehe — in the body; 'smin = asmin — in this; puruṣaḥ — spirit; paraḥ — highest*

**The observer, the permitter, the supporter, the experiencer, the Supreme Lord and the Supreme Soul as He is called, He is the highest spirit in the body. (13.23)**

### *Siddha Swami's Commentary:*

*Śrī* Krishna described the *puruṣah parah*, the Supreme Spirit, as contrasted to the beginningless Supreme Reality *(anādimat param brahma)* mentioned in text 13 of this chapter. Is there a difference between the two?

Krishna attributed the Supreme Spirit as being localized in the body of an individual being, functioning as the observer, permitter, supporter and super-experiencer. This Supreme Spirit is one and He reinforces the existence of the limited spirits who also observe, permit, support and experience.

य एवं वेत्ति पुरुषं
प्रकृतिं च गुणैः सह ।
सर्वथा वर्तमानोऽपि
न स भूयोऽभिजायते ॥१३.२४॥
ya evaṁ vetti puruṣaṁ
prakṛtiṁ ca guṇaiḥ saha
sarvathā vartamāno'pi
na sa bhūyo'bhijāyate (13.24)

*ya = yaḥ — who; evaṁ — thus; vetti — knows; puruṣaṁ — spiritual person; prakṛtiṁ — material nature; ca — and; guṇaiḥ — with the variations of material nature; saha — with; sarvathā — in whatever way; vartamāno = vartamānaḥ — existing presently, present condition; 'pi = api — also; na — not; sa = saḥ — he; bhūyo = bhūyaḥ — again; 'bhijāyate — abhijāyate — is born*

**He who knows the spiritual person and material nature, along with the variations of material nature, is not born again, regardless of his present condition. (13.24)**

### *Siddha Swami insisted on a new translation:*

**He who is fully aware of the spirit-person reality and of material nature, along with the variations of material nature, is not born again, regardless of his present condition. (13.24)**

### *Siddha Swami's Commentary:*

This holds true so long as that person remains in that awareness. If for any reason he is removed from it, either by his lack of vigilance into it or by the action of some other person, then he may again be born again. This statement of *Śrī* Krishna applies to a person who becomes aware of the limited persons and of the Supreme Spirit, as well as material nature, in the way *Śrī* Krishna described. But it must be an experience of natural, supernatural, and spiritual proportions, just as Arjuna saw the apparition of the Universal Form and the four-armed Divine Form. While having such an experience, and so long as the experience remains prominent to the vision of the *yogin*, that *yogin* cannot under any circumstance succumb to rebirth on lower planes of existence. It can only happen if he loses touch with the experience or if he becomes unlinked to the supernatural and spiritual planes of consciousness and links back into this mundane world.

The term *puruṣam* in this verse is a genus or class noun meaning all spiritual persons. These include any and all of the finite spiritual selves and the Supreme Spiritual Self, *Śrī* Krishna, as He described.

ध्यानेनात्मनि पश्यन्ति
केचिदात्मानमात्मना ।
अन्ये सांख्येन योगेन
कर्मयोगेन चापरे ॥ १३.२५॥
dhyānenātmani paśyanti
kecidātmānamātmanā
anye sāṁkhyena yogena
karmayogena cāpare (13.25)

*dhyānenātmani = dhyānena — through meditative perception + ātmani — in the spirit; paśyānti — they perceive; kecit — some; ātmānam — by the spirit; ātmanā — the spirit; anye — others; sāṁkhyena — by Sāṁkhya philosophical conclusions; yogena — by yoga practice; karmayogena — by yogic disciplined action; cāpare = ca — and + apare — others*

**Some perceive the spirit by the spirit through meditative perception of the spirit. Others do so with Sāṁkhya philosophical conclusions and others by yogic disciplined action. (13.25)**

***Siddha Swami's Commentary:***

The methods for having the supernatural and spiritual experience denoted in the previous verse are listed in this verse as direct spiritual perception, meditative perception through linking of the attention to the supernatural and spiritual levels and yoga practice along the lines of approach followed by the Samkhya yogins and yogically-disciplined actions in *karma yoga* used by those who mastered *buddhi yoga* and applied that to cultural affairs.

In brief, these methods are: *ātma* yoga *(ātmānamātmanā), dhyāna* yoga *(dhyānenātmani), jñāna yoga (sāṁkhyena yogena)* and *karma yoga (karmayogena).*

This brings to mind another statement by *Śrī* Krishna:

*śrībhagavānuvāca*
*loke'smindvividhā niṣṭhā purā proktā mayānagha*
*jñānayogena sāṁkhyānāṁ karmayogena yoginām (3.3)*

***The Blessed Lord said: In the physical world, a two-fold standard was previously taught by Me, O Arjuna, my good man. This was mind regulation by the yoga practice of the Sāṁkhya philosophical yogis and the action regulation by the yoga practice of the non-philosophical yogis. (3.3)***

*Śrī* Krishna listed only two yogas initially, namely *jñāna yoga* and *karma yoga*; which are both progressions from *buddhi yoga*. In the first case, the superior process of *jñāna yoga* was taken up by those yogins who did not have destined obligations *(karma)* for cultural activities as Arjuna did. They progressed from elementary *buddhi yoga* into *jñāna yoga*. Those with obligations progressed from *buddhi yoga* into applied *buddhi yoga* in reference to cultural activities; they performed *karma yoga* to the satisfaction of the Universal Form. *Karma yoga* is inferior to *jñāna yoga* but it is better to regard it as a preparation for *jñāna yoga*.

*Śrī* Krishna listed *ātma* yoga in this verse, citing that some persons can see the spirit by their own causeless spiritual perception, without yoga practice. Such divine persons take up material bodies from time to time but they retain spiritual perception anyway. Thus for them, yoga may be regarded as superfluous or as a reinforcement.

He listed *dhyāna* yoga to include those who cannot naturally do *ātma* yoga but who effortlessly link their attention to higher concentration forces in higher dimensions. Their psychic abilities which carry over into their material existence enable this. Such persons might exhibit psychic power even without doing yoga.

*Śrī* Krishna mentioned yoga with philosophical conclusions. This was mentioned in Chapter 3 as a course taught by *Śrī* Krishna Himself at the very beginning of the creation of human beings. He also listed *karma yoga* which was taught then as well, to the kings who had to engage in cultural activities and political affairs.

अन्ये त्वेवमजानन्तः
श्रुत्वान्येभ्य उपासते ।
तेऽपि चातितरन्त्येव
मृत्युं श्रुतिपरायणाः ॥ १३.२६ ॥
anye tvevamajānantaḥ
śrutvānyebhya upāsate
te'pi cātitarantyeva
mṛtyuṁ śrutiparāyaṇāḥ (13.26)

*anye — others; tu — but; evam — thus; ajānantaḥ — not knowing; śrutvānyebhya = śrutvā — hearing + anyebhya — from others; upāsate — they worship; te — they; 'pi = api — also; catitaranti = ca — and + atitaranti — transcend; eva — indeed; mṛtyuṁ — death; śrutiparāyaṇāḥ = śruti — hearing + parāyaṇāḥ — putting confidence in as the highest*

**But some, though they are ignorant, hear from others. They worship and by their confidence in what is heard, they also transcend death. (13.26)**

***Siddha Swami's Commentary:***

In this verse a most unusual method is itemized, which is confidence in someone who experiences the spiritual reality. *Śrī* Krishna attests to this easy method. We must note, however, that by such confidence in hearing from those who are self-realized, some faithful disciples do transcend death. There is no statement that such faithful disciples get the realization mentioned in text 24, regarding knowledge of the spirit-person reality, material nature and the variations of it. For such development, those persons would have to practice yoga, master *buddhi yoga*, go further to the completion of *jñāna yoga* and then they would have supernatural and spiritual perceptions.

यावत्संजायते किंचित्
सत्त्वं स्थावरजङ्गमम् ।
क्षेत्रक्षेत्रज्ञसंयोगात्
तद्विद्धि भरतर्षभ ॥ १३.२७
yāvatsaṁjāyate kiṁcit
sattvaṁ sthāvarajaṅgamam
kṣetrakṣetrajñasaṁyogāt
tadviddhi bharatarṣabha (13.27)

*yāvat — as for; saṁjāyate — is born; kiṁcit = kiṁcid — anything, whatever; sattvaṁ — existence; sthāvarajaṅgamam = sthāvara — stationary + jaṅgamam — moving; kṣetrakṣetrajñasaṁyogāt = kṣetra — living space + kṣetrajña — experiencer + saṁyogāt — from the synthesis; tat — that; viddhi — know; bharatarṣabha — strong man of the Bharatas*

**As for anything that is produced in this existence, be it a stationary or moving object, know, O strong man of the Bharatas, that it is produced from a synthesis of the experiencer and the living space. (13.27)**

***Siddha Swami's Commentary:***

The *samyogāt* or synthesis of the experiencer and the psychology, results in the material objects which we perceive. There are also subtle and super-subtle objects which come about in the same way. Essentially this means that all these manifestations are produced from varying degrees of fusion between the Supreme Spirit, the limited spirits and material nature's energies.

समं सर्वेषु भूतेषु
तिष्ठन्तं परमेश्वरम् ।
विनश्यत्स्वविनश्यन्तं
यः पश्यति स पश्यति ॥१३.२८॥
samaṁ sarveṣu bhūteṣu
tiṣṭhantaṁ parameśvaram
vinaśyatsvavinaśyantaṁ
yaḥ paśyati sa paśyati (13.28)

*samam — similar; sarveṣu — in all; bhūteṣu — in beings; tiṣṭhantaṁ — situated; parmeśvaram — Supreme Lord; vinaśyatsu — in disintegrations; avinaśyantaṁ — not perishing; yaḥ — who; paśyati — perceive; sa = saḥ — he; paśyati — really sees*

**The Supreme Lord is similarly situated in all beings without perishing when they disintegrate. He who perceives that, really sees. (13.28)**

***Siddha Swami's Commentary:***

*Parameśvaram* is the Supreme Lord of the world, the most superior of the individual spirits. Categorically, He cannot be superseded or out-performed. He is the destined God of the world by virtue of His existential category. He is situated in all creature forms which are gross or subtle, but He does not disintegrate when a body perishes or disappears. The limited spirit too does not disintegrate but the limited spirit suffers from an attachment to temporary forms and thus he might become distressed when a form disintegrates. The Supreme Person does not experience a distressful condition like the limited spirits.

समं पश्यन्हि सर्वत्र
समवस्थितमीश्वरम् ।
न हिनस्त्यात्मनात्मानं
ततो याति परां गतिम् ॥१३.२९॥
samaṁ paśyanhi sarvatra
samavasthitamīśvaram
na hinastyātmanātmānaṁ
tato yāti parāṁ gatim (13.29)

*samaṁ — same; paśyan — seeing; hi — indeed; sarvatra — everywhere; samavasthitam — same established; īśvaram — Lord; na — not; hinasti — degrade; ātmānātmānaṁ = ātmanā — by the soul + ātmānaṁ — the soul; tato = tataḥ — subsequently; yāti — goes; parām — supreme; gatim — destination*

**Seeing the same Lord being situated everywhere, he does not degrade the soul by his own soul. Subsequently, he goes to the supreme destination. (13.29)**

***Siddha Swami's Commentary:***

Degradation of a limited soul occurs under certain influences in the absence of certain other associations. Because a limited soul is dependent by nature, and because he or she is not absolute, the soul is susceptible to lifting or degrading influences. The soul's endeavor plays a part either to reinforce a good influence or to nullify it. Thus if one takes up *buddhi yoga* and learns how to develop and constantly use mystic vision, one is sustained by force of the Supreme Being and is not degraded. Subsequently one would go to the supreme destination, as soon as one is eligible.

प्रकृत्यैव च कर्माणि
क्रियमाणानि सर्वशः ।
यः पश्यति तथात्मानम्
अकर्तारं स पश्यति ॥१३.३०

*prakṛtyaiva = prakṛtya — by material nature + eva — indeed; ca — and; karmāṇi — actions; kriyamāṇāni — performed; sarvaśaḥ — in all cases; yaḥ — who; paśyati — he sees; tathātmānam = tathā — as regarding + ātmānam*

prakṛtyaiva ca karmāṇi
kriyāmāṇāni sarvaśaḥ
yaḥ paśyati tathātmānam
akartāraṁ sa paśyati (13.30)

*— self; akartāraṁ — non-doer; sa = saḥ — he; paśyati — truly sees*

**He who sees, that in all cases, the actions are performed by material nature, and whoever regards himself as a non-doer, truly sees. (13.30)**

***Siddha Swami's Commentary:***

In all cases, even in the actions of the Universal Form, the final act is performed by material nature, even when the supreme will motivates or reinforces. The Supreme Being and the limited spirits cannot act directly in any material creation, whether it be subtle or gross. They must use the material energy in an instrumental way for these activities. One should always keep this in mind. The shuffle in the material world between good and bad, pious and impious, religious and irreligious, involves the material energy and its regulations. Thus one should never forget this. But such information does not give one the right to go against the Supreme will without adverse consequences. Therefore one should always cooperate with the divine beings in all cultural undertakings.

यदा भूतपृथग्भावम्
एकस्थमनुपश्यति ।
तत एव च विस्तारं
ब्रह्म संपद्यते तदा ॥१३.३१॥
yadā bhūtapṛthagbhāvam
ekasthamanupaśyati
tata eva ca vistāraṁ
brahma saṁpadyate tadā (13.31)

*yadā — when; bhūtapṛthagbhāvam = bhūta — being + pṛthak — various + bhāvam — existential state; ekastham — based in one foundation; anupaśyati — he sees; tata — from that conclusion; eva — only; ca — and; vistāraṁ — extending, emanating; brahma — spiritual plane; saṁpadyate — he reaches; tadā — then*

**When a person sees that all the various states of being are based on a single foundation, and only from that everything emanates, then he reaches the spiritual plane. (13.31)**

***Siddha Swami's Commentary:***

The material world came about as a result of the admixture of the spiritual persons and the material energy. Both are involved. Material nature has the visible, perceptible reality but its display is based on energization from the powers of the spiritual persons. Arjuna did perceive a single foundation as the Universal Form, but as admitted by *Śrī* Krishna in the previous verse, the actions are in all cases performed by material nature. Sanjaya describes the Universal Form seen by Arjuna:

*tatraikasthaṁ jagatkṛtsnaṁ pravibhaktamanekadhā*
*apaśyaddevadevasya śarīre pāṇḍavastadā (11.13)*

***There the entire universe existed as one reality divided in many ways. Arjuna Pandava then saw the God of gods in that body. (11.13)***

Just as the material body is based on the conjunction of material nature and the spiritual presence of a limited spirit, so this universe is based on the fusion of material nature with the energy of the Supreme Spirit, so it seems.

अनादित्वान्निर्गुणत्वात्
परमात्मायमव्ययः ।
शरीरस्थोऽपि कौन्तेय
न करोति न लिप्यते ॥१३.३२॥
anāditvānnirguṇatvāt
paramātmāyamavyayaḥ
śarīrastho'pi kaunteya
na karoti na lipyate (13.32)

*anāditvāt = due to being without a beginning; nirguṇatvāt — due to being devoid of the influence of material nature; paramātmāyam = paramātmā — Supreme Soul + ayam — this; avyayaḥ — imperishable; śarīrastho = śarīrasthaḥ — situated in the material body; 'pi = api — even though; kaunteya — O son of Kuntī; na — not; karoti — he does; na — not; lipyate — become contaminated*

**Since this imperishable Supreme Lord is beginningless and devoid of the influence of material nature, even though He is situated in the material body, O son of Kuntī, He does not act or become contaminated. (13.32)**

***Siddha Swami's Commentary:***

The actions of the supreme do not cause the Supreme Being to become contaminated. Such actions are, in fact, carried out by material nature through supernatural maneuvers of the Supreme Being. A limited soul may also be afforded immunity from the effects of material nature but to enjoy that, he or she must exhibit perfect detachment when in linkage to any mechanism of material nature.

*Śrī* Krishna precisely described His status as the imperishable Supreme Lord, the *Paramātma* Supreme Soul Who, though He might appear to be situated in a material body as the son of *Devakī* and *Vasudeva*, was transcendental to the liabilities which form in material nature.

यथा सर्वगतं सौक्ष्म्याद्
आकाशं नोपलिप्यते ।
सर्वत्रावस्थितो देहे
तथात्मा नोपलिप्यते ॥१३.३३॥
yathā sarvagataṁ saukṣmyād
ākāśaṁ nopalipyate
sarvatrāvasthito dehe
tathātmā nopalipyate (13.33)

*yathā — as; sarvagataṁ — all-pervading; saukṣmyāt — as by subtlety; ākāśaṁ — sky; nopalipyate = na — not + upalipyate — is polluted; sarvatrāvasthito = sarvatra — all over + avasthitaḥ — situated; dehe — in the body; tathātmā = tathā — so + ātmā — soul; nopalipyate = na — not + upalipyate — affected*

**As by subtlety, the all-pervading space is not polluted, so the soul, though situated all over the body, is not affected actually. (13.33)**

***Siddha Swami's Commentary:***

Even the limited soul is not affected by the movement of material nature but the same unaffected soul may come to imagine or conceive of such affectation. Hence the need arises to free itself from the proximity to the psychic equipments through which it conceives such unreal things.

यथा प्रकाशयत्येकः
कृत्स्नं लोकमिमं रविः ।
क्षेत्रं क्षेत्री तथा कृत्स्नं
प्रकाशयति भारत ॥१३.३४॥

*yathā — as; prakāśayati — illuminates; ekaḥ — one, alone; kṛtsnaṁ — whole; lokam — world; imaṁ — this; raviḥ — sun; kṣetraṁ — living space; kṣetrī — the user of the living space; tathā*

yathā prakāśayatyekaḥ
kṛtsnaṁ lokamimaṁ raviḥ
kṣetraṁ kṣetrī tathā kṛtsnaṁ
prakāśayati bhārata (13.34)

*— so; kṛtsnaṁ — entire; prakāśayati — gives feeling; bhārata — O man of the Bhārata family*

**As the sun alone illuminates the whole world, O man of the Bharata family, so the user of the living space gives feeling to the entire psyche. (13.34)**

***Siddha Swami's Commentary:***

The limited spirit though not the Supreme Soul, does enliven his material and subtle bodies, just as the sun sheds light through outer space. This is to be realized by each and every spirit. One's power, as it is expressed in the psychic environment, causes the psychic objects to fascinate and bewitch one. This is to be realized fittingly.

क्षेत्रक्षेत्रज्ञयोरेवम्
अन्तरं ज्ञानचक्षुषा ।
भूतप्रकृतिमोक्षं च
ये विदुर्यान्ति ते परम् ॥१३.३५॥
kṣetrakṣetrajñayorevam
antaraṁ jñānacakṣuṣā
bhūtaprakṛtimokṣaṁ ca
ye viduryānti te param (13.35)

*kṣetrakṣetrajñayoḥ — of the experiencer and the living space; evam — thus; antaraṁ — difference; jñānacakṣuṣā = jñāna — perceptive knowledge + cakṣuṣā — intuitive vision; bhūtaprakṛtimokṣaṁ = bhūta — being + prakṛti — material nature + mokṣaṁ — liberation; ca — and; ye — who; viduḥ — they know; yānti — they go; te — they; param — supreme*

**Those who by intuitive perception know the difference between the living space and the experiencer, as well as the liberation of the living being from material nature, go to the Supreme. (13.35)**

***Siddha Swami's Commentary:***

*Jñānacakṣuṣā* refers to intuitive perception, developed for accurate and precise vision in *samādhi* practice of higher yoga. This is not mere knowledge or information from the *Bhagavad Gītā;* otherwise the term *cakṣuṣā* would not be mentioned. One must in higher yoga, in *jñāna yoga*, perceive the difference between one's spirit and the subtle or psychic environment otherwise known as the mind energy and the emotional spaces. These are the locations for the psychic equipments which are used and energized by the spirit.

The liberation of the spirit from material nature will come about only by perfect vision in sorting the various subtle equipments in the psychic spaces. When the spirit detaches himself or herself from the psychic tools, then there is a chance for liberation from the influence of material nature, not otherwise. And this is achieved by endeavor in higher yoga.

# CHAPTER 14

# Guṇāh Prakṛti Sambhavāh

# The Influences Produced of Material Nature *

*sattvaṁ rajastama iti guṇāḥ prakṛtisaṁbhavāḥ*
*nibadhnanti mahābāho dehe dehinamavyayam (14.5)*

***Clarity, impulsion and retardation are the influences produced of material nature. They captivate the imperishable embodied soul in the body, O strong-armed hero. (14.5)***

***Siddha Swami assigned this chapter title on the basis of verse 5 of this chapter.**

श्रीभगवानुवाच
परं भूयः प्रवक्ष्यामि
ज्ञानानां ज्ञानमुत्तमम् ।
यज्ज्ञात्वा मुनयः सर्वे
परां सिद्धिमितो गताः ॥ १४.१ ॥
śrībhagavānuvāca
paraṁ bhūyaḥ pravakṣyāmi
jñānānāṁ jñānamuttamam
yajjñātvā munayaḥ sarve
parāṁ siddhimito gatāḥ (14.1)

*śrī bhagavān — the Blessed Lord; uvāca — said; paraṁ — highest; bhūyaḥ — further; pravakṣyāmi — I will explain; jñānānāṁ — of the knowledges; jñānam — information; uttamam — the very best; yat — which; jñātvā — having experienced; munayaḥ — yogī philosophers; sarve — all; parāṁ — supreme; siddhim — perfection; ito = itaḥ — from here; gatāḥ — done*

**The Blessed Lord said: I will explain more, giving the highest information of all knowledges, the very best. Having experienced that, all the yogi philosophers went away from here to the Supreme Perfection. (14.1)**

***Siddha Swami's Commentary:***

The *parām siddhim* is that which concerns the siddha perfected yogi sages, those who mastered *buddhi yoga* and progressed on to *jñāna yoga*. These persons moved up from lower to higher dimensions gradually and with certainty, neither slipping downwards, nor going up haphazardly.

*Śrī* Krishna gave detailed information in this chapter, which He considered to be the very best education one might receive in the transcendence science. Of course information itself is just the beginning of progression. Supernatural and spiritual perception would have to be developed by yogic means, in combination with the grace of *Śrī* Krishna.

At the time of this discourse, Arjuna was not rated as a siddha but *Śrī* Krishna was encouraged by the student relationship Arjuna displayed, and thus the Lord gladly gave detailed knowledge about the course taken by the siddhas, a process Arjuna would take up later in his life.

इदं ज्ञानमुपाश्रित्य
मम साधर्म्यमागताः ।
सर्गेऽपि नोपजायन्ते
प्रलये न व्यथन्ति च ॥ १४.२ ॥
idaṁ jñānamupāśritya
mama sādharmyamāgatāḥ
sarge'pi nopajāyante
pralaye na vyathanti ca (14.2)

*idaṁ — this; jñānam — experience; upāśritya — resorting to; mama — my; sādharmyam — a nature that is similar; āgatāḥ — transformed into; sarge — at the time of the universal creation; 'pi = api — even; nopajāyante = na — not + upajāyante — they are born; pralaye — at the time of universal dissolution; na — not; vyathanti — disturbed; ca — and*

**Resorting to this experience, being transformed into a nature that is similar to My own, they are not born even at the time of the universal creation, nor are they disturbed at the time of dissolution. (14.2)**

***Siddha Swami's Commentary:***

The *sādharmyam* is a nature that is similar to *Śrī* Krishna's transcendental status. For the limited entity in this world, it is a definite upgrade. It is a movement into the realm of *Śrī* Krishna's existence, a totally different way of experiencing.

It is not stated whether every limited entity may attain such a divine status but it is clear from what *Śrī* Krishna said that those who do achieve that are not born even at the time of the universal creation and are not disturbed at the time of dissolution. This cannot mean that such persons may not appear in material bodies because *Śrī* Krishna did so at *Kurukṣetra*, but it indicates that the disturbances in the material energy do not affect the security of the perfected siddhas. Their consciousness having been shifted off this level, and not being aligned with or reliant on the subtle material force, is not adjusted as the conditioned beings are.

मम योनिर्महद्ब्रह्म
तस्मिन्गर्भं दधाम्यहम् ।
संभवः सर्वभूतानां
ततो भवति भारत ॥ १४.३ ॥
mama yonirmahadbrahma
tasmingarbhaṁ dadhāmyaham
saṁbhavaḥ sarvabhūtānāṁ
tato bhavati bhārata (14.3)

*mama — my; yoniḥ — womb; mahat — extensive; brahma — reality; tasmin — into it; garbhaṁ — essence; dadhāmi — I impregnate; aham — I; saṁbhavaḥ — origin; sarvabhūtānāṁ — of all beings; tato = tataḥ — from that; bhavati — comes into being; bhārata — O man of the Bharata family*

**The extensive mundane reality is My womb. I impregnate the essence into it. The origin of all beings comes from that reality, O man of the Bharata family. (14.3)**

***Siddha Swami's Commentary:***

Among the siddhas, some of them do not acknowledge a Supreme Person who fits the description of *Śrī* Krishna, but all do admit that regardless of the personal or impersonal connotations, the Primal Reality or Primal Creative Cause is in relation to the sum-total material energy, just as a potent man is to the womb of a female.

In the discussion with Uddhava, Lord Krishna called the charged force the *sūtram*, but here to Arjuna He used the term *garbham*, which means embryo or what is developed after an impregnation. Undoubtedly, the living beings in the universe have their origin from the initial impregnation of emotional force into the cosmos.

सर्वयोनिषु कौन्तेय
मूर्तयः संभवन्ति याः ।
तासां ब्रह्म महद्योनिर्
अहं बीजप्रदः पिता ॥ १४.४ ॥
sarvayoniṣu kaunteya
mūrtayaḥ saṁbhavanti yāḥ
tāsāṁ brahma mahadyonir
ahaṁ bījapradaḥ pitā (14.4)

*sarvayoniṣu — in all wombs; kaunteya — O son of Kuntī; mūrtayaḥ — forms; saṁbhavanti — they are produced; yāḥ — which; tāsāṁ — of them; brahmā — mundane reality; mahat — great; yoniḥ — giving; aham — I; bījapradaḥ — seed-giving; pitā — father*

**Forms are produced in all types of wombs, O son of Kuntī, I am the seed-giving father. The extensive mundane reality is the great womb. (14.4)**

***Siddha Swami's Commentary:***

The *brahma mahat* is the extensive mundane reality. This is because the material nature at large cannot be dismissed as just an illusion; it may be regarded as something temporarily manifested. It may be rated like that but actually it is more than any limited spirit can handle. And thus in comparison to a limited being, it is an extensive reality. It does have permanence but not in terms of its manifested forms.

A limited living entity cannot afford to dismiss the mundane potency as just an illusion, as *Śrīpad* Shankaracharya suggested. For a limited entity, that potency is formidable and is something that he must struggle with life after life, almost always being defeated and subdued by it. Thus *Śrī* Krishna appropriately told Arjuna of that *brahma mahat*, extensive mundane reality, which almost always defeats the limited beings who are produced in it, and which surely keeps them subdued.

सत्त्वं रजस्तम इति
गुणाः प्रकृतिसंभवाः ।
निबध्नन्ति महाबाहो
देहे देहिनमव्ययम् ॥ १४.५ ॥
sattvaṁ rajastama iti
guṇāḥ prakṛtisaṁbhavāḥ
nibadhnanti mahābāho
dehe dehinamavyayam (14.5)

*sattvaṁ — clarity; rajaḥ — impulsion; tama — retardation; iti — thus; guṇāḥ — influences; prakṛtisaṁbhavāḥ = prakṛti— material nature + saṁbhavāḥ — produced of; nibadhnanti — they captivate; mahābāho — O great-armed hero; dehe — in the body; dehinaṁ — embodied soul; avyayam — imperishable*

**Clarity, impulsion and retardation are the influences produced of material nature. They captivate the imperishable embodied soul in the body, O strong-armed hero. (14.5)**

***Siddha Swami's Commentary:***

All through the Vedic literature, the *Vedas*, the Upanishads, the *Bhagavad Gītā* and the *Purāṇas*, the imperishable *avyayam* nature of the embodied souls is affirmed, but we find that not all the living entities agree with this. Many embodied beings assert their mortality because of a helpless identification with the perishable body. Thus the imperishability of the soul must be realized through *buddhi yoga* practice.

One notation is that the consciousness experienced by the embodied being wavers and thus the embodied being lacks confidence in an immortal principle. In other words, since the embodied soul suffers from unconsciousness from time to time, he cannot be confident of the immortality which the Vedic literatures and persons like *Śrī* Krishna accredit.

Therefore to express faith in the words of Śrī Krishna, the limited entity must assume that even though he or she may pass through phases of unconsciousness, still he or she is eternal and will continue to exist regardless. It must also be assumed that even though one has a faulty and limited memory, still one will continue to exist regardless. And this is the only type of confidence one may have, at least until one can be upgraded, existentially as described in verse 2 of this chapter, regarding being transformed into a nature that is similar to Śrī Krishna's *(mama sādharmyam āgatāh).*

The captivation of the imperishable eternal soul was a subject of discussion for centuries. Many great sages and religious leaders tried to fathom the compulsions of material nature, under which the soul seems to labor and be confined. But despite all their discussions and promises, most of the human beings remain time bound in the cycle of repeated birth and death. It appears therefore that material nature has no intention of releasing the bound souls. As far as the liberated entities are concerned, many of them find that their status is constantly threatened by material nature, which endeavors to put them under its control for regulation of the social issues of their disciples.

Many spiritual leaders flaunt themselves on human society as liberators of disciples but in fact their assumption of the social life of their wards is no different from the responsibility parents must assume for the children which pass out of their bodies through the sexual openings. Thus the claim of the gurus about taking the sins of disciples is mostly a farce, for that is something that every type of guardian has to deal with, not just the spiritual teachers.

On a careful reading of what *Śrī* Krishna stated in this verse, we get the important hint, that a captivation of the embodied soul is related to with the three varying psychological states of subtle material nature. This is experienced in the mental and emotional states of the soul. These are a clear state of perception, an impulsive feeling and a retardive mood. Any of these are potential psychological contents of the mind and emotions of the limited being.

The compartment where his consciousness occurs is one but the contents of that compartment vary. According to the contents, that is the state of judgment of the limited being. And that is how material nature exercises dominance.

तत्र सत्त्वं निर्मलत्वात्
प्रकाशकमनामयम् ।
सुखसङ्गेन बध्नाति
ज्ञानसङ्गेन चानघ ॥ १४.६ ॥
tatra sattvaṁ nirmalatvāt
prakāśakamanāmayam
sukhasaṅgena badhnāti
jñānasaṅgena cānagha (14.6)

*tatra — regarding these; sattvaṁ — clarifying influence; nirmalatvāt — relatively free from perceptive impurities; prakāśakam — illuminating; anāmayam — free from disease; sukhasaṅgena = sukha — happiness + saṅgena — by attachment; badhnāti — it binds; jñānasaṅgena = jñāna — knowledge of expertise + saṅgena — by attachment; cānagha = ca — and + anagha — sinless one*

**Regarding these influences, the clarifying one is relatively free from perceptive impurities. It is illuminating and free from disease, but by granting an attachment to happiness and to expertise, it captivates a person, O sinless one. (14.6)**

***Siddha Swami's Commentary:***

We must consider that this refers mostly to the subtle body; it is not the gross form which is put to question but the subtle and causal ones.

When the subtle body is mostly powered by clarifying energy, one experiences illumination and one's perception is clear. One can make the proper decision and gage the realities encountered in material existence more accurately. Then the subtle body is relatively free from subtle diseases. However as it is with material nature, even the clarifying influences are flawed, though to the minimal degree.

These clarifying energies leave one with a sense of attachment to happiness and to expertise. One then becomes captivated by legitimate pleasures and to the skills which make one popular with other living beings. Thus in the end, the clarifying mode causes one to act in a way which promotes addictions of happiness and skillful exhibitions.

Some think that a transcendentalist need not bother with material nature, but they are being very naive and idealistic. One has to progress through the modes of nature gradually. One cannot shed these modes suddenly. Even if one is placed on the transcendental level by the grace of a divinity like *Śrī* Krishna, still one will have to return to one's normal state of mind and emotions and then work one's way up by performance of austerities. One may check the history of Arjuna in the *Mahābhārata* literature.

*Śrī* Krishna took care of His responsibility to the limited entities by explaining the nature of the various levels of development. This is an alert so that each of them might know what to expect as they develop through the modes of nature. It is not an explanation to be used to preach down to others or to think that since one has the information, one is exempt from the influences. Rather one should regard this information as an alert, a preview of what to expect as one develops spiritually.

रजो रागात्मकंविद्धि
तृष्णासङ्गसमुद्भवम् ।
तन्निबध्नाति कौन्तेय
कर्मसङ्गेन देहिनम् ॥ १४.७॥
rajo rāgātmakaṁviddhi
tṛṣṇāsaṅgasamudbhavam
tannibadhnāti kaunteya
karmasaṅgena dehinam (14.7)

*rajo = rajaḥ — impulsive influence; rāgātmakaṁ — characterized by passion; viddhi — know; tṛṣṇāsaṅgasamudbhavam = tṛṣṇā — desire + saṅga — earnest + samudbhavam — produced from; tat — this; nibadhnāti — it captivates; kaunteya — O son of Kuntī; karmasaṅgena — by attachment to activity; dehināṁ — the embodied soul*

**Know that the impulsive influence is characterized by passion. It is produced from earnest desire and attachment. O son of Kuntī, this mode captivates the embodied soul by an attachment to activity. (14.7)**

***Siddha Swami's Commentary:***

The heart of the impulsive force is passion or *rāgā* which denotes strong impulsion. It is not subjected to reason and it acts on its own. It was described by *Śrī* Krishna under the term *kāmarūpah*:

*arjuna uvāca*
*atha kena prayukto'yaṁ pāpaṁ carati pūruṣaḥ*
*anicchannapi vārṣṇeya balādiva niyojitaḥ (3.36)*
*śrībhagavānuvāca*
*kāma eṣa krodha eṣa rajoguṇasamudbhavaḥ*
*mahāśano mahāpāpmā viddhyenamiha vairiṇam (3.37)*
*dhūmenāvriyate vahnir yathādarśo malena ca*
*yatholbenāvṛto garbhas tathā tenedamāvṛtam (3.38)*
*āvṛtaṁ jñānametena jñānino nityavairiṇā*
*kāmarūpeṇa kaunteya duṣpūreṇānalena ca (3.39)*
*indriyāṇi mano buddhir asyādhiṣṭhānamucyate*
*etairvimohayatyeṣa jñānamāvṛtya dehinam (3.40)*
*tasmāttvamindriyāṇyādau niyamya bharatarṣabha*
*pāpmānaṁ prajahihyenaṁ jñānavijñānanāśanam (3.41)*

***Arjuna said: Then explain, O family man of the Vṛṣṇis, by what is a person forced to commit an evil unwillingly, just as if he were compelled to do so?***

***The Blessed Lord said: This force is craving. This power is anger. The passionate emotion is the source. It has a great consuming power and does much damage. Recognize it as the enemy in this case.***

***As the sacrificial fire is obscured by smoke, and similarly as a mirror is shrouded by dust or as an embryo is covered by a skin, so a man's insight is blocked by the passionate energy.***

***The discernment of educated people is adjusted by their eternal enemy which is the sense of yearning for various things. O son of Kuntī, the lusty power is as hard to satisfy as it is to keep a fire burning.***

***It is authoritatively stated that the senses, the mind and the intelligence are the combined warehouse of the passionate enemy. By these facilities, the lusty power confuses the embodied soul, shrouding his insight.***

***Thus regulating the senses initially, you should, O powerful man of the Bharata family, squelch this degrading power which ruins knowledge and discernment. (3.36-41)***

Even though the impulsive influence is produced from earnest desire and attachment, a question arises: What is the origin of such desire and attachment? Are these perpetually ingrained qualities of the spirit? The quest of *brahma yoga*, which is advanced *buddhi yoga*, concerns itself with this inquiry into the nature of the spirit. It is necessary to section off the spirit in order to sort between the qualities and habits of the psyche which it inhabits.

The attention of the spirit seems to be fused into the earnest desire and attachment. Thus in *brahma yoga* an attempt is made to extract the attention from such impulsive energy. If the student *yogin* can do this, then he can figure out where his core self begins and where the surrounding psyche ends. But this is not an easy achievement. It takes hours and hours of meditative research in *samādhi* practice to sort this.

The fusion of the attention into the psychic equipments and energies is the problem. A *yogin* must work hard in higher yoga to separate out the attentive energy which emanates from his core self.

Cultural activity in the material world, *karma*, cannot be a main interest of the spirit soul because this environment is a downgrade from the spiritual level. Hence *Śrī* Krishna alerted Arjuna:

*indriyāṇi parāṇyāhur indriyebhyaḥ paraṁ manaḥ*
*manasastu parā buddhir yo buddheḥ paratastu saḥ (3.42)*
*evaṁ buddheḥ paraṁ buddhvā saṁstabhyātmānamātmanā*
*jahi śatruṁ mahābāho kāmarūpaṁ durāsadam (3.43)*

***The ancient psychologists say that the senses are energetic, but in comparison to the senses, the mind is more energetic. In contrast to the mind, the intelligence is even more sensitive. But in reference, the spirit is most elevated.***

***Thus having understood what is higher than intelligence, keeping the personal energies under control of the spirit, root out, O powerful man, the enemy, the form of passionate desire which is difficult to grasp. (3.42-43)***

The only way to root out the *kāmarūpa* form of passionate desire is to first locate it, then separate the core self from it and study its alignment with the core self and make repeated attempts in the practice of higher yoga to segregate it from the self. The cultural force, *karma*, causes activity by motivations. One cannot get rid of this unless one roots its out on the subtle and causal planes.

तमस्त्वज्ञानजं विद्धि
मोहनं सर्वदेहिनाम् ।
प्रमादालस्यनिद्राभिस्
तन्निबध्नाति भारत ॥ १४.८॥
tamastvajñānajaṁ viddhi
mohanaṁ sarvadehinām
pramādālasyanidrābhis
tannibadhnāti bhārata (14.8)

*tamaḥ — depressing mode; tu — but; ajñānajaṁ — produced of insensibility; viddhi — know; mohanam — confusion; sarvadehināṁ — of all embodied beings; pramādālasyanidrābhiḥ = pramāda — inattentiveness + ālasya — laziness + nidrābhiḥ — sleep; tat — this; nibadhnāti — captivates; bhārata — O man of the Bharata family*

**But know that the depressing mode is produced of insensibility which is the confusion of all embodied beings. This captivates by inattentiveness, laziness and sleep, O man of the Bharata family. (14.8)**

***Siddha Swami's Commentary:***

*Śrī* Krishna alerted that the clarifying force, which is the best of the subtle material energies, accustoms the spirit to happiness and exhibitions of skills. This is its flaw. The passionate force habituates the self to cultural activities, encouraging the self by showing promise for development and elevation in the material world.

The last of the mundane influences comes as a dulling force. This dulls the clarity and dampens the enthusiasm which is produced from passion. This dulling force is psychological. It produces inattentiveness, laziness and sleep. It passes itself off as relaxation and uncertainty, but in fact it confuses the discernment of the living entity and makes him forget his objectives.

सत्त्वं सुखे सञ्जयति
रजः कर्मणि भारत ।
ज्ञानमावृत्य तु तमः
प्रमादे सञ्जयत्युत ॥१४.९॥
sattvaṁ sukhe sañjayati
rajaḥ karmaṇi bhārata
jñānamāvṛtya tu tamaḥ
pramāde sañjayatyuta (14.9)

*sattvaṁ — clarifying influence; sukhe — in happiness; sañjayati — causes attachment; rajaḥ — impulsive influence; karmaṇi — to action; bhārata — O Bharata family man; jñānam — experience; āvṛtya — obscuring; tu — but; tamaḥ — depressing mode; pramāde — to negligence; sañjayati — causes attachment; uta —even*

**The clarifying influence causes attachment to happiness. The impulsive one causes a need for action, O Bharata family man. But the depressing mode obscures experience and causes attachment to negligence. (14.9)**

***Siddha Swami's Commentary:***

*Śrī* Krishna graciously explained the effects of each of the three modes. These are psychological states which one may learn to observe in one's psyche, so that eventually one can learn how to deal with each of them. In *brahma yoga* practice, this is part of the course.

रजस्तमश्चाभिभूय
सत्त्वं भवति भारत ।
रजः सत्त्वं तमश्चैव
तमः सत्त्वं रजस्तथा ॥१४.१०॥
rajastamaścābhibhūya
sattvaṁ bhavati bhārata
rajaḥ sattvaṁ tamaścaiva
tamaḥ sattvaṁ rajastathā (14.10)

*rajaḥ — impulsiveness; tamaścābhibhūya = tamaḥ — depression + ca — and + abhibhūya — predominating over; sattvaṁ — clarity; bhavati — emerges; bhārata — O Bharata family man; rajaḥ — impulsiveness; sattvaṁ — clarity; tamaścaiva = tamaḥ — depression + caiva — and indeed; tamaḥ — depression; sattvaṁ — clarity; rajaḥ — impulsion; tathā — similarly*

**When predominating over impulsiveness and depression, clarity emerges, O Bharata family man. Depression rises, predominating over impulsiveness and clarity. Similarly, impulsion takes control over depression and clarity. (14.10)**

***Siddha Swami's Commentary:***

*Śrī* Krishna explained that these modes compete with one another for control of the core self. Stated from another angle, these modes compete for empowerment by the core self, since they pull energy from the self for their operations. Thus if a spirit can exercise control over the distribution of energies, he may regulate his alliance with any of these modes. He has to restrict his energy from each of the modes. The question arises as to whether this is an impractical ideal.

If the various modes compete with one another for the attention of the self, what part may the self play in rejecting any of the modes? Can the self quiet down or squelch the modes completely?

*Śrī* Krishna made it clear in this verse, that normally, when clarity emerges as prominent, it predominates over impulsiveness and depression. Thus it uses those modes to promote its interest. On the other hand, the lower modes of impulsiveness and depression may emerge supreme in any given circumstance. And they, in turn, would each predominate over the others, making them subservient to its aims.

A student *yogin* is trained to observe how this operates. Gradually he discusses with his teacher methods of mystic practice through which he may take command over the modes.

सर्वद्वारेषु देहेऽस्मिन्
प्रकाश उपजायते ।
ज्ञानं यदा तदा विद्याद्
विवृद्धं सत्त्वमित्युत ॥ १४.११ ॥
sarvadvāreṣu dehe'smin
prakāśa upajāyate
jñānaṁ yadā tadā vidyād
vivṛddhaṁ sattvamityuta (14.11)

*sarvadvāreṣu — in all openings; dehe — in the body; 'smin = asmin — in this; prakāśa — clear perception; upajāyate — is felt; jñānaṁ — true knowledge; yadā — when; tadā — then; vidyāt — it should be concluded; vivṛddhaṁ — dominant; sattvam — clarifying mode; iti — thus; uta — indeed*

**When clear perception, true knowledge, is felt in all openings of the body, then it should be concluded that the clarifying mode is predominant. (14.11)**

***Siddha Swami's Commentary:***

A body may be healthy with feelings in all its orifices, and still that body may be dominated by impulsion or depression. In that case, the lower mode would be utilizing the services of the higher one which causes the healthy condition. There must be clear perception and true knowledge for a predominance of the clarifying mode. Even in an unhealthy body, the mental and emotional energies might be under the influence of the clarifying mode. In *brahma yoga* practice, one is trained in facilitating the highest energies which material nature would offer. In that way one denies the lower modes in their attempts at predominance.

लोभः प्रवृत्तिरारम्भः
कर्मणामशमः स्पृहा ।
रजस्येतानि जायन्ते
विवृद्धे भरतर्षभ ॥ १४.१२ ॥
lobhaḥ pravṛttirārambhaḥ
karmaṇāmaśamaḥ spṛhā
rajasyetāni jāyante
vivṛddhe bharatarṣabha (14.12)

*lobhaḥ = greed; pravṛttiḥ — over-exertion; ārambhaḥ — rash undertaking; karmaṇām — of action; aśamaḥ — restlessness; spṛhā — craving; rājasī — in impulsiveness; etāni — those; jāyante — are produced; vivṛddhe — in the dominance; bharatarṣabha — strong man of the Bharatas*

**Greed, overexertion, rash undertakings, restlessness and craving, these are produced when impulsiveness is predominant, O strong man of the Bharatas. (14.12)**

***Siddha Swami's Commentary:***

A student *yogin* is trained to recognize in his own nature or psyche, the forces of greed, over-exertion, rashness, restlessness and craving along with their subsidiary and supportive potencies. They try to seize control of the psyche from time to time but since they are recognized, the student yogi may squelch them the way an alert security force stops the destructive efforts of insurgents.

**Greed** is observed in the psyche through its quest for good nutrition, sensual satisfaction and sexual attraction. Observing how his nature operates, the student *yogin* gets advisories from more advanced ascetics in how he may change, alter or at least incapacitate the lusty urges.

**Over-exertion** is sponsored by the quest for popularity which is allied to the sexual force. A student *yogin* has to make note of this and get advice on how to curb this.

**Rash undertaking** is under the auspices of the *buddhi* intellect organ which calculates how to take advantage of situations. But its underlying basis is the quest for popularity and expanded sexuality. A student yogi has to take note and make a decision to come to terms with this.

**Restlessness** comes from the assumption of duties not assigned by the Universal Form, but which might please other entities. Due to the lack of support from the Universal Personality of *Śrī* Krishna, one becomes insecure in pursuing the objective of others and so one has to abandon the association of all those who are adverse to the divine will. This is not easy to attain. A student *yogin* who is restless is usually asked by his teacher to concentrate on his brow chakra. This takes his attention away from the various cultural pursuits which baffled the intellect. When the mind relaxes its hold on the cultural objectives, he begins to listen to the teacher and then he may start the *buddhi yoga* practice.

**Craving** arises from too much exposure to sensual objects. There is a craving energy in the psyche of a living entity. It comes from the need to take in energy, either as subtle or gross nutrition. Eventually by the practice of *prāṇāyāma*, one sheds off that greed.

अप्रकाशोऽप्रवृत्तिश्च
प्रमादो मोह एव च ।
तमस्येतानि जायन्ते
विवृद्धे कुरुनन्दन ॥१४.१३॥
aprakāśo'pravṛttiśca
pramādo moha eva ca
tamasyetāni jāyante
vivṛddhe kurunandana (14.13)

*aprakāśo = aprakāśaḥ — lack of clarity; 'pravṛttiśca = apravṛttiśca = apravṛttiḥ — lack of energy + ca — and; pramādo = pramādaḥ — inattentiveness; mohā — confusion; eva — indeed; ca — and; tamasī — in depression; etāni — these; jāyante — they emerge; vivṛddhe — in the dominance; kurunandana — O dear son of the Kurus*

**Lack of clarity, lack of energy, inattentiveness and confusion emerge when depression is predominant, O dear son of the Kurus. (14.13)**

***Siddha Swami's Commentary:***

Clarity is one type of subtle material energy. The lack of it is another type of that energy. In *brahma yoga* one is trained in how to regard this. Normally one is eager to use the various psychological energies and in doing so one falls under their influence and loses whatever little or much objectivity one may have. But in *brahma yoga*, in higher meditation, one makes an indepth study of one's relationship to the various psychological states. If for instance the inattentive energy overcomes one by inducing a blank state, then one studies how that is done by that energy and one finds a way to transcend its power. This is all done in very subtle meditations.

Sometimes a student *yogin* is told to focus on a certain location within the psyche, say for instance, a focus on the location of the memory chamber or a particular image in the memory. He does this but then finds that he cannot maintain that focus and is shifted from it to something else either in the memory or in some other psychological location near the memory but outside of it. In this way, he studies the various locations and the power of the various equipments over him. Why is he not able to stop the memory from arresting his attention? This is all studied in great detail as one is guided by superior yogins.

Lack of energy is not a lack of an energy but is rather the influence of a particular type of stupefying subtle force. A *yogin* studies this power in meditation to see how it holds dominance over his attention. Can the energy that produced the lazy mood be used for an enthused psychological activity? In the practice of *prāṇāyāma* one learns how to convert a lazy energy into a productive force.

Confusion also is a type of energy. It is an admixture of certain psychological gases. A *yogin* may learn how to separate these, so that he may use them for constructive purposes.

Thus this verse gives us some idea of how the depression-producing psychic forces cause a lack of clarity, lack of energy, inattentiveness and confusion to bog down the attention.

यदा सत्त्वे प्रवृद्धे तु
प्रलयं याति देहभृत् ।
तदोत्तमविदां लोकान्
अमलान्प्रतिपद्यते ॥ १४.१४॥
yadā sattve pravṛddhe tu
pralayaṁ yāti dehabhṛt
tadottamavidāṁ lokān
amalānpratipadyate (14.14)

*yadā — when; sattve — in clarity; pravṛddhe — under the dominance of; tu — but; pralayaṁ — death experience; yāti — he goes; dehabhṛt — the embodied soul; tadottamavidāṁ = tadā — then + uttamavidāṁ — of those who know the supreme; lokān — worlds; amalan — pure; pratipadyate — he is transferred*

**When the embodied soul goes through the death experience while under the dominance of the clarifying mode, he is transferred to the pure world of those who know the Supreme. (14.14)**

***Siddha Swami's Commentary:***

*Śrī* Krishna could only give a generalization by stating that a person who passes from his material body, while his psychology is saturated with clarifying energy, would go to one of the worlds of those superior entities who know the Supreme. These are described as pure worlds, because these places are full of subtle energies from the clarifying part of material nature. The lower modes of impulsion and depression do not usually arise in such places. These are the cleanest psychological environments in the material world.

In Tibetan yoga, even in the *Tibetan Book of the Dead,* the *Bardo Thodol*, it is believed that if one were to assume a clarifying state of mind at the time of passing from the body, one would go to a pure world, to the land of the Buddhas, where one would immediately get enlightenment. Other religions give similar guarantees. Such procedures though very promising cannot create purity in the mind of a person who is usually impure, since the impure nature will remain active in the mental zones of that personality. But if one has cultivated the required purity in *buddhi yoga* practice, then certainly one has every chance of going to the pure world. *Buddhi yoga* is not limited to practitioners in India or to practitioners who believe in *Śrī* Krishna. Anyone anywhere with any belief, who practices *buddhi yoga* effectively, either through self discovery, learning from a teacher or learning from *Bhagavad Gītā,* will through that mastership attain purity of the psyche and will be attracted to the pure worlds described in this verse.

रजसि प्रलयं गत्वा
कर्मसङ्गिषु जायते ।
तथा प्रलीनस्तमसि
मूढयोनिषु जायते ॥ १४.१५ ॥
rajasi pralayaṁ gatvā
karmasaṅgiṣu jāyate
tathā pralīnastamasi
mūḍhayoniṣu jāyate (14.15)

*rajasi — in the impulsive mode; pralayam — death experience; gatvā — having gone; karmasaṅgiṣu = karmā — work + saṅgiṣu — among people who are prone; jāyate — is born; tathā — likewise; pralīnaḥ — dying; tamasi — in the depressive mode; mūḍhayoniṣu = mūḍha — ignorant; yoniṣu — in the wombs or species; jāyate — is born*

**Having gone through the death experience in the impulsive mode, the soul is born among the work-prone people; likewise when dying in the depressive mode, the soul takes birth from the wombs of the ignorant species. (14.15)**

***Siddha Swami's Commentary:***

The destination of a soul is reliant on his general consciousness. If generally one is in the clarifying mode, then one will go to a place which has that type of energy in saturation. If however one is generally dominated by impulsion, one will be attracted to people who are like that and will come out again after some time as a child of human or animal parents. A loss of consciousness at the time of death cannot in any way frustrate the appearance of the spirit in some other location according to the general demeanor he or she had while performing culturally. The essential self in the form of urges remains intact even during a coma or during any type of loss of consciousness. Those urges dictate where and how that spirit will appear in the next manifestation.

Even a human being if he or she passes from the body being habituated to depressed states, or to laziness, inattentiveness and confusion, runs the risk of having to develop as an embryo in an ignorant species, either as an animal, or vegetation or as the child of parents who are retarded and mentally-handicapped in some way or the other. It does not matter if such a person had religious bearings, for after all, we do see in this world that some who are in religious societies are retarded or mentally handicapped. That itself is evidence of their appearance in ignorant species. It is the state of mind that dictates the next formation of a body, not the religious faith of the person. Therefore elsewhere in the *Gītā*, *Śrī* Krishna spoke of self elevation by self endeavor.

*uddharedātmanātmānaṁ nātmānamavasādayet*
*ātmaiva hyātmano bandhur ātmaiva ripurātmanaḥ (6.5)*
*bandhurātmātmanastasya yenātmaivātmanā jitaḥ*
*anātmanastu śatrutve vartetātmaiva śatruvat (6.6)*

***One should elevate his being by himself. One should not degrade the self. Indeed, the person should be the friend of himself. Or he could be the enemy as well.***

***The personal energies are the friend of the person by whom those energies are subdued. But for one whose personality is not self-possessed, the personal energies operate in hostility like an enemy. (6.5-6)***

कर्मणः सुकृतस्याहुः
सात्त्विकं निर्मलं फलम् ।
रजसस्तु फलं दुःखम्
अज्ञानं तमसः फलम् ॥ १४.१६ ॥
karmaṇaḥ sukṛtasyāhuḥ
sāttvikaṁ nirmalaṁ phalam
rajasastu phalaṁ duḥkham
ajñānaṁ tamasaḥ phalam (14.16)

*karmaṇaḥ — of action; sukṛtasyāhuḥ = sukṛtasya — of well-performed + āhuḥ — the authorities say; sāttvikaṁ — of the clarifying mode; nirmalaṁ — free of defects; phalam — result; rajasaḥ — of impulsion; tu — but; phalaṁ — result; duḥkham — distress; ajñānaṁ — ignorance; tamasaḥ — of the depressing mode; phalam — consequences*

**The authorities say that the result of a well-performed action is in the clarifying mode and is free of defects. But the result of an impulsive act is distress, while the consequence of a depressive act is ignorance. (14.16)**

***Siddha Swami's Commentary:***

A student is required to study the effects of particular action so that he may understand the material world. It is not the encouragement one receives to perform an activity, that determines the result of it, but it is rather the type of energy which is used in the performing the act. This is psychological energy, found in the subtle body. Certain types of encouragement energies provide certain results of activities. This must be studied by each *yogin* in detail. This is how one studies one's nature in *buddhi yoga* practice and in the *ātma* yoga which was mentioned in Chapter Six.

Stated differently, a well-performed action is one which is approved by the Universal Form of *Śrī* Krishna. However most persons, even devotees of *Śrī* Krishna, do not have a method for gauging their actions continuously. Thus how can they know which actions are approved by the Lord? It is not a matter of doing pious activities, because as Arjuna experienced, even a pious act might be disapproved by the supreme will. Arjuna wanted to act piously by departing from the battlefield, by making overtures to stop the battle, but *Śrī* Krishna did not grant approval. Thus what is a pious act? Obviously the definition is subject to the desires of the Universal Form and His disciplinary will as it is pushed down into this world and enforced by Him through the physical actions of others and directly by His own acts when He descends.

Of note, *Śrī* Krishna described the superior actions as well-performed ones. He did not say pacifist acts or kind and loving acts. These well-performed acts are free of defects by His definition, because He considers what He has to do as the Central Figure in the Universal Form. Arjuna's acts on the battlefield of *Kurukṣetra* were seen by some in his own time as abominable acts. Even today some readers of the *Mahābhārata* history condemn such acts as reprehensible. But *Śrī* Krishna stated that these acts were free of defects, which means that this is Krishna's opinion. It means that such acts will not bear repercussions from the Universal Form of *Śrī* Krishna, but it does not mean that material nature or other limited beings may not react adversely to such acts. In the eyes of God, such acts are free of defects but that is all that can be said about it.

Impulsive acts by their very nature always end in distress. This is because an impulsion cannot cover the liabilities which will result from its actions. Once the actions are enacted, there will be liability and since the impulsion does not reveal this beforehand, the actor gets caught off guard when he or she is held accountable for the act by time and circumstances.

Depressive acts also bear repercussions but since the act occurs in a dull state of mind, one does not take the reactions seriously. And thus that person is saved for the time being from realizing the full impact of the action. Being sprayed over by ignorance, a person with a depressed psychology ignores the reactions and is thus saved from the brunt of liabilities. This is why such persons baffle jurors in a court of law.

सत्त्वात्संजायते ज्ञानं
रजसो लोभ एव च ।
प्रमादमोहौ तमसो
भवतोऽज्ञानमेव च ॥१४.१७॥
sattvātsaṁjāyate jñānaṁ
rajaso lobha eva ca
pramādamohau tamaso
bhavato'jñānameva ca (14.17)

*sattvāt — from clarity; saṁjāyate — is produced; jñānaṁ — factual knowledge; rajaso — rajasaḥ — from impulsion; lobha — greed; eva — indeed; ca — and; pramādamohau — inattentiveness and confusion; tamaso = tamasaḥ — from depression; bhavato = bhavataḥ — they come; 'jñānam = ajñānam — ignorance; eva — indeed; ca — and*

**Factual knowledge is produced from clarity. Greed comes from impulsion. Inattentiveness, confusion, and ignorance come from depression. (14.17)**

***Siddha Swami's Commentary:***

There is some awareness in all the states of consciousness, otherwise it would not be possible for anyone in a coma to revive, or for any living entity to emerge again in this world after having lost a body here and then having to endure the trance-like forgetfulness while living as sperm and embryo in the parents' bodies. Even in unconsciousness, consciousness must be present, though in dormancy. In modern medicine many anesthetics are used. By studying the effect of these, one can understand that consciousness endures through unconsciousness. The handicap is memory. In some states of consciousness, memory is unable to function and thus one does not recall anything. In these states where the memory is inactivated, the sense of being an observer may also be removed. It is a fact that sometimes when memory ceases to function, the person may still observe but he cannot recall what was experienced by him. These varying states of consciousness are studied carefully in *brahma yoga* practice, so that the *yogin* can understand the methods of the psyche.

In a state of clarity, one's energy supports observation mainly, but in impulsion one's attention is forged into consumption, which converts into the habit of greed. In depression, one's attention is sucked up by inattentiveness, confusion and ignorance. Arjuna for instance was seized by depression in Chapter One of this discourse. Thus he was in confusion and spoke from the perspective of ignorance.

ऊर्ध्वं गच्छन्ति सत्त्वस्था
मध्ये तिष्ठन्ति राजसाः ।
जघन्यगुणवृत्तस्था
अधो गच्छन्ति तामसाः ॥१४.१८॥

*ūrdhvaṁ — upward; gacchanti — they go; sattvasthā — situated in clarity; madhye — in the middle; tiṣṭhanti — they are situated; rājasāḥ — those who are impulsive; jaghanyaguṇavṛttasthā = jaghanya — lowest + guṇavṛttasthā — situated in the influence of the material energy; adho = adhaḥ — downward;*

ūrdhvaṁ gacchanti sattvasthā
madhye tiṣṭhanti rājasāḥ
jaghanyaguṇavṛttasthā
adho gacchanti tāmasāḥ (14.18)

*gacchanti — they go; tāmasāḥ — those who are retarded*

**Those who are anchored in clarity, go upward. Those who are impulsive are situated in the middle. Those who are habituated to the lowest influence of the material energy, the retarded people, go downward. (14.18)**

***Siddha Swami's Commentary:***

The human beings on this earthly planet are stationed in the middle as far as various locations one may exist in and function culturally in the material world. Thus humans are mostly influenced by the impulsive mode. The *brahma yoga* practice is designed for the slow but sure elevation upwards and away from this middle location. In *brahma yoga* there are no assumptions and the student is trained to realize himself as he is with all faults. He is then given the means to conquer his nature by deep introspection.

If one could become anchored in clarity, one would do so by endeavor because clarity is not a natural state for a human being. The human condition is one of impulsion. Thus if one could endeavor and maintain clarity, then one would go upwards to higher dimensions, where in higher association one would be elevated further. Śrī Krishna particularly used the term *sattvasthā*. And this means that no one can become upgraded unless he endeavors to be situated *(sthā)* in clarity *(sattva)*. Thus attempts to enter clarity at the time of death will not qualify one for such elevation. If sufficient endeavor was not made during life, one will again emerge as the child of a human being or some other species on an earthly planet like this one.

Habituation to the lowest influence, that of depressive energy, will cause a human being to descend to lower species of life. Habituation to the depressing energy is naturally fostered in lower life forms.

नान्यं गुणेभ्यः कर्तारं
यदा द्रष्टानुपश्यति ।
गुणेभ्यश्च परं वेत्ति
मद्भावं सोऽधिगच्छति ॥ १४.१९ ॥
nānyaṁ guṇebhyaḥ kartāraṁ
yadā draṣṭānupaśyati
guṇebhyaśca paraṁ vetti
madbhāvaṁ so'dhigacchati (14.19)

*nānyaṁ = na — not + anyam — other; guṇebhyaḥ — than the influences of material nature; kartāraṁ — the performer; yadā — when; draṣṭānupaśyati = draṣṭā — observer + anupaśyati — he perceives; guṇebhyaḥ — than the influences of material nature + ca — and; paraṁ — higher; vetti — he knows; madbhāvaṁ — my level of existence; so = saḥ — he; 'dhigacchati = adhigacchati — he reaches*

**When the observer perceives no performer besides the influences of material nature and knows what is higher than those influences, he reaches My level of existence. (14.19)**

***Siddha Swami's Commentary:***

*Śrī* Krishna kept repeating this point in so many words here and there in the *Gītā*. It is important to understand that the idea of God as the only performer in this world, is mostly self-assurance that God has the interest of His devotee as foremost. However when one splits off from these religious views and gets down to introspection, one descovers the truth, just as *Śrī* Krishna revealed it to Arjuna.

In truth, there is no other performer in the material world, except the influences of material nature, not even God. God is so detached from this situation, that to peg Him with the actions of matter is ludicrous and laughable.

One requires endeavor in higher yoga, in introspective meditation, to see exactly what is going on. As a matter of religious faith, one may feel that God is performing all the actions in this world, but such an idea has no place in the vision of reality which is perceived in higher yoga.

गुणानेतानतीत्य त्रीन्
देही देहसमुद्भवान् ।
जन्ममृत्युजरादुःखैर्
विमुक्तोऽमृतमश्नुते ॥१४.२०॥
guṇānetānatītya trīn
dehī dehasamudbhavān
janmamṛtyujarāduḥkhair
vimukto'mṛtamaśnute (14.20)

*guṇān — the influences of material nature; etān— these; atītya — transcends; trīn — three; dehī — embodied soul; dehasamudbhavān = deha — body + samudbhavān —formulated in; janmamṛtyujarāduḥkhaiḥ = janma — birth + mṛtyu — death + jarā — old age + duḥkhaiḥ — with distress; vimuktaḥ — released; 'mṛtam = amṛtam — immortality; aśnute — he attains*

**When the embodied soul transcends these three influences of material nature which are formulated in the body, he is released from birth, death, old age, and distress, and attains immortality. (14.20)**

***Siddha Swami's Commentary:***

The human body, that material form, is very important as a staging plank from which to gain liberation. This human life may provide the impulsion to strive for spiritual freedom, because this is the plane where impulsion is foremost. Even though in the subtle world, the influences of material nature are also present, the defect there is that one may have less objectivity. In the human world, because it is a hostile environment, one is more apt to face situations objectively and to try to figure where one stands in the range of these existences.

One can study the influences of material nature more objectively in a human body than in any other type of body. These influences are also in the subtle form but it is difficult to study there if one does not have a gross form. This is because the subtle body tends to absorb the experiences and one's objectivity becomes greatly relaxed in the psychic world.

Many male or female students are wonder-struck, when they find themselves in immoral situations in their dreams in the subtle world. In such encounters with other subtle beings, they sometimes engage in whimsical sexual intercourse, something that they would not have enacted on the material level. They are sometimes amazed that their discrimination stayed behind in their gross bodies when their subtle forms separated during the sleep of the gross forms. This proves that the gross body causes the discrimination to be more assertive, more definite. And this is why *Śrī* Krishna stated in this verse, that one may transcend the three influences of material nature which are formulated in the physical body *(dehasamudbhavān)*. Conversely, this means that when the subtle body is interspaced in a living physical form, one has a much better chance to use discrimination.

This is confirmed by the fact that those ascetics who practice yoga to an extent and who then lose their physical forms, are usually enticed to go to the heavenly planets, where they encounter angelic women whom they find to be sexually irresistible. After enjoying life with these females for a time, they again return to the earthly planet with much regret. They then hope to again assert or pick up their discrimination, and they work hard to by-pass such heavenly paradises where sexual energies attack them when they are helpless.

Immortality in this verse means not the immortality of the spirit but rather the spirit's break-off from having to be fused into temporary forms. When the spirit no longer has to use such forms or stated more precisely, when the spirit no longer feels a reliance on the temporary energies, then he is regarded as immortal.

अर्जुन उवाच
कैर्लिङ्गैस्त्रीन्गुणानेतान्
अतीतो भवति प्रभो ।
किमाचारः कथं चैतांस्
त्रीन्गुणानतिवर्तते ॥ १४.२१ ॥
arjuna uvāca
kairliṅgaistrīnguṇānetān
atīto bhavati prabho
kimācāraḥ kathaṁ caitāṁs
trīnguṇānativartate (14.21)

*arjuna — Arjuna; uvāca — said; kaiḥ — by what; liṅgaiḥ — by features; trīn — three; guṇān — influences; etān — these; atīto = atītaḥ — transcending; bhavati — he is; prabho — respectful Lord; kimācāraḥ = kim — what + ācāraḥ — conduct; kathaṁ — how; caitān = ca — and + etān — these; trîn — three; guṇān — influences; ativartate — he transcends*

**Arjuna said: In regards to a person who transcended the three influences of material nature, by what features is he recognized, O respectful Lord? What is his conduct? And how does he transcend the three influences? (14.21)**

***Siddha Swami's Commentary:***

This is a very good question. Praise be to Arjuna! No one wants to be cheated. How are we to identify a person who transcended the three influences? Since the transcendence is mostly an internal act, something psychic, how are we to perceive it?

श्रीभगवानुवाच
प्रकाशं च प्रवृत्तिं च
मोहमेव च पाण्डव ।
न द्वेष्टि संप्रवृत्तानि
न निवृत्तानि काङ्क्षति ॥ १४.२२ ॥
śrībhagavānuvāca
prakāśaṁ ca pravṛttiṁ ca
mohameva ca pāṇḍava
na dveṣṭi saṁpravṛttāni
na nivṛttāni kāṅkṣati (14.22)

*śrī bhagavān — the Blessed Lord; uvāca — said; prakāśaṁ — enlightenment; ca — and; pravṛttiṁ — enthusiasm; ca — and; moham — depression; eva — indeed; ca — and; pāṇḍava — O son of Pāndu; na — not; dveṣṭi — scorns; saṁpravṛttāni — presence; na — nor; nivṛttāni — absence; kāṅkṣati — yearns for*

**The Blessed Lord said: O son of Pāndu, he does not scorn nor does he yearn for the presence or absence of enlightenment, enthusiasm or depression. (14.22)**

***Siddha Swami's Commentary:***

One cannot identify such a person unless one is somewhat advanced in *buddhi yoga*, and one must have him under observation for some time. In addition one may hear of him from a reliable source.

This transcendence is denoted by total detachment when the *yogin* becomes advanced in the practice. This describes a person so advanced that he no longer has to endeavor for enlightenment. His example cannot to be followed by student yogins because they will only make progress through the exertion of efforts in *buddhi yoga*.

दासीनवदासीनो
गुणैर्यो न विचाल्यते ।
गुणा वर्तन्त इत्येव
योऽवतिष्ठति नेङ्गते ॥ १४.२३ ॥
udāsīnavadāsīno
guṇairyo na vicālyate
guṇā vartanta ityeva
yo'vatiṣṭhati neṅgate (14.23)

*udāsinavat — detached; āsīnaḥ — sitting, existing; guṇaiḥ — by the influences of material nature; yo = yaḥ— who; na — not; vicālyate — he is affected; guṇā — the mundane influences; vartanta — they operate; iti — thus (thinking that); eva — indeed; yo = yaḥ — who; 'vatiṣṭhati = avatiṣṭhati — he is spiritually situated; neṅgate = na — not + iṅgate — he becomes excited*

**Being situated in the body, but being detached, not being affected by the influences of material nature, considering that the modes are operating naturally, he who is spiritually-situated, who does not become excited, (14.23)**

***Siddha Swami's Commentary:***

*Śrī* Krishna told Uddhava about such a person who was an accomplished renunciant. This was explained in Canto 11 of *Śrīmad Bhāgavatam*. These descriptions are not to be imitated. These only give the student some idea of the advanced stages, after the efforts in *buddhi yoga* have borne success.

A student *yogin* should aspire to become a disciple of such a person but he should not interfere with that teacher. He should continue his endeavors in austerities while taking advice from such an advanced ascetic, just as King Yadu took instructions from the renunciant and Uddhava took instructions from Lord Krishna.

One should be like a good son or daughter to such a spiritual master. In that way, by his silent blessings one will complete the austerities which are mandatory in spiritual life. The purpose of associating with such a person is not to imitate or to be able to avoid the austerities but rather to develop the power to complete them.

समदुःखसुखः स्वस्थः
समलोष्टाश्मकाञ्चनः ।
तुल्यप्रियाप्रियो धीरस्
तुल्यनिन्दात्मसंस्तुतिः ॥ १४.२४ ॥
samaduḥkhasukhaḥ svasthaḥ
samaloṣṭāśmakāñcanaḥ
tulyapriyāpriyo dhīras
tulyanindātmasaṁstutiḥ
(14.24)

*samaduḥkhasukhaḥ = samā — equally regarded + duḥkha — pain + sukhaḥ — pleasure; svasthaḥ — self-situated; samaloṣṭāśmakāñcanaḥ = samā — regarded in the same way + loṣṭa — lump of clay + aśmā — stone + kāñcanaḥ — gold; tulyapriyāpriyo = tulyapriyāpriyaḥ = tulya — treated equally + priya — loved one + apriyaḥ — despised person; dhīraḥ — one who is steady of mind; tulyanindātmasaṁstutiḥ = tulya — regarded equally + nindā — condemnation + ātmā — self + saṁstutiḥ — congratulation*

**...to whom pain and pleasure are equally regarded, who is self-situated, to whom a lump of clay, a stone or gold, are regarded in the same way, by whom a loved one and a despised person are treated equally, who is steady of mind, to whom condemnation and congratulations are regarded equally, (14.24)**

***Siddha Swami's Commentary:***

Such an advanced ascetic is sometimes absent-minded, sometimes he is attentive, and sometimes he continues the mystic research. His disciples should not interfere with him or try to build a big mission around him, which might serve as a distraction for all concerned.

मानावमानयोस्तुल्यस्
तुल्यो मित्रारिपक्षयोः ।
सर्वारम्भपरित्यागी
गुणातीतः स उच्यते ॥ १४.२५ ॥
mānāvamānayostulyas
tulyo mitrāripakṣayoḥ
sarvārambhaparityāgī
guṇātītaḥ sa ucyate (14.25)

*mānāvamānayoḥ — in honor and dishonor; tulyaḥ — equally-disposed; tulyo = tulyaḥ — impartial; mitrāripakṣayoḥ — to friend or foe; sarvārambhaparityāgī = sarvā — all + ārambha — undertaking + parityāgī — renouncing; guṇatītaḥ = guṇa — mundane influence + atītaḥ — transcending; sā = saḥ — he; ucyate — is said to be*

**...who is equally disposed to honor and dishonor, who is impartial to friend or foe, who has renounced all undertakings, is said to have transcended the mundane influences. (14.25)**

***Siddha Swami's Commentary:***

The advanced ascetic having, an exemption from cultural activities, does renounce all undertakings but that does not mean that his disciples are in that category. He may advise some of his students to perform culturally and others to refrain from that, just as *Śrī* Krishna insisted that Arjuna fight on the battlefield but He told Uddhava to go to Badarinatha to do *tapasya* austerities in isolation from worldly life.

मां च योऽव्यभिचारेण
भक्तियोगेन सेवते ।
स गुणान्समतीत्यैतान्
ब्रह्मभूयाय कल्पते ॥ १४.२६ ॥
māṁ ca yo'vyabhicāreṇa
bhaktiyogena sevate
sa guṇānsamatītyaitān
brahmabhūyāya kalpate (14.26)

*māṁ — me; ca — and; yo = yaḥ — who; 'vyabhicāreṇa = avyabhicāreṇa — with unwavering; bhaktiyogena — by yogically-disciplined affection; sevate — serves; sā = saḥ — he; guṇān — the mundane influences; samatītyaitān = samatītya — transcending + etān — these; brahmabhūyāya — absorbing in spiritual existence; kalpate — is suited*

**And a person who serves Me with unwavering, yogicly-disciplined affection and who transcends these mundane influences, is suited for absorption in spiritual existence. (14.26)**

***Siddha Swami's Commentary:***

*Śrī* Krishna changed the subject suddenly by making this important statement about *bhakti yoga*. Besides the ascetics who transcended the influence of material nature, those who serve *Śrī* Krishna unwaveringly by yogically-disciplined affections also transcend the three influences. They are suited for absorption in spiritual existence. Thus there are two categories, those like the accomplished renunciant and then others who having mastered *buddhi yoga*, apply their affection or devotional love for *Śrī* Krishna, in a yogically-disciplined way. They also are rated as being transcendental to material nature. *Śrī* Krishna clarified that for one and all.

ब्रह्मणो हि प्रतिष्ठाहम्
अमृतस्याव्ययस्य च ।
शाश्वतस्य च धर्मस्य
सुखस्यैकान्तिकस्य च ॥ १४.२७ ॥
brahmaṇo hi pratiṣṭhāham
amṛtasyāvyayasya ca
śāśvatasya ca dharmasya
sukhasyaikāntikasya ca (14.27)

*brahmaṇo = brahmaṇaḥ — of spiritual existence; hi — indeed; pratiṣṭhāham = pratiṣṭhā — basis + aham — I; amṛtasyāvyayasya = amṛtasya — of the immortal + avyayasya — of the imperishable; ca — and; śāśvatasya — of the perpetual; ca — and; dharmasya — of the rules for social conduct; sukhasyaikāntikasya = sukhasya — of happiness + ekāntikasya — of the absolute; ca — and*

**...for I am the basis of the immortal, imperishable spiritual existence and of the perpetual rules of social conduct and of absolute happiness. (14.27)**

***Siddha Swami's Commentary:***

*Śrī* Krishna admitted Himself as the standard reference for spiritual advancement, ideal conduct and absolute happiness.

# CHAPTER 15

# Dvau Imau Puruṣau

# Types of Spirits*

*dvāvimau puruṣau loke kṣaraścākṣara eva ca*
*kṣaraḥ sarvāṇi bhūtāni kūṭastho'kṣara ucyate (15.16)*
*uttamaḥ puruṣastvanyaḥ paramātmetyudāhṛtaḥ*
*yo lokatrayamāviśya bibhartyavyaya īśvaraḥ (15.17)*

***These two types of spirits are in this world, namely the affected ones and the unaffected ones. All mundane creatures are affected. The stable soul is said to be unaffected.***

***But the highest spirit is in another category. He is called the Supreme Spirit, Who having entered the three worlds as the eternal Lord, supports it. (15.16-17)***

***Siddha Swami assigned this chapter title on the basis of verses 16 and 17 of this chapter.***

श्रीभगवानुवाच
ऊर्ध्वमूलमधःशाखम्
अश्वत्थं प्राहुरव्ययम् ।
छन्दांसि यस्य पर्णानि
यस्तं वेद स वेदवित् ॥ १५.१ ॥
śrībhagavānuvāca
ūrdhvamūlamadhaḥśākham
aśvatthaṁ prāhuravyayam
chandāṁsi yasya parṇāni
yastaṁ veda sa vedavit (15.1)

*śrī bhagavān — The Blessed Lord; uvāca — said; ūrdhvamūtam = urdhva — upward + mūlam — root; adhaḥśākham = adhaḥ — below + śākham — branch; aśvatthaṁ — ashvattha tree; prāhuḥ — the yogī sages say; avyayam — imperishable; chandāṁsi — Vedic hymns; yasya — of what, of which; parṇāni — leaves; yaḥ — who; taṁ — this; veda — knows; sa = saḥ — he; vedavit — knower of the Vedas*

**The Blessed Lord said: The yogi sages say that there is an imperishable Ashvattha tree which has a root going upwards and a trunk downwards, the leaves of which are the Vedic hymns. He who knows this is a knower of the *Vedas*. (15.1)**

***Siddha Swami's Commentary:***

The key point here is that the *aśvattha* tree is imperishable. It cannot be destroyed at any time by anyone, not even by God. The tree is eternal. It cannot be rooted out by anyone. In addition the tree grows inverted. While normally a tree is rooted into a gross material like soil and grows out into a more subtle material like air, this imperishable tree is rooted into a subtle dimension and grows into a gross one for development.

अधश्चोर्ध्वं प्रसृतास्तस्य शाखा
गुणप्रवृद्धा विषयप्रवालाः ।
अधश्च मूलान्यनुसंततानि
कर्मानुबन्धीनि मनुष्यलोके ॥ १५.२ ॥
adhaścordhvaṁ prasṛtāstasya śākhā
guṇapravṛddhā viṣayapravālāḥ
adhaśca mūlānyanusaṁtatāni
karmānubandhīni manuṣyaloke (15.2)

*adhaścordhvaṁ = adhaḥ — downward + ca — and + urdhvam — upward; prasṛtāh — widely spreading; tasya — of it; śākhā — branches; guṇa — mundane influence; pravṛddhā — nourished; viṣayapravālāḥ = viṣaya — attractive objects + pravālāḥ — sprouts; adhaśca = adhaḥ — below + ca — and; mūlāni — roots; anusaṁtatāni — stretched out; karmānubandhīni = karmā — action + anubandhīni — promoting; manuṣyaloke = manuṣya — of human being + loke — in the world*

**Branches spread from it, upwards and downwards. It is nourished by the mundane influences and the attractive objects are its sprouts. The roots are spread below, promoting action in the world of human beings. (15.2)**

***Siddha Swami's Commentary:***

The mundane influence which *Śrī* Krishna described as three psychological states, comprises subtle energies. The tree is nourished by these. The tree takes soil nutrients both from the upward direction in which the main root travels and from the downward direction, where some subsidiary roots expand. These downward roots foster cultural activities in the material world. The tree feeds on those cultural acts.

न रूपमस्येह तथोपलभ्यते
नान्तो न चादिर्न च संप्रतिष्ठा ।
अश्वत्थमेनं सुविरूढमूलम्
असङ्गशस्त्रेण दृढेन छित्त्वा ॥ १५.३

*na — not; rūpam — form; asyeha = asya — of it + iha— in this dimension; tathopalabhyate = tathā— thus + upalabhyate — it is perceived; nānto = nāntah = na — not + antaḥ — end; na — nor;*

na rūpamasyeha tathopalabhyate
nānto na cādirna ca saṁpratiṣṭhā
aśvatthamenaṁ suvirūḍhamūlam
asaṅgaśastreṇa dṛḍhena chittvā
(15.3)

*cādiḥ = ca — and + ādiḥ — end; na — nor; ca — and; saṁpratiṣṭhā — foundation; aśvatthaṁ — ashvattha tree; enam — this; suvirūḍhamūtam = suvirūḍha — well-developed + mūlam — root; asaṅgaśastreṇa = asaṅga — non-attachment + śastreṇa — with the axe; dṛḍhena — with the strong; chittvā — cutting down*

**Its form is not perceived in this dimension, nor its end, beginning or foundation. With the strong ax of non-attachment, cut down this Ashvattha tree with its well-developed roots. (15.3)**

***Siddha Swami's Commentary:***

This is not a gross manifestation which one can see with physical eyes, but one can, even if he or she cannot perceive this, consider it mentally and try to imagine it. This tree may be seen from the supernatural view point by highly advanced mystics and by the divine personalities.

Even though one cannot see this tree, one can feel its influence by studying how one is affected by the three types of energies in subtle material nature. Thus one can become convinced to follow *Śrī* Krishna's advice about cutting down the influence of this *aśvattha* tree. When a living being develops the required detachment, the influence of this tree is cut down only for himself or herself. Others must endeavor for conquest over those influences individually.

ततः पदं तत्परिमार्गितव्यं
यस्मिन्गता न निवर्तन्ति भूयः ।
तमेव चाद्यं पुरुषं प्रपद्ये
यतः प्रवृत्तिः प्रसृता पुराणी. ॥ १५.४॥
tataḥ padaṁ tatparimārgitavyaṁ
yasmingatā na nivartanti bhūyaḥ
tameva cādyaṁ puruṣaṁ prapadye
yataḥ pravṛttiḥ prasṛtā purāṇī (15.4)

*tataḥ — then; padaṁ — please; tat — that; parimārgitavyaṁ — to be sought; yasmin — to which; gatā — some; na — not; nivartanti — they return; bhūyaḥ — again; tam — that; eva — indeed; cādyaṁ = ca — and + ādyaṁ — primal; puruṣaṁ — person; prapadye — I take shelter; yataḥ — from whom; pravṛttiḥ — creation; prasṛtā — emerged; purāṇī — in primeval times*

**Then that place is to be sought, to which having gone, the spirits do not return to this world again. One should think: I take shelter with that Primal Person, from Whom the creation emerged in primeval times. (15.4)**

***Siddha Swami's Commentary:***

The *ādyam puruṣam*, Primal Person, is the alternative influence one leans on, if one intends to abandon the shelter of the material energy. Still, one cannot merely rely on that person in a passive way with a plan for Him to do everything required. One takes instructions from Him for the application of all of one's power in learning *buddhi yoga* and advancing along the path of development mentioned herein by *Śrī* Krishna.

निर्मानमोहा जितसङ्गदोषा
अध्यात्मनित्या विनिवृत्तकामाः ।
द्वंद्वैर्विमुक्ताः सुखदुःखसंज्ञैर्
गच्छन्त्यमूढाः पदमव्ययं तत् ॥ १५.५

*nirmāna — devoid of pride; mohā — confusion; jita — conquered; saṅga— attachment; doṣā — faults; adhyātmanityā = adhyātma — Supreme Spirit + nityā — constantly; vinivṛtta — ceased; kāmāḥ — cravings; dvandvaiḥ — by dualities;*

nirmānamohā jitasaṅgadoṣā
adhyātmanityā vinivṛttakāmāḥ
dvaṁdvairvimuktāḥ
sukhaduḥkhasaṁjñair
gacchantyamūḍhāḥ
padamavyayaṁ tat (15.5)

*vimuktāḥ — freed; sukhaduḥkha — pleasure-pain; saṁjñaiḥ — known as; gacchanti — they go; amūḍhāḥ — the undeluded souls; padam — place; avyayam — imperishable; tat = tad — that*

**Those who are devoid of pride and confusion, who have conquered the faults of attachment, who constantly stay with the Supreme Spirit, whose cravings ceased, who are freed from the dualities known as pleasure and pain, these undeluded souls go to that imperishable place. (15.5)**

***Siddha Swami's Commentary:***

*Nirmānamohā* means that one is devoid of the influence of the mental and emotional energy. This energy is usually identified as *citta* in the Sanskrit language. This energy is there perpetually but when one is able to resist it continuously as a matter of course, one is said to be *nirmānamohā* or without susceptibility *(nir)* to the mental *(māna)* and emotional *(mohā)* energies. Thus this verse is better translated as follows:

**Those who are not susceptible to the mental and emotional energy, who conquered the defect of relying on that energy, who constantly stay with the Supreme Spirit, whose cravings ceased, who are freed from the dualities known as pleasure and pain, these undeluded souls go to that imperishable place.(15.5)**

The important word is *amūḍhāh* which means undeluded in reference to the mental and emotional force and its influence upon the spirit. When one is freed from reliance on that force and can stand apart from it, one develops the ability to stay constantly in touch with the Supreme Spirit. *Śrī Patañjali Mahārṣi* explained what happens when one breaks off the reliance on the mental and emotional energies within one's psyche:

*puruṣārthaśūnyānāṁ guṇānāṁ pratiprasavaḥ*
*kaivalyaṁ svarūpapratiṣṭhā vā citiśaktiritiṁ*

***Separation of the spirit from the mento-emotional energy (kaivalyam) occurs when there is neutrality in respect to the influence of material nature, when the yogi's psyche becomes devoid of the general aims of a human being. Thus at last, the spirit is established in its own form as the force empowering the mento-emotional energy. (Yoga Sūtra, 4.34)***

The defect of the spirit is its reliance on the mental and emotional energies to which it becomes linked in the subtle material energy. Once this fault is realized, one may work to eliminate it. This work, however, is mostly done on the supernatural level; hence one needs to master *buddhi yoga* and its advanced stage which is *brahma yoga*. By such skill, one breaks the reliance on the subtle material force. This results in detachment and a simultaneous linking up with the Supreme Spirit, bringing on transference of focus to the imperishable place, the *padam avyayam*.

न तद्भासयते सूर्यो
न शशाङ्को न पावकः ।
यद्गत्वा न निवर्तन्ते
तद्धाम परमं मम ॥ १५.६ ॥

*na — not; tat — that; bhāsayate — illuminates; sūryo = sūryaḥ — the sun; na — nor; śaśāṅko = śaśāṅkaḥ — moon; na — nor; pāvakaḥ — fire; yat — which; gatvā — having gone; na — never; nivartante — they*

na tadbhāsayate sūryo
na śaśāṅko na pāvakaḥ
yadgatvā na nivartante
taddhāma paramaṁ mama (15.6)

*return; tat — that; dhāmā — residence; paramaṁ — supreme; mama — my*

**The sun does not illuminate that place, nor the moon, nor the fire. Having gone to that location, they never return. That is My supreme residence. (15.6)**

***Siddha Swami's Commentary:***

*Śrī* Krishna described the imperishable location, the anti-material sky, which might be called the reverse of this perishable place, as His supreme residence, *dhāma paramam mama*. He may be found in other dimensions in this world but the other locations are not His selected residence.

ममैवांशो जीवलोके
जीवभूतः सनातनः ।
मनःषष्ठानीन्द्रियाणि
प्रकृतिस्थानि कर्षति ॥ १५.७॥
mamaivāṁśo jīvaloke
jīvabhūtaḥ sanātanaḥ
manaḥṣaṣṭhānīndriyāṇi
prakṛtisthāni karṣati (15.7)

*mamaivāṁśaḥ = mama — my + eva — indeed + aṁśaḥ — partner; jīvaloke = jīva — individualized conditioned being + loke — in the world; jīvabhūtaḥ — individual soul; sanātanaḥ — eternal; manaḥ — mind; ṣaṣṭhānindriyāṇi = saṣṭhāni — sixth + indriyāṇi — sense, detection device; prakṛtisthāni — mundane; karṣati — draws*

**My partner is in this world of individualized conditioned beings. He is an eternal individual soul but he draws to himself the mundane senses of which the mind is the sixth detection device. (15.7)**

***Siddha Swami's Commentary:***

*Śrī* Krishna acknowledged the existence of Himself as the Supreme Person. He explained that the multiple entities are limited to their individual psyches. He accredits them as partners. Their defect or fault was stated before in verse 5 of this chapter as attachment to their mental and emotional energy. Here the same is stated more precisely as being an irresistible urge for the mundane senses of which the mind is the sixth detection device.

In the wording of *brahma yoga*, *kriyā yoga* or even kundalini yoga, the mind as described here is the *buddhi* or intellect organ, the mechanism in the head of the subtle body which imagines and analyzes. What is termed by *Śrī* Krishna as the mundane senses are the five super-subtle sensual orbs for hearing, touching, seeing, tasting and smelling. These orbs work in subordination to the intellect organ even though functionally they condition the intellect to obey their every whim.

Through reliance on the psyche, the mind and its contents of psychic energy and psychic sensing instruments, the living entity or the spirit becomes conditioned to their usages and remains stupefied in the material world, where he or she is forced to endure an haphazard and very temporary form of life.

शरीरं यदवाप्नोति
यच्चाप्युत्क्रामतीश्वरः ।
गृहीत्वैतानि संयाति
वायुर्गन्धानिवाशयात् ॥ १५.८॥

*śarīraṁ — by body; yad — which; avāpnoti — he acquires; yat — which; cāpi — and also; utkrāmatīśvaraḥ = utkrāmati — departs from + īśvaraḥ — master; gṛhītvaitāni = gṛhītvā —*

śarīraṁ yadavāpnoti
yaccāpyutkrāmatīśvaraḥ
gṛhītvaitāni saṁyāti
vāyurgandhānivāśayāt (15.8)

*taking + etāni — these; saṁyāti — he goes; vāyuḥ — wind; gandhān — perfumes; ivāśayāt = ivā — just as + āśayāt— from source*

**Regardless of whichever body that master acquires, or whichever one he departs from, he goes taking these senses along, just as the wind goes with the perfumes from their source. (15.8)**

***Siddha Swami's Commentary:***

The existential status of the spirit in this material world could not be described more aptly as was done by *Śrī* Krishna in this verse. Here the key to reincarnation is clearly extolled.

After compiling numerous cultural acts in one life, either in terms of fostering more material existence or curtailing the same, the spirit moves on to another life in the same location or somewhere else, taking along his sensual energies to the next manifestation in the same condition as in the previous existence. No change is made in the interim state. One has to go to from one life to another with the same developed or undeveloped, materially-addicted or spiritually-inclined sensual development which one cultivated.

श्रोत्रं चक्षुः स्पर्शनं च
रसनं घ्राणमेव च ।
अधिष्ठाय मनश्चायं
विषयानुपसेवते ॥ १५.९ ॥
śrotraṁ cakṣuḥ sparśanaṁ ca
rāsanaṁ ghrāṇameva ca
adhiṣṭhāya manaścāyaṁ
viṣayānupasevate (15.9)

*śrotraṁ —hearing; cakṣuḥ — vision; sparśanaṁ — sense of touch; ca — and; rāsanaṁ — taste; ghrāṇaṁ — smell; eva — indeed; ca — and; adhiṣṭhāya — governing; manaścāyaṁ = manaḥ — mind + ca — and + ayaṁ — this; viṣayān — attractive objects; upasevate — becomes addicted*

**While governing the sense of hearing, the vision, the sense of touch, the sense of taste, the sense of smell and the mind, My partner becomes addicted to the attractive objects. (15.9)**

***Siddha Swami's Commentary:***

The system of the subtle body's enjoyment facilities are beautifully described in this verse by *Śrī* Krishna. While in theory the spirit is supposed to govern *(adhiṣṭhāya)* the sensual energies which divest into five pathways, in practice the spirit becomes addicted to the attractive objects which the senses pursue. Thus *Śrī* Krishna indicated that by the use of the senses, His partner becomes a stooge to the sensual energies. Being thus conditioned to the sensual intakes, the limited spirit acts in a way that embarrasses itself and degrades his or her position as a partner of the Supreme Being.

The secret to freedom from the sensual addictions is detachment from the sensing energy itself. This is taught in the *buddhi yoga* practice.

उत्क्रामन्तं स्थितं वापि
भुञ्जानं वा गुणान्वितम् ।
विमूढा नानुपश्यन्ति
पश्यन्ति ज्ञानचक्षुषः ॥ १५.१० ॥

*utkrāmantaṁ — departing; sthitaṁ — remaining; vāpi = vā — or + api — also; bhuñjānaṁ — exploiting; vā — or; guṇānvitam — under the influence of*

utkrāmantaṁ sthitaṁ vāpi
bhuñjānaṁ vā guṇānvitam
vimūḍhā nānupaśyanti
paśyanti jñānacakṣuṣaḥ (15.10)

*material nature; vimūḍhā — idiots; nānupaśyanti = na — not + aupaśyanti — they perceived; paśyanti — they perceive; jñānacakṣuṣaḥ — vision of reality*

**The idiots do not perceive how the spirit departs or remains or exploits under the influence of material nature. But those who have the vision of reality do perceive this. (15.10)**

***Siddha Swami's Commentary:***

This text describes the freed, statically-bound or actively-bound condition of a spirit in reference to material nature. It is important to know your condition in relation to the mundane energy, for then one may work for release or, if released already, endeavor to stay apart from it.

If a spirit leaves his material body behind and continues in his psychic existence under the influence of material nature, his position in reference to that energy is not altered in the least. It is therefore stupid to feel that one became freed merely because he or she lost a gross body. The perplexity is the subtle body itself. Thus the departure from a gross form does not tell us anything about the status of the spirit in reference to the subtle one. All the same a spirit who remains in a gross body cannot do so unless he has a subtle body because the gross body cannot stay alive unless it is powered or supplied with psychic energy (kundalini power) from the subtle form. This means, therefore, that any spirit who uses a physical form must be fused into a subtle one. But it does not necessary hold true that all persons using physical forms are attached to their subtle forms. Some are detached to a greater or lesser degree according to their existential status as divine beings and according to their mastery of *buddhi yoga*. Thus someone may have a gross body and be liberated from the subtle form for the most part.

Mostly, however, those who appear to be enjoying life in a gross body are being increasingly conditioned by the sensual energies as described in the previous verse. Their exploitation of the pleasures is itself the means of their addictions to the sense objects.

When in *buddhi yoga* one develops the *jñānacakṣuṣah* (15.10), vision of reality, one is able to see the degree of fusion of a particular spirit with his or her subtle form and one can gage the person's degree of continuous, regular detachment from the psychic mundane energies. Otherwise one has to believe falsehood or truth according to prejudiced notions of one's impure intellect or what one is told by misleading or trustworthy authorities.

This verse should be understood in the context of the three previous verses, in the sense that the spirit is pursued or hunted down by the mundane senses of which the mind is labeled as the sixth detection device. This psychic energy is fused into the spirit in such a way that it follows the person wherever he may go into material bodies and out of them when they deteriorate. Thus the death of a gross form is no indication of freedom from material nature.

यतन्तो योगिनश्चैनं
पश्यन्त्यात्मन्यवस्थितम् ।
यतन्तोऽप्यकृतात्मानो
नैनं पश्यन्त्यचेतसः ॥ १५.११ ॥
yatanto yoginaścainaṁ
paśyantyātmanyavasthitam
yatanto'pyakṛtātmāno
nainaṁ paśyantyacetasaḥ (15.11)

*yatanto = yatantaḥ — endeavoring; yoginaścainaṁ = yoginaḥ — yogis + ca — and + enam — this (spirit); paśyānti — they see; ātmani — in the self; avasthitam — situated; yatanto = yatantaḥ — exertion; 'pi = api — even; akṛtātmāno — akṛtātmānaḥ = akṛta — not in order, imperfect + ātmānaḥ — self; nainaṁ = na — not + enam — this (spirit); paśyanti — they see; acetasaḥ — thoughtless ones*

**The endeavoring yogis see the spirit as being situated in itself; but even with exertion, the imperfected souls, the thoughtless ones, do not perceive it. (15.11)**

***Siddha Swami's Commentary:***

Even with exertion *(yatanto)* one cannot see the psychological organs which are known as the inner instruments or *antah karaṇa*. This is due to psychic blindness. However by the practice of *buddhi yoga* one may gain the vision (*jñāna cakṣuṣah,* 15.10). This vision is not a mental understanding or a theoretical view; it is an actual mystic perception which one develops after mastering *buddhi yoga*.

The failure of non-mystics to see the spirit as being situated in itself with an intellect and senses about it, is caused by their preoccupation with the external world. This diversion, which is naturally the urge of the intellect and senses, is curbed through the practice of *buddhi yoga*. That yoga, however, is not much liked by the conditioned beings and hence they are condemned to mystic blindness.

यदादित्यगतं तेजो
जगद्भासयतेऽखिलम् ।
यच्चन्द्रमसि यच्चाग्नौ
तत्तेजो विद्धि मामकम् ॥ १५.१२ ॥
yadādityagataṁ tejo
jagadbhāsayate'khilam
yaccandramasi yaccāgnau
tattejo viddhi māmakam (15.12)

*yat — which; ādityagatam — sun-yielding; tejo = tejaḥ — splendor; jagat — universe; bhāsayate — illuminates; 'khilam = akhilam — completely; yat — which; candramasi — in the mood; yat — which; cāgnau = ca — and + āgnau — in fire; tat — that; tejo = tejaḥ — splendor; viddhi — knows; māmakam —mine*

**That sun-yielding splendor which illuminates the universe completely, which is in the moon and which is in fire; know that splendor to be Mine. (15.12)**

***Siddha Swami's Commentary:***

*Śrī* Krishna explained the source of material light as something that ultimately originated from Him. A directive force, we may assume, must have a personal source behind it. Thus whatever is grand, great or all-pervasive must come from the Supreme Personality or from one of His parallel divinities.

गामाविश्य च भूतानि
धारयाम्यहमोजसा ।
पुष्णामि चौषधीः सर्वाः
सोमो भूत्वा रसात्मकः ॥ १५.१३ ॥

*gām — the earth; āviśya — penetrating; ca — and; bhūtāni — beings; dhārayāmi — I support; aham — I; ojasā — with potency; puṣṇāmi — I cause to thrive; cauṣadhīḥ = ca — and + auṣadhīḥ — plants; sarvāḥ — all;*

gāmāviśya ca bhūtāni
dhārayāmyahamojasā
puṣṇāmi cauṣadhīḥ sarvāḥ
somo bhūtvā rasātmakaḥ (15.13)

*somo = somaḥ — moon; bhūtvā — having influenced; rasātmakaḥ — sap-producing*

**And penetrating the earth, I support all beings with potency. And having influenced the sap-producing moon, I cause all plants to thrive. (15.13)**

***Siddha Swami's Commentary:***

This explains how the divine force of *Śrī* Krishna converts into mundane power in the material world. The nourishing forces in the universe are sometimes supportive of the desire of a limited entity. At other times, they seem to disregard him. Thus we see that a person flourishes sometimes and then clashes with the nourishing potencies at other times. Certainly the limited entities are not in control of their well-being.

अहं वैश्वानरो भूत्वा
प्राणिनां देहमाश्रितः ।
प्राणापानसमायुक्तः
पचाम्यन्नं चतुर्विधम् ॥ १५.१४॥
ahaṁ vaiśvānaro bhūtvā
prāṇināṁ dehamāśritaḥ
prāṇāpānasamāyuktaḥ
pacāmyannaṁ caturvidham (15.14)

*aham — I; vaiśvānaro = vaiśvānaraḥ — Vaiśvānara, a supernatural being, digestive heat; bhūtvā — becoming; prāṇināṁ — of the breathing beings; deham — body; āśritaḥ — entering; prāṇāpānasamāyuktaḥ = prāṇāpāna — inhaled and exhaled breath + samāyuktaḥ — combining; pacāmi — digest; annam — food; caturvidham — four kinds*

**Becoming the Vaiśvānara digestive heat, I, entering the body of all breathing beings and combining with the inhaled and exhaled breath, digest the four kinds of foodstuffs. (15.14)**

***Siddha Swami's Commentary:***

This is studied in one's body during kundalini yoga practice. Unless one can efficiently use the *Vaiśvānara* digestive heat and properly monitor the breathing of the body one uses, one cannot master yoga practice.

सर्वस्य चाहं हृदि संनिविष्टो
मत्तः स्मृतिर्ज्ञानमपोहनं च ।
वेदैश्च सर्वैरहमेव वेद्यो
वेदान्तकृद्वेदविदेव चाहम् ॥ १५.१५॥
sarvasya cāhaṁ hṛdi saṁniviṣṭo
mattaḥ smṛtirjñānam apohanaṁ ca
vedaiśca sarvairahameva vedyo
vedāntakṛdvedavideva cāham
(15.15)

*sarvasya — of all; cāhaṁ = ca — and + aham — I; hṛdi — in the central, psyche; saṁniviṣṭo = saṁniviṣṭaḥ — entered; mattaḥ — from me; smṛtiḥ — memory; jñānam — knowledge; apohanaṁ — reasoning; ca — and; vedaiśca = vedaiḥ — by the Vedas + ca — and; sarvaiḥ — by all; aham — I; eva — indeed; vedyo = vedyaḥ— to be known; vedāntakrt = vedānta — Vedānta + kṛt — maker, author; vedavit — knower of the Vedas; eva — indeed; cāham = ca — and + aham — I*

**And I entered the central psyche of all beings. From Me comes memory, knowledge and reasoning. By all the Vedas, I am to be known. I am the author of *Vedānta* and the knower of the Vedas. (15.15)**

***Siddha Swami's Commentary:***

Memory, knowledge and reasoning or analysis concern the memory and the intellect organs which are psychic mechanisms in the head of the subtle body. One should study this in the *buddhi yoga* practice or the *kriyā yoga* meditation process. The memory is a major cause for failure in meditation because it effectively interrupts higher focus and causes the self to remain preoccupied with mundane images and sounds. *Śrī* Krishna warned about the power of the memory in disrupting student yogis.

*karmendriyāṇi saṁyamya ya āste manasā smaran*
*indriyārthānvimūḍhātmā mithyācāraḥ sa ucyate (3.6)*

***A person who, while restraining his bodily limbs, sits with mind remembering attractive objects, is a deceiver. So it is declared. (3.6)***

Thus unless one masters *buddhi yoga*, one will not be able to shut down the power of the memory. This power is its ability to compel the imagination faculty (*buddhi* ) to illustrate stored impressions for preoccupation of the self. So long as one has not mastered memory control, one cannot attain *samādhi*.

As the Supreme Being, the Supreme Soul, *Śrī* Krishna is responsible for the creation of the psychic instruments which are called memory and intellect. But, the use of such instruments is a problem for the limited entities. They struggle to control these.

The *Vedas* and Vedanta give hints about such control. Each human being should study these texts and learn from a teacher how to put the *buddhi yoga* teaching into effect as a practical discipline. This is what Arjuna was trained to do by *Śrī* Krishna. Arjuna learnt it in about thirty minutes before the battle of *Kurukṣetra* but others may learn it over a number of years or a number of lives.

द्वाविमौ पुरुषौ लोके
क्षरश्चाक्षर एव च ।
क्षरः सर्वाणि भूतानि
कूटस्थोऽक्षर उच्यते ॥ १५.१६ ॥
dvāvimau puruṣau loke
kṣaraścākṣara eva ca
kṣaraḥ sarvāṇi bhūtāni
kūṭastho'kṣara ucyate (15.16)

*dvau — two; imau — these two; puruṣau — two spirits; loke — in the world; kṣaraścākṣara = kṣaraḥ — affected + ca — and + akṣara — unaffected; eva — indeed; ca — and; kṣaraḥ — affected; sarvāṇi — all; bhūtāni — mundane creatures; kūṭastho = kūṭasthaḥ — stable soul; 'kṣara — akṣara — unaffected; ucyate — is said to be*

**These two types of spirits are in this world, namely the affected ones and the unaffected ones. All mundane creatures are affected. The stable soul is said to be unaffected. (15.16)**

***Siddha Swami's Commentary:***

This refers to the limited spirits, some affected and others unaffected, all depending on their existential category and on their relationship to the material nature. The term *bhūtāni* indicates those limited spirits who are fused into subtle bodies, which have memory and intellectual mechanisms. Some of these spirits are detached from the psychic ways of perceiving and some are not. Those detached are not as affected as the others. Since the feed-back of influence from the psychic equipments is minimal. For the others, it is maximized such that they appear to be affected and they identify themselves as the psychic instruments.

उत्तमः पुरुषस्त्वन्यः
परमात्मेत्युदाहृतः ।
यो लोकत्रयमाविश्य
बिभर्त्यव्यय ईश्वरः ॥ १५.१७॥
uttamaḥ puruṣastvanyaḥ
paramātmetyudāhṛtaḥ
yo lokatrayamāviśya
bibhartyavyaya īśvaraḥ (15.17)

*uttamaḥ — higher; puruṣaḥ — spirit; tu — but; anyaḥ — another; paramātmeti = paramātmā — Supreme Spirit + iti — thus; udāhṛtaḥ — is called; yo = yaḥ — who; lokatrayam — three worlds; āviśya — entering; bibharti — supports; avyaya — eternal; īśvaraḥ — Lord*

**But the highest spirit is in another category. He is called the Supreme Spirit, Who having entered the three worlds as the eternal Lord, supports it. (15.17)**

***Siddha Swami's Commentary:***

The *Paramātma*, the Supreme Spirit, is in a separate category, because He is immune to the psychic equipments which may short-circuit the power of the limited spirits. Having entered these worlds and saturated them with His influence, that Supreme Person maintains them in His own way in conjunction with the absorbing powers of the subtle material nature.

The energy of the limited spirit, which is eternally produced, is inefficiently drained or drawn out by the psychic equipments, and thus the linkage with such a psyche is very taxing for the spirit. For the Supreme Person, this problem does not arise.

यस्मात्क्षरमतीतोऽहम्
अक्षरादपि चोत्तमः ।
अतोऽस्मि लोके वेदे च
प्रथितः पुरुषोत्तमः ॥ १५.१८॥
yasmātkṣaramatīto'ham
akṣarādapi cottamaḥ
ato'smi loke vede ca
prathitaḥ puruṣottamaḥ (15.18)

*yasmāt — since; kṣaram — affected; atīto = atītaḥ — beyond; 'ham = aham — I; akṣarāt — than the unaffected spirits; api — even; cottamaḥ = ca — and + uttamaḥ — higher; ato = ataḥ — hence; 'smi = asmi — I am; loke — in the world; vede — in the Veda; ca — and; prathitaḥ — known as; puruṣottamaḥ — Supreme Person*

**Since I am beyond the affected spirits and I am even higher than the unaffected ones, I am known in the world and in the *Vedas* as the Supreme Person. (15.18)**

***Siddha Swami's Commentary:***

*Puruṣottamah*, the Supreme Person, is glorified in the *Vedas*, and He is known in this world as God. However not every human being admits His existence. Many deny Him.

यो मामेवमसंमूढो
जानाति पुरुषोत्तमम् ।
स सर्वविद्भजति मां
सर्वभावेन भारत ॥ १५.१९॥
yo māmevamasaṁmūḍho
jānāti puruṣottamam
sa sarvavidbhajati māṁ
sarvabhāvena bhārata (15.19)

*yo = yaḥ— who; mām — me; evam — in this way; asaṁmūḍho = asaṁmūḍhaḥ — undeluded; jānāti — knows; puruṣottamam — Supreme Person; sa — he; sarvavit — all-knowing, knowledgeable; bhajati — worships; mām — me; sarvabhāvena — with all being; bhārata — O man of the Bharata family*

**In this way, he who is undeluded, who knows Me as the Supreme Person, he being knowledgeable, worships Me with all his being, O man of the Bharata family. (15.19)**

***Siddha Swami's Commentary:***

It is natural that as soon as a living being becomes convinced about the supremacy of Lord Krishna, there would ensue worship of the Lord. Even if one does not accept *Śrī* Krishna as the Supreme Person, still if one accepts that there is such a Supreme Lord, one will be inclined to worship according to the information and experience at one's disposal.

इति गुह्यतमं शास्त्रम्
इदमुक्तं मयानघ ।
एतद्बुद्ध्वा बुद्धिमान्स्यात्
कृतकृत्यश्च भारत ॥ १५.२० ॥
iti guhyatamaṁ śāstram
idamuktaṁ mayānagha
etadbuddhvā buddhimānsyāt
kṛtakṛtyaśca bhārata (15.20)

*iti — thus; guhyatamaṁ — most secret; śāstram — teaching; idam — this; uktaṁ — is declared; mayā — by me; 'nagha = anagha — O blameless man; etat — this; buddhvā — having realized; buddhimān — wise; syāt — he should become; kṛtakṛtyaśca = kṛtakṛtyaḥ — with duties accomplished + ca — and; bhārata — O descendant of Bharata*

**Thus the most secret teaching is declared by Me, O blameless man. Having realized this, O descendant of the Bharatas, one becomes a wise person, whose duties are accomplished. (15.20)**

***Siddha Swami's Commentary:***

The categorical situations of the various spirits is a most secret revelation. At first one may hear of it from *Śrī* Krishna or from some advanced being. But then one should go on to realize it, beginning with a careful study of one's psychic and spiritual existence. This is done in *brahma yoga* practice. It is important to know the category of one's spirit, as well as that of others in the psychic environment.

# CHAPTER 16

# Dvau Bhūta Sargau

# Types of Created Beings*

*dvau bhūtasargau loke'smin daiva āsura eva ca*
*daivo vistaraśaḥ prokta āsuraṁ pārtha me śṛṇu (16.6)*

***There are two types of created beings in this world, the godly type and the wicked. The godly type was explained in detail. Hear from me of the wicked, O son of Pṛthā. (16.6)***

***Siddha Swami assigned this chapter title on the basis of verse 6 of this chapter.***

श्रीभगवानुवाच
अभयं सत्त्वसंशुद्धिर्
ज्ञानयोगव्यवस्थितिः ।
दानं दमश्च यज्ञश्च
स्वाध्यायस्तप आर्जवम् ॥ १६.१ ॥

śrībhagavānuvāca
abhayaṁ sattvasaṁśuddhir
jñānayogavyavasthitiḥ
dānaṁ damaśca yajñaśca
svādhyāyastapa ārjavam (16.1)

*śrī bhagavān —the Blessed Lord; uvāca — said; abhayaṁ —fearlessness; sattvasaṁśuddhiḥ = sattva — existence, being + saṁśuddhiḥ — purity; jñānayogavyavasthitiḥ = jñāna — mental concept + yoga — application of yoga + vyavasthitiḥ — consistence; dānaṁ — charity; damaśca = damaḥ — self-restraint + ca — and; yajñaśca = yajñaḥ— worship ceremony + ca — and; svādhyāyaḥ — recitation of scripture; tapa — austerity; ārjavam — straight-forwardness*

**The Blessed Lord said: Fearlessness, purity of being, consistency in application of yoga to mental concepts, charity, self-restraint, worship ceremony, recitation of scripture, austerity and straight-forwardness, (16.1)**

***Siddha Swami's Commentary:***

This is part of the listing of those qualities which are conducive to the development of spiritual realization. If cultivated and maintained, these habits reinforce the clarifying mode of material nature and that leads to spiritual insight, from which one may develop an interest in abandoning the fondness for the psychic equipments.

As a reality unto itself and especially when referenced to the temporary forms of the material energy, the spirit is eternal. Thus it should not feel insecure. It should not be threatened by anything. But since the spirit is fused to the temporary sensing mechanisms, it may derive from that association a sense of insecurity. This results in fearfulness. By resituating itself in the clarifying mode of material nature, the spirit gains a sense of fearlessness and feels advantaged in the material creation. Then later, through mastery of *buddhi yoga*, the spirit can isolate itself even from the clarifying energy. And it then realizes its superiority. This was explained by *Śrī* Krishna:

*indriyāṇi parāṇyāhur indriyebhyaḥ paraṁ manaḥ*
*manasastu parā buddhir yo buddheḥ paratastu saḥ (3.42)*

***The ancient psychologists say that the senses are energetic, but in comparison to the senses, the mind is more energetic. In contrast to the mind, the intelligence is even more sensitive. But in reference, the spirit is most elevated. (3.42)***

**Fearlessness,** though a godly quality, does not necessarily free a person from trauma. His or her subtle body may still react adversely or with fearfulness because that is the nature of the subtle mechanism. But the spirit which is fused to the psyche should keep focused on its eternity, regardless of the actions and reactions in the psychology.

**Purity of being**, listed in Sanskrit as *sattvasamśuddhih*, means the purity of the psychic energy as well as the detachment of the spirit which is tied to a psyche. This was explained by *Śrī Patañjali* in another way:

*sattva puruṣayoḥ śuddhi sāmye kaivalyam iti*

***When there is equal purity between the intelligence energy of material nature and the spirit, then there is total separation from the mundane psychology. (Yoga Sūtra, 3.56)***

*Śrī Patañjali Mahārṣi* also used the terms *sattva* and *śuddhi*, being quite consistent with Lord Krishna. The point is that purity of being occurs only after mastership of *buddhi yoga* to such proficiency that the *yogin* has effected purity of his psychic body and the instruments within it, as well as purity of his spirit by virtue of detachment from the psychic equipments.

When this is achieved one is welcomed into the association of the siddhas, who were mentioned by Arjuna as *siddhasamghāh*:

*arjuna uvāca*
*sthāne hṛṣīkeśa tava prakīrtyā jagatprahṛṣyatyanurajyate ca*
*rakṣāṁsi bhītāni diśo dravanti sarve namasyanti ca siddhasaṁghāḥ (11.36)*

***Arjuna said: Everything is in position, O Hṛṣīkeśa, masterful controller of the senses. The universe rejoices and is delighted by Your fame. The demons being terrified, flee in all directions. All the groups of perfected souls will reverentially bow to You. (11.36)***

**Consistency in application of yoga to mental concepts** is the mastership of *jñāna yoga*, techniques which are higher than *karma yoga*. Eventually when one is done with social life, one turns to practice of *jñāna yoga*. This is very advanced *buddhi yoga*. It starts with learning *buddhi yoga* and then one takes up *karma yoga*, because one must complete certain social tasks in promoting righteous lifestyle as instructed by *Śrī* Krishna. When one has done enough of that and gains the approval of *Śrī* Krishna, one takes to *jñāna yoga*. But for consistency in that, one must practice for some time and be free from the cultural associations which keep one tied to social activities. It is doubtful as to whether anyone can become liberated without mastership of *jñāna yoga*. In fact if one cannot practice this, then it indicates that one will remain hooked up to the cultural stipulations in this world.

**Charity** is required all through life since one cannot live anywhere and not make contact with other beings. Even in the case of those yogins who are elevated to higher realms where they meet only higher beings who cannot possibly need anything from them, there is still the urge for charity. It is satisfied there by living in a way which is approved by the higher yogins. One's gift to the spiritual teacher is the taking up of disciplines which causes one to remain in their association. That is the disciple's charity to his teachers.

**Self restraint** is practiced in all phases of yoga but it is demonstrated differently according to the advancement of a particular ascetic. *Damah* means to be restrained from mixing into the cultural life of the world. It is to be restrained from involvements without alienating other entities who desire that one be committed to material existence for one reason or another. The involvements from many previous lives created impressions and formative energies, which try to lure an ascetic to return to the world to reap benefits of his former pious activities. He must see this and resist it, awarding it to providence freely so that it might be given to others for their usage. An example is sexual indulgence. If for instance, a certain *yogin* is due, by his previous pious life, to be in a sexual relationship with a well-to-do respected lady, even in a morally approved way, he may sidestep that and award the pious result to some other man. In that way he restrains himself from taking a benefit which was due to him by the laws of consequence. This is what is meant by *damah*.

**Worship ceremony** is like a bridge construction which was never completed, reaching only half way across a deep and very wide gorge. Many persons take such an uncompleted bridge and at the end of it, they wonder as to its completion. They become baffled to find that it will not take them across the dimensions which span from this world to the other imperishable location, which *Śrī* Krishna called His special abode.

**Recitation of scripture** does not in itself take one across the chasm either but it helps one to develop the determination required to perform the austerities through which one might bridge the chasm. The most important part of the scriptures is the descriptions of the lives of those ascetics who completed the austerities and actually left this place, crossing to the imperishable location.

**Austerity** is an essential part of the journey from this world to the transcendental place, but the problems arise with austerity because of performance of the wrong disciplines. Gradually an ascetic reforms his mistaken efforts and by advice from superior yogins, he comes to take up the correct path of *buddhi yoga* in its lower and higher stages.

**Straightforwardness** comes after one attains purification of the psyche through the mastership of kundalini yoga, to eliminate negative psychic energy or prana from the subtle body and replace it with positive psychic energy which fosters clarification of consciousness and development of the supernatural insight, termed as *jñānacakṣuṣah* in the *Bhagavad Gītā*.

अहिंसा सत्यमक्रोधस्
त्यागः शान्तिरपैशुनम् ।
दया भूतेष्वलोलुप्त्वं
मार्दवं ह्रीरचापलम् ॥१६.२॥

ahiṁsā satyamakrodhas
tyāgaḥ śāntirapaiśunam
dayā bhūteṣvaloluptvaṁ
mārdavaṁ hrīracāpalam (16.2)

*ahiṁsā — nonviolence; satyam — recognition of reality; akrodhaḥ — absence of anger; tyāgaḥ — abandonment of consequences; śāntiḥ — spiritual security; apaiśunam — absence of destructive criticism; dayā — compassion; bhūteṣu — in beings; aloluptvam — freedom from craving; mārdavaṁ — gentleness; hrīḥ — modesty; acāpalam — absence of fickleness*

**...nonviolence, recognition of reality, absence of anger, abandonment of consequences, spiritual security, absence of destructive criticism, compassion for the beings, freedom from craving, gentleness, modesty, absence of fickleness, (16.2)**

***Siddha Swami's Commentary:***

**Nonviolence** cannot be exercised fully without a waiver from cultural activity from the Universal Form, from *Śrī* Krishna. In any type of cultural participation, there would be violence in one way or another to one life form or another. Only when one has exited from this dimension, can one rid oneself of the need for violence. Ascetics should all practice nonviolence as much as they can afford. One should move away from societies in which violence is highlighted and found to be necessary for the upkeep of the people. But one must work individually to remove the psychic need to be in environments where violence must be perpetrated for survival of one's body in those locations.

The cultivation of nonviolence is related to diet. If for instance one needs a certain vitamin for bodily survival, then one should try to acquire that from vegetarian sources. But if one lives in an area where that vitamin is only available from animal bodies, then one should consider relocating to a place where a vegetative produce yields that type of diet. In this way an effort will be made to decrease mandatory violence for survival purposes. Providence will take note of the endeavor. Thus in a future time, one will be transferred to a place where sordid activities are not part of the day to day existence.

Even if a vitamin is available from an animal body as well as from a vegetative form, the acquirement of it from animal flesh involves a greater degree of suffering to the creature concerned. It also involves a certain callousness towards the creature killed for the sake of one's belly. Thus one should decrease the violence perpetrated for diet by selecting the least hazardous course for nutritional needs.

The **recognition of reality** comes about through purification of the psychic equipments. These equipments carry in them certain prejudices. As soon as one becomes detached within the psyche, one sees internal opposition to the prejudices and one can make a decision to curb them by practicing *kriyā yoga*. *Kriyā yoga* concerns performance of effective, non-imaginative mystic actions which effect changes in the subtle body, changes which enable control of memory activation and the imagination faculty.

**Absence of anger** is the removal of the mento-emotional energies which seek out fulfillments in the material world. These energies are prone to frustration since they are not always coordinated with reality. In the mento-emotional psyche, there are many energies of expression which are totally impractical in terms of their expression, fulfillment and expansion in the subtle or gross material world. When such energies are expressed, they convert into frustration if the expressions do not find accommodations in the subtle or gross world. Hence, through *buddhi yoga* and *brahma yoga,* one must become distanced from these energies, so that one does not become victimized in trying to express them for fulfillments.

*Śrī* Krishna laid out the formula for anger previously, when He said:

*dhyāyato viṣayānpuṁsaḥ saṅgasteṣūpajāyate*
*saṅgātsaṁjāyate kāmaḥ kāmātkrodho'bhijāyate (2.62)*
*krodhādbhavati saṁmohaḥ saṁmohātsmṛtivibhramaḥ*
*smṛtibhraṁśādbuddhināśo buddhināśātpraṇaśyati (2.63)*

***The act of considering sensual objects, creates in a person, an attachment to them. From attachment comes craving. From this craving, anger is derived.***

***From anger, comes delusion. From this delusion, the conscience vanishes. When he loses judgment, his discerning power fades away. Once the discernment is affected, he is ruined. (2.62-63)***

He also stated elsewhere:

*śrībhagavānuvāca*
*kāma eṣa krodha eṣa rajoguṇasamudbhavaḥ*
*mahāśano mahāpāpmā viddhyenamiha vairiṇam (3.37)*

***The Blessed Lord said: This force is craving. This power is anger. The passionate emotion is the source. It has a great consuming power and does much damage. Recognize it as the enemy in this case. (3.37)***

One must carefully study these explanations of *Śrī* Krishna. Then one must meditate steadily and find out the truth of the matter. One must derive from a yoga master the technique for removing these energies from the nature. If these cannot be removed, then one must take steps to remove oneself from the parts of the psyche in which such unruly energies developed.

External expressions of anger are not the problem. It is the internal energies which sponsor, endorse and produce this. Thus one should go deeply within and find out the sources of such powers.

The **abandonment of consequences** is the preliminary practice for attaining true *sannyāsa*, which is the abandonment of opportunities in the material world. *Śrī Patañjali Mahārṣi*, our teacher, informed that the *prakṛti* material energy may serve us in two instances, either to provide experiences or to inspire liberation. Some of the experiences themselves are the spur for liberation. It may be said that some of the experiences are worth while and that some are entertaining. Others are definitely degrading. Thus the need for liberation arises in those living entities who have a higher view of themselves. Such souls try to turn away from the material nature in all its shapes and forms, but initially they are unable to get out.

At first one must aim to abandon the consequences which arrive in time as destined results of previous activities. Some of these one may avoid while others have a force which buffets rejection. Gradually when one learns the art of avoidance, and develops the ability to step aside from the opportunities for actions, as well as from the results yielded from previous action. To do this one requires the assistance of *Śrī* Krishna, the Person Who is Central in the Universal Form.

**Spiritual security** or *śāntih* is achieved after one scaled down the expenditure of psychic energy. Due to too much involvement with others, one expends more energy than one can afford on the psychological plane. One does this to impress others and to become important or loved in the world. Hence after finding that one has drained his or her emotions, one seeks ways of curtailing the involvements which demand so much expenditure of mental and emotional force.

As soon as one reduces the expenditure, especially of the emotional energies, one finds that one feels much better psychologically. Additionally, one must stay away from the places and persons which extract more energy than is safe for one's well being. One must link up to those who are not parasitic or demanding of too much attention. One must link to the higher persons who are linked to *Śrī* Krishna, the Lord of the world. From them one may get uplifting associations which replace normal worldly association which is degrading.

The **absence of destructive criticism** occurs when one has become removed from so much challenging association in the world. The more one spreads out with many, many people of this world, the more it becomes necessary to consider the circumstances of others and to make remarks concerning their various positions in the world. *Śrī* Krishna listed isolation as a requirement for yoga practice. To be successful one has to move away from worldly association. As soon as one does this, one will begin advancing into higher association, leaving aside the ordinary persons of this world.

*Śrī* Krishna explained to Arjuna the concerns of the Universal Form, as *dharma* righteous lifestyle. One should leave that sort of business to the God and helping in that task only if He so desires, as He did with Arjuna. Otherwise one should not be overly concerned with the progress of human history. One's main business is spiritual advancement, mastership of *buddhi yoga* as *Śrī* Krishna taught it. To get out of the way of the Universal Form, is also a service to God, just as to help Him clear the way for righteous lifestyle, is the service of *karma yoga*. To get out of His way is *jñāna yoga*, which is one of the two disciplines which He taught initially. One must either help Him or act in a way which does not oppose Him.

**Compassion for the beings** serves the purpose to free the *yogin* from selfishness. In that action, the *yogin*'s nature sheds its need to scramble for resources. However, a preoccupation with compassion is not recommended. One should administer compassion by the dictates of the Universal Form of *Śrī* Krishna and not otherwise, for then one might run the risk of resisting the divine will which levies its concerns for the beings in disciplinary and affectionate ways according to its discretion. The concern of the Supreme Being may be termed as divine love or it may be called divine harassment, but in either case it is the administration of divine affection to the limited beings. Hence one should not act with compassion whimsically or upon demand by others but should be inspired by the supreme will. In that way one would remain compatible to the Supreme Being.

**Freedom from craving** is attained through mastership of *buddhi yoga*. This is because the root of craving is the subtle and causal bodies combined. In these subtle and super-subtle forms, energies sponsor the cravings which are manifested in the gross and subtle worlds. These energies may be de-existed or squelched completely by mastership of *pratyāhār* sensual energy withdrawal and containment practice. This is done in higher yoga only. Attempts at the conquest of vice through *yama* restraints and *niyama* approved behaviors are external and thus these are ineffective methods which work on occasion and fail miserably at other times when strong urges overpower and control the sense of discrimination in the intellect. Religious principles, regulative principles, morality and such rules of behavior and values of social interactions are external means of controlling the urges but these cannot bring about a total elimination. Hence the need exists for *buddhi yoga* to root out the urges in their psychic locales. *Śrī* Krishna hinted that the senses, mind and intelligence were places of habitation of the lusty power. Here is what He said:

*indriyāṇi mano buddhir asyādhiṣṭhānamucyate*
*etairvimohayatyeṣa jñānamāvṛtya dehinam (3.40)*

***It is authoritatively stated that the senses, the mind and the intelligence are the combined warehouse of the passionate enemy. By these facilities, the lusty power confuses the embodied soul, shrouding his insight. (3.40)***

The craving energies emerged fromcertain parts of the subtle material nature. They can be retrogressed back into non-existence, although their potential will still remains. At least their de-existence would put their potential out of commission for the particular *yogin* who can control his nature. Material nature, the subtle aspect of it, has cosmic potential for manifestation and one must get himself or herself into a psychic position from which one might choose which of the her expressions one is compatible with. This can only be done in higher yoga practice.

**Gentleness** is achieved in higher yoga when one gets continuous association with great yogins and with the divine beings. After escaping from lower association in the world of human beings, a student *yogin* becomes gentle. He or she no longer makes so many efforts in a struggle to procure one's basic needs and find placement in environments which are shared by immature living beings. Looking back, a student yogi reviews his or her past in the world of the embodied souls who struggle with one another for pleasures and commodities. Finished with that, one becomes gentle as a son or daughter of the great persons in the divine world.

**Modesty** becomes important to those student yogins who no longer want to expose themselves to social interactions. They desire to remain with the *siddhas*. Realizing that exposure sponsors and aggravates the consequential results of their former actions, they assume a modest posture, so as to lay low in the realm of subtle material nature. This gives them the ability to apply for an exemption from cultural acts, something which they might achieve by the grace of the Universal Form. Unless one is modest, one cannot avoid the consequences of one's actions from this and many, many past lives. And if one remains exposed to material nature, it will of necessity tag one for reactions, and one would not be able to a decrease the amount of time spent responding to challenges of destiny, which are based on one's past.

**Absence of fickleness** happens on the high end of yoga practice, after one gains exemption from cultural activities and begins to dedicate oneself to a consistent *buddhi yoga* practice, above everything else. This means that the student *yogin* is freed from the cultural associations which bar him from yoga austerities. He remains constant in practice and his advancement begins to consolidate. Great yogins enter his subtle body and show him the advanced *kriyā yoga* techniques. He is able to escape from the routine type of life endured by most human beings and so he progresses rapidly. The fulfillment gained from association with advanced beings who have material bodies and those advanced persons who do not have any, is such that he no longer feels the need to be near to human beings. Thus he can sincerely honor the requirement for isolation while practicing *buddhi yoga*.

तेजः क्षमा धृतिः शौचम्
अद्रोहो नातिमानिता ।
भवन्ति संपदं दैवीम्
अभिजातस्य भारत ॥ १६.३ ॥
tejaḥ kṣamā dhṛtiḥ śaucam
adroho nātimānitā
bhavanti saṁpadaṁ daivīm
abhijātasya bhārata (16.3)

*tejaḥ — vigor; kṣamā — forbearance; dhṛtiḥ — strong-mindedness; śaucam — purity; adroho = adrohaḥ — freedom from hatred; nātimānitā = na — not + ātimānitā — conceit; bhavanti — they are; saṁpadaṁ — nature; daivīm — godly; abhijātasya — of those born; bhārata — O desendant of Bharata*

**...vigor, forbearance, strong-mindedness, purity, freedom from hatred, and the freedom from conceit; these are the talents of those born with the godly nature, O descendent of Bharata. (16.3)**

***Siddha Swami's Commentary:***

**Vigor** is the result of celibacy through yoga practice by mastering kundalini energy. It comes from a reformed pranic force in the subtle body. When the *yogin* breaks off from sexual needs, he begins to see himself as a son of Lord Shiva. In the case of the yoginis, they take shelter of Lord Shiva and Goddess *Durgā* as daughters only. These are daughters without needs for sexual intercourse. In such a relationship with the Lord, they get shelter from the miseries of righteous or irreligious lifestyle. Both the righteous and unrighteous people in this world are subjected to miseries, even though the irresponsible people get more harassment. But when at last one gives up the envy of Lord Shiva and Goddess *Durgā*, the chief parents of this subtle and gross world, then one is freed from the responsibilities and their psychological or emotional stresses.

By relinquishing sexual needs, one conserves vigor. The reserved energy can then be used to energize the subtle body. This results in higher perception and the development of higher preferences.

**Forbearance** comes after leaving one's consequences as a donation to others and as something discarded into the material world for use by others. Due to many, many lives in the cultural environments of this world, each living entity has innumerable pious and sinful reactions coming to him in providence. These forces cannot be wished away by desire. They cannot be removed from the material energy. Hence, as soon as one gets a waiver from the Universal Form, one donates these reactionary energies to nature, so that others might utilize them as they are released into manifestation. When this is done, development of a forbearance energy occurs in the subtle body, which allows the student *yogin* to take on the duties of higher yogins, who left the subtle existence. Those higher yogins, having left the subtle existence, cannot help some of their students who have not advanced very far in higher yoga. Thus some of their duties may be taken up by student yogins who can see or hear them in the higher subtle world. These student yogins act as substitute teachers for those higher teachers.

In order to do this, they have to take recourse in a forbearance energy which comes from the Supreme Person. This energy allows one to teach without jeopardizing one's advancement. Those who teach but who are not protected by that forbearance energy, regress and fall down, losing their foothold in yoga. Thus forbearance is a necessary energy if one is required to teach others on behalf of anybody.

**Strong-mindedness** is the result of gravitating towards superior beings and breaking off from the shared enjoyments with human beings. So long as the student *yogin* takes pleasure in association with human beings through varied social interactions, he cannot be single-minded. Human existence means a varied life for sense enjoyment either through approved behavior or by reckless life. In either case an attachment to such association causes weak-mindedness towards real spiritual practice. Those who are piously inclined and who support responsible life in the human community, take pride in elementary religion and walk around with chips on their shoulders in a self-righteous mood. They fail to see that they too are weak-minded since their main objective is material opulence and outward bodily appearance with status consciousness. Their absorption with this causes them to be weak-minded towards *buddhi yoga* practice even though they are enthusiastic about temple worship, religious festivals and the related observances. These facets of spiritual life are not deep enough to affect their inner psyche.

**Purity** in this application means purity of intent in dealing with others. To master this one must break off from social intercourses, develop mastership of the kundalini energy which sponsors selfishness, and then link up with the Universal Form. Actions committed with good intentions but which run contrary to the Supreme Will are psychically impure, but the actor is usually forced to commit these under the opinion that they will be beneficial. This purity means that the actor has lost interest in any and everybody in the material world and only takes up tasks which are endorsed by the Supreme Personality. The *yogin*'s main duty is his own psychic purity and everything else is secondary. But such secondary acts are done under the watchful gaze of the Supreme Person only.

**Freedom from hatred** occurs when the student *yogin* develops dispassion towards one and all in this world except for the advanced teachers and the Supreme Person. So long as one has social interests on the lower levels with persons of equal or lower status, one will exhibit hatred on occasion because this is the way of material nature. As soon as one develops dispassion, which is disinterest in the social concerns of this world, one loses the tendency for hatred. These are advancements in higher yoga. These attributes develop as one practices, as a matter of course.

**Freedom from conceit** comes when one knows for sure, that one's existence is completely unnecessary in this world. Even great devotees of *Śrī* Krishna sometimes fall down to the level of conceit. It is said that *Bhīmasena*, the elder brother of Arjuna, boasted that he alone could rid the world of the Kauravas, his rival cousins. He said he could do this in a few days or less, but such a feat was hardly possible for him, because his great uncle Bhishma along with the veteran warrior and teacher *Droṇa* were on the side of their opponents. For a limited entity, conceit of any sorts is superfluous and unnecessary. But it is hard to realize this. One must first rid oneself of the need to participate in the social affairs of this world. Here it is not so much a matter of good or bad, beneficial or unbeneficial; it is whatever providence endorses for the time being. Only providence is indispensible. And one can never know for sure what providence may endorse or for how long providence will support a particular scheme.

*Śrī* Krishna listed these qualities as talents born of the godly nature. These are exhibited when the highest influence in material nature predominates in the psyche of an individual soul. It is not the soul that is being discussed here but instead its conjunction with material nature, under the best conditions. One must learn in higher yoga how to fuse the self with material nature under such ideal conditions. This saves one from incurring responsibility for reckless acts under the lower dominance.

*Śrī* Krishna addressed Arjuna as *Bhārata* which means a notable descendant of King Bharata, an ancient king of India. The idea is that from the social viewpoint, Arjuna should be under the highest influence of material nature, with exhibition of godly qualities. So long as one is required to act socially, one must be particular to remain under the higher influences and that will save one from irresponsible acts. Thus one will qualify for the grace of Krishna.

दम्भो दर्पोऽतिमानश्च
क्रोधः पारुष्यमेव च ।
अज्ञानं चाभिजातस्य
पार्थ संपदमासुरीम् ॥ १६.४॥

dambho darpo'timānaśca
krodhaḥ pāruṣyameva ca
ajñānaṁ cābhijātasya
pārtha saṁpadamāsurīm (16.4)

*dambho = dambhaḥ — deceit; darpo = darpaḥ — arrogance; 'timānaśca = atimānaśca = atimānaḥ — conceit + ca — and; krodhaḥ — anger; pāruṣyam — abusive language; eva — indeed; ca — and; ajñānaṁ — lack of knowledge; cābhijātasya = ca — and + abhijātasya — of those born; pārtha — son of Pṛthā; saṁpadam — tendency; āsurīm — those with a wicked nature*

**Deceit, arrogance, conceit, anger, abusive language, and lack of knowledge are the tendencies of those born with a wicked nature, O son of Pṛthā. (16.4)**

***Siddha Swami's Commentary:***

**Deceit** is part of the energy of privacy. Privacy itself is farcical because everything which is conceived of, is sensed by others. One may hide one's thought for instance from another person who is grossly aware for the most part, but that same idea would be known to someone with psychic sensitivity. There are many beings on the supernatural level who have the required ability to pry into any or all of one's affairs. Hence there is really no such thing as privacy.

In *brahma yoga*, one begins to understand this, when one associates with great yogins and with divine beings who are met on higher planes. Still when one returns to the gross level, the level of the human beings, one may find it necessary to hide some features of one's actions. These actions should be ones which will yield advancement in the *buddhi yoga* practice. If a student yogi finds that others object to his practice or are disturbed by it, he should try to hide it, so as to be peaceful and agreeable to others. In that way the need for privacy is maintained on the normal level in a constructive way for spiritual advancement.

This is related to celibacy. If one does not develop celibacy through *prāṇāyāma* techniques and if one does not become an *ūrdhva retā* yogi, whose semen flows upward instead of downward through the genitals, one will use privacy for sexual engagements and that will ruin yoga. One should escape from the association of persons who degrade one's identity as a son or daughter of Lord Shiva without sexual needs. So long as there are sexual needs, one cannot get rid of the need for privacy. And as such, one will not be able to rid oneself of conceit.

**Arrogance** is sponsored by the lower modes of material nature, when they gain the upper hand over the higher clarifying mode. Then those lower energies use the clarifying mode, but since they are unable to maintain it, they fail at their endeavor when it peters out or fades from view. The key to this is higher yoga, to gain understanding of how the various modes manifest in one's psyche.

If the energy ingested into the psyche through eating and breathing comes from the lower modes, then the psyche will be dark internally. This will be experienced in meditation practice. When one is able to change this, then there will be psychic light in the head of the subtle body and one will begin to perceive the status of the various parts of the kundalini energy. It happens gradually and comes as a consequence of a consistent yoga practice. There may be revelation from time to time, just as Arjuna experienced when gazing at the Universal Form and four-armed Form of *Śrī* Krishna, but if one has not practiced sufficiently, then even a revelation will not stay. One will resume the old dark mentality which is saturated with energy from the lower modes.

**Conceit** is also known as vanity, when a person feels that he is more than he really is. This has to do with having inappropriate social associations. But so long as one is in the material world, such association is unavoidable. Thus *Śrī* Krishna gave isolation from this, as a prerequisite for yoga practice. One must get away from the type of environment which necessitates a conceited mentality. One must, of course, recognize the conceit-energy in one's nature.

The obsession in *brahma yoga* is self purification, the removal of impurities, in the psychic body of the self. One must become industrious at this, making this the number one priority. It is personal conquest over the psychic self energies.

**Anger** was listed by *Śrī* Krishna as part of the expression of the *kāma* craving energy, as being emitted from the *rajo* passionate emotion. This is what He said:

*śrībhagavānuvāca*
*kāma eṣa krodha eṣa rajoguṇasamudbhavaḥ*
*mahāśano mahāpāpmā viddhyenamiha vairiṇam (3.37)*

***The Blessed Lord said: This force is craving. This power is anger. The passionate emotion is the source. It has a great consuming power and does much damage. Recognize it as the enemy in this case. (3.37)***

One has to trace out these energies and their origins in the head of the subtle body, in the kundalini chakra system of psychic energy distribution and in the causal body. One must then root out these energies if at all possible. One must discuss this with an able *yogin* and get the mystic means for their suppression or removal.

**Abusive language** for a *yogin* is different from the moral principle of ordinary people who avoid curses and abuses. Their idea is to keep from exhibiting feelings of hatred, anger, vexation and frustration in public and to suppress the same if they arise.

In yoga we are concerned with the energy which may be converted into anger, hatred, vexation and frustration. This is the *kāma* craving energy and the *rajo* passionate emotion. In yoga we want to curb this energy so that it does not have to be suppressed or denied in the nature. The type of association one keeps is of great importance in cultivating purity of the psyche. If one stays with worldly people too closely, one is bound to become degraded in due course.

**Lack of knowledge** is a main impetus for someone to become a *yogin*. He is inspired to perform austerities because he wants to perceive the truth. He no longer wants to remain in intellectual and mental darkness. To remove the ignorance which veils his intellect, a person should learn *buddhi yoga*. Through its austerities for self purification, the psychic senses become clarified. Then he or she may perceive the truths.

*Śrī* Krishna attributed deceit, arrogance, conceit, anger, abusive language, and lack of knowledge as the tendencies of those born in this world with a wicked nature. But that does not mean that the spirit itself has that nature. The meaning is that since a spirit is fused into a psyche which has wicked tendencies, that person becomes responsible for the actions promoted by his nature. Such a person can be purified if he takes to the instructions which are recommended by *Śrī* Krishna in the *Bhagavad Gītā*.

दैवी संपद्विमोक्षाय
निबन्धायासुरी मता ।
मा शुचः संपदं दैवीम्
अभिजातोऽसि पाण्डव ॥१६.५॥
daivī saṁpadvimokṣāya
nibandhāyāsurī matā
mā śucaḥ saṁpadaṁ daivīm
abhijāto'si pāṇḍava (16.5)

*daivī — godly; saṁpad — talent; vimokṣāya — to liberation; nibandhāyāsurī = nibandhāyā — to bondage + āsurī – wicked tendency; matā — considered to be; mā — not; śucaḥ —worry, saṁpadaṁ — nature; daivīm — godly; abhijāto = abhijātaḥ — born; 'si = asi — you are; pāṇḍava — son of Pāndu*

**The godly talent is conducive to liberation. It is considered that the wicked tendencies facilitate bondage. Do not worry. You are endowed with the godly nature, O son of Pāndu. (16.5)**

***Siddha Swami's Commentary:***

Even though the godly talents are conducive to liberation, each or more than one of them combined does not give a soul liberation unless that is his or her intention. One must become liberated by deliberate intention and by working with those talents under strict supervision of a *mahāyogin* or under the direction of Lord Shiva or Lord Krishna or one of their divinities.

On the other hand, any of the wicked tendencies or any combination of these would take a person downwards in the mundane evolutionary cycle. *Śrī* Krishna assured of Arjuna's godly nature, but the same *Śrī* Krishna advised Arjuna earlier in this text to abandon kind sentiments for relatives. Those were loving sentiments of concern for the Kauravas. Thus Arjuna, even though godly by nature, had to be directed in how to use his good qualities.

द्वौ भूतसर्गौ लोकेऽस्मिन्
दैव आसुर एव च ।
दैवो विस्तरशः प्रोक्त
आसुरं पार्थ मे शृणु ॥१६.६॥
dvau bhūtasargau loke'smin
daiva āsura eva ca
daivo vistaraśaḥ prokta
āsuraṁ pārtha me śṛṇu (16.6)

*dvau — two; bhūtasargau = bhūta — being + sargau — two created types; loke — in the world; 'smin = asmin — in this; daiva — godly; āsura — wicked; eva — indeed; ca — and; daivo = daivah — godly type; viṣṭaraśaḥ — in detail; prokta — explained; āsuraṁ — wicked: pārtha — son of Pṛthā; me — from me; śṛṇu — hear*

**There are two types of created beings in this world, the godly type and the wicked. The godly type was explained in detail. Hear from me of the wicked, O son of Pṛthā. (16.6)**

***Siddha Swami's Commentary:***

These are the beings or psychological compartments used by the individual living entities, the spirits. One may acquire a godly or wicked type of psyche for usage in this world. If a cultured gentleman mounts a wild horse, it will throw him to the ground. It will not allow him mastership, merely because of his cultured nature. And if a wicked person mounts a tame domestic animal, it will more than likely serve his every need, according to its domesticity. Thus those spirits who have psyches with wicked tendencies become responsible for irreligious activities, regardless of whether they like it or not. They can however reform their psychology by austerity and godly association.

प्रवृत्तिं च निवृत्तिं च
जना न विदुरासुराः ।
न शौचं नापि चाचारो
न सत्यं तेषु विद्यते ॥१६.७॥
pravṛttiṁ ca nivṛttiṁ ca
janā na vidurāsurāḥ
na śaucaṁ nāpi cācāro
na satyaṁ teṣu vidyate (16.7)

*pravṛttiṁ — what to do; ca — and; nivṛttiṁ — what not to do; ca — and; janā — people; na — not; viduḥ — they know; āsurāḥ — wicked; na — neither; śaucaṁ — cleanliness; nāpi = na — nor + api — also; cācāro = cācāraḥ = ca — and + ācāraḥ — good conduct; na — nor; satyam — realism; teṣu — in them; vidyate — is found*

**The wicked people do not know what to do and what not to do. Neither cleanliness or even good conduct, nor realism is found in them. (16.7)**

***Siddha Swami's Commentary:***

This is because they do not have access to a higher grade of pranic or psychic energy. Because they rely on dark psychic energies, they do not get the insight which allows a proper assessment of reality. Thus they are misled. However in time, after repeated frustration and seeing others who are making great decisions, they aspire for more clarity. Eventually they perform austerities to curb their psyche and to allow them to stay with superior personalities.

असत्यमप्रतिष्ठं ते
जगदाहुरनीश्वरम् ।
अपरस्परसंभूतं
किमन्यत्कामहैतुकम् ॥१६.८॥
asatyamapratiṣṭhaṁ te
jagadāhuranīśvaram
aparasparasaṁbhūtaṁ
kimanyatkāmahaitukam (16.8)

*asatyam — unreal; apratiṣṭhaṁ — without a foundation; te — they; jagat — the world; āhuḥ — they say; anīśvaram — without a Supreme Lord; aparasparasaṁbhūtaṁ = aparaspara — without a series of causes + saṁbhūtaṁ — produced; kim — what?; anyat — other cause; kāmahaitukam = kāma — sexual urge + haitukam — caused*

**They say that the universe is unreal, without a foundation, without a Supreme Lord, without a series of causes. They explain, saying, "Sexual urge is the cause. What other basis could there be?" (16.8)**

***Siddha Swami's Commentary:***

*Kāma,* which is lust and craving, is highlighted by sexual urge. This is a cause but it is not the supreme cause. However when one is enthused by the passionate force, one feels that that power as being supreme, and one conducts himself or herself in a passionate way, ignoring other causes which transcend the lusty urges. One develops a strong belief in the lusty energy as being all-powerful.

एतां दृष्टिमवष्टभ्य
नष्टात्मानोऽल्पबुद्धयः ।
प्रभवन्त्युग्रकर्माणः
क्षयाय जगतोऽहिताः ॥ १६.९ ॥
etāṁ dṛṣṭimavaṣṭabhya
naṣṭātmāno'lpabuddhayaḥ
prabhavantyugrakarmāṇaḥ
kṣayāya jagato'hitāḥ (16.9)

*etāṁ — this; dṛṣṭim — view; avaṣṭabhya — holding; naṣṭātmāno = naṣṭātmānaḥ = naṣṭa — lost + ātmānaḥ — to their spiritual selves; 'lpabuddhayaḥ = alpabuddhayaḥ = alpa — negligible + buddhayaḥ— intelligence; prabhavanti — they become; ugrakarmāṇaḥ = ugra — cruel + karmāṇaḥ — acts; kṣayāya — to destruction; jagato = jagataḥ — of the world; 'hitāḥ = ahitāḥ — enemies*

**Holding this view, men who lost track of their spirituality, who have negligible intelligence, who commit cruel acts, become enemies for the destruction of the world. (16.9)**

***Siddha Swami's Commentary:***

When one falls under the dominance of the two lower modes, one loses his or her sharp intellectual perception. One feels that morality has no place in the behavioral performance of human beings. Having such conclusions, one commits irreligious acts for which one is held accountable. Such accountability leads to judgment from which punishment is derived. From punishment, one comes to self reflection from which repentance develops. And from repentance one develops a desire for self reform.

काममाश्रित्य दुष्पूरं
दम्भमानमदान्विताः ।
मोहाद्गृहीत्वासद्ग्राहान्
प्रवर्तन्तेऽशुचिव्रताः ॥ १६.१०
kāmamāśritya duṣpūraṁ
dambhamānamadānvitāḥ
mohādgṛhītvāsadgrāhān
pravartante'śucivratāḥ (16.10)

*kāmam — lusty urge; āśritya — relying; duṣpūraṁ — non-fulfilling; dambhamānamadānvitāḥ = dambha — hypocrisy + māna — pride + mada — intoxicated + anvitāḥ — possessed by; mohāt — from delusion; gṛhītvā — having accepted; 'sadgrāhān = asadgrāhān = asad (asat) — unrealistic + grāhān — views; pravartante — they proceed; 'śucivratāḥ = aśucivratāh = aśuci — impure + vratāḥ — objectives*

**Being reliant on the non-fulfilling lusty urge, possessed of hypocrisy, pride, and intoxication, having accepted unrealistic views, through delusion, they proceed with impure objectives. (16.10)**

***Siddha Swami's Commentary:***

The lusty urge, like many other motivations which come from the lower psychological influences, is exhausting and non-fulfilling but it holds advantage over many living entities because it promises pleasure. The proper usage of it is the begetting of progeny. However since such begetting leads to many years of responsibility for the children produced, human beings desire to have the pleasure only.

To use the sexual function for pleasure and to circumvent its begetting purpose, one has to exhibit hypocrisy and pride. To do this easily, one has to use various means of intoxication. This is sponsored by the dulling and enthusing psychological energies.

चिन्तामपरिमेयां च
प्रलयान्तामुपाश्रिताः ।
कामोपभोगपरमा
एतावदिति निश्चिताः ॥ १६.११ ॥

*citām — worry; aparimeyāṁ — endless; ca — and; pralayāntām — ending at death; upāśritāḥ — clinging; kāmopabhogaparamā = kāma — lust + upabhoga — enjoyment + paramā — highest aim; etāvat — so much; iti*

cintāmaparimeyāṁ ca
pralayāntāmupāśritāḥ
kāmopabhogaparamā
etāvaditi niścitāḥ (16.11)

*— thus; niścitāḥ — convinced*

**And clinging to endless worries which end at the time of death, with lusty enjoyment as the highest aim, being convinced that this is all there is, (16.11)**

***Siddha Swami's Commentary:***

Any living entity who falls under the enthusing influence of material nature will be subjected to endless worries. That person's intellect will flicker rapidly as it invents various schemes for procuring *kāma upabhoga*, lusty enjoyments. Such a person is forced from within the psyche, to live as if there will be no other life. He or she tries to fulfill all possible desires in one life. This causes endless anxieties.

आशापाशशतैर्बद्धाः
कामक्रोधपरायणाः ।
ईहन्ते कामभोगार्थम्
अन्यायेनार्थसंचयान् ॥ १६.१२ ॥
āśāpāśaśatairbaddhāḥ
kāmakrodhaparāyaṇāḥ
īhante kāmabhogārtham
anyāyenārthasaṁcayān (16.12)

*āśāpāśaśataiḥ = āśāpāśa — frustrating expectations + śataiḥ — by a hundred; baddhāḥ — bound; kāmakrodhaparāyaṇāḥ = kāma — craving + krodha — anger + parāyaṇāḥ — cherishing; īhante — they strive to acquire; kāmabhogārtham = kāma — craving + bhoga — pleasure + artham — fulfillment; anyāyenārthasañcayān = anyāyena — with any other + artha — money + sañcayān — huge sums*

**...bound by hundreds of frustrating expectations, cherishing craving and anger, using any means, they strive to acquire huge sums of money for the fulfillment of craving and pleasure. (16.12)**

***Siddha Swami's Commentary:***

Though a subtle power, the two lower modes of material nature point the individual spirit influencing, in a downward direction towards manifestation of desires which involve gross matter. A student *yogin* is advised to reverse this downward sense of determination. It begins with *pratyāhār* practice, in causing the sensual energies to revert back into the mind chamber from which they were originally emitted.

इदमद्य मया लब्धम्
इदं प्राप्स्ये मनोरथम् ।
इदमस्तीदमपि मे
भविष्यति पुनर्धनम् ॥ १६.१३
idamadya mayā labdham
idaṁ prāpsye manoratham
idamastīdamapi me
bhaviṣyati punardhanam (16.13)

*idam — this; adya — today; mayā — by me; labdham — obtained; idaṁ — this; prāpsye — I will fulfill; manoratham — fantasy; idam — this; astīdam = asti — it is + idam — this; api — also; me — mine; bhaviṣyati — will be; punaḥ — again, also; dhanam — wealth*

**Thinking: "This was obtained by me today, I will fulfill this fantasy. This is it. This wealth will also be mine. (16.13)**

***Siddha Swami's Commentary:***

Subtle material nature concerns itself with desire and fulfillment of the same, in an endless effort to reveal the imprints of subtle impressions and motivate the agents and materials for manifesting these. Thus a student *yogin* has to struggle against this vast mundane power which has the upper hand against all those who are not detached from it. The most important desire is for liberation from material nature itself. When a person thinks of this, he or she is diverted into a plan for helping others. Following the various religious and social schemes for the exhibition of compassion, one loses the objective of liberation and pansies around in the creation, pretending to be a savior of major or minor significance. All this is enacted under the influence of material nature.

असौ मया हतः शत्रुर्
हनिष्ये चापरानपि ।
ईश्वरोऽहमहं भोगी
सिद्धोऽहं बलवान्सुखी ॥१६.१४॥
asau mayā hataḥ śatrur
haniṣye cāparānapi
īśvaro'hamahaṁ bhogī
siddho'haṁ balavānsukhī (16.14)

*asau — that; mayā — by me; hataḥ — was killed; śatruḥ — enemy; haniṣye — I will kill; cāparān = ca — and + aparān — others; api — as well as; īśvaro = īśvaraḥ — controller; 'ham = aham — I; aham — I; bhogī — enjoyer; siddho = siddhaḥ — successful; 'ham = aham — I; balavān — powerful; sukhī — happy*

**"That enemy was killed by me, I will kill others as well. I am the controller. I am the enjoyer. I am successful, powerful and happy. (16.14)**

***Siddha Swami's Commentary:***

In material existence, one may certainly become a successful, powerful and happy controller and enjoyer. However, that is not the issue for student yogins. For them it is a question of who or what sponsored the status, power and psychology. One must be sponsored by the right type of person and by the right type of energy. And in the least, one must be endorsed by the highest type of mental and emotional force in the creation, namely, the *sattva guṇa* clarifying power of material nature. For association one should have a great *yogin*, a person who mastered his psychology and who has spiritual vision, whose subtle head is filled with light, not mental darkness. One's success, power and happiness should be based on self conquest, having little or nothing to do with the external gross or subtle worlds.

आढ्योऽभिजनवानस्मि
कोऽन्योऽस्ति सदृशो मया ।
यक्ष्ये दास्यामि मोदिष्य
इत्यज्ञानविमोहिताः ॥१६.१५॥
āḍhyo'bhijanavānasmi
ko'nyo'sti sadṛśo mayā
yakṣye dāsyāmi modiṣya
ityajñānavimohitāḥ (16.15)

*āḍhyo = ādhyaḥ — rich; 'bhijanavān = abhijanavān — upper class; asmi — I am; ko = kaḥ — who; 'nyo = anyaḥ — other; 'sti = asti — there is; sadraśo = sadraśaḥ — like; mayā — me; yakṣye — I will perform religious ceremony; dāsyāmi — I will give in, donate; modiṣya — I will make merry; iti — thus is said; ajñānavimohitāḥ = ajñāna — ignorance + vimohitāḥ — those who are deluded*

**"I am rich and upper class. Who is there besides me? I will perform religious ceremony. I will donate. I will make merry." This is what is said by those who are deluded by ignorance. (16.15)**

***Siddha Swami's Commentary:***

Each of the three influences of material nature, sponsors, creates and then endorses a particular type of portrait for the individual entity. A student must first be trained to recognize his condition. Then later he must be trained to admit faults and to work to elevate the self step by step. Material nature is not a power that can be transcended quickly. It takes years, if not lives, to elevate oneself to higher and higher levels. Student yogins who are hasty and feel entitled to a quick elevation, usually become frustrated in yoga and give up the quest. But those who understand what they are up against, work steadily day after day, accumulating days and then years of steady practice to develop the strength to challenge nature's dominance.

The external environment, though daunting, is not the problem. The problem is the psychology used by the self and the self's own way of relating to those psychological energies. When one masters this, one may be recognized as a *yogin*.

अनेकचित्तविभ्रान्ता
मोहजालसमावृताः ।
प्रसक्ताः कामभोगेषु
पतन्ति नरकेऽशुचौ ॥ १६.१६ ॥
anekacittavibhrāntā
mohajālasamāvṛtāḥ
prasaktāḥ kāmabhogeṣu
patanti narake'śucau (16.16)

*anekacittavibhrāntā = aneka — many + citta — idea + vibhrāntā — carried away; mohajālasamāvṛtāh = moha — delusion + jāla — entanglement + samāvṛtāḥ — occupied by; prasaktāḥ — being attached; kāmabhogeṣu = kāma — craving + bhogeṣu — in enjoyments; patanti — they fall; narake — in hellish condition; 'śucau = aśucau — unclean*

**Being carried away by many ideas, being occupied by entangling delusions, being attached by cravings and enjoyments, they fall into an unclean, hellish condition. (16.16)**

***Siddha Swami's Commentary:***

One has to be careful since the downward pull of material nature causes one to take lower life forms which limit one's perception of liberation. In fact, in many lower forms the thought of liberation arises only as an idea to take on a more advantageous form, like that of one's predator. For instance, if one is in a caterpillar body, one may develop the desire to take the form of a wasp. One's need for liberation then surfaces as an inspiration to leave the caterpillar species to assume the species which has the power to exploit caterpillar bodies by stinging and then eating them. Thus the impulse for liberation is used improperly in the lower species.

Even in the human species, the urge for liberation is absorbed by the survival instinct. For instance, a poor man might desire to become as rich as the person who employs him at a meager wage. Or a servile woman might desire to be like the lordly lady who supervises her services. A visitor to a temple, a pilgrim, might desire to be a *pujārī*, a ceremonial priest who officiates. These are all perverted uses of the liberation tendency. But when one submits to a great *yogin*, one gets the proper idea about being liberated internally from the subtle influences of material nature, in terms of controlling the psyche.

A man who falls into a psychologically unclean condition, whereby he becomes habituated to the lower two modes of material nature, should understand his condition, get a method from a reliable teacher, and make efforts to liberate himself from the grip of bad habits. When he makes such endeavor, he will realize certain things about his nature. Thus he may no longer find it too difficult and time-consuming to reform his psyche.

आत्मसंभाविताः स्तब्धा
धनमानमदान्विताः ।
यजन्ते नामयज्ञैस्ते
दम्भेनाविधिपूर्वकम् ॥ १६.१७॥
ātmasaṁbhāvitāḥ stabdhā
dhanamānamadānvitāḥ
yajante nāmayajñaiste
dambhenāvidhipūrvakam (16.17)

*ātmasaṁbhāvitāḥ — self-conceited; stabdhā — stubborn; dhanamānamadānvitāḥ = dhanamāna — arrogance of having money + mada — pride + anvitāḥ — possessed with; yajante — they worship in ceremony; nāmayajñaiḥ — with religious ceremony in name only; te — they; dambhenāvidhipūrvakam = dambhena — with hyprocrisy + avidhipurvakam — with reference to Vedic injunction*

**Self-conceited, stubborn, possessed of pride and the arrogance of having money, with hypocrisy and without reference to Vedic injunctions, they worship in ceremonies that are religious in name only. (16.17)**

***Siddha Swami's Commentary:***

Whatever religion it may be, if it is not concerned with reforming the self from dependence on the lower modes of material nature, it is actually useless. Religion for status purposes, for instance, is a sheer waste of time. Religion for showing higher education such as the knowledge of Sanskrit pronunciation is also a waste of time. Religion for converting piety or good acts into prosperity is another waste of time. Religion for the sake of setting oneself apart from sinners is a waste of time. But that religion which is used to understand how to reform the self from ungodly ways and how to elevate the self so that it is no longer susceptible to nature's dominance, is supreme religion, which is the proper use of one's time.

One limited being cannot be responsible for liberating other limited ones, even though such a limited soul might assist the Supreme Person in that upliftment. Thus one should not become preoccupied as a teacher of others. One should instead help the Supreme Person to reform one's psychology. That should be the prime objective.

अहंकारं बलं दर्पं
कामं क्रोधं च संश्रिताः ।
मामात्मपरदेहेषु
प्रद्विषन्तोऽभ्यसूयकाः ॥ १६.१८॥
ahaṁkāraṁ balaṁ darpaṁ
kāmaṁ krodhaṁ ca saṁśritāḥ
māmātmaparadeheṣu
pradviṣanto'bhyasūyakāḥ (16.18)

*ahaṁkāraṁ — misplaced self-identity; balam — brute force; darpaṁ — arrogance; kāmaṁ — craving; krodhaṁ — anger; ca — and; saṁśritāḥ — clinging to; mām — me; ātmaparadeheṣu = ātma — self + para — other + deheṣu — in bodies; pradviṣanto = pradviṣantaḥ — disliking; 'bhyasūyakāḥ = abhyasūyakāḥ — those who are envious*

**Clinging to a misplaced self-identity, brute force, arrogance, craving and anger, those who are envious dislike Me, in their own bodies and in those of others. (16.18)**

***Siddha Swami's Commentary:***

Negativity towards the Supreme Person, towards God, comes about because of the assumption that it is His duty to facilitate one's quest for happiness. If one thinks that God should ease all frustrations and provide all fulfillments, one is bound to detest the Supreme Person, since in all cases of individual entities, there are disappointments. But it occurs because one does not understand the way of reality. In the lower modes, one is dominated by an insight which does not allow one to gage the reality and one adopts many unrealistic views. Thus one becomes hostile to the Supreme Being.

Even though most human beings and animals do not directly perceive the Supreme Person they do perceive His influence as destiny, as the circumstances of life around them. These are circumstances which they attempt to control in their favor but which only serve their purposes from time to time. Thus those who dislike the Supreme Being do so by posing in opposition to destiny. And thus they develop resentful feelings which are manifested in their minds and emotions as defiance and tendencies for vices and criminal activities.

तानहं द्विषतः क्रूरान्
संसारेषु नराधमान् ।
क्षिपाम्यजस्रमशुभान्
आसुरीष्वेव योनिषु ॥ १६.१९
tānahaṁ dviṣataḥ krūrān
saṁsāreṣu narādhamān
kṣipāmyajasramaśubhān
āsurīṣveva yoniṣu (16.19)

*tān — them; aham — I; dviṣataḥ — those who are despising; krūrān — those who are cruel; saṁsāreṣu — in the cycles of rebirth; narādhamān — lowest of humans; kṣipāmi — I hurl; ajasram — constantly; aśubhān — the vicious; āsurīṣu — into the wicked people; eva — indeed; yoniṣu — in the wombs*

**I constantly hurl the despising cruel, vicious, lowest of humans into the cycles of rebirth in the wombs of wicked people. (16.19)**

***Siddha Swami's Commentary:***

By mystic acts, the Supreme Person puts those who are adverse to Him, at a great distance existentially. This means that they go down to lower life forms or remain as human beings with a dark mentality based on a stronger and more thorough dominance from the two lower modes. In rare cases, some agents of the Supreme Person might curse someone and on the strength of their divine power, send a soul headlong into a lower species or to a lower realm, at a distance existentially. Such souls stay down for some time and then move upwards again as their attitudes change.

Before one can move close to the Supreme Person, one has to become compatible to Him. This begins by psychological reform to change the nature of the one's mind and emotions. One cannot attain the association of the Supreme Person if one does not effect changes in one's mental and emotional energies.

आसुरीं योनिमापन्ना
मूढा जन्मनि जन्मनि ।
मामप्राप्यैव कौन्तेय
ततो यान्त्यधमां गतिम् ॥ १६.२० ॥
āsurīṁ yonimāpannā
mūḍhā janmani janmani
māmaprāpyaiva kaunteya
tato yāntyadhamāṁ gatim (16.20)

*āsurīṁ — the wicked people; yonim — womb; āpannā — entering; mūḍhā — the blockheads; janmani janmani — in birth, in birth again; mām — me; aprāpyaivā = aprāpya — associating + eva — indeed; kaunteya — O son of Kuntī; tato = tataḥ — thence; yānti — they traverse; adhamāṁ — lowest; gatim — route of transmigration*

**Thus, O son of Kuntī, entering the wombs of the wicked people, the blockheads, after not associating with Me in birth after birth, traverse the lowest route of transmigration. (16.20)**

***Siddha Swami's Commentary:***

Since the living entitles are hitched to a set of psychological equipments, they are to an extent limited to what such equipments allow them to perceive. Thus if one gets into a lower species of life, one will develop lowly priorities, which to one's senses, may appear as a high order of preferences. If for instance one enters the species of the big cats, like the lions and tigers, one's intellect will be inclined to analyzing methods of catching herbivores like deer and cattle. Using the intellect in that way, one will feel superior to other life forms which are not obsessed with such methods of killing other species for food. Thus even though the same intellect may be used for earning one's way to liberation and divine association, one will have no idea of such usage.

A living entity who has a leonine form in one life time, will take with him his intellect, mind space, emotional and sensual energies, along with his memory when he transmigrates to any other life form. Even if he attains the form of a human being, he will still do so with the same intellect he used in the lower species. One must know that there is no change in the psychological equipments even though there might be a change in the gross body. The subtle body adapts to any new gross form one takes but that subtle form is not changed for a new one. It is therefore important to take up the task of reforming the subtle form, since it is the same form one will use through the duration of the creation.

One remains in a lower form or goes to an even lower species, through the method of becoming addicted to the senses of the subtle body. For then, whatever is shown to one by such senses, becomes one's basis for the next transmigration. Unless one can curb the subtle body so that its quest for lower gratifications is eliminated, one will have to enter lower life forms.

त्रिविधं नरकस्येदं
द्वारं नाशनमात्मनः ।
कामः क्रोधस्तथा लोभस्
तस्मादेतत्त्रयं त्यजेत् ॥ १६.२१ ॥
trividhaṁ narakasyedaṁ
dvāraṁ nāśanamātmanaḥ
kāmaḥ krodhastathā lobhas
tasmādetattrayaṁ tyajet (16.21)

*trividhaṁ — threefold; narakasyedaṁ = narakasya — of hell + idam — this; dvāraṁ — avenues; nāśanam — destructive of, degrading towards; ātmanaḥ — of the self; kāmaḥ — craving; krodhaḥ — anger; tathā— as well; lobhaḥ — greed; tasmāt — therefore; etat — this; trayam — three-fold; tyajet — should abandon*

**Craving, anger and greed are the three avenues of hell which degrade the soul. Therefore one should abandon this threefold influence. (16.21)**

***Siddha Swami's Commentary:***

Craving, anger and greed are the adverse forms taken by the mento-emotional energy. This mento-emotional energy is experienced by a bewildered person as sensual force which causes impulsions. The conversion of the mento-emotional energy into impulses for cravings, anger and greed must be observed by student yogins. Thus they can understand the psychic chemistry of the psyche. From this education, they may learn how not to allow the energies to be converted.

*Śrī* Krishna requested that we abandon those energies, but that is easier said than done. It requires mastership of *buddhi yoga*.

एतैर्विमुक्तः कौन्तेय
तमोद्वारैस्त्रिभिर्नरः ।
आचरत्यात्मनः श्रेयस्
ततो याति परां गतिम् ॥ १६.२२ ॥
etairvimuktaḥ kaunteya
tamodvāraistribhirnaraḥ
ācaratyātmanaḥ śreyas
tato yāti parāṁ gatim (16.22)

*etair (etaiḥ) — by these; vimuktaḥ — released; kaunteya — son of Kuntī; tamodvārais = tamo (tamaḥ) — depression + dvāraiḥ — by avenues; tribhir (tribhiḥ) — by three; naraḥ — a person; ācaratyātmanaḥ = ācarati — he serves + ātmanaḥ — of the self; śreyaḥ — best interest; tato (tataḥ) — then; yāti — goes; parāṁ — supreme; gatim — destination*

**Being released from these three avenues of depression, O son of Kuntī, a person serves his best interest and then goes to the highest destination. (16.22)**

***Siddha Swami's Commentary:***

*Tamo dvāraih* refers to the avenues of sensuality which cause one to think that a downward descent in the evolutionary cycle is in one's highest interest. Through showing one lower and more basic methods of living, the psychology becomes adapted to abominable sensual intakes, and thus one goes downward. Let us take for example the form of a vulture. The sense of taste in the body of that creature dictates that rotten flesh be considered a delicacy. This same sensual energy may be used in a human form of life. Hence *Śrī* Krishna advocated release from the lower taste, so that one may get a hint about progression to higher taste and values.

यः शास्त्रविधिमुत्सृज्य
वर्तते कामकारतः ।
न स सिद्धिमवाप्नोति
न सुखं न परां गतिम् ॥ १६.२३ ॥
yaḥ śāstravidhimutsṛjya
vartate kāmakārataḥ
na sa siddhimavāpnoti
na sukhaṁ na parāṁ gatim (16.23)

*yaḥ — who; śāstravidhim — scriptural injunction; utsṛjya — discarding; vartate — he follows; kāmakārataḥ — impulsion, inclination; na — not; sa = saḥ — he; siddhim — perfection; avāpnoti — attains; na — nor; sukhaṁ — happiness; na — nor; parāṁ — highest; gatim — destination*

**Whosoever discards the scriptural injunctions, and follows the impulsive inclinations, does not get perfection or happiness or the supreme destination. (16.23)**

***Siddha Swami's Commentary:***

The scriptural injunctions in the *Bhagavad Gītā* and in its supportive literature are designed for restriction of the sensuality, for the purpose of causing the subtle body to develop higher taste and higher values. If one does not follow these injunctions either naturally or by disciplinary means, then one will of necessity go downwards. The same sensuality which may develop divine habits may also exhibit and crave ungodly propensities. One has to be careful. One must restrict the self from what is degrading and also point the self in the direction of what is elevating.

तस्माच्छास्त्रं प्रमाणं ते
कार्याकार्यव्यवस्थितौ ।
ज्ञात्वा शास्त्रविधानोक्तं
कर्म कर्तुमिहार्हसि ॥ १६.२४ ॥
tasmācchāstraṁ pramāṇaṁ te
kāryākāryavyavasthitau
jñātvā śāstravidhānoktaṁ
karma kartumihārhasi (16.24)

*tasmāt — therefore; śāstram — scripture; pramāṇaṁ — recommendation; te — your; karyākāryavyavasthitau = kārya — duty + akārya — non-duty + vyavasthitau — setting; jñātvā — knowing; śāstravidhānoktaṁ = śāstravidhāna — scriptural rules + uktaṁ — prescribed; karma — action; kartum — to perform; ihārhasi = ihā — here in this world + arhasi — you can*

**Therefore, setting your standard of duty and non-duty by scriptural recommendation, knowing the scriptural rules prescribed, you should perform actions in this world. (16.24)**

***Siddha Swami's Commentary:***

Arjuna wanted to abandon the duties assigned to him by the Universal Form of *Śrī* Krishna. This is because Arjuna's senses found those duties to be unpalatable. But *Śrī* Krishna lectured extensively to convince Arjuna that the decision of the senses is not to be followed in all cases. Unless the senses are disciplined through *buddhi yoga*, they are apt to influencing the intellect to make wrong decisions, for short term happiness, and long term distress.

To rein in the senses, one must become familiar with scriptural injunctions. One must try to follow these. One must also accept a spiritual master who is expert at discerning what is duty and what is neglect of duty according to the view of *Śrī* Krishna.

# CHAPTER 17

## Trividhā Bhavati Śraddhā

## Three Types of Confidences*

*śrībhagavānuvāca*
*trividhā bhavati śraddhā dehināṁ sā svabhāvajā*
*sāttvikī rājasī caiva tāmasī ceti tāṁ śṛṇu (17.2)*

***The Blessed Lord said: According to innate tendency, there are three types of confidences of the embodied souls. These are clarifying, motivating and depressing. Hear about this. (17.2)***

***Siddha Swami assigned this chapter title on the basis of verse 2 of this chapter.**

अर्जुन उवाच
ये शास्त्रविधिमुत्सृज्य
यजन्ते श्रद्धयान्विताः ।
तेषां निष्ठा तु का कृष्ण
सत्त्वमाहो रजस्तमः ॥ १७.१ ॥
arjuna uvāca
ye śāstravidhimutsṛjya
yajante śraddhayānvitāḥ
teṣāṁ niṣṭhā tu kā kṛṣṇa
sattvamāho rajastamaḥ (17.1)

*arjuna — Arjuna; uvāca — said; ye — who; śastravidhim — scriptural injunction; utsṛjya — disregarding; yajante — they perform religiously-motivated ceremony and austerity; śraddhayānvitāḥ — with full confidence; teṣāṁ — of them; niṣṭhā — position; tu — but; kā — what; kṛṣṇa — O Krishna; sattvaṁ — clarity; āho — is it?; rajaḥ — impulsion; tamaḥ — depression*

**Arjuna said: Concerning those who disregard scriptural injunction, but who with full confidence perform religiously-motivated ceremonies and austerities, what indeed, is their position, O Krishna? Is it clarity, impulsion or depression? (17.1)**

***Siddha Swami's Commentary:***

It all depends on which person or energy inspired and directed the performer. It is not true that all those people who disregard the scriptural injunctions are doing so under a bad influence. Some may do so under divine sanction as well. Witness the case of Rishi *Yajñavalka* who fell out with his teacher, adopted questionable austerities and composed the White *Yajur Veda* as inspired by the sun-god. Even though *Yajñavalka* discarded what was considered to be the scriptural injunctions, still he was successful in spiritual life and composed authoritative Vedic texts.

It is unwise, however, to disregard scriptural injunctions. Persons like *Yajñavalka* are super-human and come from their past lives with much scriptural adherence. Hence their seeming disregard for scriptural injunctions does not degrade them. Most others, however, will have no such luck.

श्रीभगवानुवाच
त्रिविधा भवति श्रद्धा
देहिनां सा स्वभावजा ।
सात्त्विकी राजसी चैव
तामसी चेति तां शृणु ॥ १७.२ ॥
śrībhagavānuvāca
trividhā bhavati śraddhā
dehināṁ sā svabhāvajā
sāttvikī rājasī caiva
tāmasī ceti tāṁ śṛṇu (17.2)

*śrī bhagavān — The Blessed Lord; uvāca — said; trividhā — three types; bhavati — there is; śraddhā — confidence; dehināṁ — of the embodied souls; sā — anyone; svabhāvajā — produced from innate tendency; sāttvikī — clarifying; rājasī — motivating; caiva — and indeed; tāmasī — depression; ceti = ca — and + iti — thus; tāṁ — this; śṛṇu — hear*

**The Blessed Lord said: According to innate tendency, there are three types of confidences of the embodied souls. These are clarifying, motivating and depressing. Hear about this. (17.2)**

***Siddha Swami's Commentary:***

The bottom line in religion is innate tendency, *svabhāva*. Whatever a person does is based on such innate tendency or is produced *(jā)* from such nature. Therefore purification of the psyche has all significance. You may love God, but what is quality of that affection? It will be based on your innate tendency. Religious life, therefore, begins with psychic purity.

In common experience one sometimes finds that a well-formed, luscious fruit is rotten internally, while a deformed fruit may be sweet internally. Thus we should not gage a person by his or her external religious format.

सत्त्वानुरूपा सर्वस्य
श्रद्धा भवति भारत ।
श्रद्धामयोऽयं पुरुषो
यो यच्छ्रद्धः स एव सः ॥ १७.३ ॥
sattvānurūpā sarvasya
śraddhā bhavati bhārata
śraddhāmayo'yaṁ puruṣo
yo yacchraddhaḥ sa eva saḥ (17.3)

*sattvānurūpā = sattva — essential nature + anurūpā — according to; sarvasya—of every person; śraddhā — confidence; bhavati — becomes manifest; bhārata — O man of the Bharata family; śraddhāmayaḥ — made of faith, trend of confidence; 'yaṁ = ayaṁ — this; puruṣo = puruṣaḥ — human being; yo = yaḥ — who; yacchraddhah = yac (yad) —which + chraddhaḥ (śraddhaḥ) — faith; sa = saḥ — he; eva — only: saḥ — he*

**Confidence becomes manifest according to the essential nature of the person, O man of the Bharata family. A human being follows his trend of confidence. Whatever type of faith he has, that he expresses only. (17.3)**

***Siddha Swami's Commentary:***

A person's confidence is derived from the inner nature. Whatever he expresses naturally will represent the inner constitution. In *brahma yoga*, the whole idea is to study yourself internally so that you can effect changes to elevate your nature.

यजन्ते सात्त्विका देवान्
यक्षरक्षांसि राजसाः ।
प्रेतान्भूतगणांश्चान्ये
यजन्ते तामसा जनाः ॥ १७.४ ॥
yajante sāttvikā devān
yakṣarakṣāṁsi rājasāḥ
pretānbhūtagaṇāṁścānye
yajante tāmasā janāḥ (17.4)

*yajante — they worship; sāttvikā — clear-minded people; devān — supernatural rulers; yakṣarakṣāṁsi = yakṣa — passionate sorcerers + rakṣāṁsi — to cannibalistic powerful humans; rājasāḥ — impulsive people; pretān — the departed spirits; bhūtagaṇāṁścānye = bhūtagaṇān — hordes of ghosts + ca — and + anye — others; yajante — they petition; tāmasā = retarded; janāḥ — people*

**The clear-minded people worship the supernatural rulers. The impulsive ones worship the passionate sorcerors and the cannibalistic humans. The others, the retarded people, petition the departed spirits and the hordes of ghosts. (17.4)**

***Siddha Swami's Commentary:***

The association of the different types of living beings existed from time immemorial and it will continue forever. It is described that even those who have no coverings of forms as we are familiar with, do associate with one another in compact clusters, like beads of golden effulgence tightly packed together without spaces. This was seen by great yogins who go to the edge of the subtle material existence.

Mostly, on the basis of their psychological energy, the spirits in this type of world congregate together and form different types of gross, subtle or super-subtle communities. Both in the physical world and in the astral regions, we find living entities congregating together on the basis of the type of psychological energy they utilize.

Some siddhas remain isolated by themselves for practice purposes but even they associate in higher realms with greater yogins. An ascetic siddha who is alone might be associating with others, just as the recorder of my ideas, associated with me mentally within his own psyche and jots down whatever I desire to say in this book.

This verse about the various worshipful associations, means that the clear-minded people worship those who use subtle bodies which are filled with clear light, while the impulsive persons worship those powerful persons whose subtle forms have much passionate energy. And the others heed those powerful persons whose subtle forms have a darkish energy. The word *devān* indicates those persons who reached a status whereby they are satisfied living as sunlight or moonlight. They are not required to take on gross bodies as we are obliged. Other persons like the Yakshas may become satisfied taking on astral bodies which have much impulsive energy within it. We experience such bodies when we dream. Those persons live in dream bodies and may not be required to enter into this gross level of life.

But the retarded people become attached to disembodied spirits who want to take gross life but cannot for one reason or the other, being deprived by the laws of nature.

अशास्त्रविहितं घोरं
तप्यन्ते ये तपो जनाः ।
दम्भाहंकारसंयुक्ताः
कामरागबलान्विताः ॥१७.५॥
aśāstravihitaṁ ghoraṁ
tapyante ye tapo janāḥ
dambhāhaṁkārasaṁyuktāḥ
kāmarāgabalānvitāḥ (17.5)

*aśāstravihitaṁ = aśāstra — not of scripture + vihitaṁ — recommended; ghoraṁ — terrible; tapyante — they endure; ye — who; tapo = tapaḥ — austerity; janāḥ — people; dambhāhaṁkārasaṁyuktāḥ = dambha — deceit + ahaṁkāra — misplaced identity + saṁyuktāḥ — enthused with; kāmarāgabalānvitāḥ = kāma — craving + rāga — rage + bala — brute force + anvitāḥ — possessed with*

**People who endure terrible austerities which are not recommended in the scripture, people who are enthused with deceit and misplaced identity, who are possessed with craving, rage and brute force, (17.5)**

***Siddha Swami's Commentary:***

This is part of the description of criminally-minded persons who are distressed with destiny and who feel that they can uproot the natural order of things. Of course it is not possible for a limited being to change the way material nature operates. In fact, even the Supreme Being rarely interferes with the laws of nature. And when and if He does, we find that nature quickly resumes its course. Even though there were many incarnations of Godhead, parallel divinities of the Supreme God, still we find that the material world courses as normal just as if God had not altered it in the least.

It is pointless to become dissatisfied with material nature. Instead one should study how it operates and make the best use of it. One should try to figure out where one is located in the scheme of nature. If one does not like material existence, an alternative exists in the way of liberation, the path of the siddhas. One may learn this and practice it to perfection. Otherwise there is no other recourse but to go along with nature, willingly or unwillingly.

A paltry attempt to disrupt nature or disrupt a minor display in nature, will do one no good. If one dislikes the current arrangement, one should take up the study of history to come to an understanding regarding the repetition of events. For instance, if one thinks that a certain river should flow away from the sea and should be emptied instead on a mountain top, one should study if that is a possibility. Can it done? Will nature support such a course? In that way one can understand one's position and make a proper decision. Modern science has made many efforts to rock the boat of nature, but is it worth the endeavor? And how long will the same nature allow the human beings the advantages which they cull out in the modern age? When will a meteor hit this planet and end the human civilization here? Or when will the sun suddenly send out burning rays which will wipe out humanity? In studying such possibilities, one may come to the proper conclusion regarding the worth of challenging nature.

कर्शयन्तः शरीरस्थं
भूतग्राममचेतसः ।
मां चैवान्तःशरीरस्थं
तान्विद्ध्यासुरनिश्चयान् ॥ १७.६ ॥
karśayantaḥ śarīrasthaṁ
bhūtagrāmamacetasaḥ
māṁ caivāntaḥśarīrasthaṁ
tānviddhyāsuraniścayān (17.6)

*karśayantaḥ — torturing, troubling; śarīrasthaṁ — within the body; bhūtagrāmam — collection of elements; acetasaḥ — senseless; māṁ — me; caivantaḥ = ca — and + eva — indeed + antaḥ — within; śarīrasthaṁ — within the body; tān — them; viddhi — know; āsura — wicked + niścayān — intentions*

**...those who torture the collection of the elements which comprise the body, who also trouble Me within the body, know that they have wicked intentions. (17.6)**

***Siddha Swami's Commentary:***

One should perform austerities as instructed by a great *yogin* who mastered his psychology. The reason is this: Such a person knows the correct restraints for bringing about enlightenment. Let us take the example of Lord Buddha. For final austerities, he did not take a teacher. He went and did whatever austerities ascetics were practicing in the area where he lived. But after some time, he realized that those austerities did not result in enlightenment. Therefore he abandoned those methods and found what he called the Middle Path. It was a moderate way of austerities which did not disturb the collection of elements which comprise the body. Thus those who become students of Buddha had the advantage of his direction and guidance, to avoid the extreme measures which do not result in enlightenment.

There is another aspect. That is motive. What is your motive for performing austerities? Is it political? For instance in the *Purāṇas* we hear of *Dhruva*, a boy prince, who had some political ambitions and who took up austerities for these purposes.

Is it romance that is bothering you? We hear of *Āgnīdra*, another prince, who wanted a celestial woman to become his wife. Is it envy? We hear of *Viśvāmitra* who became competitive towards the sage *Vasiṣṭha*. Is it supernatural power? We hear of *Rāvaṇa* who got the better of many beings of light, the *devas*. Is it because you want to take revenge upon the killer of your relative? *Hiranyakāśipu* performed austerities to get the power to challenge his brother's victor.

Despite the many reasons a person could take up austerities, the only authorized reason given in the *Gītā* is purification of the psyche. Some who begin austerities with a bad motive, become purified of it as they progress with the austerities. That was the case of Prince Dhruva. Others become more resentful and more crazy, such as *Rāvaṇa* and *Kumbhakaraṇa*.

By the grace of material nature and the Supreme Being, we have this human body. In fact any of these bodies, human, animal or vegetable, are acquired only by the grace of the two powers, namely material nature and the Supreme Being. Thus to an extent we have to respect both material nature and the Supreme Being.

We are obligated to both. If any of us act in a way that shows utter disregard for either of these powers, we will reap adverse consequences.

It may be asked why material nature or even God allows any of us to offend either of them. And the answer is: It is allowed for the sake of our education. We are ignorant for the most part. The only way we can learn is by the allowance to be defiant. If there was another way, we would have taken it a long time ago. Our very nature is this ignorance which must be dispelled by taking the course of *buddhi yoga*.

आहारस्त्वपि सर्वस्य
त्रिविधो भवति प्रियः ।
यज्ञस्तपस्तथा दानं
तेषां भेदमिमं शृणु ॥ १७.७॥
āhārastvapi sarvasya
trividho bhavati priyaḥ
yajñastapastathā dānaṁ
teṣāṁ bhedamimaṁ śṛṇu (17.7)

*āhāraḥ — food; tu — but; api — as well; sarvasya — of all; trividho = trividhaḥ — three kinds; bhavati — is; priyaḥ — likes; yajñaḥ — religious ceremony; tapaḥ — austerity; tathā — as; dānaṁ — charity; teṣāṁ — of them; bhedam — difference; imaṁ — this; śṛṇu — hear*

**But food as well, which is liked by all, is of three kinds as are religious ceremony, austerity and charity. Hear of the difference between them. (17.7)**

***Siddha Swami's Commentary:***

In every field of learning has theoretical and practical parts. Teachers take recourse to both methods. The theoretical part is a way of introducing the experience of the teacher to the student. Whatever is explained in theory which the student has not experienced, gives an idea of what one should aspire to perceive. *Śrī* Krishna in this course on *buddhi yoga* gave some information about various topics, telling us things that we may accept from Him on a matter of trust, until we acquire direct insight into those aspects.

In this type of world, our means of perception, what we perceive and even the conclusions we may draw, are based on material nature, which has three segments to it. Usually we think of it as something solid. Usually we feel we have bright objects, colorful objects and dark objects, such as daylight, orange tinged sunlight and night, or yellow objects, reddish objects and mud colored objects.

When *Śrī* Krishna spoke of the three aspects or divisions of material nature, he was not discussing gross segmentation, but rather subtle division of the energy. Because we are presently confused, we think that our psychological energy is spiritual. But that energy is material also, even though it is subtle. In His vocabulary, the material nature is a subtle phenomenon.

He divided material nature into types of psychological energy which affect us to produce clarity of perception, force of impulsion and force of intoxication to dull our perception and decrease motivation.

आयुःसत्त्वबलारोग्य-
सुखप्रीतिविवर्धनाः ।
रस्याः स्निग्धाः स्थिरा हृद्या
आहाराः सात्त्विकप्रियाः ॥ १७.८॥

*āyuḥsattvabalārogya = āyuḥ — duration of life + sattva — spiritual well-being + bala— strength + ārogya — health; sukhaprītivivardhanāḥ = sukha — happiness + prīti — satisfaction + vivardhanāḥ — increasing; rasyāḥ — juicy; snigdhāḥ — milky;*

āyuḥsattvabalārogya-
sukhaprītivivardhanāḥ
rasyāḥ snigdhāḥ sthirā hṛdyā
āhārāḥ sāttvikapriyāḥ (17.8)

*sthirā — sustaining; hṛdyā — palatable; āhārāḥ — foods; sāttvikapriyāḥ — dear to the clear-minded people*

**Foods which increase the duration of the life, the spiritual well-being, strength, health, happiness and satisfaction, which are juicy, milky, sustaining and palatable, are eatables which are dear to the clear-minded people. (17.8)**

***Siddha Swami's Commentary:***

There are general guidelines for life in the highest of the influences, the clarifying energy. It is a matter of which influences give us the highest, most clear and true perception, since on the basis of perception, we make decisions, endeavor and act.

Even though Arjuna was accredited by *Śrī* Krishna as being born with godly nature, still that does not restrict or bar anyone of a lower nature from elevation. In fact, the presence of Arjuna or any other godly person is the hint given to those below, about the possibility of upgrading their existence.

One may not have a taste for the food which the elevated beings prefer but still from being in their association, one may begin to cultivate their higher selection. This is the point. For indeed, even those who are generally categorized as being in the clarifying influence do fall lower if they are careless and do not take steps to reinforce the selection. Arjuna himself became degraded just seeing his relatives on a war field. *Śrī* Krishna lifted Arjuna up mentally and emotionally and thus Arjuna regained his footing and progressed onwards.

कट्वम्ललवणात्युष्ण-
तीक्ष्णरूक्षविदाहिनः ।
आहारा राजसस्येष्टा
दुःखशोकामयप्रदाः ॥१७.९॥
kaṭvamlalavaṇātyuṣṇa-
tīkṣṇarūkṣavidāhinaḥ
āhārā rājasasyeṣṭā
duḥkhaśokāmayapradāḥ (17.9)

*kaṭvamlalavaṇātyuṣṇa = kaṭv (kaṭu) — pungent + amla — sour + lavaṇa — salt; atyuṣṇa — peppery; tīkṣṇarūkṣavidāhinaḥ = tīkṣṇa — acidic + rūkṣa — dry + vidāhinaḥ — overheated; āhārā — foods; rājasasyeṣṭā = rajasasya — of the passionate people + iṣṭā — desired; duḥkhaśokāmayapradāḥ = duḥkha — pain + śoka — misery + āmaya — sickness + pradāḥ — causing*

**Foods which are pungent, sour, salty, peppery, acidic, dry and overheated, are desired by the passionate people. These foods cause pain, misery and sickness. (17.9)**

***Siddha Swami's Commentary:***

Food or anything ingested into the body and digested by it, has a subtle counterpart which affects the material body and the subtle one. A student *yogin* must study the psychological effects of different types of foods. He must take steps to eliminate from his diet, foods which lower consciousness, which cause bad dreams, which increase sensuality and sexuality and which hinder progress in meditation.

Whatever adversely affects the consciousness may be regarded as an intoxicant. For instance, a simple liquid like black tea, China tea or coffee may have an effect on the consciousness in the form of sleep deprivation. One may learn to use these fluids to keep the body awake or to remove its sluggishness. Sugary foods may cause the body to be energetic until their effect wears off and the body enters an energy deficit in terms of irritability or depression. Thus food is a form of intoxication, though mild in comparison to narcotics like opium or hashish.

The student *yogin* should study this. He or she need not blindly accept anything. Even common household spices like peppers and condiments may cause alterations in the consciousness which restrict a person in his or her selection. Whatever assists one in the objectives of yoga, in self purification, should be eaten and what hinders yoga should be avoided. That is the best rule to follow. One must make a careful study of one's diet and not be so addicted to any type of food, whereby one cannot objectively observe its effects on spiritual progress.

यातयामं गतरसं
पूति पर्युषितं च यत् ।
उच्छिष्टमपि चामेध्यं
भोजनं तामसप्रियम् ॥ १७.१० ॥
yātayāmaṁ gatarasaṁ
pūti paryuṣitaṁ ca yat
ucchiṣṭamapi cāmedhyaṁ
bhojanaṁ tāmasapriyam (17.10)

*yātayāmaṁ — stale; gatarasaṁ — tasteless; pūti — rotten; paryuṣitaṁ — left over; ca — and; yat = yad — which; ucchiṣṭam — rejected; api — also; cāmedhyam = ca — and + amedhyaṁ — unfit for religious ceremony; bhojanaṁ — food; tāmasapriyam.— cherished by the depressed people*

**Food which is stale, tasteless, and rotten, which was left over, as well as that which is rejected or unfit for religious ceremony, is cherished by the depressed people. (17.10)**

***Siddha Swami's Commentary:***

It is very important that one become sensitive to the needs of the elevated souls and to the Deities who are installed in the home or temple. Persons who offer food to Deities should follow the stipulations for the food to be offered in the worshipful, ceremonial way. And an ascetic should not eat any type of food which would be rejected by the *devas*, the supernatural controllers who inhabit the Universal Form of *Śrī* Krishna.

Those who follow the path of *buddhi yoga* should never eat any flesh of any sort, neither from animals nor fish. One should not eat eggs. Such things are unnecessary for the sake of survival, since the human body can subsist quite satisfactorily on vegetable, nut and fruit products. One may take milk and milk products but one should not inconvenience cows just to get their milk. If one takes milk from cows they should be treated as very dear animals and one should provide them with ample fodder.

Stale food should not be taken by an ascetic since such food has a negative energy which will affect the mind in a degrading way. Tasteless, rotten foods should also not be taken. These should be regarded as food for lower animals, insects and micro-organisms. Eating is linked to association. If one associates with highly elevated persons who are careful in their lifestyle and religious principles, one will naturally eat the proper foods.

अफलाकाङ्क्षिभिर्यज्ञो
विधिदृष्टो य इज्यते ।
यष्टव्यमेवेति मनः
समाधाय स सात्त्विकः ॥ १७.११ ॥
aphalākāṅkṣibhiryajño
vidhidṛṣṭo ya ijyate
yaṣṭavyameveti manaḥ
samādhāya sa sāttvikaḥ (17.11)

*aphalākāṅkṣibhiḥ = aphalā — no benefits + kāṅkṣibhiḥ — desiring; yajño = yajñaḥ — a religious discipline or ceremony; vidhidṛṣṭo = vidhidṛṣṭaḥ = vidhi — scripture + dṛṣṭaḥ — observing; ya — who; ijyate — is offered; yaṣṭavyam — to be sacrificed; eveti = eva — indeed + iti — thus; manaḥ — mind; samādhāya — concentrating; sa — it; sāttvikaḥ — realistic*

**A religious discipline or ceremony in observance of the scripture, by those who do not desire a benefit and who, while concentrating, think, "This is to be sacrificed," is a ceremony of the realistic type. (17.11)**

***Siddha Swami's Commentary:***

Advanced students of *brahma yoga* may be absent from many religious ceremonies because of their need for isolation to complete yoga austerities. But they should not be against such ceremonies, knowing fully well the usefulness and productiveness in the lives of others.

Those who are sincere in the performance of religious ceremonies, should work to free themselves of motives, reaching the stage where they perform ceremonies for the reason stated by *Śrī* Krishna in this verse, that is for the cause of duty as human beings, who are off-shoots of the Supreme Lord. So long as one is involved in cultural activities, on the course of *pravṛttih marga* or cultural acts for righteous development, one should perform the religious ceremonies with fire sacrifices and Deity worship. All this should be done in the highest mode of goodness.

Even though in a Vedic religious ceremony, the main objective is to sacrifice something to the Supreme Lord or to His agent, still that does not mean that a life should be taken. Persons who are elevated should not participate, condone or promote the taking of life in any religious sacrifice. Something must be sacrificed and thus one's time is the first aspect to be offered. One's cleanliness is offered. One's endeavor in acquiring the ingredients and articles for the ceremony is offered. One's attentiveness is offered. One's affection for the specific Deity is offered. But one should not attempt to offer the life of a creature.

Those who feel that some life must be taken should scale down their need to be satisfied in that way, by offering a coconut or a cucumber or some other type of vegetative life. In fact, in such a ceremony if a knife is put to the coconut or vegetable, a sensitive devotee will feel as if a life was taken. Unless one has that sort of sensitivity, one cannot experience what it is like to be in the clarifying influence, through which one perceives what is divine.

अभिसंधाय तु फलं
दम्भार्थमपि चैव यत् ।
इज्यते भरतश्रेष्ठ
तं यज्ञं विद्धि राजसम् ॥ १७.१२ ॥
abhisaṁdhāya tu phalaṁ
dambhārthamapi caiva yat
ijyate bharataśreṣṭha
taṁ yajñaṁ viddhi rājasam (17.12)

*abhisandhāya — kept in mind; tu — but; phalam — benefit; dambhārtham — for the sake of outsmarting the deity; api — also; caiva — and indeed; yat = yad — which; ijyate — is offered; bharataśreṣṭha — best of the Bhāratas; tam — this; yajñaṁ — disciplined worship; viddhi — know; rājasam — impulsive*

**But when a benefit is kept in mind and when the motive is to outsmart the deity, know, O best of the Bharatas, that the disciplinary worship offered is based on impulsion. (17.12)**

***Siddha Swami's Commentary:***

Religious development includes honesty to admit where one is situated in the development of higher principles. Pretending to be at a higher stage will not help the devotee. In fact, that will degrade him and cause disgrace. Thus if one is on a lower level, one must recognize that condition and then get instructions from a trustworthy senior on how to advance. If one cannot stop the tendency for outsmarting the Deity, one should realize the defect and get advice on how to upgrade the psyche.

Many devotees worship from the passionate, impulsive level but who carefully hide their tendencies in order to be recognized as great and pure devotees of *Śrī* Krishna or some other Deity. That is not good for progression.

विधिहीनमसृष्टान्नं
मन्त्रहीनमदक्षिणम् ।
श्रद्धाविरहितं यज्ञं
तामसं परिचक्षते ॥ १७.१३ ॥
vidhihīnamasṛṣṭānnaṁ
mantrahīnamadakṣiṇam
śraddhāvirahitaṁ yajñaṁ
tāmasaṁ paricakṣate (17.13)

*vidhihīnam — scripture neglected; asṛṣṭānnaṁ = asṛṣṭa — not offered + annam — food; mantrahīnam — Vedic hymn not recited; adakṣiṇam — no fee for the priest; śraddhāvirahitaṁ — confidence lacking; yajñaṁ — disciplinary worship; tāmasaṁ — depressive; paricakṣate — they regard*

**When scripture is neglected, food is not offered, Vedic hymns not recited, a fee not given to the priest, and confidence is lacking, regard that disciplinary worship as depressive. (17.13)**

***Siddha Swami's Commentary:***

Even though this kind of worship is depressive, certainly, this is still an effort at worship. Those who perform this devilish type of worship and who do so non-willfully, merely because they came up from the animal world and entered the human species with much ignorance, have hope for elevation by higher guidance and association.

Others who do this deliberately and who have neglected good advice from more elevated and cultured people, set the stage for their own ruination in hellish life by advocating and performing such ceremonies.

देवद्विजगुरुप्राज्ञ-
पूजनं शौचमार्जवम् ।
ब्रह्मचर्यमहिंसा च
शारीरं तप उच्यते ॥ १७.१४ ॥
devadvijagurupraājña-
pūjanaṁ śaucamārjavam
brahmacaryamahiṁsā ca
śārīraṁ tapa ucyate (17.14)

*devadvijagurupraājña = deva — supernatural ruler + dvija = those who are qualified by sacred thread ceremony + guru — spiritual teacher + prājña — wise man; pūjanaṁ — reverential respect; śaucam — purity; ārjavam — straightforwardness; brahmacaryam — celibacy; ahiṁsa — non-violence; ca — and; śārīraṁ — body; tapa — austerity; ucyate — is said to be*

**Reverential respect of the supernatural rulers, of those who are qualified by the sacred thread ceremony, of the spiritual teacher, and of the wise man, purity, straightforwardness, celibacy and non-violence, are said to be austerity of the body. (17.14)**

***Siddha Swami's Commentary:***

This tells us how to control the material body. The body prefers certain conditions but a human being should show that he is greater than the animals by exercising control over the material form. The body should be made to **offer formal respect to the supernatural rulers, the duly-qualified brahmins, the spiritual teacher and any wise man** even if he is from a seemingly inferior race or family.

Sometimes the body willingly offers such respect. Othertimes it resists and assumes a stiffness and reluctance. Even then, when the body is unwilling it should be made to offer due obeisance.

External **purity** of the body by means of bath to remove sweat and other pollutants from the form is necessary for a human being, even though for the animals it is not required. Basic hygiene is required in terms of prompt evacuation of urine and stools. Usually the animals excrete everywhere and anywhere, because for them there is no restriction as to the place for evacuation. The human being has the special responsibility to pass waste in particular places and he or she must make a special effort to be prompt in the evacuation of airy, watery or solid waste from the body.

**Straightforwardness** is required for developing honesty and for removing oneself from trickery and deception. Such effort does wonders for purifying the subtle body which has energies in it to sponsor either honesty or dishonesty.

**Celibacy** is required. Without celibacy one cannot develop and experience the higher senses of the subtle body. And without such experience one cannot have faith in the world of the *devas* and of the Supreme Being. To achieve celibacy, one has to master yoga practice.

**Non-violence** is required since that is the epitome of morality. One who masters non-violence is the most moral of the human beings. The highest type of non-violence is the coordination of one's cultural activities with those of the Universal Form of *Śrī* Krishna. This might entail physical or even psychological disciplinary acts on behalf of *Śrī* Krishna, but it is non-violence in the spiritual sense, since the Supreme Being only acts to protect the spiritual integrity of the living beings.

Of the various parts of this austerity of the body, the most essential and pivotal one is celibacy. One who masters celibacy adopts a junior attitude towards Lord Shiva and other *mahāyogins*, and towards *Śrī* Krishna, the Central Figure in the Universal Form. Assuming an attitude of dependency on those Lords, the devotee gets perfect guidance and develops the required qualities. A true celibate would not disrespect the supernatural rulers, the brahmins, the spiritual master or any other person who proves himself to be a wise man.

In the history of the *Purāṇas*, we find that the demoniac persons became hostile to the *devas* or to the Supreme Being. Usually there is some type of competitive attitude towards the masculine authority of the superior personalities. Thus if one remains as a celibate, one will not have to compete for any of the spouses of the superior personalities. This is to be kept in mind by student yogins. And in any case, one can hardly master those celestial or divine females. Thus it is best to keep oneself as a dependent son or daughter of the great authorities.

अनुद्वेगकरं वाक्यं
सत्यं प्रियहितं च यत् ।
स्वाध्यायाभ्यसनं चैव
वाङ्मयं तप उच्यते ॥ १७.१५॥
anudvegakaraṁ vākyaṁ
satyaṁ priyahitaṁ ca yat
svādhyāyābhyāsanaṁ caiva
vāṅmayaṁ tapa ucyate (17.15)

*anudvegakaraṁ — not causing distress; vākyaṁ — speech; satyam — truthful; priyaḥitam — agreeable and beneficial; ca — and; yat = yad — which; svādhyāyābhyāsanaṁ = svādhyāya — recitation of scripture + abhyāsanaṁ — practice, regularity; caiva — and indeed; vāṅmayaṁ — speech-made; tapa — discipline; ucyate — is called*

**Speech which does not cause distress and is truthful, agreeable and beneficial, as well as regular recitation of the scriptures is the discipline of speech. (17.15)**

***Siddha Swami's Commentary:***

The curbing of the impulse of speech is part of the effort of *pratyāhār* practice to curb the impulses of the subtle body. It actually begins in the causal body when the cramped potentially-violent energies are released into the mind chamber. These released impressions burst into pictures and sounds when the imagination faculty is hit by them. From this display within the mind, comes speech and other expressions from the body.

The regular recitation of the scriptures and the repetition of special sounds which remind one of the divinities, and the supreme energy, *brahman*, orients the subtle and causal bodies to higher association, thus squelching the lower tendencies which those forms are capable of exhibiting.

In *brahma yoga*, the student is trained to track the source energies of his or her speech through the subtle form into the causal body, through its mouth which is the memory chamber. From the causal body, impressions travel out through the memory and hit the imagination orb, where they are translated into visions and language. The reverse also occurs, whereby visions and language are reduced to micro-impressions which enter the memory and fall lower into the causal body for storage in what modern psychologists call the sub-conscious mind. Student *brahma yogis* must be trained to track such energies. Then they will be able to practice the austerity of speech *(vāk mayam tapa)* by the process of *pratyāhār* which is the 5th stage of yoga.

मनःप्रसादः सौम्यत्वं
मौनमात्मविनिग्रहः ।
भावसंशुद्धिरित्येतत्
तपो मानसमुच्यते ॥ १७.१६ ॥
manaḥprasādaḥ saumyatvaṁ
maunamātmavinigrahaḥ
bhāvasaṁśuddhirityetat
tapo mānasamucyate (17.16)

*manaḥprasādaḥ = manah — mind + prasādaḥ — peace; saumayatvaṁ — gentleness; maunam — silence; ātmavinigrahaḥ — self-restraint; bhāvasaṁśuddhiḥ = bhāva — being + saṁśuddhiḥ — purity; iti — thus, etat = etad — this; tapo = tapaḥ — discipline; mānasam — of the mind; ucyate — is called*

**Peace of mind, gentleness, silence, self restraint, and purity of being, this is called discipline of mind. (17.16)**

***Siddha Swami's Commentary:***

*Tapo mānasam*, discipline of mind, is the *buddhi yoga* practice which was taught to Arjuna in this *Bhagavad Gītā*. There is no substitute for it. It is not *bhaktih*, devotion to *Śrī* Krishna, but it may be facilitated by devotion to *Śrī* Krishna. One may be more willing to commit oneself to that practice, if one has devotion to *Śrī* Krishna. *Bhakti* or devotion does not substitute for *buddhi yoga* practice nor does *buddhi yoga* practice substitute for *bhaktih* but the two may be related if one is a devotee of *Śrī* Krishna.

The first part of *buddhi yoga* results in *prasādah* or peace of mind. This comes about by mastership of *pratyāhār* sensual energy withdrawal and containment in the psyche. Without this one cannot escape from the *kāma* craving energy.

**Gentleness** comes about by withdrawal from social affairs. But one cannot do this without a waiver from the Supreme Person, to authoritatively move away from social interactions. This may be illustrated by studying Arjuna. He did desire to be gentle at *Kurukṣetra*, but the same *Śrī* Krishna did not allow him. Since the Universal Form has many disciplinary duties, He will of necessarily be engaging His principal agents in scolding tasks, where gentleness has no place. Thus, unless one is freed from such social interaction, one cannot be gentle consistently. In this world, most persons are acting in a defiant manner towards God Almighty, and thus there is a need for divine chastisement.

**Silence** is part of the *buddhi yoga* practice. This comes about after mastership of *pratyāhār*. When one masters the sensual energies and controls them from going outwards into the gross and subtle material world, one is left with one's psyche. At that point one begins to perceive the various parts of the inner psychic world. This consists of mental space, imagination faculty, analytical faculty, sense of identity and psychic energy for mental endeavor and emotional exchange.

By going to a silent place to practice, the student yogi becomes aware of the internal vibrations which disrupt psychic silence and which keep the psychic equipments operating only in their lower pursuits. He learns from a yogi guru how to stop the disruptive internal noises and how to lean on the higher inner sounds or vibrations which foster higher mystic perceptions. Unless there is silence, *buddhi yoga* practice cannot be achieved. First there must be external silence. A yogi should be in a place where human noises are decreased mostly if not altogether. Then the *yogin* must work for inner silence, because after one gets outer silence, one encounters a noisy environment on the inside. In the mind, the memory releases impressions which have noisy content when they are expanded by the imagination faculty.

It is to be realized and seen internally by each *yogin*, that after the senses are closed off to the external world and deprived of their objectives in the gross environment, they will seek out objects in the subtle world. Then after they are deprived of these objects, the mind will internalize, seeking objects from the memory. In conjunction with the imagination faculty, the memory will torment the student yogins. Thus all of them will have to get help from superior ascetics who will show the way to master the mind by *buddhi yoga* practice. It was described by *Śrī* Krishna in this *Gītā*, but still one will need a teacher to help in the struggle to get control of the inner world.

The term *ātmavinigrahah* is interesting. *Grahah* means seizing, grasping, taking or receiving. Now if we add *vini* to that word as a prefix, then we get the exact opposite. Thus when the *ātma* or **self** becomes **restrained** from the indulgence, that is the culmination of yoga. *Bhāvasamśuddhi* is a related condition where the **self** becomes **purified**. The entire psyche, which consists mostly of psychic instruments and their energy intake or power supplies, must become purified. Otherwise the self, which is fused with these equipments, will be affected in an adverse way. All this must be realized and mastered by *buddhi yoga* practice.

श्रद्धया परया तप्तं
तपस्तत्त्रिविधं नरैः ।
अफलाकाङ्क्षिभिर्युक्तैः
सात्त्विकं परिचक्षते ॥१७.१७॥
śraddhayā parayā taptaṁ
tapastattrividhaṁ naraiḥ
aphalākāṅkṣibhiryuktaiḥ
sāttvikaṁ paricakṣate (17.17)

*śraddhayā — with faith; parayā — with the highest; taptam — performed; tapaḥ — austerity; tat = tad — this; trividham — three-fold; naraih — by people; aphalākāṅkṣibhiḥ — by those who do not aspire for a benefit; yuktaiḥ — by those disciplined in yoga; sāttvikaṁ — realilstic; paricakṣate — they consider*

**When this threefold austerity is performed with the highest faith by yogicly-disciplined people who do not aspire for a benefit, the authorities consider it to be realistic. (17.17)**

***Siddha Swami's Commentary:***

This three-fold austerity of body, speech and mind cannot be performed by persons proficiently unless they master the *buddhi yoga* discipline. The term *yuktaih* means by those who are disciplined in the same *buddhi yoga* which *Śrī* Krishna explained to Arjuna in the preceding chapters, especially in Chapter Two. Much of this concerns mystic control, which is mastered through higher yoga.

Such devotees of *Śrī* Krishna have the highest faith, *śraddhayā parayā* because of their direct experiences of the subtle and super-subtle realities.

सत्कारमानपूजार्थं
तपो दम्भेन चैव यत् ।
क्रियते तदिह प्रोक्तं
राजसं चलमध्रुवम् ॥ १७.१८ ॥
satkāramānapūjārthaṁ
tapo dambhena caiva yat
kriyate tadiha proktaṁ
rājasaṁ calamadhruvam (17.18)

*satkāramānapūjārthaṁ = satkāra — reputation + māna — respect + pūjā — reverence + arthaṁ — for the sake of; tapo = tapaḥ — austerity; dambhena — with trickery; caiva — and indeed; yat = yad — which; kriyate — performed; tat — this; iha — in this world; proktaṁ — is declared; rājasaṁ — impulsive; calam — shifty; adhruvam — temporary*

**Austerity which, in this world is performed with trickery for the sake of reputation, respect and reverence, is declared to be impulsive, shifty and temporary. (17.18)**

***Siddha Swami's Commentary:***

Such austerity is of the passionate nature, even if performed in the religious field, even if done by a devotee of *Śrī* Krishna. It is the nature of the motivation which determines the type of propensity. Many who become *sannyāsis* and *pujārīs* in great religious societies, do so for the sake of acquiring respect and reverence from others. They pose as devotees of *Śrī* Krishna or some other divinity and advise the public to offer respect and reverence because of their position as established, well-known devotees. This is all done from the position of impulsion.

मूढग्राहेणात्मनो यत्
पीडया क्रियते तपः ।
परस्योत्सादनार्थं वा
तत्तामसमुदाहृतम् ॥ १७.१९ ॥
mūḍhagrāheṇātmano yat
pīḍayā kriyāte tapaḥ
parasyotsādanārthaṁ vā
tattāmasamudāhṛtam (17.19)

*mūḍhagrāheṇātmano = mūḍha — foolish + grāheṇa = by mistaken ideas + ātmano (ātmanaḥ) — of the self; yat = yad — which; pīḍayā — with torture; kriyāte — is performed; tapaḥ — austerity; parasyotsādanārthaṁ = parasya — of someone else + utsādana — harming + artham — purpose; vā — or; tat — that; tāmasam — depressive; udāhṛtam — said to be*

**Austerity performed with foolish, mistaken ideas, and with torture or for the purpose of harming someone else, is said to be depressive. (17.19)**

***Siddha Swami's Commentary:***

Even though austerity is efficiently used only for curbing the psyche, still many persons can only see a use for it to take revenge or to intensify a grudge towards others. This is because from the animal perspective, the idea of purification of the psyche does not arise in one's intellect.

Animals are taught about austerity through their hunger impulse. When they cannot find food for many days, they get some idea of austerity. But when at last they do locate their prey, they greedily pursue it. Thus they learn that austerities sponsor the enthusiasm for eating greedily. Later on when an animal transmigrates into the human species, it continues this profile for austerity. All such habits may be studied carefully by the students of *brahma yoga* practice.

दातव्यमिति यद्दानं
दीयतेऽनुपकारिणे ।
देशे काले च पात्रे च
तद्दानं सात्त्विकं स्मृतम् ॥ १७.२० ॥
dātavyamiti yaddānaṁ
dīyate'nupakāriṇe
deśe kāle ca pātre ca
taddānaṁ sāttvikaṁ smṛtam (17.20)

*dātavyam — to be given; iti — thus; yat — which; dānaṁ — gift; dīyate — is given; 'nupakāriṇe = anupakāriṇe — to one who has not done a prior favor; deśe — in proper place; kāle — at the proper time; ca — and; pātre — to as worthy person; ca — and; tat — that; dānaṁ — gift; sāttvikaṁ — virtuous; smṛtam — remembered as*

**A gift given to one who has not done a prior favor, in the proper place and time and to a worthy person, is remembered as being virtuous. (17.20)**

***Siddha Swami's Commentary:***

This kind of gift is presented by the inspiration of the Universal Form of *Śrī* Krishna. A limited entity can hardly know what to give and what not to give unless he or she takes direction from the divine personages. This is because of limited perception of the past. *Śrī* Krishna informed Arjuna that the limited souls like Arjuna were unable to remember former lives. As such, it is only possible for them to act perfectly when they are inspired by the Divinity.

This sort of perfect action cannot be figured out intellectually or by emotional sensing. One must instead tune into the mind of the Universal Form to determine what to do and what not to do. This is achieved by mastership of *buddhi yoga*, by psychic purity, which permits one's nature to be absorbent towards the Supreme Being.

यत्तु प्रत्युपकारार्थं
फलमुद्दिश्य वा पुनः ।
दीयते च परिक्लिष्टं
तद्दानं राजसं स्मृतम् ॥ १७.२१ ॥
yattu pratyupakārārthaṁ
phalamuddiśya vā punaḥ
dīyate ca parikliṣṭaṁ
taddānaṁ rājasaṁ smṛtam (17.21)

*yat — which; tu — but; pratyupakārārthaṁ — for a compensation; phalam — a result; uddiśya — pointing to, hoping; vā — or; punaḥ — alternately; dīyate — is given; ca — and; parikliṣṭaṁ — grudgingly; tat — that; dānaṁ — gift; rājasaṁ — impulsive; smṛtam — mentally noted*

**But the gift which is given grudgingly for a compensation or alternately hoping for a reward, is mentally noted as being impulsive. (17.21)**

***Siddha Swami's Commentary:***

Both in this verse and in the previous one, *Śrī* Krishna used the term *smṛtam* which means *remembered as* as or *mentally noted as*. This hint for yogis, that in the matter of giving either under the inspiration of God or as otherwise impelled for reward that creates an obligation for someone else, there will be a mental note of the occurence in the mind of the person. This type of giving either as divinely inspired or as impelled by passion, will contribute to the formation of one's sense of conscience. In other words, one will use this to determine the value of the person to whom the gift is presented, at a later date.

In the material world, the minute one becomes a donor to anyone, there might be an energy of obligation levied on oneself or on the recipient of the gift. Such matters are psychological and students should take up the study of this in yoga meditations.

अदेशकाले यद्दानम्
अपात्रेभ्यश्च दीयते ।
असत्कृतमवज्ञातं
तत्तामसमुदाहृतम् ॥ १७.२२ ॥
adeśakāle yaddānam
apātrebhyaśca dīyate
asatkṛtamavajñātaṁ
tattāmasamudāhṛtam (17.22)

*adeśakāle — at the wrong place and time; yat — which; dānam — gift; apātrebhyaśca = apātrebhyaḥ — to a unworthy person + ca — and; dīyate — is given; asatkṛtam — without paying respect; avajñātaṁ — without due consideration; tat = tad — that; tāmasam — depressive mode; udāhrtam — is said to be*

**That gift which is given in the wrong place and time, to an unworthy person, without paying respect, without due consideration, is said to be of the depressive mode. (17.22)**

***Siddha Swami's Commentary:***

A person who recently moved into the human species from the animal incarnations, might act in an awkward way, due to unfamiliarity with the constraints and patterns of human behavior. But in time, such a person would adjust and become cultured. Of course this may take many, many lives as a human being.

ओं तत्सदिति निर्देशो
ब्रह्मणस्त्रिविधः स्मृतः ।
ब्राह्मणास्तेन वेदाश्च
यज्ञाश्च विहिताः पुरा ॥ १७.२३ ॥
oṁ tatsaditi nirdeśo
brahmaṇastrividhaḥ smṛtaḥ
brāhmaṇāstena vedāśca
yajñāśca vihitāḥ purā (17.23)

*oṁ — Om; tat = Tat; sat = Sat; iti — pronouncement; nirdeśo = nirdeśaḥ — designation; brahmaṇaḥ — of spiritual reality; trividhaḥ — three-fold; smrtah — is known; brahmaṇaḥ — by the brahmins; tena — by this; vedāsca = vedāh — of the Vedas + ca — and; yajñāśca = yajñāḥ — religious disciplines and ceremony + ca — and; vihitāḥ — prescribed; purā — anciently*

**The pronouncement *Om Tat Sat* is known as the threefold designation of spiritual reality. By this expression, the brahmins, the *Vedas,* and the prescribed religious disciplines and ceremonies were ordained in ancient times. (17.23)**

***Siddha Swami's Commentary:***

*Om tat sat* means: This is the reality. We located It. We will focus on It and attain eternity.

This was the attitude of the sages in the time of the Upanishads. They were speaking of their contact with the *brahman* spiritual world.

तस्मादोमित्युदाहृत्य
यज्ञदानतपःक्रियाः ।
प्रवर्तन्ते विधानोक्ताः
सततं ब्रह्मवादिनाम् ॥१७.२४॥
tasmādomityudāhṛtya
yajñadānatapaḥkriyāḥ
pravartante vidhānoktāḥ
satataṁ brahmavādinām (17.24)

*tasmāt — hence; om — the sound Om; iti — thus; udāhṛtya — uttering; yajñadānatapaḥkriyāḥ = yajña — sacrifice + dāna — charity + tapaḥ — austerity + kriyāḥ — acts; pravartante — they begin; vidhānoktāḥ = vidhāna — prescription + uktāḥ — said; satatam — always; brahmavādinām — of the spiritual masters*

**Hence as prescribed in the *Vedic* scriptures, acts of sacrifice, charity, and austerity always begin by the spiritual masters while uttering the sound *Om*. (17.24)**

***Siddha Swami's Commentary:***

*Brahmavādinām* refers to those spiritual masters who become so proficient in higher yoga, that they reach into the spiritual reality and remain connected with it by their continued austerities and mystic reach. The saying of *Om* was the way of contacting the spiritual plane. It was also a signal event for those able yogins who could instantly switch themselves away from this subtle and gross material world to the spiritual levels.

तदित्यनभिसंधाय
फलं यज्ञतपःक्रियाः ।
दानक्रियाश्च विविधाः
क्रियन्ते मोक्षकाङ्क्षिभिः ॥१७.२५॥
tadityanabhisaṁdhāya
phalaṁ yajñatapaḥkriyāḥ
dānakriyāśca vividhāḥ
kriyānte mokṣakāṅkṣibhiḥ (17.25)

*tat — Tat; iti — saying; anabhisaṁdhāya — without an interest; phalam — benefit; yajñatapaḥkriyāḥ = yajña — sacrifice + tapaḥ — austerity + kriyāḥ — actions; dānakriyāśca = dānakriyāḥ — acts of charity + ca — and; vividhāḥ — various types; kriyānte — are performed; mokṣakāṅkṣibhiḥ — by those who desire liberation*

**While saying Tat without an interest in a benefit, acts of sacrifice, austerity and various types of charity are performed by those who are desirous of liberation. (17.25)**

***Siddha Swami's Commentary:***

This is further confirmation that *Om tat sat* was used by the advanced yogis ascetics, those who were desirous of liberation, the *mokṣakāṅkṣibhih* personalities.

Here *Śrī* Krishna addresses the needs of the rishis of the Upanishadic era. They also had material needs. They had to act to get food and shelter but they were not focused down into the material world. Hence their acquirement of basic necessities did not become an obsession for them. It was just a routine. They acted culturally but without impulsion and were freed from forming obligations in themselves or in others.

The period of the Upanishads is very important even to modern yogins, since the foundation of yoga practice was laid at that time by the Vedic rishis. From them, we received the hint for higher yoga.

सद्भावे साधुभावे च
सदित्येतत्प्रयुज्यते ।
प्रशस्ते कर्मणि तथा
सच्छब्दः पार्थ युज्यते ॥१७.२६॥

*sadbhāve = sad (sat) — reality + bhāve — in meaning; sādhubhāve = sādhu — excellence + bhāve — in meaning; ca — and; sat — reality, that which is productive of reality; iti — thus; etat*

sadbhāve sādhubhāve ca
sadityetatprayujyate
praśaste karmaṇi tathā
sacchabdaḥ pārtha yujyate (17.26)

*= etad — this; prayujyate — is used; praśaste — is praiseworthy; karmāṇi — in action; tathā— also; sacchabdaḥ = sat — Sat + śabdaḥ — word; pārtha — son of Pṛthā; yujyate — is used*

**The word Sat is used to mean reality and excellence and also for a praiseworthy act, O son of Pṛthā. (17.26)**

***Siddha Swami's Commentary:***

*Sat* was said by those great rishis who reached the spiritual plane and who figured how to act in the material world in a way conducive to continued contact with the spiritual level. Great satisfaction was derived from that contact by the able yogi sages of ancient times.

यज्ञे तपसि दाने च
स्थितिः सदिति चोच्यते ।
कर्म चैव तदर्थीयं
सदित्येवाभिधीयते ॥ १७.२७॥
yajñe tapasi dāne ca
sthitiḥ saditi cocyate
karma caiva tadarthīyaṁ
sadityevābhidhīyate (17.27)

*yajñe — in sacrifice; tapasi — in austerity; dāne — in charity; ca — and; sthitiḥ — steady application; sat — realism; iti —thus; cocyate = ca — and + ucyate — is designated; karma — action; caiva — and indeed; tadarthīyaṁ — for the purpose of that; sat — realistic; iti — thus; evābhidhīyate = eva — indeed + abhidhīyate — is designated*

**Steady application in sacrifice, austerity and charity, is also called *Sat*. An action which is supportive of this purpose is also designated as *Sat*. (17.27)**

***Siddha Swami's Commentary:***

To be realistic one must not expect to get out of the material world by one's endeavor. Self endeavor may cause one to get in touch with the spiritual reality or *Sat*, but it will not get one out of this place. For getting out, one depends on the will of the Supreme God. And it is not a matter of influencing Him by performance of any type of devotional service, or by austerities. He will make up His mind all by Himself. If He has no intention of releasing a particular person from this place, the person's desires or services will not cause release. It is important to accept this.

Hence one should aim for the ability to get in touch with spiritual reality always and leave the rest to God. One should not waste valuable time thinking of ways and means of influencing God, for God cannot be influenced by any limited being. Whatever one is destined to do, one will have to do, and wherever one is destined to live, one will have to reside there. But one may take the initiative to be desirous of liberation in the sense of keeping in constant touch with the divinities and their spiritual locale.

Thus this advice of *Śrī* Krishna for steady application in sacrifice, austerity and charity with actions which are supportive of spiritual elevation, is vital for all yogins.

अश्रद्धया हुतं दत्तं
तपस्तप्तं कृतं च यत् ।
असदित्युच्यते पार्थ
न च तत्प्रेत्य नो इह ॥ १७.२८॥

*aśraddhayā — with a lack of faith; hutaṁ — oblation; dattaṁ —offered; tapaḥ — austerity; taptaṁ — performed; kṛtaṁ — done; ca — and; yat — which; asat — unrealistic; iti — thus; ucyate — is called; pārtha — son of*

aśraddhayā hutaṁ dattaṁ
tapastaptaṁ kṛtaṁ ca yat
asadityucyate pārtha
na ca tatpretya no iha (17.28)

*Prthà; na — no; ca — and; tat — that; pretya — hereafter; no = naḥ — to us; iha — here*

**An oblation offered with a lack of faith and austerity performed in the same way is called asat, unrealistic, O son of Pṛtha. And that has no value to us here or in the hereafter. (17.28)**

***Siddha Swami's Commentary:***

One has to get in touch with the higher personalities and then maintain contact with them at all costs. This is vital. Faith in God, faith in His agents, is very important. Association with great persons is very important. In fact, one cannot make spiritual progression unless one falls under the influences of the great persons who are in touch with the Divine Lord. We must all remain in divine association, maintaining favorable, loving contact with the proper respect for those above us. No one should become haughty to *Śrī* Krishna or to any of His agents. Everyone in the yoga schools should remain very humble to the spiritual teachers, to Lord Shiva and to Lord Krishna as well as to any of their agents or parallel divinities. That alone is sufficient for spiritual life.

# CHAPTER 18

## Sarva Guhyatamam

## The Most Secret of All Information*

*sarvaguhyatamaṁ bhūyaḥ śṛṇu me paramaṁ vacaḥ*
*iṣṭo'si me dṛḍhamiti tato vakṣyāmi te hitam (18.64)*

***Hear again of My supreme discourse, the most secret of all information. You are surely loved by Me. Hence I speak for your benefit. (18.64)***

**Siddha Swami assigned this chapter title on the basis of verse 64 of this chapter.*

अर्जुन उवाच
संन्यासस्य महाबाहो
तत्त्वमिच्छामि वेदितुम् ।
त्यागस्य च हृषीकेश
पृथक्केशिनिषूदन ॥ १८.१ ॥
arjuna uvāca
saṁnyāsasya mahābāho
tattvamicchāmi veditum
tyāgasya ca hṛṣīkeśa
pṛthakkeśiniṣūdana (18.1)

*arjuna — Arjuna; uvāca — said; saṁnyāsasya — of the rejection of opportunity; mahābāho — O strong-armed hero; tattvam — fact; icchāmi — I want; veditum — to know; tyāgasya — of the rejection of consequences; ca — and; hṛṣīkesa — O Hṛṣīkeśa; pṛthak — distinguish; keśiniṣūdāna — slayer of Keshi*

**Arjuna said: Regarding the rejection of opportunity, O strong-armed hero, I want to know the fact. And regarding the rejection of consequences, O Hṛṣīkeśa, distinguish these, O slayer of Keshi. (18.1)**

***Siddha Swami's Commentary:***

Rejection of consequences is actually for the *karma* yogis, while rejection of opportunity is for the *jñāna* yogis. Here *Śrī* Krishna instructed both types of yogis. The *jñāna* yogis learn how to reject opportunities for cultural life, because they are no longer interested in acquiring knowledge about how to better exist in the subtle or gross material world. Having lost interest in this situation, they are ready to leave aside all sorts of opportunities for a better type of life in a better species of existence.

On the other hand, *karma* yogis are interested only in righteous lifestyle here, As stipulated by the Universal Form of *Śrī* Krishna for ideal cultural interaction. Thus the *karma* yogis do not want to reject the opportunities. They welcome the chance to participate, since by those actions they facilitate their social careers. Students may recall a verse in this discourse, when *Śrī* Krishna alerted Arjuna about the value of social opportunities:

*svadharmamapi cāvekṣya na vikampitumarhasi*
*dharmyāddhi yuddhācchreyo'nyat kṣatriyasya na vidyate (2.31)*
*yadṛcchayā copapannaṁ svargadvāramapāvṛtam*
*sukhinaḥ kṣatriyāḥ pārtha labhante yuddhamīdṛśam (2.32)*

***And considering your assigned duty, you should not look for alternatives. In fact, for the son of a king, there is no other duty which is better than a righteous battle.***

***And by a stroke of luck, the gate of heaven is opened. Thrilled are the warriors who get such a battle opportunity, O son of Pṛthā. (2.31-32)***

*Śrī* Krishna even described in plain terms the social promotions Arjuna would derive from exploiting the opportunity for battle which was presented by providence. This is what Krishna said:

*hato vā prāpsyasi svargaṁ jitvā vā bhokṣyase mahīm*
*tasmāduttiṣṭha kaunteya yuddhāya kṛtaniścayaḥ (2.37)*

***Either be killed and achieve the angelic world or having conquered, enjoy the nation. Therefore stand up and be decisive, O son of Kunti. (2.37)***

Arjuna could not reject the opportunity without adverse consequences. He had no license as a *jñāna* yogi. He was not exempt from cultural activities. Only a *jñāna* yogi who has the exemption may reject the opportunities. Thus he does not have to deal with future consequences. What would such a *jñāna yogin* do with reactions that come to him from his previous social involvements? The answer is that he is trained to deal with them in a terminal way so as to close off his cultural accounts. He is also trained in *kriyā* and *brahma yoga* to neutralize the impressions which arise from the memory and which, if not smothered, will cause him to go back for social activity. He is trained in how to arrest the urges or motivations within his psyche which would weaken his determination and cause him to again become involved in the social world.

Arjuna sought to reject the opportunity for battle. After *Śrī* Krishna made it clear that He did not approve that option, Arjuna wanted to know what the preference. *Śrī* Krishna explained that Arjuna's only approved action was to reject the consequences which would come from taking the opportunity to fight, an opportunity forced on by the Central Figure of the Universal Form, Who is *Śrī* Krishna Himself.

Arjuna did not want to be in opposition to the Universal Form. Therefore he wanted to get a clearance from *Śrī* Krishna, such that he would not be liable for violent acts on the war field.

श्रीभगवानुवाच
काम्यानां कर्मणां न्यासं
संन्यासं कवयो विदुः ।
सर्वकर्मफलत्यागं
प्राहुस्त्यागं विचक्षणाः ॥ १८.२ ॥
śrībhagavānuvāca
kāmyānāṁ karmaṇāṁ nyāsaṁ
saṁnyāsaṁ kavayo viduḥ
sarvakarmaphalatyāgaṁ
prāhustyāgaṁ vicakṣaṇāḥ (18.2)

*śrī bhagavān — the Blessed Lord; uvāca — said; kāmyānāṁ — prompted by craving; karmaṇāṁ — of actions; nyāsaṁ — renunciation; saṁnyāsaṁ —rejection of opportunity; kavayo = kavayaḥ — authoritative speakers; viduḥ — know; sarvakarmaphalatyāgaṁ = sarva — all + karma — action + phala — benefit + tyāgaṁ — abandonment; prāhuḥ — they declare; tyāgaṁ — rejection of consequences; vicakṣaṇāḥ — the clear-sighted person*

**The Blessed Lord said: The authoritative speakers know the rejection of opportunity as renunciation of actions which are prompted by craving. The clear-sighted seers declare the abandonment of the results of benefit-motivated action as the rejection of consequences. (18.2)**

***Siddha Swami's Commentary:***

All actions in the material world are prompted by craving or at least they are sponsored or handled at some point by the craving force, *kāmyānām*. It is a question of whose craving. Is it the craving of the Universal Form? Or is it the craving of the limited selves who pretend that they have autonomy to act as they please?

Action has by its very nature, the passionate force as its content. This cannot be avoided. Thus the authoritative speakers state that the rejection of opportunities which are prompted by individual craving, is a form of *sannyāsa*. The other higher form of it is the rejection even of opportunities randomly assigned by the Universal Form but which an ascetic can safely ignore by virtue of an exemption from the Universal Lord.

A spiritual seeker understands this *Bhagavad Gītā* step by step, gradually, over a long period of time of study and application of *buddhi yoga*, not otherwise. At first he is only allowed to reject some consequences of his actions. And then as he progresses, he will get an exemption from *Śrī* Krishna. If Arjuna was unable to claim one, then we can understand and accept that it will be nearly impossible for anyone else to get such a waiver from cultural acts. The Supreme Being is very reluctant to release anyone from the cultural involvements, but rather He causes everyone to face the reacting energies in proportion to the person's previous participations in social affairs.

त्याज्यं दोषवदित्येके
कर्म प्राहुर्मनीषिणः ।
यज्ञदानतपःकर्म
न त्याज्यमिति चापरे ॥ १८.३ ॥
tyājyaṁ doṣavadityeke
karma prāhurmanīṣiṇaḥ
yajñadānatapaḥkarma
na tyājyamiti cāpare (18.3)

*tyājyaṁ — to be abandoned; doṣāvat — full of fault; iti — thus; eke — some; karma — action; prāhur = prāhuḥ — they declare; manīṣaṇaḥ — philosophers; yajñadānatapaḥkarma = yajña — sacrifice + dāna — charity + tapaḥ — austerity + karma — action; na — not; tyājyam — be abandoned; iti — thus; cāpare = ca — and + apare — others*

**Some philosophers declare that action is to be abandoned, since it is full of faults. Some others say that acts of sacrifice, charity and austerity are not to be abandoned. (18.3)**

***Siddha Swami's Commentary:***

Usually those philosophers who advocate abandonment of action, do so on the basis of tracing adverse consequences to actions. They presume that if one does not act, there would be no reaction forthcoming. They also surmise that good actions lead to bad actions eventually. Thus they say that all actions are potentially damaging, since no one can guarantee that a good action from the past will not produce the energy for a future bad action which rebounds on the performer as bad consequences.

Seeing the world as being essentially *doṣavat* or full of faults, they recommend an abandonment of action in this world. Contrary to these philosophers, others advocate acts of sacrifice, charity and austerity for the good of the world, for the sake of righteousness as they define it or as their scriptures legislate it.

निश्चयं श्रृणु मे तत्र
त्यागे भरतसत्तम ।
त्यागो हि पुरुषव्याघ्र
त्रिविधः संप्रकीर्तितः ॥ १८.४ ॥
niścayaṁ śṛṇu me tatra
tyāge bharatasattama
tyāgo hi puruṣavyāghra
trividhaḥ saṁprakīrtitaḥ (18.4)

*niścayaṁ — view; śṛṇu — hear; me — my; tatra — here, on this matter; tyāge — in the abandonment of consequences; bharatasattama — best of the Bharatas; tyāgo (tyāgaḥ) — abandonment of consequences; hi — indeed; puruṣavyāghra — tiger among men; trividhaḥ — three-fold; saṁprakīrtitaḥ — designated*

**Hear my view on this matter of abandonment of the consequences of action, O best of the Bharatas. The abandonment of consequences, O tiger among men, is designated as being threefold. (18.4)**

***Siddha Swami's Commentary:***

*Śrī* Krishna gave His view on the matter, an opinion that ranks highly if we regard Him as the Supreme Being. He stressed again and again that each type of endeavor and each type of confidence should be categorized according to the energy which comprises it. He listed three types of influences.

यज्ञदानतपःकर्म
न त्याज्यं कार्यमेव तत् ।
यज्ञो दानं तपश्चैव
पावनानि मनीषिणाम् ॥ १८.५ ॥
yajñadānatapaḥkarma
na tyājyaṁ kāryameva tat
yajño dānaṁ tapaścaiva
pāvanāni manīṣiṇām (18.5)

*yajñadānatapaḥkarma = yajña — sacrifice + dāna — charity + tapaḥ — austerity + karma — action; na — not; tyājyaṁ — to be abandoned; kāryam — to be performed; eva — indeed; tat = tad — this; yajño = yajñaḥ — sacrifice; dānaṁ — charity; tapaścaiva = tapaḥ — austerity + caiva — and indeed; pāvanāni — purificatory acts; manīṣiṇāṁ — for the wise men*

**Acts of sacrifice, charity, and austerity are not to be abandoned but should be performed. Sacrifice, charity and austerity are purificatory acts even for the wise men. (18.5)**

***Siddha Swami's Commentary:***

*Śrī* Krishna does not support the abandonment of acts of sacrifice, charity and austerity. He advocates those as purificatory even for the wise men. This is because no limited being is independent. There is an eternal social situation which requires some participation, no matter how little, by all others in the creation environments. In fact, even the Supreme Person feels obligated. He stated:

*na me pārthāsti kartavyaṁ triṣu lokeṣu kiṁcana*
*nānavāptamavāptavyaṁ varta eva ca karmaṇi (3.22)*
*yadi hyahaṁ na varteyaṁ jātu karmaṇyatandritaḥ*
*mama vartmānuvartante manuṣyāḥ pārtha sarvaśaḥ (3.23)*

***For Me, O son of Pṛthā, there is nothing specific that must be done in the three divisions of the universe. And there is nothing that I have not attained or should acquire, and yet I function in cultural activities.***

***If perchance, I did not perform attentively, then all human beings, O son of Pṛthā, would follow Me in all respects. (3.22-23)***

एतान्यपि तु कर्माणि
सङ्गं त्यक्त्वा फलानि च ।
कर्तव्यानीति मे पार्थ
निश्चितं मतमुत्तमम् ॥ १८.६ ॥
etānyapi tu karmāṇi
saṅgaṁ tyaktvā phalāni ca
kartavyānīti me pārtha
niścitaṁ matamuttamam (18.6)

*etāni — these; api — also; tu — but; karmāṇi — actions; saṅgaṁ — attachment; tyaktvā — giving up; phalāni — results; ca — and; kartvyānīti = kartvyāni — to be done + iti — thus; me — my; pārtha — O son of Pṛthā; niścitaṁ — definitely; matam — opinion; uttamam — highest*

**But these actions are to be performed by giving up attachment to results, O son of Pṛthā. This is definitely My highest opinion. (18.6)**

***Siddha Swami's Commentary:***

This is the basic requirement for those performing *karma yoga*. They must practice giving up attachment to the consequences of action. Actions are themselves binding because of the performer's attachment to the results. The actor feels a certain fulfillment or satisfaction in the results. In *brahma yoga*, the students are trained to orient the self to live without looking forward to consequences. In the time of Arjuna this training was given as part of *karma yoga*. More recently though, *karma yoga* is misunderstood. Thus many who come for *brahma yoga* practice must be trained in *karma yoga* before they can become student *brahma yogins*.

नियतस्य तु संन्यासः
कर्मणो नोपपद्यते ।
मोहात्तस्य परित्यागस्
तामसः परिकीर्तितः ॥१८.७॥
niyatasya tu saṁnyāsaḥ
karmaṇo nopapadyate
mohāttasya parityāgas
tāmasaḥ parikīrtitaḥ (18.7)

*niyatasya — of obligation; tu — but; saṁnyāsaḥ — renunciation; karmaṇo (karmaṇaḥ) — of action; nopapadyate = na — not + upapadyate — it is proper; mohāt — from delusion; tasya — of it; parityāgaḥ— rejection; tāmasaḥ — influence of depression; parikīrtitaḥ — is said to be*

**But renunciation of obligatory actions is not proper. The rejection of it on the basis of delusion, is said to occur by the influence of depression. (18.7)**

***Siddha Swami's Commentary:***

This is part of the answer to a question Arjuna asked before:

*arjuna uvāca*
*ye śāstravidhimutsṛjya yajante śraddhayānvitāḥ*
*teṣāṁ niṣṭhā tu kā kṛṣṇa sattvamāho rajastamaḥ (17.1)*

***Arjuna said: Concerning those who disregard scriptural injunction, but who with full confidence perform religiously-motivated ceremonies and austerities, what indeed, is their position, O Krishna? Is it clarity, impulsion or depression? (17.1)***

Obligatory actions, *niyatasya karmaṇo*, are those assigned by the Universal Form. However, people are normally trained to regard the obligations as what is recommended by parents, priests, and scripture. The normal way or traditional way is very faulty but it is functional in so far as human beings, even their leaders, are unable to decipher the supreme will. The scriptures are in place because most of the human leaders are unable to keep in contact with the Supreme Personality.

In all respects, a human being should try to stick to obligatory actions, either those recommended in scripture or those which are told by the Supreme Person or by His agent. It is a good habit to live by the ways of the scripture.

Generally, the rejection of the scriptural recommendations occurs under the influence of the lower modes of material nature, the depressing or dulling force. This force causes the consciousness not to perceive the most beneficial course. It inspires a way of life which leads downwards. Still, not all rejection of scriptural recommendations is faulty. Some of it is based on clarification about the proper interpretation of scriptural rules. Arjuna is an example of a person who was conversant with scriptural rules, as explained in Chapter One of this discourse. But Arjuna was misinterpreting these and *Śrī* Krishna provided him with the proper sense of priorities.

दुःखमित्येव यत्कर्म
कायक्लेशभयात्त्यजेत् ।
स कृत्वा राजसं त्यागं
नैव त्यागफलं लभेत् ॥१८.८॥

*duḥkham — difficult; ityeva = iti — thus + eva — indeed; yat = yad — which; karma — action; kāyakleśabhayāt = kāya — body + kleśa — suffering + bhayāt — from fear; tyajet— should abandon; sa =*

duḥkhamityeva yatkarma
kāyakleśabhayāttyajet
sa kṛtvā rājasaṁ tyāgaṁ
naiva tyāgaphalaṁ labhet (18.8)

*saḥ — he; kṛtvā — having performe;: rājasaṁ — impulsive influence; tyāgaṁ — renunciation; naiva = na — not + eva — indeed; tyāgaphalam — result of renunciation; labhet — should obtain*

**He who abandons action because of difficulty or because of a fear of bodily suffering, performs impulsive renunciation. He would not obtain the desired result of that renunciation. (18.8)**

***Siddha Swami's Commentary:***

For the purposes of *brahma yoga*, a student should learn from the teacher how to sort the various energies in the psyche. These must be traced to their subtle causes and then controlled. They must not be allowed to come into manifestation as random motivations. This all takes meticulous training in higher meditations.

Any type of motivation will cause a result. Thus a student is shown how to trace the psychological energy which drove him to act in a certain way. Once this is mastered, *brahma yoga* may begin in earnest. The question remains of how to get a certain result. The answer is this: Study the way of operation of the subtle energies and subtle equipments in the psyche.

कार्यमित्येव यत्कर्म
नियतं क्रियतेऽर्जुन ।
सङ्गं त्यक्त्वा फलं चैव
स त्यागः सात्त्विको मतः ॥१८.९॥
kāryamityeva yatkarma
niyataṁ kriyāte'rjuna
saṅgaṁ tyaktvā phalaṁ caiva
sa tyāgaḥ sāttviko mataḥ (18.9)

*káryam — to be done; ityeva = iti — thus + eva — indeed; yat — which; karma — action; niyataṁ — disciplinary manner; kriyāte — is performed; 'rjuna = arjuna — Arjuna; saṅgaṁ — attachment; tyaktvā — abandoning; phalaṁ — result; caiva — and indeed; sa = saḥ — it; tyāgaḥ — renunciation; sāttviko = sāttvikaḥ — of the clarifying mode; mataḥ — is considered*

**O Arjuna, when an action is done in a disciplinary manner, because it is to be performed, and with renunciation of the attachment to the results, it is considered to be in the clarifying mode. (18.9)**

***Siddha Swami's Commentary:***

This is an action which is assigned by the Universal Form. The actor does not have to know of the Universal Power; he or she may not be aware of the Supreme Lord. Still if the act was done in a disciplinary manner, because it should be performed and with renunciation of attachment to results, it will be accredited as being complimentary and supportive of the divine will. The actor will in fact become more and more compatible to *Śrī* Krishna, if he or she continues doing such acts in a detached mood.

न द्वेष्ट्यकुशलं कर्म
कुशले नानुषज्जते ।
त्यागी सत्त्वसमाविष्टो
मेधावी छिन्नसंशयः ॥१८.१०॥
na dveṣṭyakuśalaṁ karma
kuśale nānuṣajjate
tyāgī sattvasamāviṣṭo
medhāvī chinnasaṁśayaḥ (18.10)

*na — not; dveṣṭi — hates; akuśalaṁ — disagreeable; karma — action; kuśale — is agreeable; nānuṣajjate = na — not + anuśajjate — is attached; tyāgī — renouncer; sattvasamāviṣṭo = sattva — clarity + samāviṣṭo (samāviṣṭah) — filled with; medhāvi — wise man; chinnasaṁśayaḥ = chinna — removed + saṁśayaḥ — doubt*

**The renouncer who is filled with clarity, the wise man whose doubts are removed, does not hate disagreeable action, nor is he attached to agreeable performance. (18.10)**

***Siddha Swami's Commentary:***

The removed doubts are those concerning one's involvement and one's rights in this world. When one realizes in fact that one has no rights in this world and that this is the world created, monitored and ended by the Supreme Being for His own purposes, one no longer has any doubts about anything. Then one only has to look to the Supreme Person for instructions. When one loses a personal interest in the world, one can take up the mission of the Supreme Being and be a person who represents Him.

Disagreeable actions and agreeable performances are all irrelevant to the advanced *yogin* because he has no interest in this world. It is not his world. It is not his responsibility. It was not created for his pleasure. And it was not created just to aggravate him. Thus he becomes freed from prejudices.

न हि देहभृता शक्यं
त्यक्तुं कर्माण्यशेषतः ।
यस्तु कर्मफलत्यागी
स त्यागीत्यभिधीयते ॥१८.११॥
na hi dehabhṛtā śakyaṁ
tyaktuṁ karmāṇyaśeṣataḥ
yastu karmaphalatyāgī
sa tyāgītyabhidhīyate (18.11)

*na — not; hi — indeed; dehabhṛtā — by the body-supported; śakyaṁ — possible; tyaktuṁ — to abandon; karmāṇi — actions; aśeṣataḥ — completely; yaḥ—who; tu — but; karmaphalatyāgī = karma — action + phala — result + tyāgī — renouncer; sa = saḥ — he; tyāgīti = tyāgī — renunciate + iti — thus; abhidhīyate — is called*

**Indeed it is not possible for the body-supported beings to abandon actions completely. But whosoever is the renouncer of the results of actions is called a renunciate. (18.11)**

***Siddha Swami's Commentary:***

So long as one is not advanced enough to end the reliance on the material body and on subtle forms of the material energy, one cannot abandon actions. And one cannot gain from God an exemption for cultural activity because one does not qualify for it. One has to be very advanced in the *buddhi yoga, brahma yoga* practice, before the Supreme Person would even consider allowing one an exemption from cultural involvement.

Thus to be practical, one should practice to abandon the results of actions, especially the favorable ones to which one is helplessly addicted. In that way one may build up a resistance to the pleasures which are pursued by the subtle body.

अनिष्टमिष्टं मिश्रं च
त्रिविधं कर्मणः फलम् ।
भवत्यत्यागिनां प्रेत्य
न तु संन्यासिनां क्वचित् ॥१८.१२॥
aniṣṭamiṣṭaṁ miśraṁ ca
trividhaṁ karmaṇaḥ phalam
bhavatyatyāginām̐ pretya
na tu saṁnyāsināṁ kvacit (18.12)

*aniṣṭam — undesired; iṣṭaṁ — desired; miśraṁ — mixed; ca — and; trividham — three types; karmaṇaḥ — of action; phalam — result; bhavati — it is; atyāgināṁ — of those who do not renounce results; pretya — departing; na — not; tu — but; saṁnyāsināṁ — of the renouncers; kvacit — any at all*

**Undesired, desired and mixed are the three types of results of actions that occur for the departing souls who do not renounce results. But for the renouncers of opportunity, there is no result at all. (18.12)**

***Siddha Swami's Commentary:***

All intelligent human beings should ponder on the life they are currently enduring. They should realize that this life will come to an end for this body and the personality will have to move on to the hereafter. It is therefore a question of what sort of existence will be endured after being relinquished or permanently disconnected from the body.

Questions should be asked: Where will I be living after my person leaves this body? What sort of place will it be? Will it be as flimsy and uncertain as the subtle states I endured in dreams? Will I be able to reenter this world as an infant of a woman, just as I did in this life? Will I remember my past life or will I again enter and be in ignorance of any past identity?

Each spirit who leaves a body has accrued undesired, desired and mixed consequences which are due to that person, as dished out to him or her by the time factor. One cannot control how time will administer those results. One may get a desired result in the childhood of the next body and not be able to enjoy it fully in that state. Sometimes we see that a person, who developed a large, successful industrial enterprise, takes birth in the house of a wealthy man and lives in palatial buildings but due to the infant form, he cannot appreciate the opulence. Hence the time factor might reward a personality at a time when he or she cannot enjoy a particular result.

Sometimes when one looks for a benefit, when one is in need of something that one is qualified for by a past life, it is withheld by providence. Thus a *yogin,* after observing all such ups and downs of material existence, forms the conclusion that providence is not designed to serve any limited entity. This gives one the courage to abandon the part of one's nature which hankers for advantages.

Eventually after sufficient harassment by destiny and after being trained sufficiently by great yogins, one develops a nature that allows one to abandon opportunities. One loses the taste to exploit opportunities but one also realizes that it is necessary, in fact mandatory, that one serve in the world at the behest of the Supreme Personality. *I may not want to act on my own but I know that if God wants to act, that is His prerogative. And if God wants me to act on His behalf then He has every right to command me. It is His opportunity, not mine. I am nothing but His servant. I do not have the right to refuse His commands.*

When one assumes that mood consistently, no results come to one, because the results cannot cling to someone who lost the exploitive mentality. But still a devotee may be required to take opportunities as an agent of the Supreme Being, as commanded by providence or as inspired from within by God.

In advancing from being a *tyāgi* to being a *sannyāsi*, one must first become expert at abandoning the results of actions. Then one must take on a mood to give up the need for opportunities. In the advanced stage one must realize that the opportunities are God's opportunities. Thus there is no need to give them up. One instead sheds the false sense of identity which causes one to confiscate or to attempt to take what belongs to the Supreme Being. Once this is done, one can then be free to serve the Supreme Person if He requires.

It is a matter of proprietorship. In this world, one assumes that one may take possession of animate and inanimate parts of this creation. One does not take into account the Supreme Person Who is in fact the only proprietor. Thus one works to derive a profit. From such a profit, one might offer something in charity and become known as a good man.

Nature encourages this by giving one a good reputation and by causing the formulation of piety energies in one's aura. Thus one takes to being a *tyāgi* or a person who works for profit and who donates some of the benefit to others who are not as proficient or skilled at exploitation as oneself. Later one begins to understand that the opportunities presented by nature for exploitation are full of peril and disaster. They are all risky. Thus one becomes attracted to the idea of abandoning the opportunities altogether. When one masters this, then one sees that this creation was never really an available world. It was always under the control of the Supreme Person. It was always His property only. At all stages, one made attempts at theft. This is why one got adverse consequences no matter how well one conducted an activity or no matter how much piety one accrued by giving in charity.

But then something else comes to mind, regarding one's identity. Is the self a commodity of the Supreme Being? Should the self be a servant of the Supreme Being? Is the self under the control of the Supreme Person? Is there any possibility of independence from the control of the Supreme Person? Of course, the answer is that the self is a commodity of the Supreme Person, and independence is a sure figment of imagination. When this is realized, one truly becomes a surrendered soul.

पञ्चैतानि महाबाहो
कारणानि निबोध मे ।
सांख्ये कृतान्ते प्रोक्तानि
सिद्धये सर्वकर्मणाम् ॥१८.१३॥
pañcaitāni mahābāho
kāraṇāni nibodha me
sāṁkhye kṛtānte proktāni
siddhaye sarvakarmaṇām (18.13)

*pañcaitāni = pañca — five + tāni — these; mahābāho — O mighty-armed man; kāraṇāni — factors; nibodha — learn; me — from me; sāṁkhye — in Sāṁkhya philosophy; krtānte — in conclusion, in doctrīne; proktāni — declared; siddhaye — in accomplishment; sarvakarmaṇām — of all actions*

**Learn from Me, O mighty-armed man, of the five factors declared in the Sāṁkhya doctrine for the accomplishment of all actions: (18.13)**

***Siddha Swami's Commentary:***

It is important to take lessons from the senior yogins, even from those who departed this world long, long ago. All the great yogis who left are either currently taking bodies again, or they have gone to higher or lower worlds. They are still in existence. Hence we may still learn from them, either from their writings or from their inspirations, which may enter our psyche as we qualify for the instructions.

What was already mapped out, need not be mapped again, unless the instructor was faulty. In so far as the ancient teachers spoke truthfully and accurately, we need not create separate ideas. But we should realize the truths which they expounded.

अधिष्ठानं तथा कर्ता
करणं च पृथग्विधम् ।
विविधाश्च पृथक्चेष्टा
दैवं चैवात्र पञ्चमम् ॥१८.१४॥

*adhiṣṭhānaṁ — location; tathā — as well as; kartā — the agent; karaṇaṁ — the instrument; ca — and; prthagvidham — various kinds; vividhāśca = vividhāḥ — various + ca — and; pṛthakceṣṭa —*

adhiṣṭhānaṁ tathā kartā
karaṇaṁ ca pṛthagvidham
vividhāśca pṛthakceṣṭā
daivaṁ caivātra pañcama (18.14)

*movements; daivam — destiny; caivātra = ca — and + eva — indeed + atra — here in this case; pañcamam — the fifth*

**The location, the agent, the various instruments, the various movements, and destiny, the fifth factor. (18.14)**

***Siddha Swami's Commentary:***

For the purpose of *brahma yoga*, these five factors are within the psyche. These should be regarded and dealt with in reference to their effects within the psyche of the *yogin* as follows:

*Adhiṣṭhānam* or the **location** is the subtle and causal bodies. For *brahma yogins*, the location is not physical but it is so for others, even for *karma* yogins. In the case of Arjuna, it was a physical location, *Kurukṣetra*, a place in India. But for the *brahma yogi*ns, the advanced *buddhi yogins*, *jñāna yogins*, there is no concern with physical locations. We are concerned with the subtle and causal bodies.

*Kartā* or the **agent** in this case is the attentive energy of the self. This attentive energy is the factor which sanctions the promptings of the subtle energies and causes them to be developed into subtle and then physical actions. This attentive energy is known as *ahankāra* which is sometimes translated into other languages to mean false ego. It is the sense of identity in material nature. Unless this sense of identity is restricted in its involvement with the subtle body, there can be no effective control of that form.

Some argue that the agent is the spirit itself and not its attention merely. This argument does not hold for the purposes of *brahma yoga*, because the attention is to an extent, a power unto itself. Student yogins struggle to control this independent attention which operates automatically as it is prompted by the organs in the subtle body and by the *citta* energy in the causal form. The sensitivity of the attention needs to be curbed. For now it is too sensitive to the organs of the subtle body and to the memories. Hence it is a botheration.

*Karaṇam*, the **various instruments**, are the organs in the subtle body, which are the intellect, the mind chamber with its sensitivity, the senses which emit from the mind chamber, the imagination orb which is a technical part of the intellect, and the memory which is the linking point between the subtle and causal forms.

At the point where the subtle body connects to the causal form, there is a nexus junction which is the mouth to the subtle body. This is experienced as the memory in the psychic domain. Unless these instruments are curbed from their impulsive operations, there cannot be success in the spiritual quest. *Śrī Patañjali* alerted us to this as follows:

*yogaḥ cittavṛtti nirodhaḥ*

***The skill of yoga is demonstrated by the conscious non-operation of the vibrational modes of the mento-emotional energy. (Yoga Sūtra, 1.2)***

*Pṛthakceṣṭā* or the **various movements** are the exchanges between the energies and instruments in the psyche. In higher yoga, the student must know when the memory passes information to the *buddhi* organ's imagination faculty. He must note how the imagination faculty converts that energy of memory into pictures and sounds for consideration by the analytical faculty. He must understand how the senses pass information to the intellect and how the attention is influenced helplessly to endorse these psychological movements.

*Daivam* or **destiny** is observed in higher yoga as the mandatory forces in the psychic environment which the *yogin* cannot adjust and which can force him to act impulsively. As he advances he gets these forces under control. His problem is not the external environment. It is the internal psychic energy which he struggles to regulate during meditation.

शरीरवाङ्मनोभिर्यत्
कर्म प्रारभते नरः ।
न्याय्यं वा विपरीतं वा
पञ्चैते तस्य हेतवः ॥१८.१५॥
śarīravāṅmanobhiryat
karma prārabhate naraḥ
nyāyyaṁ vā viparītaṁ vā
pañcaite tasya hetavaḥ (18.15)

*śarīravāṅmanobhiḥ = śarīra — body + vān(vās) — speech + manobhiḥ — with mind; yat = yad — whatever; karma — project; prārabhate — he undertakes; naraḥ — a human being; nyāyyaṁ — moral; vā — or; viparītam — immoral; vā — or; pañcaite = pañca — five + ete — these; tasya — of it; hetavaḥ — factors*

**As for whatever project a human being undertakes with body, speech and mind, regardless of it being moral or immoral, these are its five factors. (18.15)**

***Siddha Swami's Commentary:***

No matter what a person does in this world, he must be using psychological equipments and mostly he does so by impulsion. If however he stops and takes up the practice of *buddhi yoga*, there is a chance for psyche control. Mastery of the five factors within is the key to liberation from the impulsive nature.

तत्रैवं सति कर्तारम्
आत्मानं केवलं तु यः ।
पश्यत्यकृतबुद्धित्वान्
न स पश्यति दुर्मतिः ॥१८.१६॥
tatraivaṁ sati kartāram
ātmānaṁ kevalaṁ tu yaḥ
paśyatyakṛtabuddhitvān
na sa paśyati durmatiḥ (18.16)

*tatraivaṁ = tatra — here, in this case + evam — thus; sati — in reality, correctly; kartāram — agent; ātmānaṁ — self; kevalam — only; tu — but; yaḥ — who; paśyati — he regards; akṛtabuddhitvāt = akṛta — undone, defective + buddhitvāt — due to intellect; na — not; sa = saḥ — he; paśyati — he perceives; durmatiḥ — idiot*

**In that case, whosoever regards himself as the only agent, does not perceive correctly. This is due to the defective intellect of the idiot. (18.16)**

***Siddha Swami's Commentary:***

Anyone who regards himself as the only agent is a lunatic. Unfortunately most limited entities in this world are in that category. It is by mastership of *buddhi yoga*, that one is freed from being a mad man or mad woman. All limited entities who have not mastered their psyches, possess defective intellects which are incapable of perceiving truth; hence *buddhi yoga* is needed to adjust the intellect.

यस्य नाहंकृतो भावो
बुद्धिर्यस्य न लिप्यते ।
हत्वापि स इमाँल्लोकान्
न हन्ति न निबध्यते ॥१८.१७॥
yasya nāhaṁkṛto bhāvo
buddhiryasya na lipyate
hatvāpi sa imām̐llokān
na hanti na nibadhyate (18.17)

*yasya — regarding who; nā'haṁkṛto = na — not + ahaṁkṛto (ahaṁkṛtaḥ) — falsely assertive; bhāvaḥ — attitude: buddhiḥ— intellect; yasya — of whom; na — not; lipyate — is clouded; hatvā — having slain + api — even; sa = saḥ — he; imān — these; lokān — people; na — not; hanti — he slays; na — not; nibadhyate — is implicated*

**Regarding the person whose attitude is not falsely assertive, whose intellect is not clouded, even after slaying these people, he would not slay or be implicated. (18.17)**

***Siddha Swami's Commentary:***

This is possible for a person who mastered *buddhi yoga*, whose psychology no longer operates in the impulsive way.

ज्ञानं ज्ञेयं परिज्ञाता
त्रिविधा कर्मचोदना ।
करणं कर्म कर्तेति
त्रिविधः कर्मसंग्रहः ॥१८.१८॥
jñānaṁ jñeyaṁ parijñātā
trividhā karmacodanā
karaṇaṁ karma karteti
trividhaḥ karmasaṁgrahaḥ (18.18)

*jñānaṁ — experience; jñeyaṁ — the item of research; parijñātā — the experience; trividhā — three aspects; karmacodanā = karma — action + codanā — impetus for; karaṇaṁ — instrument; karma — action; karteti = kartā — agent + iti — thus; trividhaḥ — three; karmasaṁgrahaḥ = karma — action + saṁgrahaḥ — parts*

**Experience, the item of research, and the experiencer are the three aspects which serve as the impetus for action. The instrument, the action itself, and the agent are three parts of an action. (18.18)**

***Siddha Swami's Commentary:***

For *brahma yogins*, these are psychological equations, which are understood on the psychic plane during meditation. The experience is a psychic energy which comes into the psychology after contacting other psychic phenomena. The real interest is the need for experience. What is the need-energy? Where is it in the psyche? How can it be controlled? Can it be curbed at all? Why is it that even after having a certain experience and after forming definite conclusions about it, one is again forced to go through the same experience and form the same conclusions about it again and again? Where does the need-energy originate? Does it come out of the causal body or the subtle body? If it comes from the causal form, how is it transferred into the subtle body?

What is the item of research? Is that something psychic? How far is it from the self? Is it a variety of the same type of energy of which the psychology consists? Who is the experiencer? Or what is the experiencer? Where is the spirit located? Is the attention the controller of both the spirit from which it emanates and the psychic equipments which prompts it to give energy for mental and emotional operations?

*Śrī* Krishna listed the experience, the item of research and the experiencer as the aspects which serve as impetus. The control of these would give the person involved more control over his or her actions in the gross or subtle environments.

Within the psyche, the instrument which is the *buddhi* intellect organ, as well as the action it takes and the attention of the spirit or the spirit's interest are the three factors which work in joint operation to produce a psychic action, which is followed by a physical action or by an action which stops other actions. These factors must be studied in meditation during *buddhi yoga* practice.

ज्ञानं कर्म च कर्ता च
त्रिधैव गुणभेदतः ।
प्रोच्यते गुणसंख्याने
यथावच्छृणु तान्यपि ॥१८.१९॥

*jñānaṁ — experience; karma — action; ca — and; kartā — agent; ca — and; tridhaiva = tridha — three types + eva — indeed; guṇabhedataḥ — categorized by the influences of material nature; procyate — is stated; guṇasaṁkhyāne — in the*

jñānaṁ karma ca kartā ca
tridhaiva guṇabhedataḥ
procyate guṇasaṁkhyāne
yathāvacchṛṇu tānyapi (18.19)

*Sāṁkhya analysis of the influences of material nature; yathāvat — correctly; śṛṇu — hear; tāni — these; api — as well*

**In the Sāṁkhya analysis of the influence of material nature, it is stated that experience, action, and the agent are of three types as categorized by the influence of material nature. Hear correctly of these as well. (18.19)**

***Siddha Swami's Commentary:***

Essentially the student *yogin* has to study his psychology. He must carefully sort the various influences, knowing how to recognize each of them and how to situate himself quickly in the highest one. If this is not achieved, higher yoga will never be within reach.

The experiential energy in the psyche is the sensuous force through which all sensing is conducted. If this is in a lower mode, one will form incorrect opinions about objects. The actions are motivated by pranic or psychic force. If these forces are in the lower modes, the actions themselves will be faulty and will bring adverse consequences to the performer. The performer is for the most part the agent's sense of identity while functioning through the intellect. If this joint operation is under the lower modes, then whatever is done will be faulty and will implicate the personality.

सर्वभूतेषु येनैकं
भावमव्ययमीक्षते ।
अविभक्तं विभक्तेषु
तज्ज्ञानं विद्धि सात्त्विकम् ॥ १८.२० ॥
sarvabhūteṣu yenaikaṁ
bhāvamavyayamīkṣate
avibhaktaṁ vibhakteṣu
tajjñānaṁ viddhi sāttvikam (18.20)

*sarvabhūteṣu — in all beings; yenaikaṁ = yena — by which + ekam — one; bhāvam — being; avyayam — imperishable; īksate — one perceives; avibhaktaṁ — undivided; vibhakteṣu — in the divided; tat — that; jñānaṁ — experience; viddhi — know; sāttvikaṁ — clarifying*

**That experience by which one perceives one imperishable being in all beings, undivided in the divided, know it to be an experience in clarity. (18.20)**

***Siddha Swami's Commentary:***

In *brahma yoga* practice, this experience occurs at the tail end of one's austerities, when one understands that the limited self is merely a reflection of the Supreme Being and nothing else. In the material world, the limited self may be regarded as paramount or most essential, but in reference to the spiritual reality at large, the limited self is just a minute reflection.

When a mirror is used to reflect sunlight into a cave, the residents of the cave may very well regard that reflected light as very important. Being over-powered and distressed by the darkness, any bit of light no matter how small assumes importance. The fact is, however, that in reference to the sun, the reflected light is insignificant.

In the psychological darkness of the psyche, the limited self serves as a power source, but in terms of the Supreme Being, that self is insignificant. Thus *Śrī* Krishna explained that there is one imperishable being in all the psyches, undivided in the divided, transcending the limited unique reflections of self which came to be known as the *jīva*. One should realize this in higher meditation.

पृथक्त्वेन तु यज्ज्ञानं
नानाभावान्पृथग्विधान् ।
वेत्ति सर्वेषु भूतेषु
तज्ज्ञानं विद्धि राजसम् ॥१८.२१॥
pṛthaktvena tu yajjñānaṁ
nānābhāvānpṛthagvidhān
vetti sarveṣu bhūteṣu
tajjñānaṁ viddhi rājasam (18.21)

*pṛthaktvena — with difference; tu — but; yat — which; jñānaṁ — experience; nānābhāvān = nānā — different + bhāvān — beings; pṛthagvidhān — of different kinds: vetti — realizes; sarveṣu — in all; bhūteṣu — in beings; tat — that; jñānaṁ — experience; viddhi — know; rājasam — of the impulsive mode*

**But that experience by which one realizes different beings of different kinds with differences in all beings, should be known as experience in the impulsive mode. (18.21)**

***Siddha Swami's Commentary:***

Thus the human perspective is in the mode of passion, the impulsive mode. It is deluding and causes one to feel essential and important. It sponsors a lack of research into the Absolute Truth.

यत्तु कृत्स्नवदेकस्मिन्
कार्ये सक्तमहैतुकम् ।
अतत्त्वार्थवदल्पं च
तत्तामसमुदाहृतम् ॥१८.२२॥
yattu kṛtsnavadekasmin
kārye saktamahaitukam
atattvārthavadalpaṁ ca
tattāmasamudāhṛtam (18.22)

*yat = yad — which; tu — but; kṛtsnavat — appears as the whole; ekasmin — in one; kārye — in order of action; saktam — attached; ahaitukam — without due cause; atattvārthavat — without a valid purpose; alpaṁ — petty; ca — and; tat = tad — that; tāmasam — of the depressive influence; udāhṛtam — is said to be*

**But that experience which appears to be the whole vision, being attached to one procedure without due cause, without a valid purpose, being petty, that is said to be of the depressive influence. (18.22)**

***Siddha Swami's Commentary:***

When one only sees one's own perspective and does not accommodate any other, especially when one is unaware of the other psyches and of the all-pervading influence of the Supreme Being, one is under the depressive influence. A student should research this to understand how he or she can be shifted into or under the various influences.

नियतं सङ्गरहितम्
अरागद्वेषतः कृतम् ।
अफलप्रेप्सुना कर्म
यत्तत्सात्त्विकमुच्यते ॥१८.२३॥
niyataṁ saṅgarahitam
arāgadveṣataḥ kṛtam
aphalaprepsunā karma
yattatsāttvikamucyate (18.23)

*niyatam — controlled; saṅgarahitam = saṅga— attachment + rahitam — free from; arāgadveṣataḥ — without craving or repulsion; kṛtam — performed; aphalaprepsunā = aphala — without result + prepsunā — desire to get; karma — action; yat = yad — which; tat = tad — such; sāttvikaṁ — of the clarifying influence; ucyate — is said*

**Action which is controlled, which is free from attachment, which is performed without craving or repulsion, without desire for results, such action is said to be of the clarifying influence. (18.23)**

***Siddha Swami's Commentary:***

This type of action, having two aspects, an internal and external display, is based on an internal attitude of detachment with clarity as to the various influences which affect the psyche. When the promptings in the nature are properly regulated, and when the energies which motivate the subtle equipments are in the clarifying mode, then one may act being free from attachment, without craving or repulsion and without desire for results.

यत्तु कामेप्सुना कर्म
साहंकारेण वा पुनः ।
क्रियते बहुलायासं
तद्राजसमुदाहृतम् ॥१८.२४॥
yattu kāmepsunā karma
sāhaṁkāreṇa vā punaḥ
kriyāte bahulāyāsaṁ
tadrājasamudāhṛtam (18.24)

*yat = yad — which; tu — but; kāmepsunā = kāma — craving + ipsunā — desiring to get; karma — action; sāhaṁkāreṇa — with false assertion; vā — or; punaḥ = punar — alternatively; kriyāte — is performed; bahulāyāsaṁ = bahula — much + āyāsaṁ effort; tat — that; rājasam — of the impulsive influence; udāhṛtam — is said to be*

**But that action which is performed with a wish for cravings, with false assertion or alternately with much effort, that is said to be of the impulsive influence. (18.24)**

***Siddha Swami's Commentary:***

Such actions are done with impure motivating forces from within. These energies are to be cleansed or removed from the psyche through kundalini yoga. Then one should master *buddhi yoga* to gain power to compel the psyche to remain in the clarifying energy. A vigorous effort in kundalini yoga practice pays off when the kundalini chakra becomes cleaned out, when full celibacy is achieved so that the seminal fluid moves upward naturally and the subtle seminal gases move into the head going towards the *brahmarandra* crown chakra. Mastership of kundalini yoga is vital as a preliminary step.

अनुबन्धं क्षयं हिंसाम्
अनपेक्ष्य च पौरुषम् ।
मोहादारभ्यते कर्म
यत्तत्तामसमुच्यते ॥१८.२५॥
anubandhaṁ kṣayaṁ hiṁsām
anapekṣya ca pauruṣam
mohādārabhyate karma
yattattāmasamucyate (18.25)

*anubandhaṁ — consequence; kṣayaṁ— damage; hiṁsām — violence; anapekṣya — regardless of; ca — and; pauruṣam — practical power; mohāt — from misconception; ārabhyate — is undertaken; karma — action; yat — which; tat — that; tāmasam — of the depressive mode; ucyate — is said to be*

**That action which is undertaken from a misconception, regardless of the consequence, the damage and the violence, and without considering one's practical power, is said to be of the depressive mode. (18.25)**

***Siddha Swami's Commentary:***

There is nothing as sure for ruination as the over-estimation of one's practical power, *pauruṣam*. This misconception may be removed by a careful study of the psychology in *brahma yoga* practice. Under the dulling influence of subtle material nature, a person forms the wrong view of the limited self and feels that he or she is the all in all.

The limited self is great but there are so many of them that it is safe to say that they are countless. But beyond these selves is the Supreme Being, Who is truly great. All of this should be realized by mystic perception in higher yoga.

मुक्तसङ्गोऽनहंवादी
धृत्युत्साहसमन्वितः ।
सिद्ध्यसिद्ध्योर्निर्विकारः
कर्ता सात्त्विक उच्यते ॥१८.२६॥
muktasaṅgo'nahaṁvādī
dhṛtyutsāhasamanvitaḥ
siddhyasiddhyornirvikāraḥ
kartā sāttvika ucyate (18.26)

*muktasaṅgo = muktasaṅgaḥ — freed from attachment; 'nahaṁvādi = anahaṁvādi — free from self praise, free from vanity; dhṛtyutsāhasamanvitaḥ = dhṛty (dhṛti) — consistence + utsāha — perseverance + samanvitaḥ — possessed with; siddhyasiddhyoḥ — in success or failure; nirvikāraḥ — unaffected; kartā — performer; sāttvika — in the clarifying mode; ucyate — is rated to be*

**A performer who is free from attachment, free from vanity, who is consistent and perseverant, and who is unaffected in success or failure, is rated to be in the clarifying mode. (18.26)**

***Siddha Swami's Commentary:***

The energy of the limited self, though being emitted since time immemorial and though a power in its own right, is very limited. In higher meditations, one should assess one's power and come to one's senses about one's relevance.

In the end, one will see that one is not that essential. Of course the limited spirit, as limited as he or she may be, is still eternal, at least in reference to material nature, in reference to the subtle and causal bodies which it uses currently. But still there is a higher power, the Supreme Being, Who is the essential reality.

रागी कर्मफलप्रेप्सुर्
लुब्धो हिंसात्मकोऽशुचिः ।
हर्षशोकान्वितः कर्ता
राजसः परिकीर्तितः ॥१८.२७॥
rāgī karmaphalaprepsur
lubdho hiṁsātmako'śuciḥ
harṣaśokānvitaḥ kartā
rājasaḥ parikīrtitaḥ (18.27)

*rāgī — prone to impulsiveness; karmaphalaprepsuḥ = karma — action + phala — result + prepsuḥ — craving; lubdho = lubdhaḥ — greedy; hiṁsātmako hiṁsātmakaḥ — violent nature; 'śuciḥ = aśuciḥ — unclean; harṣaśokānvitaḥ = harṣa — joy + śoka — sorrow + anvitaḥ — prone to; kartā — performer; rājasaḥ — of the impulsive mode; parikīrtitaḥ — is declared*

**A performer who is prone to impulsiveness, who craves the results of action, who is greedy, violent by nature, unclean and who is prone to joy or sorrow, is declared to be under the impulsive mode. (18.27)**

***Siddha Swami's Commentary:***

First of all the unity of the psyche which permits someone to mistake him or herself for the psychic equipments in the subtle body, must be eradicated. This is done by a careful study of the parts of the psychology in *buddhi yoga* practice. One has to sort oneself from one's attention powers. The attention must be sorted from the intellect; the intellect from the senses. The memory must be sorted from the imagination or conceptualization faculty. And that is just the preliminary course.

When a limited entity feels that he or she is one personality, comprised of memory, intellectual powers, sensual powers, will power and physical potency, then he or she is in illusion, being influenced by the impressive and depressive modes of material nature. But these impressive and depressive modes are actually types of enticing subtle energies. They are to be recognized for what they really are.

अयुक्तः प्राकृतः स्तब्धः
शठो नैष्कृतिकोऽलसः ।
विषादी दीर्घसूत्री च
कर्ता तामस उच्यते ॥ १८.२८॥
ayuktaḥ prākṛtaḥ stabdhaḥ
śaṭho naiṣkṛtiko'lasaḥ
viṣādī dīrghasūtrī ca
kartā tāmasa ucyate (18.28)

*ayuktaḥ — undisciplined; prākṛtaḥ — vulgar; stabdhaḥ — stubborn; śaṭho = śaṭhaḥ — wicked; naiṣkṛtiko = naiṣkṛtikaḥ — deceitful; 'lasaḥ = alasaḥ — lazy; viṣādī — depressed; dīrghasūtrī — neglectful; ca — and; kartā — performer; tāmasa — in the depressive mood; ucyate — is said to be*

**A performer who is undisciplined, vulgar, stubborn, wicked, deceitful, lazy, depressed and neglectful, is said to be in the depressive mode. (18.28)**

***Siddha Swami's Commentary:***

It is important to understand that when the *Gītā* is regarded from the perspective of *brahma yoga*, it is used as a treatise on the psychology of the individual soul. Indiscipline, vulgarity, stubbornness, wicked tendency, deceitfulness, laziness, depression and neglectfulness are types of psychological energy. The *brahma yogi* is concerned to remove these by restricting his psyche from their energy intakes. In traditional religion, an attempt is made to remove these by changing habits. In *brahma yoga*, the method is to remove these energies from the psyche and replace them with energies from the highest mode. That is the difference in approach between *brahma yoga* and traditional religious methods.

बुद्धेर्भेदं धृतेश्चैव
गुणतस्त्रिविधं शृणु ।
प्रोच्यमानमशेषेण
पृथक्त्वेन धनंजय ॥ १८.२९॥
buddherbhedaṁ dhṛteścaiva
guṇatastrividhaṁ śṛṇu
procyamānamaśeṣeṇa
pṛthaktvena dhanaṁjaya (18.29)

*buddheḥ — intellect; bhedaṁ — difference; dhṛteḥ — determination; caiva — and indeed; guṇataḥ — according to the influences of material nature; trividham — three types; śṛṇu — hear; procyamānam — explained; aśeṣena — thoroughly; pṛthaktvena — distinctly; dhanaṁjaya — a conqueror of wealthy countries*

**Now, O conqueror of wealthy countries, hear of the three types of intellect and also of determination, explained thoroughly and distinctly, according to their distinctions under the influences of material nature. (18.29)**

***Siddha Swami's Commentary:***

While in traditional religion this knowledge is sufficient and one hopes for the day when one would permanently move into the higher mode and then into the divine consciousness, in *brahma yoga* the student is required to begin working in the psyche for those changes. The student personally learns how to control his or her own psyche. It is not done by God or by the spiritual teacher. The teacher shows how, explains how and sometimes even enters into the psyche of the student to show in detail how the controlling should be executed but the student must achieve this.

Some devotees of Krishna feel satisfied with this information, which to them was provided by *Śrī* Krishna to save the devotees from having to do painstaking and very uncertain mystic research in higher yoga. They study *Bhagavad Gītā* very meticulously and learn how to explain this to others. Even though they have not experienced this in higher yoga, they take it upon themselves to broadcast this to the entire world, feeling that they do *Śrī* Krishna a great service while saving humanity in the process.

However for the purpose of *brahma yoga*, a student should not become a preacher. His mission should be to practice higher yoga, to realize all this by direct mystic perception. He may, if *Śrī* Krishna empowers him to be a guru, take up the services of teaching after he completes the *buddhi yoga* course as described in the *Gītā*.

प्रवृत्तिं च निवृत्तिं च
कार्याकार्ये भयाभये ।
बन्धं मोक्षं च या वेत्ति
बुद्धिः सा पार्थ सात्त्विकी ॥१८.३०॥
pravṛttiṁ ca nivṛttiṁ ca
kāryākārye bhayābhaye
bandhaṁ mokṣaṁ ca yā vetti
buddhiḥ sā pārtha sāttvikī (18.30)

*pravṛttiṁ — endeavor; ca — and; nivṛttiṁ — non-endeavor; ca — and; kāryākārye = kārya — what should be done + akārya — what should not be done; bhayābhaye — what is dangerous and what is safe; bandhaṁ — restriction; mokṣaṁ — freedom; ca — and; yā — which; vetti — discerns; buddhiḥ — intellectual insight; sā — if, partha — son of Pṛthā; sāttvikī — in the clarifying mode*

**That intellectual insight which discerns when to endeavor and when not to strive, what should be done and what should not be done, what is dangerous and what is safe, what brings restrictions and what gives freedom, that O son of Pṛthā, is in the clarifying mode. (18.30)**

***Siddha Swami's Commentary:***

Intellectual insight is a big item on the list of accomplishments for *brahma yogins*. It has to do with objectively finding the intellectual organ in the head of the subtle body. Once located, one should purify that organ by changing the energy which strikes it and the energy which empowers it. This is mystic yoga practice.

यया धर्ममधर्मं च
कार्यं चाकार्यमेव च ।
अयथावत्प्रजानाति
बुद्धिः सा पार्थ राजसी ॥१८.३१॥
yayā dharmamadharmaṁ ca
kāryaṁ cākāryameva ca
ayathāvatprajānāti
buddhiḥ sā pārtha rājasī (18.31)

*yayā — by which; dharmam — right; adharmaṁ — wrong; ca — and; kāryam — duty; cākāryam = ca — and + akāryam — neglect; eva — indeed; ca — and; ayathāvat — mistakenly; prajānāti — is identified; buddhiḥ — intellectual insight; sā — it; pārtha — son of Pṛthā; rājasī — in the impulsive mode*

**That intellectual insight by which right and wrong, duty and neglect are mistakenly identified, is, O son of Pṛthā, in the impulsive mode. (18.31)**

***Siddha Swami's Commentary:***

The intellect is an organ in the subtle body. That particular tool cannot be changed for another. A limited spirit remains with the same intellect organ throughout the duration of the creative cycle. Hence it is a matter of changing the inner workings of the organ, particularly of changing the type of energy which powers the organ. This is taught in *brahma yoga*, which is different to conventional religion.

अधर्मं धर्ममिति या
मन्यते तमसावृता ।
सर्वार्थान्विपरीतांश्च
बुद्धिः सा पार्थ तामसी ॥१८.३२॥
adharmaṁ dharmamiti yā
manyate tamasāvṛtā
sarvārthānviparītāṁśca
buddhiḥ sā pārtha tāmasī (18.32)

*adharmaṁ — wrong method; dharmam — right method; iti — thus; yā — which; manyate — it considered; tamasāvṛtā = tamasa — ignorance + āvṛtā — absorbed by; sarvārthān — all values; viparītāṁśca = viparītān — perverted + ca — and; buddhiḥ — intellectual insight; sā — it; pārtha — son of Pṛthā; tāmasī — in the depressive mode*

**That intellectual insight which is absorbed by ignorance, which considers the wrong method as the right one and perceives all values in a perverted way, is O son of Pṛthā, of the depressive mode. (18.32)**

***Siddha Swami's Commentary:***

The depressive influence is perceived plainly when the body is drowsy or intoxicated under alcohol or any other depressive drug. It is perceived in its maximum influence when someone falls into a coma, whereby they cannot move any limb of the body, or be aware of any intellectual or perceptive functions.

Appropriate sleep is a positive use of the depressive mode. Tiredness is a positive signal from the depressive energy for the body to go into a state of rest. Even the astral bodies rest, because they too become tired and need rejuvenation. After the death of a body, a priest may wish that the departed soul should rest in peace. This refers to the resting of the subtle body which becomes tired after a lifetime in union with a gross form. Thus the depressive mood has usefulness. However, if it is allowed to function beyond that capacity, it hampers the vision of the spirit.

धृत्या यया धारयते
मनःप्राणेन्द्रियक्रियाः ।
योगेनाव्यभिचारिण्या
धृतिः सा पार्थ सात्त्विकी ॥१८.३३॥
dhṛtyā yayā dhārayate
manaḥprāṇendriyakriyāḥ
yogenāvyabhicāriṇyā
dhṛtiḥ sā pārtha sāttvikī (18.33)

*dhṛtyā — by determination; yayā — by which; dhārayate — it holds; manaḥprāṇendriyakriyāḥ = manaḥ — mind + prāṇa — energizing breath + indriyakriyāḥ — senses; yogenāvyabhicāriṇyā = yogena — by yoga practices + avyabhicāriṇyā — unwavering, constant; dhṛtiḥ — determination; sā — it; pārtha — son of Pṛthā; sāttvikī — of the clarifying influence*

**The determination which holds the mind, the energizing breath, and the senses by constant yoga expertise, that O son of Pṛthā, is of the clarifying influence. (18.33)**

***Siddha Swami's Commentary:***

There is much evidence that *Śrī* Krishna propagated the *buddhi yoga* techniques as the main hub of the *Bhagavad Gītā*. This is proven by a careful study of the Sanskrit terms and by Krishna's frequent use of the term yoga.

For the determination to be realistic, one must express it in a way that is acceptable to material nature. In each of the modes of nature, there are different conditions of operation or ways in which a particular aspect may be achieved. This verse should be translated as follows:

**The determination which holds the mind, the energizing energy, and the senses by constant yoga expertise, that O son of Pṛthā, is of the clarifying influence.**

*Prāṇa* in this verse is the energizing energy on the subtle plane. It is not merely the energizing breath. There is a relationship between breath and the energizing energy. The breath is one of the components of that energy.

It is by *buddhi yoga* practice, and that alone, that one develops the determination to hold the mind, the pranic energy and the senses in check, so that one can proceed with an objective without having distractions. The energy taken in by the mind determines how often the mind will focus and unfocus. Hence it is important to monitor and properly select that energy. This is learned in higher yoga, beginning with proper sitting posture, āsana, proper pranic intake, *prāṇāyāma*, sensual energy restriction and containment, *pratyāhār*, and then linking of the attention to higher concentration forces, *dhāranā*. This is *buddhi yoga*, not *bhakti* or *bhakti yoga*. But *buddhi yoga* once perfected should be applied to all other divine pursuits.

यया तु धर्मकामार्थान्
धृत्या धारयतेऽर्जुन ।
प्रसङ्गेन फलाकाङ्क्षी
धृतिः सा पार्थ राजसी ॥१८.३४॥
yayā tu dharmakāmārthān
dhṛtyā dhārayate'rjuna
prasaṅgena phalākāṅkṣī
dhṛtiḥ sā pārtha rājasī (18.34)

*yayā — by which; tu — but; dharmakāmārthān = dharma — duty + kāma — pleasure + arthān — wealthy; dhṛtyā — with determination; dhārayate — it holds; 'rjuna = arjuna — Arjuna; prasaṅgena — with attachment; phalākāṅkṣī — desiring results; dhṛtiḥ— determination; sā —it; pārtha — son of Pṛthā; rājasī — impulsion*

**But the determination by which one holds duty, pleasure, and wealth with attachment and with desire for results, is an impulsion, O son of Pṛthā. (18.34)**

***Siddha Swami's Commentary:***

So long as the mind takes in passionate energy, it will follow the passionate course either directly or indirectly, either in a vulgar way or with sophistication. To adjust this permanently, one has to change the type of energy invested by the mind.

Duty, pleasure and wealth, *dharmakāmārthān*, is the objective of cultural life in the material world. These aspects are left aside when one pursues *brahma yoga*.

यया स्वप्नं भयं शोकं
विषादं मदमेव च ।
न विमुञ्चति दुर्मेधा
धृतिः सा पार्थ तामसी ॥१८.३५॥
yayā svapnaṁ bhayaṁ śokaṁ
viṣādaṁ madameva ca
na vimuñcati durmedhā
dhṛtiḥ sā pārtha tāmasī (18.35)

*yayā — by which; svapnaṁ — sleep; bhayaṁ — fear; śokaṁ — sorrow; viṣādaṁ — despair; madam — pride; eva — indeed; ca — and; na — not; vimuñcati — abandons; durmedhā — idiot; dhṛtiḥ — determination; sā — it; pārtha — son of Pṛthā; tāmasī — of the depressive mode*

**That determination by which an idiot does not abandon sleep, fear, sorrow, despair and pride, is of the depressing mode. (18.35)**

***Siddha Swami's Commentary:***

Students are to be taught that sleep, fear, sorrow, despair and pride are types of psychic energy. If even a good man falls under the influence of these potencies, he will have to act in the negative ways which are sponsored by them. Thus it is important to avoid ingestion of these subtle energies. One should learn in yoga how to restrict the psyche to a higher grade of energy.

सुखं त्विदानीं त्रिविधं
शृणु मे भरतर्षभ ।
अभ्यासाद्रमते यत्र
दुःखान्तं च निगच्छति ॥ १८.३६ ॥
sukhaṁ tvidānīṁ trividhaṁ
śṛṇu me bharatarṣabha
abhyāsādramate yatra
duḥkhāntaṁ ca nigacchati (18.36)

*sukhaṁ — happiness; tu — but; idānīṁ — now; trividhaṁ — types; śṛṇu — hear; me — from me; bharatarṣabha — O strong man of the Bharatas; abhyāsāt — from habit; ramate — enjoys; yatra — where, through which; duḥkhāntaṁ — end of sorrow; ca — and, or; nigacchati — one comes to*

**But now hear from Me, O strong man of the Bharatas, regarding the three types of happiness which one either enjoys from habit or through which one comes to the end of sorrow. (18.36)**

***Siddha Swami's Commentary:***

Most of the human beings enjoy happiness through habit. These habits were introduced to them during the fusion with the causal and subtle bodies, particularly with the subtle body, and thereafter with many material forms.

There is another strange type of happiness which causes a living entity to come to the end of sorrows, *duhkhāntam*. In the *buddhi yoga* practice, one becomes habituated to that promotional joy which causes one to come to the end of sorrows.

यत्तदग्रे विषमिव
परिणामेऽमृतोपमम् ।
तत्सुखं सात्त्विकं प्रोक्तम्
आत्मबुद्धिप्रसादजम् ॥ १८.३७॥
yattadagre viṣamiva
pariṇāme'mṛtopamam
tatsukhaṁ sāttvikaṁ proktam
ātmabuddhiprasādajam (18.37)

*yat = yad — which; tat — that; agre — initially; viṣam — poison; iva — like; pariṇāme — in changing; 'mṛtopamam = amṛtopamam = amṛta — nectar + upamam — likeness; tat = tad — that; sukham — happiness; sāttvikaṁ — of the clarifying mode; proktam — is said to be; ātmabuddhiprasādajam = ātmabuddhi — spiritual discernment + prasāda — clarity + jam — produced by*

**That which initially is like poison but which changes into an experience like nectar, and which is felt through the clarity of spiritual discernment, is said to be happiness in the clarifying mode. (18.37)**

***Siddha Swami's Commentary:***

*Ātma buddhi prasādajam* is a state attained in the advanced course of *buddhi yoga*. This course begins like poison because initially one has to face the internal psyche, leaving aside the sensuous pursuits to which one was habituated. Those were the external sensual enjoyments which came through hearing pleasing sounds from the external world, touching smooth surfaces like the skin of the opposite sex, seeing sensually-attractive shapes, tasting palatable foods and smelling nice odors.

The sensual restrictions seem like poison when one first begins the *pratyāhār* sense withdrawal practice. Therefore many devotees hate yoga and chide it as being void, tasteless and lacking any type of *bhakti* or devotional happiness. However in the end, if one masters *pratyāhār,* one moves on to *dhāranā*, linkage of the attention to higher persons and energies. Then what began as poison, turns into nectar.

When the student *yogin* gains clarity and can differentiate clearly between his attention and intellect, then he gets *prasāda,* the happiness which is derived from that separation.

विषयेन्द्रियसंयोगाद्
यत्तदग्रेऽमृतोपमम् ।
परिणामे विषमिव
तत्सुखं राजसं स्मृतम् ॥ १८.३८॥
viṣayendriyasaṁyogād
yattadagre'mṛtopamam
pariṇāme viṣamiva
tatsukhaṁ rājasaṁ smṛtam (18.38)

*viṣayendriyasaṁyogāt = viṣaya — attractive objects + indriya — sense organs + saṁyogāt — from contact; yat — which; tat — that; agre —in the beginning; 'mṛtopamam = amṛtopamam = amṛta — nectar + upamam — likeness; pariṇāme — changes into; viṣam — poison; ivā — like; tat — that; sukham — happiness; rājasaṁ — impulsion; smṛtam — recognized as*

**That happiness which in the beginning seems like nectar and which comes from the contact between the sense organs and attractive objects, which changes as if it were poison, is recognized as an impulsion. (18.38)**

***Siddha Swami's Commentary:***

This happiness is from an impulsion based on fusion between the self and the psychological equipments in the subtle body. But when the self learns to segregate from those equipments, it breaks away from sensual reliance and is freed. *Śrī Patañjali Mahārṣi* said:

*tadā draṣṭuḥ svarūpe avasthānam*

***Then the perceiver is situated in his own form. (Yoga Sūtra, 1.3)***

Initially the self considers itself to be under the influence of the sensual energies, but when the self endeavors for it and does become segregated, it realizes itself by itself and derives a different and pure happiness.

*Śrī Patañjali* warned that when the self is not segregated, it is in conformity with the mento-emotional energy. It is then a stooge.

*vṛtti sārūpyam itaratra*

***At other times, there is conformity with the mento-emotional energy.***

***(Yoga Sūtra, 1.4)***

यदग्रे चानुबन्धे च
सुखं मोहनमात्मनः ।
निद्रालस्यप्रमादोत्थं
तत्तामसमुदाहृतम् ॥ १८.३९॥
yadagre cānubandhe ca
sukhaṁ mohanamātmanaḥ
nidrālasyapramādotthaṁ
tattāmasamudāhṛtam (18.39)

*yat — which; agre — in the beginning: cānubandhe = ca — and + anubandhe — in consequence; ca — and; sukham — happiness; mohanam — bewildering; ātmanaḥ — of the person; nidrālasyapramādotthaṁ = nidrā — sleep + ālasya — laziness + pramāda — confusion + uttham — comes from; tat = tad — that; tāmasam — depressive mode; udāhṛtam — said to be*

**And that happiness which in the beginning and in consequence is bewildering to the person, which comes from sleep, laziness and confusion, is said to be of the depressive mode. (18.39)**

***Siddha Swami's Commentary:***

The energies of material nature occur on the psychological plane as well as on the gross physical level. Those on the psychological plane occur in a human psyche as mental power or will power and as sensual energy and emotional force. One can derive happiness from sleep, laziness and confusion. Thus one can become habituated to either or all of these.

न तदस्ति पृथिव्यां वा
दिवि देवेषु वा पुनः ।
सत्त्वं प्रकृतिजैर्मुक्तं
यदेभिः स्यात्त्रिभिर्गुणैः ॥ १८.४० ॥
na tadasti pṛthivyāṁ vā
divi deveṣu vā punaḥ
sattvaṁ prakṛtijairmuktaṁ
yadebhiḥ syāttribhirguṇaiḥ (18.40)

*na — not; tat — that; asti — there is; pṛthivyāṁ — on earth; vā — or; divi — in the supernatural world; deveṣu — among the supernatural rulers; vā — or; punaḥ = punar — even; sattvaṁ — something substantial; prakṛtijaiḥ — produced by material nature; muktaṁ — freed, without; yat — which; ebhiḥ — by these; syāt — it can exist; tribhiḥ — by three; guṇaiḥ — by influence of modes*

**There is no object on earth or even in the subtle mundane domains, that can exist without these three modes which were produced from material nature. (18.40)**

***Siddha Swami's Commentary:***

No attempt is made in *brahma yoga* to deny the possibility of the influences of material nature, or to negate that power or claim that the Supreme Being alone is the full power. In *brahma yoga* the student is trained to recognize the strength of material nature. He learns to gage its influence and to research the possibility of escaping from it.

ब्राह्मणक्षत्रियविशां
शूद्राणां च परंतप ।
कर्माणि प्रविभक्तानि
स्वभावप्रभवैर्गुणैः ॥ १८.४१ ॥
brāhmaṇakṣatriyaviśāṁ
śūdrāṇāṁ ca paraṁtapa
karmāṇi pravibhaktāni
svabhāvaprabhavairguṇaiḥ (18.41)

*brāhmaṅakṣatriyaviśāṁ = brāhmaṇa — priestly teacher + kṣatriya — ruling sector + viśāṁ— productive managers; śudrāṇāṁ — of the working class; ca — and; paraṁtapa — scorcher of the enemy; karmāṇi — activities; pravibhaktāni — allotted; svabhāvaprabhavaiḥ = svabhāva — own nature + prabhavaiḥ — by being produced; guṇaiḥ — by the modes of material nature*

**The activities of the priestly teachers, the ruling sector, the productive managers and the working class, are allotted by the modes of material nature which arise from natural tendencies. (18.41)**

***Siddha Swami's Commentary:***

All the social configurations and profiles are formed by combination of the energies of material nature. These potencies are subtle in origin.

शमो दमस्तपः शौचं
क्षान्तिरार्जवमेव च ।
ज्ञानं विज्ञानमास्तिक्यं
ब्रह्मकर्म स्वभावजम् ॥ १८.४२ ॥

*śamo = śamaḥ — tranquility; damaḥ — restraint; tapaḥ — austerity; śaucaṁ— cleanliness; kṣāntiḥ — patience; ārjavam — straightforwardness; eva — indeed; ca — and; jñānaṁ — knowledge;*

śamo damastapaḥ śaucaṁ
kṣāntirārjavameva ca
jñānaṁ vijñānamāstikyaṁ
brahmakarma svabhāvajam (18.42)

*vijñānaṁ — discrimination; āstikyaṁ — a belief in God; brahmakarma — work of a priestly teacher; svabhāvajam — based on natural tendencies*

**Tranquility, restraint, austerity, cleanliness, patience, straightforwardness, knowledge, discrimination and a belief in God, are the work of a priestly teacher based on his natural tendencies. (18.42)**

***Siddha Swami's Commentary:***

These higher qualities are sponsored by, developed and fostered in the highest level of material nature. Despite some condemnation of material nature, it does foster a belief in God. This is because it reflects the power of the Supreme Being. And ultimately it is empowered by Him.

शौर्यं तेजो धृतिर्दाक्ष्यं
युद्धे चाप्यपलायनम् ।
दानमीश्वरभावश्च
क्षात्रंकर्म स्वभावजम् ॥ १८.४३ ॥
śauryaṁ tejo dhṛtirdākṣyaṁ
yuddhe cāpyapalāyanam
dānamīśvarabhāvaśca
kṣātraṁkarma svabhāvajam (18.43)

*śauryaṁ — heroism; tejo = tejaḥ — majesty; dhṛtiḥ — determination; dākṣyaṁ— expertise; yuddhe — in battle; cāpi — and also; apalāyanam — lack of cowardice; dānam — charitable disposition; īśvarabhāvaśca = īśvarabhāvaḥ — governing tendency + ca — and; kṣātraṁ— of the ruling human being; karma — action; svabhāvajam — based on natural tendency*

**Heroism, majesty, determination, expertise, lack of cowardice in battle, charitable disposition, and governing tendency are the actions of a ruling human being, based on natural tendency. (18.43)**

***Siddha Swami's Commentary:***

This is the 2nd in the categories of occupation and tendency for human beings. These persons are more inclined to *karma yoga*, while those listed in the previous verse, are more inclined to *jñāna yoga*. Both are advised to take up the practice of *buddhi yoga*.

कृषिगोरक्ष्यवाणिज्यं
वैश्यकर्म स्वभावजम् ।
परिचर्यात्मकं कर्म
शूद्रस्यापि स्वभावजम् ॥ १८.४४ ॥
kṛṣigorakṣyavāṇijyaṁ
vaiśyakarma svabhāvajam
paricaryātmakaṁ karma
śūdrasyāpi svabhāvajam (18.44)

*kṛṣigaurakṣyavāṇijyaṁ = kṛṣi — agriculture + gaurakṣya — cow tending + vāṇijyaṁ — trading; vaiśyakarma — action of the productive manager; svabhāvajam — based on natural tendency; paricaryātmakaṁ = paricaryā — service + ātmakaṁ — of natural tendency; karma — action; śudrasyāpi = śudrasya — working class + api — also; svabhāvajam — based on natural tendency*

**Agriculture, cow-tending and trading are the productive manager's activity based on natural tendency. Service actions are produced of a working class person based on natural tendency. (18.44)**

***Siddha Swami's Commentary:***

The general energy in the psyche dictates the general tendency of a human being. *Buddhi yoga* practice allows the human to view itself objectively, to recognize its category according to the influences which prevail in its nature, and to plan out and execute preferences for higher development.

स्वे स्वे कर्मण्यभिरतः
संसिद्धिं लभते नरः ।
स्वकर्मनिरतः सिद्धिं
यथा विन्दति तच्छृणु ॥ १८.४५ ॥
sve sve karmaṇyabhirataḥ
saṁsiddhiṁ labhate naraḥ
svakarmanirataḥ siddhiṁ
yathā vindati tacchṛṇu (18.45)

*sve sve — his own, his own, consistent; karmaṇi — in action; abhirataḥ — content; saṁsiddhiṁ — perfection; labhate — attain; naraḥ — human being; svakarmanirataḥ = svakarma — own duty + nirataḥ — satisfied; siddhiṁ — perfection; yathā — as the means; vindati — finds; tat — that; śṛṇu — hear*

**A human being attains perfection by being content in the consistent execution of his duty. Hear of the means through which a duty-satisfied person finds perfection.(18.45)**

***Siddha Swami's Commentary:***

This is so because a human being is under the gaze of *Śrī* Krishna, the Central Person in the Universal Form. If one does not complete the duties which are assigned by providence, one cannot be happy and one certainly cannot attain perfection. For perfection a human being must secure the cooperation of the Supreme Being, of *Śrī* Krishna. Thus if one does not cooperate with Him, if one is defiant towards Him, one certainly cannot make spiritual progression.

Even though many duties assigned by the Universal Form might be unpalatable, and some might only be for social maintenance, still the completion of such tasks brings on the grace of the Supreme Being, and that in turn sponsors spiritual advancement.

यतः प्रवृत्तिर्भूतानां
येन सर्वमिदं ततम् ।
स्वकर्मणा तमभ्यर्च्य
सिद्धिं विन्दति मानवः ॥ १८.४६ ॥
yataḥ pravṛttirbhūtānāṁ
yena sarvamidaṁ tatam
svakarmaṇā tamabhyarcya
siddhiṁ vindati mānavaḥ (18.46)

*yataḥ — from whom; pravṛttiḥ — origin; bhūtānāṁ — of beings; yena — by whom; sarvam — all; idam — this; tatam — is pervaded; svakarmaṇā — through his duty; tam — his; abhyarcya — worshipping; siddhiṁ — perfection; vindati — he finds; mānavaḥ — human being*

**Through the performance of his own duty, a human being finds perfection by worshipping the Person from Whom the beings originate and by Whom all this is pervaded. (18.46)**

***Siddha Swami's Commentary:***

This formula if followed by any human being, will cause his or her compatibility with the Supreme Person and from that will develop spiritual progression. Even though the Supreme Lord, *Śrī* Krishna, has social concerns for righteous lifestyle, He does sponsor spiritual progression which removes one from those social duties. Thus if one complies with a social obligation stipulated by Him, one will in the course of time, find perfection through worship and honor of *Śrī* Krishna, the Supreme Lord. Through His association one would be instructed in the *buddhi yoga* practice which was taught to Arjuna and eventually one would attain liberation.

श्रेयान्स्वधर्मो विगुणः
परधर्मात्स्वनुष्ठितात् ।
स्वभावनियतं कर्म
कुर्वन्नाप्नोति किल्बिषम् ॥ १८.४७॥
śreyānsvadharmo viguṇaḥ
paradharmātsvanuṣṭhitāt
svabhāvaniyataṁ karma
kurvannāpnoti kilbiṣam (18.47)

*śreyān — better; svadharmo = svadharmaḥ — own duty; viguṇāḥ — imperfectly; paradharmāt — than another's duty; svanuṣṭhitāt = su + anuṣṭhitāt — well performed, perfectly; svabhāvaniyataṁ = svabhāva — own nature + niyatam — restricted; karma — action; kurvan — performing; nāpnoti = na — not + āpnoti — he acquires; kilbiṣam — sin, fault*

**Better to attend to one's own duty imperfectly than to heed another's perfectly. By performing actions which are restricted by one's own nature, one does not acquire fault. (18.47)**

***Siddha Swami's Commentary:***

In all respects one has to work through one's acquired nature. One cannot adopt the nature of another person, even of one's guru or of a divine being like *Śrī* Krishna. Whatever nature one acquired *(svabhāva)*, one will have to deal with its reform, to purify and upgrade it. One should work through the impediments placed before one by providence, and take hints and help from the Supreme Being and His agents.

Certainly there would be faults in the performance of one's duty which is assigned by providence, but still those faults would not be categorized as radical departures from the supreme will. Thus one should stick to purifying oneself step by step rather than rushing after something which is due to another.

सहजं कर्म कौन्तेय
सदोषमपि न त्यजेत् ।
सर्वारम्भा हि दोषेण
धूमेनाग्निरिवावृताः ॥ १८.४८॥
sahajaṁ karma kaunteya
sadoṣamapi na tyajet
sarvārambhā hi doṣeṇa
dhūmenāgnirivāvṛtāḥ (18.48)

*sahajaṁ — inborn; karma — action; kaunteya — son of Kunti; sadoṣam — with fault; api — even; na — not; tyajet — should abandon; sarvārambhā — all undertakings; hi — indeed; doṣeṇa — with defect; dhumenāgniḥ = dhumena — with smoke + āgniḥ — fire; ivāvṛtaḥ = iva — like + āvṛtaḥ — is shrouded*

**One should not abandon inborn duty, O son of Kuntī, even if it is faulty. Indeed, all undertakings are with defect, even as fire is shrouded with smoke. (18.48)**

***Siddha Swami's Commentary:***

Material nature is defective but it does facilitate elevation. Thus one should not develop the idea that duties in this world may be abandoned whimsically or negated altogether. It is important to get clearance from the Universal Form before one renounces duty.

असक्तबुद्धिः सर्वत्र
जितात्मा विगतस्पृहः ।
नैष्कर्म्यसिद्धिं परमां
संन्यासेनाधिगच्छति ॥ १८.४९॥

*asakta — unattached + buddhiḥ — intellect; sarvatra — in all applications; jitātmā — self-conquered; vigataspṛhah = vigata — disappeared + spṛhaḥ = yearnings; naiṣkarmya — exemption*

asaktabuddhiḥ sarvatra
jitātmā vigataspṛhaḥ
naiṣkarmyasiddhiṁ paramāṁ
saṁnyāsenādhigacchati (18.49)

*from activities + siddhim — perfection; paramāṁ — supreme; saṁnyāsenādhigacchati = saṁnyāsena — by renunciation of opportunities + adhigacchati — he attains*

**He whose intellect is unattached in every application, who is self-controlled, whose yearnings disappeared, by the renunciation of opportunities, attains supreme perfection of being exempt from action. (18.49)**

***Siddha Swami's Commentary:***

This comes after mastery of *buddhi yoga*, when the intellect is weaned from its attachment to the sensual energies and memory. Then the yearnings in relation to the subtle and gross material worlds, disappear due to detachment from the memory. Because the attentive power of the self became detached from the intellect, the memory and sensual energies can no longer command the intellect and so the self becomes freed from mental and sensual dominance.

In this case the renunciation of opportunities, *sannyāsa*, is done by the self on behalf of itself, even though on behalf of the Supreme Self, that very same renounced person may again act in the social field, taking up opportunities as instructed by the Universal Form. One who serves God and who also has personal needs will inevitably enjoy for himself or herself and for God. But one who serves God and who has no personal needs will serve God and leave aside his own needs, due to having outgrown those impulsions by mastership of *buddhi yoga*.

At first when a *yogin* renounces opportunities, he or she might do so without understanding the role of the Supreme Being, without understanding that there can be no absolute independence for a limited being. As the *yogin* advances, he or she comes to understand that even though participation in this world is not a necessity for every limited person, it is for the Supreme Being. And since all are under the Supreme Being as dependents, no one can be completely exempt from service to the Supreme Personality.

One should be detached for one's own sake and to keep spiritual integrity, but if the Supreme Person requires services one should cooperate without hesitation. A loyal butler may have no appetite, but if requested by his master, he may taste and give an opinion freely. Thus one who lost interest in the material world and its cultural affairs, would serve in the same cultural setting if the Supreme Person or an elevated soul requested him to do so.

सिद्धिं प्राप्तो यथा ब्रह्म
तथाप्नोति निबोध मे ।
समासेनैव कौन्तेय
निष्ठा ज्ञानस्य या परा ॥१८.५०॥
siddhiṁ prāpto yathā brahma
tathāpnoti nibodha me
samāsenaiva kaunteya
niṣṭhā jñānasya yā parā (18.50)

*siddhiṁ — perfection; prāpto = prāptaḥ — attained; yathā — as; brahma — spirituality; tathāpnoti = tathā — thus + āpnoti — attains; nibodha — learn; me — from me; samāsenaiva = samāsena — in brief + eva — indeed; kaunteya — son of Kuntī; niṣṭhā — state; jñānasya — of experience; yā — which; parā — highest*

**Learn from Me briefly, O son of Kuntī, how a person who attained perfection, also reaches a spirituality which is the highest. (18.50)**

***Siddha Swami's Commentary:***

There is a distinction between perfection, *siddhim*, and attainment of the highest spirituality, *brahma parā*. Perfection means that one has fine tuned the psychic equipments which are in the subtle body. After this is attained, one aspires for a new accomplishment, namely to transfer away from the subtle equipments like intellect, mind energy, sensual energy, and memory.

बुद्ध्या विशुद्धया युक्तो
धृत्यात्मानं नियम्य च ।
शब्दादीन्विषयांस्त्यक्त्वा
रागद्वेषौ व्युदस्य च ॥ १८.५१ ॥
buddhyā viśuddhayā yukto
dhṛtyātmānaṁ niyamya ca
śabdādīnviṣayāṁstyaktvā
rāgadveṣau vyudasya ca (18.51)

*buddhyā — with intellect; viśuddhayā — with purified; yukto = yuktaḥ — yogically disciplined; dhṛtyātmānaṁ = dhṛtyā — with firmness + ātmānaṁ — self; niyamya — controlling; ca — and; śabdādīn = śabda — sound + ādīn — beginning with, and others; viṣayān — attractive sensations; tyaktvā — abandoning; rāgadveṣau = rāga — craving + dveṣau — hatred; vyudasya — rejecting; ca — and*

**Being yogicly-disciplined with purified intelligence and controlling the soul, firmly abandoning sound and other attractive sensations, rejecting craving and hatred, (18.51)**

***Siddha Swami's Commentary:***

The mastership of *buddhi yoga* results in a purified intellect organ in the subtle body. From this one begins to control the relationship between the soul and its attentive powers. One is able to segregate the soul from its sense of identity which was derived from the subtle material energy.

In the training of *buddhi yoga*, one is taught how to abandon sound and the other attractive sensations, which are surfaces, shapes, flavors and odors. These are to be abandoned, including mantras given to one by spiritual masters. But one takes up other sounds which come into the psyche from the spiritual zone. These sounds are not uttered by anyone on this side of existence but are heard coming in from the sky of consciousness, the chit akasha.

In the mastery of *prāṇāyāma* which is a part of *buddhi yoga*, one is able to reject craving and hatred because one manages to do so by driving out the lower psychic energies which sponsor creature existence in the material world.

विविक्तसेवी लघ्वाशी
यतवाक्कायमानसः ।
ध्यानयोगपरो नित्यं
वैराग्यं समुपाश्रितः ॥ १८.५२ ॥
viviktasevī laghvāśī
yatavākkāyamānasaḥ
dhyānayogaparo nityaṁ
vairāgyaṁ samupāśritaḥ (18.52)

*viviktasevī = vivikta — is isolated + sevī — living at; laghvasi = laghv (laghu)— lightly + āsī — eating; yatavākkāyamānasaḥ = yata — controlled + vāk (vāc) — speech + kāya — body + mānasaḥ — mind; dhyānayogaparo = dhyāna — meditation + yoga — yoga + paro (paraḥ) — devoted to; nityam — always; vairāgyam — dispassion; samupāśritaḥ — resorting to*

**...living in isolation, eating lightly, controlling speech, body and mind, always being devoted to yogic meditation, resorting to dispassion, (18.52)**

***Siddha Swami's Commentary:***

Living in isolation is a basic requirement for those who practice *buddhi yoga* seriously. It is in isolation that one develops inner perfection of the psychic equipments and learns from an able spiritual master how to sort between oneself and the intellect, sensual energy, mental energy, emotional force and memory.

One is required to eat lightly. This is part of kundalini yoga to cause the life force to be attracted to the head of the subtle body, for the development of perfect celibacy. The austerity of controlling speech, body and mind is the regulation of verbal expression, bodily movements and mental considerations. These are controlled effectively and consistently only when the psychic equipments are curbed from their impulsions. This happens only when the energies used on the psychic plane, are exchanged for higher potencies. This is mastered at first by *prāṇāyāma*, but it is completed by the higher yoga practices of *pratyāhār*, *dhāranā*, *dhyāna* and *samādhi*. It takes much dedication to yogic meditation, *dhyānayogaparo*, before one can consistently cause permanent changes in one's nature. This is mastered in *dhyāna* yoga which is part of the *buddhi yoga* practice. It involves dispassion which is cultivated in the psyche by curbing the intellect's involvement with the memory and sensual energy. The intellect's automatic reception of messages from the senses and memory must be completely curbed.

अहंकारं बलं दर्पं
कामं क्रोधं परिग्रहम् ।
विमुच्य निर्ममः शान्तो
ब्रह्मभूयाय कल्पते ॥ १८.५३ ॥
ahaṁkāraṁ balaṁ darpaṁ
kāmaṁ krodhaṁ parigraham
vimucya nirmamaḥ śānto
brahmabhūyāya kalpate (18.53)

*ahaṁkāraṁ — without a misplaced initiative, without a false assertion; balaṁ — brute force; darpaṁ — arrogance; kāmaṁ — cravings; krodhaṁ — anger; parigraham — possessions; vimucya — freeing oneself; nirmamaḥ— unselfish; śānto = śāntaḥ — peaceful; brahmabhūyāya = brahma — spirit + bhūyāyā — to that level, existential; kalpate — is suited*

**...freeing oneself from a false assertion, from the application of brute force, from arrogance, from craving and from possessiveness, being unselfish and peaceful, one is suited to the spiritual level. (18.53)**

***Siddha Swami's Commentary:***

By completion of the *buddhi yoga* practice, one is able to free the self from the false sense of identity which it derived from fusion with the psychic equipments, as well as to free the self from the need for application of brute force, arrogance, cravings and from possessiveness, selfishness and disturbing mentality. When all this is achieved, one becomes suited to the spiritual level and one is rated as a *siddha*, a perfect being.

ब्रह्मभूतः प्रसन्नात्मा
न शोचति न काङ्क्षति ।
समः सर्वेषु भूतेषु
मद्भक्तिं लभते पराम् ॥ १८.५४ ॥
brahmabhūtaḥ prasannātmā
na śocati na kāṅkṣati
samaḥ sarveṣu bhūteṣu
madbhaktiṁ labhate parām (18.54)

*brabmabhūtaḥ — being absorbed in spiritual existence; prasannātmā = prasanna — peaceful + ātmā — self, spirit; na — not; śocati — laments; na — no; kāṅkṣati — hankers for something; samaḥ — impartial; sarveṣu — in all; bhūteṣu — in the beings; madbhaktiṁ — devotion to me; labhate — attains; parām — supreme*

**One who is absorbed in the spiritual existence, who has a peaceful spirit, who does not lament or hanker for anything, who is impartial to all beings, attains the supreme devotion to Me. (18.54)**

***Siddha Swami's Commentary:***

Note how *Śrī* Krishna made a distinction between devotion and supreme devotion, *madbhaktim parām*. Why make such a differentiation? And why indicate that only those who mastered *buddhi yoga* could have the supreme devotion?

भक्त्या मामभिजानाति
यावान्यश्चास्मि तत्त्वतः ।
ततो मां तत्त्वतो ज्ञात्वा
विशते तदनन्तरम् ॥१८.५५॥
bhaktyā māmabhijānāti
yāvānyaścāsmi tattvataḥ
tato māṁ tattvato jñātvā
viśate tadanantaram (18.55)

*bhaktyā — by devotion; mām — to me; abhijānāti— he realizes; yāvān — how great: yaścāsmi = yaḥ — who + ca — and + asmi — I am; tattvataḥ — in reality; tato = tataḥ — then; mām — me; tattvato = tattvataḥ — in truth; jñātvā— having known; viśate — enters; tadanantaram — immediately*

**By devotion to Me, he realizes how great I am and who I am in reality. Then having known Me in truth, he enters My association immediately. (18.55)**

***Siddha Swami's Commentary:***

Despite any credits attributed to the gopis of *Vṛndāvana* by *Śrī* Krishna, by Uddhava and by Shuka, still here, *Śrī* Krishna spoke of those who mastered *buddhi yoga*. Hence why should the students of that skill be ridiculed in the society of devotees?

सर्वकर्माण्यपि सदा
कुर्वाणो मद्व्यपाश्रयः ।
मत्प्रसादादवाप्नोति
शाश्वतं पदमव्ययम् ॥१८.५६॥
sarvakarmāṇyapi sadā
kurvāṇo madvyapāśrayaḥ
matprasādādavāpnoti
śāśvataṁ padamavyayam (18.56)

*sarvakarmāṇi — in all actions; api — furthermore; sadā — always; kurvāṇo = kurvāṇaḥ — performing; madvyapāśrayaḥ — taking reliance in me; matprasādāt — from my grace; avāpnoti — gets; śāśvataṁ — eternal; padam — abode; avyayam — imperishable*

**Furthermore, know that while performing all actions, he whose reliance is always on Me, gets by My grace, the eternal imperishable abode. (18.56)**

***Siddha Swami's Commentary:***

While the previous verses from 51 through 55 described the status and awards given to the *jñāna* yogis who master the *buddhi yoga* practice, this verse is an assurance for the *karma* yogins, the *tyāgis* like Arjuna. *Śrī* Krishna guarantees for them the eternal imperishable abode.

चेतसा सर्वकर्माणि
मयि संन्यस्य मत्परः ।
बुद्धियोगमुपाश्रित्य
मच्चित्तः सततं भव ॥१८.५७॥

*cetasā — by thought; sarvakarmāṇi — all actions; mayi — on Me; saṁnyasya — devoted to me; matparaḥ — devoted to Me; buddhiyogam — disciplining the intellect by yoga practice; upāśritya — relying on;*

cetasā sarvakarmāṇi
mayi saṁnyasya matparaḥ
buddhiyogamupāśritya
maccittaḥ satataṁ bhava (18.57)

*maccittaḥ — thinking of Me; satataṁ — constantly; bhava — be*

**Renouncing by thought, all actions to Me, being devoted to Me, relying on the process of disciplining the intellect by yoga, be constantly thinking of Me. (18.57)**

***Siddha Swami's Commentary:***

This verse should be translated as follows:

**Renouncing by emotional and mental control, all actions to Me, being devoted to Me, relying on the process of disciplining the intellect by yoga, be constantly thinking of Me.**

Those who do *karma yoga* will have to complete the course of *buddhi yoga*, before they attain the eternal, imperishable abode. This is directly given in the word *buddhiyogam*. To understand the previous verse, we must know that the *karma yogin* will get the grace of *Śrī* Krishna in the form of the ability to take up and complete the course of *buddhi yoga*. When that is done, they will attain the eternal, imperishable abode. If we delete the *buddhi yoga* process, the guarantee for the *karma* yogins like Arjuna will be null and void.

मच्चित्तः सर्वदुर्गाणि
मत्प्रसादात्तरिष्यसि ।
अथ चेत्त्वमहंकारान्
न श्रोष्यसि विनङ्क्ष्यसि ॥१८.५८॥
maccittaḥ sarvadurgāṇi
matprasādāttariṣyasi
atha cettvamahaṁkārān
na śroṣyasi vinaṅkṣyasi (18.58)

*maccittaḥ — thinking of Me; sarvadurgāṇi — all difficulties; matprasādāt — from my grace; tariṣyasi — you will surpass; atha — but; cet = ced — if; tvam — you; ahaṁkārān — false assertion; na — not; śroṣyasi — you will listen; vinaṅkṣyasi — you will be lost*

**Thinking of Me, you will, by My grace, surpass all difficulties. But if by false assertion, you do not listen, you will be lost. (18.58)**

***Siddha Swami's Commentary:***

This instruction is undoubtedly an individual one given to Arjuna alone. It concerns Arjuna's hesitation to fight a civil war at *Kurukṣetra*. But this advice may be taken by all spiritual students. Each of us, if we think of what *Śrī* Krishna said to Arjuna, will by Krishna's grace, surpass the difficulties which confront us as destiny unfolds. But if we do not listen, we will be lost, because Krishna knows what will occur in this world. He knows the path out of the enigmas of this world. In all respects, every human being should try to study the *Bhagavad Gītā*, get to know *Śrī* Krishna and apply the advice that is relevant to their level of advancement.

यदहंकारमाश्रित्य
न योत्स्य इति मन्यसे ।
मिथ्यैष व्यवसायस्ते
प्रकृतिस्त्वां नियोक्ष्यति ॥१८.५९॥

*yat — which; ahaṁkāram — false assertive attitude; āśritya — relying on; na — not; yotsya — I will fight; iti — thus; manyase — you think; mithyaiṣa = mithya — mistaken + eṣa — this; vyavasāyaḥ — determination; te*

yadahaṁkāramāśritya
na yotsya iti manyase
mithyaiṣa vyavasāyaste
prakṛtistvāṁ niyokṣyati (18.59)

*— your; prakṛtiḥ — material nature; tvāṁ — you; niyokṣyāti — you will be forced*

**While relying on a false assertive attitude, you may think, "I will not fight." But that determination is mistaken. Your material nature will force you. (18.59)**

***Siddha Swami's Commentary:***

*Śrī* Krishna alerted that Arjuna's affiliation with material nature *(prakṛtih tvām)* would cause Arjuna to fight anyway, sooner or later, when Arjuna would be cornered by destiny and be forced to defend himself in the future. If he did not fight as offered, he would be taunted by enemies until he was forced by intimidation to take up arms against them. It was just a matter of time.

Since Arjuna was not an expert *karma yogin* and since he was not given an exemption from those cultural activities by *Śrī* Krishna, he relied on the energy of material nature, which encouraged him to avoid settling the political affairs at that time. But the same material energy, when converted in the future, would nevertheless force the same Arjuna to fight under different circumstances which would be even more unpalatable to Arjuna.

स्वभावजेन कौन्तेय
निबद्धः स्वेन कर्मणा ।
कर्तुं नेच्छसि यन्मोहात्
करिष्यस्यवशोऽपि तत् ॥ १८.६० ॥
svabhāvajena kaunteya
nibaddhaḥ svena karmaṇā
kartuṁ necchasi yanmohāt
kariṣyasyavaśo'pi tat (18.60)

*svabhāvajena — of your own natural tendencies; kaunteya — son of Kuntī; nibaddhaḥ — bound; svena — by your own; karmāṇa — obligation; kartuṁ — to perform; necchasi = na — not + icchasi — you want; yan = yad — which; mohāt — from delusion; kariṣyasi — you will do; avaśo = avaśaḥ — against your own will; 'pi = api — also, even; tat = tad — that*

**By your natural tendencies, being bound by obligations, O son of Kuntī, that which you do not want to perform due to delusion, you will do even if it is against your will. (18.60)**

***Siddha Swami's Commentary:***

Evidence is given here that it was Arjuna's affiliation with material nature, which would cause Arjuna to fight in the future, though it encouraged hesitancy at the time. This is qualified by the terms *svabhāvena*, which means of your own natural tendencies *(bhāva)*. Such aspects cannot be curbed by the limited persons except by mastery of *buddhi yoga*.

ईश्वरः सर्वभूतानां
हृद्देशेऽर्जुन तिष्ठति ।
भ्रामयन्सर्वभूतानि
यन्त्रारूढानि मायया ॥ १८.६१ ॥
īśvaraḥ sarvabhūtānāṁ
hṛddeśe'rjuna tiṣṭhati
bhrāmayansarvabhūtāni
yantrārūḍhāni māyayā (18.61)

*īśvaraḥ — Lord; sarvabhūtānām — of all beings; hṛddeśe = hṛd — central psyche + deśe — in the place; 'rjuna = arjuna — Arjuna; tiṣṭhati — is situated; bhrāmayan — cause to transmigrate; sarvabhūtāni — all beings; yantrārūḍhāni = yantra — spinning machine + ārūḍhāni — fixed to; māyayā — by mystic power*

**The Lord of all beings is situated in the central psyche, O Arjuna, causing all beings to transmigrate by His mystic power, just as if they were fixed to a spinning machine. (18.61)**

***Siddha Swami's Commentary:***

One must either do as told by material nature, through its impulsive urges, or one may act as commanded by superior personalities, who are led by the Supreme Lord, the Master of all beings. In either case, one is impelled in one way or the other and cannot act freely.

A so-called free act, such as Arjuna's desire not to fight the battle, is actually conducted by the material nature through its control of the psyche of the limited being. As Arjuna could not see how he was being compelled by material nature, so many limited persons cannot understand how they are controlled. When told to do something by a higher authority, either by *Śrī* Krishna Himself or by one of Krishna's agents, people generally feel as if they are being forced against their will. But that feeling is really the opposition raised by the energies of material nature. One must sort the potencies in the psyche through the meditations which are taught in *buddhi yoga*. Then one will know what to do and what not to do for advancement.

तमेव शरणं गच्छ
सर्वभावेन भारत ।
तत्प्रसादात्परां शान्तिं
स्थानं प्राप्स्यसि शाश्वतम् ॥१८.६२॥
tameva śaraṇaṁ gaccha
sarvabhāvena bhārata
tatprasādātparāṁ śāntiṁ
sthānaṁ prāpsyasi śāśvatam (18.62)

*tam — to him; eva — only; śaraṇaṁ — shelter; gaccha — go; sarvabhāvena — with all your being; bhārata — O descendant of Bharata; tatprasādāt — from that grace; parāṁ — supreme; śāntiṁ — security; sthānaṁ — place; prāpyasi — you will attain; śāśvatam — eternal*

**With your whole being, go only to Him for shelter, O descendant of Bharata. You will attain the supreme security and the eternal place by His grace. (18.62)**

***Siddha Swami's Commentary:***

Many devotees of *Śrī* Krishna as well as student yogins, took shelter and continue to do so, in this idea of the Supreme Lord being situated in the central psyche. Some say that He is situated in the heart. However most of these persons accept this as a matter of faith in what *Śrī* Krishna told Arjuna, as well as a matter of their own insecurity and need to be in direct touch with the Supreme Being. However until one is able to master *buddhi yoga*, it would not be possible for one to take shelter with such a Supreme Lord. This is true merely because He is not available to those who have little or no perception on the causal level.

*Śrī* Krishna advised Arjuna to go to that Supreme Lord who is in the central psyche, and by whose mystic power the souls move here and there in these creations. But that Lord is not a physical manifestation. One cannot go to him physically or mentally by imagination of his location in the central psyche. One has to have mystic vision of the causal body, before one can reach Him. Thus this statement and the one in the previous verse, does not apply to most devotees.

इति ते ज्ञानमाख्यातं
गुह्याद्गुह्यतरं मया ।
विमृश्यैतदशेषेण
यथेच्छसि तथा कुरु ॥ १८.६३ ॥
iti te jñānamākhyātaṁ
guhyādguhyataraṁ mayā
vimṛśyaitadaśeṣeṇa
yathecchasi tathā kuru (18.63)

*iti — thus; te — to you; jñānam — information; ākhyātaṁ — was explained; guhyāt — than secret; guhyataraṁ — more secret; mayā — by me; vimṛśyaitat = vimṛśya — having considered + etat — this; aśeṣena — fully; yathecchasi = yathā — as + icchasi — you desire, you please; tathā — in the way; kuru — act*

**The information that is more secret than secret was explained by Me to you. Having considered this fully, you may act as you please. (18.63)**

***Siddha Swami's Commentary:***

This information about one's affiliation to material nature and its forces which may cause one to act in one way now and in a contrary way in the future, as well as the alternative influence coming from the Supreme Lord Who is situated in the central psyche, is more secret than secret. It is the most private information that may be given to anyone about himself or herself. After getting this information one should learn *buddhi yoga*.

In Arjuna's case the Supreme Lord was located physically as the chariot driver. That same Lord was located within his psyche. That same Lord was located as the Central Person in the apparition of the Universal Form. And that same Lord manifested the divine four-handed form to Arjuna as well. But others do not have those facilities. For others, it will be their spiritual teacher, this *Bhagavad Gītā* discourse, and their advancement through *buddhi yoga* practice. It is that advancement which will bring others to directly perceive their affiliation with material nature and their relationship with the Supreme Being.

सर्वगुह्यतमं भूयः
शृणु मे परमं वचः ।
इष्टोऽसि मे दृढमिति
ततो वक्ष्यामि ते हितम् ॥ १८.६४ ॥
sarvaguhyatamaṁ bhūyaḥ
śṛṇu me paramaṁ vacaḥ
iṣṭo'si me dṛḍhamiti
tato vakṣyāmi te hitam (18.64)

*sarvaguhyatamaṁ — of all, the most secret; bhūyaḥ — again; śṛṇu — hear; me — of me; paramaṁ — supreme; vacaḥ — discourse; iṣṭo = iṣṭaḥ — loved; 'si = asi — you are; me — of me; dṛḍham — surely; iti — this; tato = tataḥ — hence; vakṣyāmi — I will speak; te — your; hitam — benefit*

**Hear again of My supreme discourse, the most secret of all information. You are surely loved by Me. Hence I speak for your benefit. (18.64)**

***Siddha Swami's Commentary:***

This is Arjuna's personal qualification in his relationship with *Śrī* Krishna. We admire Arjuna for this.

मन्मना भव मद्भक्तो
मद्याजी मां नमस्कुरु ।
मामेवैष्यसि सत्यं ते
प्रतिजाने प्रियोऽसि मे ॥ १८.६५ ॥

*manmanā — be mindful of me; bhava — be; madbhakto = madbhaktaḥ — devoted to me; madyājī — sacrifice to Me; māṁ — to me; namaskuru — do bow; mām — to me; evaiṣyasi =*

manmanā bhava madbhakto
madyājī māṁ namaskuru
māmevaiṣyasi satyaṁ te
pratijāne priyo'si me (18.65)

*eva — in this way + eṣyasi — you will come; satyaṁ — in truth; te — to you; pratijāne — I promise; priyo = priyaḥ — dear; 'si = asi — you are; me — of me*

**Be mindful of Me, be devoted to Me. Sacrifice to Me. Do bow to Me. In this way you will in truth come to Me. I promise for you are dear to Me. (18.65)**

***Siddha Swami's Commentary:***

*Śrī* Krishna issued a promise to Arjuna, because of Arjuna's dearness *(priyah)* to Krishna. This cannot be used by anyone else, unless such persons are told the same by *Śrī* Krishna.

सर्वधर्मान्परित्यज्य
मामेकं शरणं व्रज ।
अहं त्वा सर्वपापेभ्यो
मोक्षयिष्यामि मा शुचः ॥१८.६६॥
sarvadharmānparityajya
māmekaṁ śaraṇaṁ vraja
ahaṁ tvā sarvapāpebhyo
mokṣayiṣyāmi mā śucaḥ (18.66)

*sarvadharmān — all traditional conduct; parityajya — abandoning; mām — in me; ekam — alone; śaraṇaṁ — refuge; vraja — lake; aham — I; tvā — you; sarvapāpebhyo = sarvapāpebhyaḥ — from all sins, of faults; mokṣayiṣyāmi — I will cause you to be freed; mā — not; śucaḥ — worry*

**Abandoning all traditional conduct, take refuge in Me alone. I will cause you to be freed of all faults. Do not worry. (18.66)**

***Siddha Swami's Commentary:***

This pledge by *Śrī* Krishna is given to Arjuna alone. No one should confiscate this pledge for himself or herself or for disciples or any other person. This pledge is to be appreciated, as a promise given to the dear friend of *Śrī* Krishna, the dear devotee Arjuna.

इदं ते नातपस्काय
नाभक्ताय कदाचन ।
न चाशुश्रूषवे वाच्यं
न च मां योऽभ्यसूयति ॥१८.६७॥
idaṁ te nātapaskāya
nābhaktāya kadācana
na cāśuśrūṣave vācyaṁ
na ca māṁ yo'bhyasūyati (18.67)

*idaṁ — this; te — of you; nātapaskāya = na — not + atapaskāya — to one who does not perform austerity; nābhaktāya = na — not + abhaktāya — to one who is not devoted; kadācana — at any time; na — not; cāśuśrūṣave = ca — and + aśuśrūṣave — one who does not desire to hear; vācyaṁ — what is to be said; na — not; ca — and; mām — me; yo = yaḥ— who; 'bhyasūyati = abhyasūyati — is critical*

**This should not be told by you to anyone who does not perform austerity or is not devoted at anytime, or does not desire to hear what is said or is critical of Me. (18.67)**

***Siddha Swami's Commentary:***

*Śrī* Krishna prohibited Arjuna from giving this guarantee to others who did not qualify according to these stipulations. *Śrī* Krishna never said that this was to be given out to others by modern spiritual masters. Arjuna alone was given the instruction to restrict the persons whom he would share the relationship with *Śrī* Krishna. The restrictions given in this verse are:

1. The person must perform austerity as *Śrī* Krishna explained in the *Bhagavad Gītā*.
2. The person must be devoted to *Śrī* Krishna and must not offend *Śrī* Krishna's Universal Form. He or she must not resist or be defiant to the Universal Form.

3. The person must desire to hear of *Śrī* Krishna from authorized sources which are consistent with this discourse with Arjuna.
4. The person must not be critical of *Śrī* Krishna but must be submissive to what *Śrī* Krishna stated.

य इदं परमं गुह्यं
मद्भक्तेष्वभिधास्यति ।
भक्तिं मयि परां कृत्वा
मामेवैष्यत्यसंशयः ॥१८.६८॥
ya idaṁ paramaṁ guhyaṁ
madbhakteṣvabhidhāsyati
bhaktiṁ mayi parāṁ kṛtvā
māmevaiṣyatyasaṁśayaḥ (18.68)

*ya — who; idam — this; paramam — supreme; guhyam — secret; madbhakteṣu — to my devotees; abhidhāsyati — he will explain; bhaktiṁ — devotion; mayi — to me; parām — highest; kṛtvā — having performed; mām — me; evaiṣyati = eva — indeed + eṣyati — he will come; asaṁśayaḥ — without a doubt, certainly*

**Whosoever, having performed the highest devotion to Me, will explain this supreme secret to My devotees, will certainly come to Me. (18.68)**

***Siddha Swami's Commentary:***

After speaking personally and directly to Arjuna, *Śrī* Krishna spoke to those persons who are His greatest devotees by virtue of having performed the highest devotion to Him *(bhaktim mayi parām)*. He guaranteed that they would come to Him, if they explained this supreme secret about the influence of material nature. This supreme secret mentioned is not devotional service or devotion to *Śrī* Krishna but rather what was explained to Arjuna in texts 50 through 62, which includes the way to reach a spirituality which is the highest:

*siddhiṁ prāpto yathā brahma tathāpnoti nibodha me*
*samāsenaiva kaunteya niṣṭhā jñānasya yā parā (18.50)*

***Learn from Me briefly, O son of Kuntī, how a person who attained perfection, also reaches a spirituality which is the highest. (18.50)***

न च तस्मान्मनुष्येषु
कश्चिन्मे प्रियकृत्तमः ।
भविता न च मे तस्माद्
अन्यः प्रियतरो भुवि ॥१८.६९॥
na ca tasmānmanuṣyeṣu
kaścinme priyakṛttamaḥ
bhavitā na ca me tasmād
anyaḥ priyataro bhuvi (18.69)

*na — not; ca — and; tasmān — than this person; manuṣyeṣu — among human beings; kaścit — anyone; me — of me; priyakṛttamaḥ = priyaḥ — pleasing + kṛttamaḥ — more in performance; bhavitā — he will be; na — not; ca — and; me — to me; tasmāt — than this person; anyaḥ — other; priyataro = priyataraḥ — more dear; bhuvi — on earth*

**And no one among human beings is more pleasing to Me in performance than he. And no one on earth will be more dear to Me than he, (18.69)**

***Siddha Swami's Commentary:***

It is clear here that anyone who is very dear to *Śrī* Krishna and explains the secrets mentioned in texts 50 through 62 to student devotees of *Śrī* Krishna, is the most dear person to the Lord.

अध्येष्यते च य इमं
धर्म्यं संवादमावयोः ।
ज्ञानयज्ञेन तेनाहम्
इष्टः स्यामिति मे मतिः ॥१८.७०॥
adhyeṣyate ca ya imaṁ
dharmyaṁ saṁvādamāvayoḥ
jñānayajñena tenāham
iṣṭaḥ syāmiti me matiḥ (18.70)

*adhyeṣyate — he will study; ca — and; ya — who; imaṁ — this; dharmyaṁ — sacred; saṁvādam — conversation; āvayoḥ — of ours; jñānayajñena — by the sacrifice of his knowledge; tenāham = tena — by him + aham — I; iṣṭaḥ — loved; syām — I should be; iti — thus; me — my; matiḥ — opinion*

**I would be loved by the devotee who by sacrifice of his knowledge, will study this sacred conversation of ours. This is My opinion. (18.70)**

***Siddha Swami's Commentary:***

Whosoever forgoes the material existence, switches off the normal track of pursuing status and prosperity in the material world and takes to studying and applying what *Śrī* Krishna taught in the *Bhagavad Gītā*, will be loving *Śrī* Krishna and will become accelerated in spiritual progression by the Lord's grace.

श्रद्धावाननसूयश्च
श्रृणुयादपि यो नरः ।
सोऽपि मुक्तः शुभाँल्लोकान्
प्राप्नुयात्पुण्यकर्मणाम् ॥१८.७१॥
śraddhāvānanasūyaśca
śṛṇuyādapi yo naraḥ
so'pi muktaḥ śubhāṁllokān
prāpnuyātpuṇyakarmaṇām (18.71)

*śraddhāvān — with confidence; anasūyaśca = anasūyaḥ — without ridiculing + ca — and; śṛṇuyāt — he should hear; api — even; yo = yaḥ — who; naraḥ — the person; so = saḥ — he; 'pi = api — also; muktaḥ — freed; śubhān — happy; lokān — worlds; prāpnuyāt — he should attain; puṇyakarmaṇām = punya — pious + karmaṇām — of actions*

**Even the person who hears with confidence, without ridiculing is freed. He should attain the happy worlds where persons of pious actions reside. (18.71)**

***Siddha Swami's Commentary:***

*Śrī* Krishna will give a privileged future life to those who merely hear with confidence and do not ridicule the *Bhagavad Gītā* discourse. Such persons would in the future be freed. But their first attainment would be the association with the pious persons who live in the happy heavenly worlds.

कच्चिदेतच्छ्रुतं पार्थ
त्वयैकाग्रेण चेतसा ।
कच्चिदज्ञानसंमोहः
प्रनष्टस्ते धनंजय ॥१८.७२॥
kaccidetacchrutaṁ pārtha
tvayaikāgreṇa cetasā
kaccidajñānasaṁmohaḥ
pranaṣṭaste dhanaṁjaya (18.72)

*kaccit — has it?; etat — this; śrutaṁ — was heard; pārtha — son of Pṛthā; tvayaikāgreṇa = tvayā — by you + ekāgreṇa — by one-pointed; cetasā — by mind; kaccit — has it?; ajñānasaṁmohaḥ = ajñāna — ignorance + saṁmohaḥ — confusion; pranaṣṭaḥ — removed; te — your; dhanaṁjaya — conqueror of wealthy countries*

**Was this heard by you, O son of Pṛthā, with a one-pointed mind? Was your ignorance and confusion removed, O conqueror of wealthy countries? (18.72)**

***Siddha Swami's Commentary:***

Arjuna asked questions. He got full answers from the Lord of the creation, *Śrī* Krishna.

अर्जुन उवाच
नष्टो मोहः स्मृतिर्लब्धा
त्वत्प्रसादान्मयाच्युत ।
स्थितोऽस्मि गतसंदेहः
करिष्ये वचनं तव ॥ १८.७३ ॥
arjuna uvāca
naṣṭo mohaḥ smṛtirlabdhā
tvatprasādānmayācyuta
sthito'smi gatasaṁdehaḥ
kariṣye vacanaṁ tava (18.73)

*arjuna — Arjuna; uvāca — said; naṣṭo = naṣṭaḥ — removed; mohaḥ — confusion; smṛtiḥ — memory; labdhā — retrieved; tvat prasādān = tvat — your + prasādān (prasādāt) — from grace; mayācyuta = mayā — by me + acyuta — O unaffected one; sthito = sthitāḥ — standing; 'smi = asmi — I am; gatasaṁdehaḥ = gatā — gone, cleared away + saṁdehaḥ — doubt; kariṣye — I will execute; vacanaṁ — instruction; tava — your*

**Arjuna said: Through Your grace, the confusion is removed, memory is retrieved by Me, O unaffected one. I stand clear of doubts. I will execute Your instruction. (18.73)**

***Siddha Swami's Commentary:***

Arjuna is convinced of *Śrī* Krishna's supremacy and of the value of following *Śrī* Krishna's directives in day to day affairs. Arjuna agreed to do what *Śrī* Krishna instructed.

संजय उवाच
इत्यहं वासुदेवस्य
पार्थस्य च महात्मनः ।
संवादमिममश्रौषम्
अद्भुतं रोमहर्षणम् ॥ १८.७४ ॥
saṁjaya uvāca
ityahaṁ vāsudevasya
pārthasya ca mahātmanaḥ
saṁvādamimamaśrauṣam
adbhutaṁ romaharṣaṇam (18.74)

*saṁjaya — Sanjaya; uvāca — said; iti — thus; aham — I; vāsudevasya — of the son of Vasudeva; pārthasya — of the son of Pṛthā; ca — and; mahātmanaḥ — great souled one; saṁvādam — talk; imam — this; aśroṣam — I heard; adbhutaṁ — amazing; romaharṣaṇam — causing hair to stand on end*

**Sanjaya said: In this way, I heard this talk of the son of Vasudeva and the great-souled son of Pṛthā. It is amazing. It causes the hairs to stand on end. (18.74)**

***Siddha Swami's Commentary:***

Sanjaya appraised Arjuna as a *mahātmanah*, a great soul. *Śrī* Krishna's conversation and revelation to Arjuna was wonderful indeed. It caused Sanjaya's hairs to stand on end.

व्यासप्रसादाच्छ्रुतवान्
एतद्गुह्यमहं परम् ।
योगं योगेश्वरात्कृष्णात्
साक्षात्कथयतः स्वयम् ॥ १८.७५ ॥
vyāsaprasādācchrutavān
etadguhyamahaṁ param
yogaṁ yogeśvarātkṛṣṇāt
sākṣātkathayataḥ svayam (18.75)

*vyāsaprasādāt = vyāsa — Vyasa + prasādāt — from grace; śrutavān — one who heard; etad — this; guhyam — secret; aham — I; param — supreme; yogaṁ — yoga; yogeśvarāt = yoga — yoga + īśvarāt — from the Lord; kṛṣṇāt — from Krishna; sākṣāt — directly; kathayataḥ — explaining; svayam — himself*

**By the grace of Vyasa, I am the one who heard this secret information of the supreme yoga from the Lord of yoga, Krishna, who Himself explained it directly. (18.75)**

***Siddha Swami's Commentary:***

Sanjaya praised his guru, his spiritual master, for giving him the opportunity to hear the *Bhagavad Gītā* and to see the vision of the Universal Form. It was a prize attainment for Sanjaya to have heard this directly from the mouth of *Śrī* Krishna as it was bestowed on the dear Arjuna.

राजन्संस्मृत्य संस्मृत्य
संवादमिममद्भुतम् ।
केशवार्जुनयोः पुण्यं
हृष्यामि च मुहुर्मुहुः ॥१८.७६॥
rājansaṁsmṛtya saṁsmṛtya
saṁvādamimamadbhutam
keśavārjunayoḥ puṇyaṁ
hṛṣyāmi ca muhurmuhuḥ (18.76)

*rājan — king; saṁsmṛtya saṁsmṛtya — remembering repeatedly; saṁvādam — talk; imam — this; adbhutam — amazing; keśavārjunayoḥ — of Keśava and Arjuna; puṇyaṁ — holy; hṛṣyāmi — I rejoice; ca — and; muhuḥ muhuḥ — again and again*

**O King, remembering repeatedly, this amazing and holy talk between Keśava and Arjuna, I rejoice again and again. (18.76)**

***Siddha Swami's Commentary:***

Sanjaya shared the glories of the Universal Form and four-handed Divine Form with King *Dhṛtarāṣṭra*. Sanjaya became spiritually excited remembering the apparitions.

तच्च संस्मृत्य संस्मृत्य
रूपमत्यद्भुतं हरेः ।
विस्मयो मे महान्राजन्
हृष्यामि च पुनः पुनः ॥१८.७७॥
tacca saṁsmṛtya saṁsmṛtya
rūpamatyadbhutaṁ hareḥ
vismayo me mahānrājan
hṛṣyāmi ca punaḥ punaḥ (18.77)

*tat — this; ca — and; saṁsmṛtya saṁsmṛtya — remembering repeatedly; rūpam— form; atyadbhutaṁ — super-fantastic; hareḥ — of Hari; vismayo = vismayaḥ — astonished; me — my; mahān — great; rājan — O King; hṛṣyāmi — I excitedly rejoice; ca — and; punaḥ punaḥ — again and again*

**And remembering repeatedly that super-fantastic form of Hari, my astonishment is great, O King, and I excitedly rejoice again and again. (18.77)**

यत्र योगेश्वरः कृष्णो
यत्र पार्थो धनुर्धरः ।
तत्र श्रीर्विजयो भूतिर्
ध्रुवा नीतिर्मतिर्मम ॥१८.७८॥
yatra yogeśvaraḥ kṛṣṇo
yatra pārtho dhanurdharaḥ
tatra śrīrvijayo bhūtir
dhruvā nītirmatirmama (18.78)

*yatra — wherever; yogeśvaraḥ — the Lord of yoga; kṛṣṇo = kṛṣṇaḥ — Kṛṣṇa; yatra — wherever; pārtho = pārthaḥ — son of Pṛthā; dhanurdharaḥ — bowman; tatra — there; śrīḥ — splendor; vijayo = vijayaḥ — victory; bhūtiḥ — prosperity; dhruvā — surely; nītiḥ — morality; matiḥ — opinion; mama — my*

**Wherever there exists the Lord of yoga, Krishna, wherever there is the son of Pṛthā, the bowman, there would surely be splendor, victory, prosperity and morality. This is my opinion. (18.78)**

***Siddha Swami's Commentary:***

Wonderful indeed is *Śrī* Krishna, the Lord of yoga, and the dear Arjuna! Who can stand against them?

*OM TAT SAT*

# Concluding Remarks

Siddha Swami *Nityānānda* gave many *techniques* in this text and many clarifications for those on the path of kundalini yoga, *buddhi yoga*, *rāja yoga*, *kriyā yoga*, *ātma yoga*, *brahma yoga*, and all such procedures which deal with reforming the inner nature and making it fit for subtle, super-subtle and spiritual perceptions. I am hopeful that I assisted him to get this information out to those who are in need of it.

When I was in England in 2004, Siddha Swami asked me to do this commentary. At first I was hesitant because I completed two commentaries already. The first was my own and the second was more or less the dictates of *Śrī Bābāji Mahāśaya*. I felt that was enough. However, under the prompting of Siddha Swami, I took up this writing. Sometimes he was in my subtle head dictating what should be written and what angle the verse should be regarded from. Sometimes he was sitting beside me using a body made of sunlight.

Now that this is completed, I feel happy to serve him as a human microphone. I lost nothing. In fact, I gained immensely and got clarification on some of my own experiences in the *kriyā yoga* and *brahma yoga* approaches to self-realization.

Siddha Swami is well known in the siddha loka places which I visited thus far. He is jovial. He is a great accomplished master without pretence or arrogance. He once told me that those who perform *agnihotra* fire sacrifices and other types of religious ceremony with fussing and colors, are being childish. He compared them to persons who while sitting on an ant hill, extract sugar-cane juice while being covered with stinging ants.

"Of course," he said, "they get some juice from the cane, but later, time will tell, when the ants position themselves on their bodies and the leading ant gives the signal. At that time, they will wiggle all over in pain."

"Advise everyone," he told me, "to learn *kriyā yoga* immediately. Then advance into *brahma yoga*. That is the real juice."

# Regarding the English Translation

The writer took assistance from many translations of the *Gītā*. Notably are Winthrop Sargeant's *The Bhagavad Gītā* (State University of New York Press) from which we noted his exact grammar-oriented Sanskrit vocabulary. We also noted the translation of *Śrīla* Bhaktivedanta Swami's *Bhagavad Gītā As It Is* (Bhaktivedanta Book Trust) and *Śrīdhara* Deva Gosvami's *The Hidden Treasure of the Sweet Absolute* (*Śrī* Chaitanya Saraswat Math, India) as well as *Śrī* Swami Sachidananda's *The Living Gītā* (Henry Holt and Co., New York) and Dr. Ramanand Prasad's *Bhagavad Gītā* (Motilal Banarsidass Publishers, India), as well as many others.

# Indexed Names of Arjuna

anagha — blameless one, good man, 3.3

anagha — sinless one, 14.6

Arjuna -- third son of King Pāndu and Queen Kuntī, cousin of Lord Krishna, 1.4; 2.1,4,54; 2.68; 3.1,7,36; 4.4,5,9,37; 5.1; 6.16,32,33,37; 6.46; 7.16; 8.1,16; 10.32,37,39,42; 11.1,36,50,51,54; 13.1; 18.73,76

bhaktaḥ — devoted person, 4.3

bhārata — man of the Bharata family, descendant of Bharata, 2.18,30; 3.25; 4.7,42; 7.27; 11.6; 13.3,34; 14.3,8,9,10; 15.19,20; 16.3; 17.3; 18.36,62

bharatarṣabha — powerful son (strong man) of the Bharatas, bullish man of the Bharata family, 7.11,16; 8.23; 13.27; 14.12

bharataśreṣṭha — best of the Bharatas, 17.12

dehabhṛtām vara — best of the embodied souls, 8.4

dhanaṁjayaḥ — conqueror of wealthy countries, 1.15; 7.7;.11.14; 18.29,72

dhanurdharaḥ — bowman, 18.78

guḍākeśa — the thick-haired baron, conqueror of sleep, 1.24, 11.7

kapidhvajaḥ — the man with a monkey insignia (*Hanumān*), 1.20

kaunteya — son of Kuntī (Pṛthā),1.27; 2.14,21,60; 3.37; 5.22; 6.35; 7.8; 8.16; 9.7,10,23,27,31; 13.2; 14.4; 16.20,22; 18.50,60

kurunandana — dear son of the Kurus,2.41,48; 6.43, 14.13

kurupravīra — great hero of the Kurus, 11.48

kurusattama — best of the Kurus., 4.31

kuruśreṣṭha — best of the Kuru clan, 10.19

mahābāho — powerful man, 3.28,43; 5.3; 10.1; 14.5; 18.13

pāṇḍava — son of Pāndu, 1.14; 4.35; 6.2; 11.13,55; 12.1; 14.21,22; 16.5; 17.1, 18.1,9,34,61

paraṁtapa — burner of enemy forces, scorcher of enemies, 4.2,5; 11.51

pārtha — son of Pṛthā (Kuntī), 1.25,26; 2.3,32,39,42,55,72; 3.16,22,23; 4.11,33; 6.40; 7.1,10; 8.8,14,19,22,27; 9.32; 10.24; 11.5,9; 12.7; 16.4,6; 17.26,28; 18.6,31,33,72,78

puruṣarṣabha — bull among men, 2.15

puruṣavyāghra — tiger among men, 18.4

sakhā — friend, 4.3

savyasācin — ambidextrous archer, 11.33

tāta — ideal one, 6.40

# Indexed Names of Krishna

acyuta, infallible one, 11.42
adhyātma, Supreme Spirit, 15.5
ādidevaḥ, first God, 11.38
ādidevamajaṁ, Primal God, 10.12
ādikartre, original creator, 11.37
ādyaṁ, primal person, 11.31
ajam, birthless, 10.12
akṣaraṁ, imperishable basis of energies, 11.37
akṣaraṁ paramaṁ, indestructible Supreme Person, 11.18
anādimadhyāntam, Person without beginning, middle or ending, 11.19
ananta deveśa, infinite Lord of the gods, 11.37
anantabāhuṁ, Person with unlimited arms, 11.19
anantarūpa, Person of Infinite Form, 11.38
anantavīryam, Person with infinite manly power, 11.19
anumantā, permitter, 13.23
aprameyam, one who is boundless, 11.42
apratimaprabhāva, person of incomparable splendor, 11.43
asat, sum total temporary existence, 11.37
atyadbhutaṁ hareḥ, super-fantastic form of Hari, 18.77
bhagavān (śrī bhagavān), the Blessed Lord, 2.2,11,55; 3.3,37; 4.1,5;
5.2; 6.1,35,40; 7.1; 8.3; 9.1; 10.1,14,17,19;
11.5,32,47,52; 12.2; 13.2; 14.1,22; 15.1; 16.1; 17.2; 18.2
bhartā, supporter, 13.23
bhavantam, Your lordship, 11.31
bhavānugrarūpo, respected person of terrible form, 11.31
bhoktā, experiencer, 13.23
bhūtabhāvana, one who sustains the existence of all others, 10.15
bhūteśa, Lord of created beings, 10.15
caturbhujena, person with four arms, 11.46
devadeva, God of the gods, 10.15
devam, God, 11.11,14,15,44,45
devavara, best of the gods, 11.31
deveśa (deva-īśa), Lord of all lords, 11.25,45
dīptahutāśavaktraṁ,
Person with the blazing oblation-eating mouth, 11.19
govinda, chief of cowherds, 1.32, 2.9
hariḥ, Hari, the God Vishnu, 11.9; 18.77
hṛṣīkeśa, Master of the sense organs, 1.15,18,24; 18.1
īśam īḍyam, Lord who is to be praised, 11.44
īśvaraḥ, Lord, 4.6

jagannivāsa (jagat-nivāsa),
refuge of the worlds, 11.25
resort of the world, 11.37
shelter of the world, 11.45
jagatpate, Lord of the universe, 10.15
janārdana, motivator of human beings, 1.38;43; 3.1; 11.51
kālo (kālah), time-limit, 11.32
kamalapatrākṣa, Person whose eyes are shaped like lotus petals,11.2
keśava, pretty-haired one, 2.54; 10.14; 11.35; 13.29; 15.17;18.61,75,76
keśiniṣūdāna, slayer of Keshi, 18.1
kṛṣṇa, person with blackish complexion 1.28,31; 6.34,37,39;
11.35,41; 17.1; 18.75,78
kṣetrajñam (sarva), experiencer of all living spaces, 13.3
mādhava, descendant of Madhu, 1.36
madhusūdana, slayer of Madhu,1.34; 2.1; 6.33; 8.2
mahābāho, mighty-armed Person, 11.23
mahātma, great personality, 11.20,37
mahātmanaḥ, great personality, 11.12
mahāyogeśvaro, the great master of yoga, 11.9
maheśvara, Supreme Lord, 5.29,13.23
mahīpate, Lord of the earth 1.21
paraṁ brahma, supreme reality, 10.12
paraṁ dhāma,
supreme refuge, 10.12
ultimate sanctuary, 11.38
paraṁ nidhānam, ultimate shelter, 11.18
paramātmā, Supreme Soul, Supreme Spirit, 13.32,15.17
parameśvara, Supreme Lord, 11.3; 13 28
pavitraṁ paramaṁ, 10.12
prabho (prabhuḥ), respected Lord, 5.14; 11.4; 14.21
prapitāmahaḥ, father of Brahmā, 11.39
pūjyaḥ guruḥ garīyān, gravest spiritual master, 11.43
puruṣaḥ paraḥ, highest spirit, 13.23
puruṣaḥ purāṇaḥ, most ancient spirit, 11.38
puruṣaṁ śāśvataṁ divyam, eternal divine person, 10.12
puruṣottama, Supreme Person, 11.3; 10.15; 15.18,19
rūpaṁ, God-form, 11.45
sahasrabāho, O thousand-armed person, 11.46
sanātanas puruṣo, most ancient person,11.18
śaśisūryanetram, Person who has sun and moon as eyes , 11.19
śāśvatadharmagoptā, eternal guardian of law, 11.18
sat, sum total permanent life, 11.37
svatejasā viśvamidaṁ tapantam,
Person heating this universe with splendor, 11.19
tatparaṁ, that which is beyond, 11.37
upadraṣṭā, observer, 13.23
vārṣṇeya, clansman of the Vṛṣṇis, 1.40

vāsudevasya, of the son of Vasudeva, 7.19; 11.50; 18.74
vibhum (vibhuḥ), Almighty God, whose influence spreads everywhere, 5.15; 10.12
viṣṇo, Lord Viṣṇu, 11.24,30
viśvamūrte,person of universal dimensions, 11.46
viśvarūpa, form of everything, 11.16
viśvasya paraṁ nidhānam, supreme refuge of all the worlds, 11.38
viśveśvara, Lord of all, 11.16
yādava, family man of the Yadus, 11.41
yogeśvara,
    Lord of yoga disciplines, 18.75,78
    Master of yoga technique, 11.4
*yogin*, mystic master, 10.17

# Names, Places and Things


Ādityas, 10.21
Agni, 10.23; 11.39
Airāvata, 10.27
Ananta, 10.29
Anantavijaya, 1.16
Arjuna,
--see Indexed Names of Arjuna
Aryamā, 10.29
Ashvattha, 10.26
Asita, 10.13
Aśvatthāmā, 1.8
Bhīma, 1.4,10,15
Bhishma, 1.8,10,25; 2.4; 11.26,34
Bhrigu, 10.25
Brahmā, 3.10; 8.16-19; 9.7; 10.33; 11.15,37,39
Brihaspati, 10.24
Cekitāna, 1.5
Chitraratha, 10.26
Dānavāḥ, 10.14
Danu, 10.14
Devadatta, 1.15
Devala, 10.13
Dhātā, 10.33
Dhṛṣṭadyumna, 1.17
Dhṛṣṭaketu, 1.5
Dhṛtarāṣṭra, 1.1,19,20,23
Dhṛti, 10.34
Diti, 10.30
Draupadī,1.6,18
Droṇa, 1.25; 2.4; 11.26,34
Drupada, 1.3,4,18
Duryodhana, 1.2,12
dvijottama, 1.7
Gāṇḍīva, 1.29
Gayatri, 10.35
Hanumān (kapi), 1.20
Hari, 11.9; 18.77
Himalayas, 10.25
Ikṣvāku, 4.1
Indra, 10.22
Jahnu, 10.31
Jayadratha, 11.34
Kamadhuk, 10.28
Kandarpa, 10.28
kapi, 1.20
Kapila, 10.26
Karṇa, 1.8; 11.34
Kāśi, 1.5,17
Kīrti, 10.34
Krishna,
- see Indexed Names of Krishna
Kṣamā, 10.34
Kubera, 10.23
Kuntī, 1.16; 13.2
Kuntibhoja, 1.5
Kuru, 1.12,25
kurukṣetre, 1.1
Manipushpaka, 1.16
Manu, 4.1
Marīci, 10.21
Medhā, 10.34
Meru, 10.23
Nakula, 1.16
Nārada, 10.13
narapuṁgavaḥ, 1.5
Pāñcajanya, 1.15
Pandava, 1.2
Pāndu, 1.1,3
Paundra, 1.15
Pavāka, 10.23
Prahlāda, 10.30
Purujit, 1.5
Rāma, 10.31
Rudra, 10.23
Sādhya, 11.22
Sahadeva, 1.16
Śaibya, 1.5
Sāma Veda chants, 10.35
Sāṁkhya, 5.5
Sanjaya, 1.1,2,24; 18.74
Śāśaṅka, 11.39
Sātyaki, 1.17
Shankara, 10.23
Shiva, 10.23
Śikhandī, 1.17
Skanda, 10.24
Smṛti, 10.34
Somadatta, 1.8
Śrī, 10.34
Subhadra, 1.6,18
Sughosha, 1.16
Uccaihśrava, 10.27
Ushana, 10.37
Uttamauja, 1.6
Vaiśvāanara, 15.2
Vajra, 10.28
Vāk, 10.34
Varuṇa, 10.29; 11.39
Vasava, 10.22
Vasudeva, 7.19; 10.37
Vasuki, 10.28
Vasus,11.22
Vāyu, 11.39
Vikarṇa, 1.8
Vinata, 10.30
Virāṭa, 1.4,17
Vishnu, 10.21; 11.9,24,30
Vishvadevas, 11.22
Vitteśaḥ, 10.23
Vivasvat, 4.1,4
Vṛṣṇis, 1.40, 10.36
Vyāsa, 10.13
Vyāsa, 10.37; 18.75
Yakshas, 10.23
Yama, 10.29, 11.39
Yudhamanyu, 1.6
Yudhishthira,1.16
Yuyudhāna, 1.4

# Index To Verses: Selected Sanskrit Words

## A


ā, 8.16
abhāvayataḥ, 2.66
abhāvo, 2.16
abhipravṛttaḥ, 4.20
abhyāsena, 6.35,44; 8.8;12.9
abhyasūyanto, 3.32
abhyutthānam, 4.7
abuddhayaḥ, 7.24
acalapratiṣṭhaṁ, 2.70
ācaratyātmanaḥ, 16.22
ācāryam, 1.2
ācāryopāsanaṁ, 13.8
acchedyo, 2.24
acetasaḥ, 3.32
acintya, 2,25; 8.9
acireṇādhigacchati, 4.39
adharma, 1.39,40; 4.7; 18.32
ādhāyātmanaḥ, 8.12
adhibhūtaṁ, 8.1,4
adhidaivaṁ, 8.1
adhipatyam, 2.8
adhiṣṭhānam, 3.40; 18.14
adhiṣṭhāya, 4.6
adhiyajñaḥ, 7.30; 8.2,4
adhyātma, 7.29; 13.12
adhyeṣyate, 18.70
ādidevamajaṁ, 10.12
ādityavaj, 5.16
ādityavarṇaṁ, 8.9
ādyantavantaḥ, 5.22
agatāsūṁś, 2.11
aghāyurindriyārāmo, 3.16
āgnidagdha, 4,19
agnirjyotirahaḥ, 8.24
ahaṁ sarvasya, 10.8
ahaṁkāraṁ,16.18
ahaṁkāraṁ balaṁ , 18.53
ahaṁkāravimūḍhā, 3.27
āhārāḥ, 17.8
ahiṁsā, 10.5; 16.2
ahoratra, 8.17
ajānantaḥ, 7.24
ajñānaṁ, 3.26
ajñānasaṁbhūtaṁ, 4.42
ajñānenāvṛtaṁ, 5.15
ajo, 4.6
akarmakṛt, 3.5
akarmaṇi, 4.18
akartāram, 4.13
ākāśaṁ, 13.33
akhilam, 7.29
ākhyāhi me ko bhavānugrarūpo, 11.31
akīrtikaram, 2.2
akṣara, 3.15; 8.3,11,21; 15.18
akṣayam, 5.21
alpamedhasām, 7.23
ambhasi, 2.67
amṛta, 2.15; 9.19
anabhisnehas,2.57
anādimatparaṁ, 13.13
anāditvānnirguṇa, 13.32
anahaṁkāra, 13.9
anāmayam, 2.51
anantaṁ, 11.11
ananyacetāḥ, 8.14
ananyamanasaḥ, 9.13
anapekṣya, 18.25
anāryajuṣṭam, 2.2
anāśino, 2.18
anasūyantaḥ, 3.31
anāvṛttim, 8.23
anekacittavibhrāntā, 16.16
anekajanma, 6.45
anekavaktra, 11.10
aniṣṭamiṣṭaṁ, 18.12
anīśvaram, 16.8
aṇīyāṁsam, 8.9
annādbhavanti, 3.14
antakāle, 8.5
antarātmanā, 6.47
anubandhaṁ, 18.25
anucintayan, 8.8
anudvegakaraṁ, 17.15
anusmaran, 8.13
anuśocanti, 2.11
anuśocitum, 2.25
anuśuśruma, 1.43
apahṛta, 2.44
apāne juhvati, 4.29
aparaṁ bhavato, 4.4
apare niyatāhārāḥ, 4.30
apareyamitastvanyāṁ, 7.5
aprameyasya, 2.18
apratiṣṭho, 6.38
apunarāvṛttiṁ, 5.17
āpūryamāṇam, 2.70
arāgadveṣataḥ, 18.23
ārjavam, 16.1
arpitamanobuddhir, 8.7
ārurukṣormuner, 6.3
asaktir, 13.10
asaṁśayaṁ, 6.35; 7.1; 8.7
asaṁyatātmanā, 6.36
asaṅgaśastreṇa, 15.3
asatas, 2.16
asito devalo vyāsaḥ, 10.13
aśraddadhānāḥ,4.40; 9.3
aśraddhayā, 17.28
aśru, 2.1
asvargyam, 2.2
aśvinau, 11.6
atīndriyam, 6.21
ātiṣṭhottiṣṭha, 4.42
atisvapna, 6.16
ātmabuddhiprasāda, 18.37
ātmānaṁ mat , 9.34
ātmanātmānaṁ, 6.5; 13.29
ātmanyevātmanā, 2.55
ātmasaṁbhāvitāḥ, 16.17
ātmasaṁsthaṁ, 6.25
ātmasaṁyamayogā, 4.27
ātmaśuddhaye, 5.11
ātmatṛptaśca, 3.17
ātmaupamyena, 6.32
ātmavān, 2.45
ātmavantaṁ, 4.41
ātmavaśyair, 2.64
ātmikā, 2.43
avabodhasya, 6.17
avadhyaḥ, 2.30
avaśaṁ, 9.8
avaśiṣyate, 7.2
avatiṣṭhate, 6.18
avibhaktaṁ, 13.17; 18.20
avidhipūrvakam, 9.23
avidvāṁas, 3.25
avināśi, 2.17
āvṛtam, 3.38,39
āvṛttiṁ, 8.23
avyaktaḥ, 2.25,28; 7.24; 12.3

avyaktāsaktacetasām, 12.5
avyavasāyinām, 2.41
avyaya,2.17; 7.24
avyayātmā, 4.6
ayajñasya, 4.31
āyuḥsattvabalārogya, 17.8
ayuktasya, 2.66

# B

bahumataḥ, 2.35
bahūnāṁ janma, 7.19
bahūni me vyatītāni, 4.5
bahuśākhā, 2.41
bahuvidhā, 4.32
balavaddṛḍham, 6.34
balavānsukhī, 16.14
bandhurātmātmanas, 6.6
Bhagavānmayā, 10.17
Bhagavānvyaktiṁ, 10.14
bhaikṣyam, 2.5
bhakta, 9 23,31; 12.1,20
bhaktiṁ mayi, 18.68
bhaktimānme, 12.19
bhaktimānyaḥ sa, 12 17
bhaktiyogena, 14.26
bhakto'si me sakhā, 4.3
bhaktyā, 8.10,22; 9.29; 11.54; 18.55
bhartā bhoktā , 13.23
bhāṣā, 2.54
bhasmasātkurute, 4.37
bhāvamāśritāḥ, 7.15
bhavantaḥ, 1.11
bhavārjuna, 2.45; 6.46
bhavato, 4.4
bhāvayatā, 3.11
bhinnā, 7.4
bhogā, 1.32; 2.5
bhogaiśvarya, 2.44
bhojanaṁ, 17.10
bhoktā, 9.24
bhoktāraṁ, 5.29
bhoktṛtve, 13.21
bhrāmayansarva, 18.61
bhraṁśāt, 2.63
bhruvoḥ, 5.27; 8.10
bhūmirāpo'nalo, 7.4
bhuñjānaṁ, 15.10
bhuñjate, 3.13
bhuñjīya, 2.5
bhuṅkte, 3.12; 13.22
bhūtabhartṛ, 13.17
bhūtabhāvana, 9.5; 10.15
bhūtabhāvodbhava, 8.3
bhūtabhṛnna, 9.5
bhūtagrāmaḥ, 8.19
bhūtagrāmamimaṁ, 9.8
bhūtamaheśvaram, 9.11
bhūtānāmīśvaro'pi, 4.6
bhūtaprakṛti, 13.35
bhūtapṛthag, 13.31
bhūtasargau, 16.6
bhūteśa, 10.15
bhūtvā, 3.30; 8.19
bījaṁ, 7.10
bījamavyayam, 9.18
boddhavyaṁ, 4.17
brahma, 8.13
brahma brahma , 8.24
brahmabhūto,5.24
brahmabhuvanāl, 8.16
brahmabhūyāya, 14.26; 18.53
brahmacārivrate, 6.14
brahmacaryaṁ, 8.11
brahmacaryama, 17.14
brahmāgnau, 4.24,25
brahmakarma, 18.42
brahmākṣarasamud, 3.15
brahmaṇaḥ, 6.38
brāhmaṇakṣatriya, 18.41
brahmāṇamīśaṁ, 11.15
brahmaṇastri, 17.23
brahmanirvāṇaṁ,2.72; 5.24-26
brahmaṇo hi, 14.27
brahmaṇo mukhe , 4.32
brahmaṇyādhāya, 5.10
brahmārpaṇaṁ, 4.24
brahmasaṁsparśam, 6.28
brahmavādinām, 17.24
brahmavidbrahmaṇi, 5.20
brāhmī sthitiḥ, 2.72
brahmodbhavaṁ, 3.15
buddhibhedaṁ, 3.26
buddhigrāhyamatī , 6.20
buddhiḥ, 2.44
buddhimānmanuṣyeṣu, 4.18
buddhimānsyāt, 15.20
buddhimatām, 7.10
buddhināśo, 2.63
*buddhi*, 2.41,66; 13.6
buddhirbuddhimatām, 7.10
buddhirjñānama, 10.4
buddhirvyatitariṣyati, 2.52
buddhisaṁyogaṁ, 6.43
buddhiyoga, 2.49; 18.57
buddhiyuktā, 2.50,51
buddhvā, 3.43
budhā, 4.19; 10.8

# C

cakraṁ, 3.16
calamadhruvam, 17.18
cañcalatvātsthitiṁ, 6.33
cāndramasaṁ, 8.25
caratāṁ, 2.67
caturbhujena, 11.46
cāturvarṇyaṁ mayā , 4.13
caturvidhā, 7.16
cendriyagocarāḥ, 13.6
cetasā , 8.8
chandāṁsi, 15,1
chinna. 5.25; 18.10
cintayet, 6.25

# D

daiva, 4.25; 16.6
daivī, 7.14
dakṣiṇāyanam, 8.25
dambha,16.17; 17.5
daṁṣṭrākarālāni, 11.25, 27
dānakriyāśca, 17.25
dānavāḥ, 10.14
darśanakāṅkṣiṇaḥ, 11.52
darśayātmānamavyayam, 11.4
dehabhṛtāṁ, 8.4
dehasamudbhavān, 14.20
devabhogān, 9.20
devadvijaguru, 17.14
devān, 3.11; 7.23
devarṣirnāradas, 10.13
dhāma, 8.21
dhārayāmyaham, 15.13
dhārayan, 5.8; 6.13
dhārayate, 18.33
dharma, 1.39; 2.7
dharmakṣetre, 1.2
dharmamadharmaṁ, 18.31
dharmasaṁsthā, 4.8
dharmātmā, 9.31
dharmyaṁ, 9.2; 12.20
dhāryate, 7.5
dhātāhaṁ viśvato , 10.33
dhātāram, 8.9
dhīmatām, 6.42
dhṛtigṛhītayā, 6.25
dhruva, 2.27; 12.3; 18.78
dhūmena, 3.38; 18.48
dhūmo rātristathā, 8.25

dhyānātkarma,12.12
dhyānenātmani, 13.24
dhyāyanta, 12.6
dhyāyataḥ, 2.62
dīpaḥ, 6.19
dīrghasūtrī, 18.28
diśaścānavalokayan, 6.13
divya, 1.14 ; 11.5
doṣa, 1.42; 2.7
dravyas, 4.28, 33
dṛḍhavratāḥ, 7.28, 9.14
dṛṣṭvā lokāḥ, 11.23
dṛṣṭvā rūpaṁ , 11.49
dṛṣṭvādbhutaṁ, 11.20
dṛṣṭvedaṁ, 11.51
duḥkhadoṣā, 13.9
duḥkhahā, 6.17
duḥkhālayam, 8.15
duḥkhaśokāmaya, 17.9
duḥkheṣvanudvigna , 2.56
durāsadam, 3.43
duratyayā, 7.14
durbuddher, 1.23
durgatiṁ, 6.40
durlabhataraṁ, 6.42
durmatiḥ, 18.16
durnigrahaṁ,6.35
duṣkṛtino, 7.15
duṣprāpa, 6.36
duṣpūreṇānalena, 3.39
dvaṁdvamoha, 7.27,28
dvaṁdvātīto, 4.22
dvārāṇi, 8.12
dveṣṭyakuśalaṁ, 18.10
dvididhā, 3.3
dvijottama, 1.7

## E

ekabhaktirviśiṣyate , 7.17
ekākī, 6.10
ekākṣaram, 8.13
ĕśvaraṁ, 11.3

## G

gahanā karmaṇo, 4.17
gāmāviśya, 15.13
gandharva, 10.26; 11.22
gāṇḍīvaṁ, 1.29
garbhas, 3.38
garīyase, 11.37
gatāḥ, 8.15
gataprāṇā, 10.9
gatasaṅgasya, 4.23
gatāsūn, 2.11
gatim, 8.13,21
gāyatrī, 10.33
glānirbhavati, 4.7
grasiṣṇu, 13.17
guhyādguhyataraṁ, 18.63
guhyamadhyātma, 11.1
guhyamahaṁ, 18.75
guhyatamam, 9.1; 15.20
guṇabhedataḥ, 18.19
guṇabhoktṛ, 13.15
guṇakarma, 3.28,29; 4.13
guṇamayī, 7.14
guṇasaṁkhyāne, 18.19
guṇātītaḥ, 14.25
gurūn, 2.5

## H

hānir, 2.65
hantāraṁ, 2.19
hanyamāne, 2.20
hareḥ, 18.77
hariḥ, 11.9
hatam, 2.19
hitakāmyayā, 10.1
hṛdayadaurbalyaṁ, 2.3
hṛddeśe'rjuna, 18.61
hṛtsthaṁ, 4.42
hutam, 4.24

## I

icchā dveṣa,7.27; 13.6
īkṣaṇam, 2.1
indriyāgniṣu, 4.26
indriyagrāmaṁ, 6.24
indriyāṇi mano, 3.40
indriyāṇīndriyā, 2.58, 68
indriyārāmaḥ, 3.16
indriyārtheṣu, 13.9
indriyasyendriyasy, 3.34
iṣṭakāmadhuk, 3.10
iṣṭānbhogānhi, 3.12
īśvaraḥ sarvabhūtānāṁ' 18.61
ivāmbhasi, 2.67

## J

jagadavyaktamūrtinā, 9.4
jagadbhāsayate , 15.12
jagadviparivartate, 9.10
jagannivāsa, 11.25,45
jāgarti, 2.69
jagataḥ, 8.26
jagatkṛtsnaṁ, 11.7,13
jagatpate, 10.15
jaghanyaguṇa, 14.18
jāgrato, 6.16
janakādayaḥ, 3.20
jānan, 8.27
jānāti, 15.19
janma, 2.27
janmabandha, 2.51
janma *karma* ca me, 4.9
janmakarmaphala, 2.43
janmamṛtyujarā, 13.9
janmāni, 4.5
jarāmaraṇamokṣāya, 7.29
jātidharmāḥ, 1.42
jijñāsurapi, 6.44
jitasaṅgadoṣā, 15,5
jitātmanaḥ, 6.7
jīvabhūta, 7.5; 15.7
jñānacakṣuṣa, 13.35; 15.10
jñānadīpena, 10.11
jñānadīpite, 4.27
jñānāgnidagdha, 4.19
jñānāgniḥ, 4.37
jñānaṁ jñeyaṁ , 13.18
jñānamāvṛtya, 3.40; 14.9
jñānamupāśritya, 14.2
jñānamuttamam, 14.1
jñānanirdhūta, 5.17
jñānārthadarśanam, 13.12
jñānasaṅgena, 14.6
jñānāsinātmanaḥ, 4.42
jñānatapasā, 4.10
jñānavānmāṁ, 7.19
jñānāvasthitacetasaḥ, 4.23
jñānavijñāna, 3.41; 6.8
jñānayajña, 4.33; 9.15; 18.70
jñānayoga,3.3; 16.1
jñānī, 3.38,39; .6.46; 7.18
jñāninastattva, 4.34
jñātavyamavaśiṣyate, 7.2
jñeyo'si niyatātmabhiḥ,8.2
juhvati, 4.26,27
jvaraḥ, 3.30
jyotir, 8.24

## K

kālena, 4.2, 38
kalevaram, 8.5
kalmaṣāḥ, 4.30; 5.17
kalpakṣaye, 9.7
kalyāṇakṛtkaścid, 6.40
kāmabhoga, 16.12,16
kāma, 2.5,62; 7.22
kāmahaitukam, 16.8
kāmaistaistairhṛta, 7.20
kāmakāmā, 2,70; 9.21
kāmakārataḥ, 16.23

kāmakāreṇa, 5.12
kāmakrodhaṁ, 5.26
kāmamāśritya, 16.10
kāmarūpa, 3.39,43
kāmātmānaḥ, 2.43
kāmopabhoga, 16.11
kāmyānāṁ, 18.2
kāṅkṣantaḥ, 4.12
kapidhvajaḥ, 1.20
kāraṇaṁ guṇasaṅgo, 13.22
kāraṇamucyate, 6.3
karmabandhaṁ, 2.39
karmabandhana, 3.9; 9.28
karmabhirna sa, 4.14
karmajā, 4.12
karmajaṁ, 2.51
karmajānviddhi, 4.32
karmākhilaṁ, 4.33
karmānubandhīni, 15.2
karmaṇyabhirataḥ, 18.45
karmaṇyakarma, 4.18
karmāṇyaśeṣataḥ, 18.11
karmaṇyatandritaḥ, 3.23
karmaphala, 4.14; 6.1; 18.27
karmaphalahetur, 2.47
karmaphala, 5.14
karmaphalāsaṅgaṁ, 4.20
karmasamādhinā, 4.24
karmasaṁgrahaḥ, 18.18
karmasaṁjñitaḥ, 8.3
karmasaṁnyāsāt, 5.2
karmasaṅga, 3.26; 14.7,15
karmayoga, 3.3'7; 13.24; 5.2
kārpaṇya, 2.7
karśayantaḥ, 17.6
kartāraṁ, 14.19
kāryakāraṇa, 13.21
kāryākārye, 18.30
kaśmalam, 2.2
kauśalam, 2.50
kavim. 8.9
kāyakleśabhayāt , 18.8
kāyaśirogrīvaṁ, 6.13
keśavārjunayoḥ, 18.76
kevalairindriyairapi, 5.11
khaṁ mano buddhir, 7.4
kiṁ tadbrahma , 8.1
kirīṭinaṁ 11.17,46
kīrtayanto, 9.14
klaibyaṁ , 2.3
kleśo'dhikataras, 12.5
kraturahaṁ, 9.16
kriyā, 1.41
kriyābhirna, 11.48
*kriyā*māṇāni, 3.27; 13.30
kriyāviśeṣabahulāṁ, 2.43
krodho, 2.62
kṛpaṇāḥ, 2.49
kṛpayāviṣṭam , 2.1
kṛṣigorakṣya, 18.44
kṛṣṇaḥ, 8.25
kṛtāñjalirabhāṣata, 11.14
kṛtsnakarmakṛt,4.18
kṛtsna, 7.6,29
kṛtsnavin, 3.29
kṣāntirārjavam, 13.8
kṣaraścākṣara, 15.16
kṣātraṁkarma, 18.43
kṣayāya jagato'hitāḥ, 16.9
kṣetrajña iti tadvidaḥ, 13.3
kṣetrakṣetrajña, 13.,27
kṣetrakṣetrajñayor, 13.3,35
kṣetraṁ kṣetrajñam 13.1
kṣetraṁ kṣetrī tathā , 13.34
kṣīṇakalmaṣāḥ, 5.25
kṣipraṁ hi mānuṣe, 4.12
kṣudraṁ, 2.3
kuladharmāḥ , 1.39,42,43
kulaghnānāṁ, 1.41,42
kulasya, 1.41
kurukṣetre , 1.1
kurunandana, 2.41
kutaḥ, 2.66
kūṭastho, 6.8; 15.16


## L


lāghavam, 2.35
lipyate, 5.6
loka, 2.5; 7.25
lobhopahata cetasaḥ, 1.37
lokamaheśvaram, 10.3
lokasaṁgraham, 3.25
lokastadanuvartate, 3.21
lokatrayamāviśya, 15.17
loke janma, 6.42
luptapiṇḍodaka, 1.41


## M


madarpaṇam, 9.26
madasrayah, 7.1
madbhakta, 7.23; 11.55; 12.14; 13.19
madbhakteṣu, 18.68
madbhaktiṁ, 18.54
madbhāva, 4.10; 10.6; 14.19
mādhavaḥ, 1.14
madvyapāśrayaḥ,18.56
madyājī, 9.25,34; 18.65
madyogamāśritaḥ, 12.11
mahadyonir, 14.4
mahāpāpmā, 3.37
mahārathāḥ, 2.35
maharṣī, 10.2,6
mahāśano, 3.37
mahatā, 4.2
mahātmā, 7.19; 8.15; 9.13; 11.12; 18.74
mahatpāpaṁ, 1.44
mahāyogeśvaro, 11.9
maheśvara, 9.11; 13.23
mama māyā, 7.14
mama yo vetti,10.7
māmāśritya, 7.29
māmevānuttamāṁ, 7.18
māmupāśritāḥ, 4.10
manaḥ,6.26; 15.7,9; 17.16
mānasa, 1.46; 17.16
mānāvamānayoḥ, 6.7
manave, 4.1
manīṣiṇām, 18.5
manmanā, 9.34; 18.65
manmayā, 4.10
manogatān,2.55
mantra,9.16; 17.13
manuṣya, 3.23; 7.3; 15.2
manyate, 3.27
mārdavaṁ, 16.2
martyalokaṁ, 9.21
matkarma, 11.54; 12.10
matparaḥ, 6.14; 18.57
matparāyaṇaḥ, 9.34
matprasādāt , 18.58
mātrāsparśās,2.14
matsaṁsthām, 6.15
matsthāni, 9.4
matvā, 3.28
maunamātmaḥ, 17.16
mayādhyakṣeṇa, 9.10
māyayā, 4.6; 7.15
mayi buddhiṁ, 12.8
mayi saṁnyasya , 12.6; 18.57
mayyarpitamano, 8.7
mayyāveśitacetasām, 12.7
mayyāveśya, 12.2
mitrāripakṣayoḥ, 14.25
modiṣya, 16.15
moghaṁ, 3.16
moghāśā, 9.12
mohādārabhyate, 18.25

mohakalilaṁ, 2.52
mohanaṁ, 14.8; 18.39
mohayasi, 3.2
mohinīṁ, 9.12
mohitam, 7.13
mokṣakāṅkṣibhiḥ, 17.25
mokṣaparāyaṇaḥ, 5.28
mokṣayiṣyāmi, 18.66
mokṣyase, 9.1,28
mriyate, 2.20
mṛtyusaṁsāra, 9.3
mucyante, 3.31
mūḍhā, 9.11
mūḍhagrāheṇā, 17.19
mūḍhayoniṣu, 14.15
muhurmuhuḥ, 18.76
muhyati(-yanti),5.15; 8.27
mukhe, 4.32
mukta, 5.28
muktasaṅga, 3.9; 18.26
muktasya, 4.23
mukto yaḥ , 12.16
mumukṣubhiḥ, 4.15
muniḥ, 2.56
munirbrahma, 5.6
munirmokṣa, 5.28
mūrdhny, 8.12
mūrtayaḥ, 14.4

# N

nābhaktāya, 18.67
naiṣkarmya, 3.4; 19.49
naiṣṭhikīm, 5.12
namaskṛtvā, 11.35
namaskuru, 9.34
nānāvarṇākṛtīni, 11.5
narādhama, 7.15; 16.19
narakāya, 1.41,42
nāsābhyantara, 5.27
nāsikāgraṁ, 6.13
nāśitamātmanaḥ, 5.16
nātyaśnatastu,6.16
navadvāre, 5.13
nāvam, 2.67
nibaddhaḥ, 18.60
nibadhnanti, 4.41
nibadhyate, 4.22
nibandhāyāsurī, 16.5
nibodha, 18.13
nidhanaṁ,3.35
nidhanāni, 2.28
nidrālasyapramād, 18.39
nigrahaṁ, 6.34
niḥspṛhaḥ, 2.71; 6.18
niḥśreyasakarāv, 5.2
nirahaṁkāraḥ, 2.71; 12.13
nirāhārasya. 2.59
nirāśīr,3.30; 4.21; 6.10
nirāśrayaḥ, 4.20
nirdeśo, 17.23
nirdhūta, 5.17
nirdoṣaṁ, 5.19
nirdvandvo, 2.45; 5.3
nirguṇaṁ, 13.15
nirmamo, 2.71; 12.13
nirmānamohā, 15.5
nirmuktā, 7.28
nirudhya, 8.12
nirvāṇam, 2.72; 6.15
nirvedaṁ, 2.52
niryogakṣema, 2.45
niścayena, 6.23
niṣṭhā, 3.3
nistraiguṇyaḥ, 2.45
nītirmatirmama, 18.78
nityābhiyuktānāṁ, 9.22
nityajātaṁ, 2.,26
nityaśaḥ, 8.14
nityasaṁnyāsī, 5.3
nityasattvastho, 2.45
nityatṛpto, 4.20
nityavairiṇā,3.39
nityayukta, 7.17; 8.14; 12.2
nivartate, 2.59; 8.25
nivṛttāni, 14.22
niyamya, 3.7,41; 6.26; 18.51
niyatāhārāḥ, 4.30
niyata, 6.15; 8.2;18.7,9
niyojitaḥ, 3.36
niyokṣyati, 18.59
nyāyyaṁ, 18.15

# O

*Om*, 8.13

# P

pacantyātmakāraṇāt, 3.13
padmapatram, 5.10
paṇḍitāḥ, 2.11; 4.19; 5.4,18;
pāpakṛttamaḥ, 4.36
pāpayonayaḥ, 9.32
pāpmānaṁ, 3.41
paradharmā, 3.35; 18.47
paradharmo, 3.35
paraṁ bhūyaḥ , 14.1
paraṁ brahma , 10.12
parāṁ gatim, 6.45
paraṁ janma, 4.4
paramāṁ, 8.13
paramāpnoti, 3.19
paramātmā, 6.7
paramātmety, 15.17
paramavyayam, 7.13
parameśvara, 11.3; 13.28
paramparāprāptam, 4.2
parāṇyāhur, 3.42
parastasmāttu, 8.20
parastāt, 8.9
parataraṁ, 7.7
parāyaṇāḥ, 4.29; 5.17
paricakṣate, 17.17
paridevanā, 2.28
parigrahaḥ, 4.21
parijñātā, 18.18
parikīrtitaḥ, 18.7,27
pariṇāme, 18.38
paripanthinau, 3.34
paripraśnena, 4.34
parisamāpyate, 4.33
paritrāṇāya, 4.8
parjanyāt, 3.14
paryavatiṣṭhate, 2.65
paśya me yogam, 11.8
paśyāmi devāṁ, 11.15
paśyāmi viśveśvara, 11.16
paśyañśṛṇvan, 5.8
paśyantyātmany, 15.11
paśyato, 2.69
patanti, 1.41
patraṁ puṣpaṁ , 9.26
paurvadehikam, 6.43
pavitraṁ,4.38; 9.2; 10.12
phalahetavaḥ, 2.49
phala,2.47; 7.23; 17.21
piṇḍa, 1.41
pitāmahaḥ, 9.17
pitaro, 1.41
pitāsi, 11.43
pitṝnyānti, 9.25
prabhāṣeta, 2.54
prabhavaḥ, 7.6
prabhureva, 9.24
prahasann, 2.10
prāhu, 18.2,3
prajāḥ, 3.10
prajahihyenaṁ, 3.41
prajāpatiḥ, 3.10
prajñā, 2.11,57,58,61,67,68
prakāśa, 7.25,14.6,11,22
prakāśayati, 5.16; 13.34
prakṛteḥ, 3.27,29,33; 9.8
prakṛtijair, 3.5; 18.40

prakṛtiṁ, 9.8; 13.1
prakṛtiraṣṭadhā, 7.4
prakṛtisaṁbhavā, 13.20; 14.5
prakṛtisthāni, 15.7
pralayaṁ, 14.14
pralaya, 7.6; 9.18; 14.2
pralīyante, 8.18,19
pramāda, 11.41; 14.9,17
pramāṇaṁ, 3.21
pramāthīni, 2.60
prāṇakarmāṇi, 4.27
prāṇam,1.33; 8.12
praṇamya, 11.14
prāṇānprāṇeṣu, 4.30
prāṇāpāna, 5.27; 15.14
pranaṣṭaste, 18.72
praṇaśyāmi, 6.30
praṇaśyati, 2.63; 9.31
praṇavaḥ, 7.8
prāṇāyāma, 4.29
prāṇendriyakriyāḥ, 18.33
prāṇe'pānaṁ, 4.29
praṇipātena, 4.34
prapadyante, 4.11; 7.19,20
prapadyate,7.19
prapannam, 2.7
prasāda, 2.64,65; 11.43
prasaktāḥ, 16.16
prasaṅgena, 18.34
prasannacetaso, 2.65
prasannātmā, 18.54
praśānta, 6.7,14,27
prasīda deveśa , 11.45
pratiṣṭhita, 2.57,58,61; 3.15; 6.11
pratyavāyaḥ, 2.40
pravakṣyāmi, 4.16
pravakṣye, 8.11
pravartante'śuci, 16.10
pravartitaṁ, 3.16
praveṣṭuṁ, 11.54
pravilīyate, 4.23
pravṛtti, 14.12;15.4; 16.7; 18.30,46
prayāṇakāle, 7.30; 8.2
prītamanāḥ, 11.49
prītiḥ, 1.35
priya, 5.20; 9.29; 10.1; 11.44;17.15; 18.69
priyaḥ priyāyārhasi , 11.44
priyo hi jñānino, 7.17
proktavān, 4.4
pṛthagvidham, 18.14
pūjanaṁ, 17.14
pūjārhāu, 2.4
punarāvartino'rjuna, 8.16
punarbrāhmaṇāḥ, 9.33
punardhanam, 16.13
punarjanma, 4.9; 8.15,16
punaryogaṁ, 5.1
puṇyakarmaṇām, 7.28
puṇyakṛtām, 6.41
puṇyaphalam, 8.28
puṇyo gandhaḥ , 7.9
purāṇamanuśāsitāram, 8.9
purātanaḥ, 4.3
pūrṇa, 2.1
puruṣaḥ, 8.4,22
puruṣottama, 8.1; 15.18,19
pūrvābhyāsena, 6.44
pūrvaiḥ,4.15
puṣpitāṁ, 2.42

# R

rādhanamīhate, 7.22
rāgadveṣau, 2.64, 3.34; 18.51
rahasi, 4.3; 6.10
rajaḥ karmaṇi, 14.9
rājarṣayaḥ, 4.2
rājavidyā, 9.2
rajoguṇa, 3.37
ramanti, 10.9
ramate, 5.22
ratāḥ, 5.25, 12.4
rātri, 8.17,18,25
ripurātmanaḥ, 6.5
ṛksāma, 9.17
romaharṣa, 1.29; 18.74
ṛṣibhirbahudhā, 13.4
ruddhvā, 4.29
rudhirapradigdhān, 2.5
rūpaṁ paraṁ, 11.47
rūpamaiśvaram, 11.9
rūpamatyadbhutaṁ, 18.77

# S

śabdabrahm, 6.44
śabdādīnviṣayān, 4.26
śabdaḥ khe, 7.8
sacarācaram, 9.10
sacchabdaḥ, 17.26
sadbhāve, 17.26
sādharmyamāgatāḥ, 14.2
śādhi, 2.7; 7,30
sādhu,4.8; 6.9
sadityevābhidhīyate, 17.27
sahasra, 7.3; 11.5,46
sahayajñāḥ, 3.10
śakyo'vāptum, 6.36
samabuddhirviśiṣyate, 6.9
samadarśana,5.18; 6.29
samādha, 2.43,53; 12.9; 17.11
samādhisthasya, 2,54
samaduḥkha, 2.15; 14.24
samagraṁ, 4.23
samāhitaḥ, 6.7
samantataḥ, 6.24
samatītāni, 7.26
saṁbhavaḥ, 3.14; 14.3
saṁbhavāmi, 4.6,8
saṁchinna, 4.41
saṁgraham, 3.20,25
saṁgrāmaṁ, 2.33
samīkṣya, 1.27
saṁjāyate, 2.62
saṁjñake, 8.18
saṁjñārthaṁ , 1.7
saṁkalpa, 6.2,24
saṁkara, 1.41,42; 3.24
sāṁkhya,2.39; 3.3; 5.4,5; 13.25
saṁmohaṁ, 7.27
sammūḍha, 2.7
saṁniyamyendriya, 12.4
saṁnyāsa,3.4; 5.1; 9.28, 18.1
saṁnyāsī, 6.1; 18.12
saṁnyasyādhyātma, 3.30
saṁpadvimokṣāya, 16.5
saṁpadyate, 13.31
saṁpaśyan, 3.20
saṁprekṣya, 6.13
samṛddhavegāḥ, 11.29
śaṁsasi, 5.1
saṁśaya, 4.40; 8.5,6
saṁsiddhi, 3.20; 6.43; 8.15
saṁsparśajā, 5.22
saṁstabhyātmānam,3.43
saṁsthāpana, 4.8
saṁśuddhakilbiṣaḥ,6.45
saṁtariṣyasi, 4.36
saṁtuṣṭa, 3.17; 4.22; 12.14
samupāśritaḥ, 18.52
saṁvādamimamad, 18.76
saṁyamī, 2.69
saṁyamya, 2.61; 3.6; 4.26; 6.14;8.12
saṁyatendriyaḥ,4.39
śanaiḥ śanair, 6.25
sanātana, 2.24; 4.31;

7.10; 8.20
sanātanastvaṁ, 11.18
saṅgavivarjitaḥ, 12.18
sañjayatyuta, 14.9
śānti, 2.66; 4.39
śaraṇaṁ, 18.62,66
śarīravāṅmano, 18.15
sarvabhāvena, 15.19
sarvabhūtānāṁ, 5.29; 12.13
sarvabhūtāni, 7.27; 9.7
sarvadharmānpari, 18.66
sarvajñāna, 3.32
sarvakāmebhyo, 6.18
sarvakarma, 12.11; 18.2
sarvaloka, 5.29
sarvāṇīndriya, 4.27
sarvasaṁkalpa 6.4
sarvatokṣiśiro, 13.14
sarvayoniṣu, 14.4
śaśisūryayoḥ, 7.8
śāśvataṁ, 18.56
śāśvate, 8.26
sasvato, 2.20
sataḥ, 2.16
satataṁ, 9.14
satkāramānapūjā, 17.18
śatruvat, 6.6
sattvamityuta, 14.11
sāttvikaṁ nirmalaṁ, 14.16
sāttvikapriyāḥ, 17.8
saukṣmyād, 13.33
saumyavapur, 11.50
siddhānāṁ, 7.3
siddhasaṁghāḥ, 11.36
siddhāvasiddhau, 4.22
siddhi, 3.4; 4.12; 12.10
siddhyasiddhyoḥ, 2.48; 18.26
śiṣyas, 2.7
śītoṣṇasukha, 2.14; 6.7
smaran, 8.5,6
smarati, 8.14
smṛti, 2.63; 15.15; 18.73
somapāḥ, 9.20
sparśanaṁ, 15.9
sparśānkṛtvā, 5.27
śraddhā, 7.20; 17.3
śraddhāvāṁ, 4.39; 6.47
śraddhāvirahitaṁ, 17.13
śraddhayānvitāḥ, 17.1
śraddhayopeto, 6.37
śreya,3.11; 4.33; 12.12; 18.47
śrīmatāṁ, 6.41
śrīrvijayo, 18.78
sṛjāmyaham, 4.7
śrotavyasya, 2.52
śrotrādīnīndriyāṇy, 4.26
sṛtī, 8.27
śrutiparāyaṇāḥ, 13.26
śrutivipratipannā, 2.53
srutva, 2.29; 13.26
stena, 3.12
sthāne hṛṣīkeśa, 11.36
sthāvarajaṅgamam, 13.27
sthirabuddhira, 5.20
sthiramāsanam, 6.11
sthitadhīḥ, 2.54, 56
sthitaprajña, 2.54,55
sthitaścalati, 6.21
striyo vaiśyāstathā, 9.32
stutibhiḥ, 11.21
śubhāśubha, 2.57; 9.28
śubhāṁllokān, 18.71
śucīnāṁ, 6.41
sudurlabhaḥ, 7.19
suduṣkaram, 6.34
suhṛnmitrāryudāsīna, 6.9
sukhaduḥkha, 2.14; 13.21; 15.5
sukhamātyantikaṁ, 6.20
sukhasaṅgena, 14.6
sukhī, 5.23
śuklaḥ, 8.24
śuklakṛṣṇe, 8.26
sukṛtaduṣkṛte, 2.50
sukṛtino'rjuna, 7.16
sūkṣmatvāttada, 13.16
sulabhaḥ, 8.14
suniścitam, 5.1
surendralokam, 9.20
susukhaṁ, 9.2
sūtre maṇigaṇā, 7.7
suvirūḍhamūlam, 15.3
svabāndhavān, 1.36
svabhāva, 2.7; 5.14; 18,41,42,47,60
svacakṣuṣā, 11.8
svadharmam, 2.31
svādhyāyā 17.15
svādhyāyajñāna, 4.28
svajanaṁ, 1.36, 44
svakaṁ rūpaṁ, 11.50
svakarmaniratаḥ, 18.45
svāmavaṣṭabhya, 9.8
svanuṣṭhitāt, 3.35; 18.47
śvapāke, 5.18
svargadvāram, 2.32
svargalokaṁ, 9.21
svargaparā, 2.43
svasyāḥ, 3.33
svatejasā viśvam , 11.19
svayamevātmanā, 10.15

# T

tadbhāvabhāvitaḥ, 8.6
tadviddhi, 4.34
tamasaḥ, 8.9
tapasvibhyo,6.46
tapobhirugraiḥ, 11.48
tapoyajñā, 4.28
tasmādyogī, 6.46
tatraikāgraṁ, 6.12
tattvadarśinaḥ, 4.34
tattvataḥ, 4.9; 6.21; 7.3
tattvavit, 3.28
tejasvinām, 7.10
tejobhirāpūrya, 11.30
tejomayaṁ, 11.47
tejorāśiṁ sarvato, 11.17
titikṣasva, 2.14
traiguṇya, 2.45
trailokya, 1.35
tribhiḥ, 7.13
trīnguṇānativartate, 14.21
trividhaṁ,16.21
tulyanindāstutir, 12.19
tulyapriyāpriyo, 14.24
tyāgaphalaṁ, 18.8
tyāgītyabhidhīyate,18.11
tyajatyante, 8.6
tyaktasarva, 4.21
tyaktvātmaśuddhaye, 5.11

# U

udaka, 1.41
udbhava, 8.3
uddharedātmanā, 6.5
upadhāraya, 7.6
upahata, 2.7
upāyataḥ, 6.36
ūrdhvaṁ, 14.18; 15.1
utkrāmantaṁ, 15.10
utsīdeyurime lokā, 3.24
uttamam, 4.3
uttaram, 6.11
uttarāyaṇam, 8.24

# V

vādinaḥ, 2.42
vahnir, 3.38

vairāgya, 6.35; 13.9
vakṣyāmyaśeṣataḥ, 7.2
varṇasaṁkaraḥ, 1.40,42
vartamāno, 6,31
vartmānuvartante, 3.23; 4.11
vāsudevastathoktvā, 11.50
vaśyātmanā, 6.36
vedāntakṛdvedavid, 15.15
vedavādaratāḥ, 2.42
vibhāga, 4.13
vibhuḥ, 5.15
vibhūti, 10.7,16
vicālayet, 3.29
viddhy, 3.37; 4.13
vidheyātmā, 2.64
viduryānti, 13.35
vidvān, 3.26
vidyādduḥkha, 6.23
vidyāvinaya, 5.18
vigatajvaraḥ, 3.30
vigatakalmaṣaḥ, 6.28
vigataspṛhaḥ, 2.56; 18.49
viguṇaḥ, 3.35
vijānataḥ, 2.46
vijānīto, 2.19
vijitātmā jitendriyaḥ , 5.6
vijitendriyaḥ, 6.8
vijñāna, 9.1; 18.42
vijñātumicchāmi, 11.31
vimohayati, 3.40
vimokṣaṇāt, 5.23
vimokṣyase, 4.32
vimūḍho, 6.38
vimuñcati, 18.35
vināśam, 2.17
vināśastasya, 6.40
vinaśyati, 4.40; 13.28
vindatyātmani, 5.21
viniyamya, 6.24
viniyataṁ, 6.18
vipaścitaḥ, 2.60
vipratipannā, 2.53
visargaḥ, 8.3
viṣayān, 2.62,64
viṣayapravālāḥ, 15.2
viṣayendriya, 18.37
viṣīdantam, 2.1,10
viśiṣṭā, 1.7
viśiṣyate, 3.7; 6.9
visṛjāmyaham, 9.7
vistareṇātmano, 10.18
viśuddhātmā, 5.6,7
viśuddhayā, 18.51
viśuddhaye, 6.12
viśvamanantarūpa, 11.38
viśvatomukham, 9.15; 10.33; 11.11
vītarāgabhaya, 2.56; 4.10
vitatā brahmaṇo, 4.32
vivasvataḥ, 4.4
viviktadeśa, 13.11
vivṛddha, 14.11,13
viyogaṁ, 6.23
viyuktānāṁ, 5.26
vratāḥ, 4.28
vṛjinaṁ, 4.36
vyāharan, 8.13
'vyakto'vyaktāt, 8.20
vyāmiśreṇeva, 3.2
vyapāśrayaḥ, 3.18
vyatitariṣyati, 2.52
vyavasāyātmikā, 2.41,43,44

# Y

yadā yadā hi, 4.7
yadrājyasukha, 1.44
yadṛccha, 2.32; 4.22
yajanta iha devatāḥ , 4.12
yajjñātvā, 13.13;14.1,12,16,35
yajjuhoṣi, 9.26
yajñabhāvitāḥ, 3.12
yajñakṣapita, 4.30
yajñānayajñāśca, 4.28
yajñārthāt, 3.9
yajñaśiṣṭāmṛtabhujo, 4.31
yajñaśiṣṭāśinaḥ, 3.13
yajñatapasāṁ, 5.29
yajñavido, 4.30
yajñenaivopajuhvati, 4.25
yaṁ yaṁ vāpi , 8.6
yānti devavratā, 9.25
yantrārūḍhāni, 18.61
yatacetasām, 5.26
yatacitta, 4.21; 6.19
yatamānas, 6.45
yatātmānaḥ, 5.25
yatendriyamano, 5.28
yathaidhāṁsi, 4.37
yatīnāṁ, 5.26
yoga, 2.48; 4.1,2; 6.2
yogabalena, 8.10
yogabhraṣṭo, 6.41
yogāccalitamānasaḥ, 6.37
yogadhāraṇām, 8.12
yogāgnau, 4.27,28
yogaḥ proktaḥ, 4.3
yogakṣemaṁ, 9.22
yogaṁ yogeśvarāt, 18.75
yogamaiśvaram, 9.5; 11.8
yogamātmanaḥ, 6.19
yogamavāpsyasi, 2.53
yogamāyāsamāvṛtaḥ, 7.25
yogārūḍha, 6.3,4
yogasaṁjñitam, 6.23
yogasaṁnyasta, 4.41
yogasaṁsiddhaḥ, 4.38
yogasaṁsiddhiṁ, 6.37
yogasthaḥ, 2.48
yogasya, 6.44
yogavittamāḥ, 12.1
yogayukta, 5.6; 6.29; 8.27
yogenāvyabhicāriṇyā, 18.33
yogeśvara, 11.4; 18.75,78
yogī, 3.3; 4.25; 5.11; 6.15,19,32,42,47; 8,14,23
yogī vigatakalmaṣaḥ , 6.28
yogī yuñjīta satatam, 6.10
yonijanmasu, 13.22
yonirmahadbrahma, 14.3
yudhyasva, 2.18; 3.30
yuga, 8.17
yugasahasrāntāṁ, 8.17
yujyasva, 2.50
yukta āsīta matparaḥ, 6.14
yuktacetasaḥ, 7.30
yuktaḥ, 3.26
yuktāhāravihārasya, 6.17
yuktatamo, 6.47
yuñjan, 6.15; 7.1

# Index to Translation


## A

A--letter, 10.33
abandonment of
consequences, 18.4
Abode of Universe, 11.25
absorber God, 13.17
absorption, 14.26
abusive language, 16.4
accomplishment, factors,
18.3
**Action/activity,**
abandonment?,
18.5, 11
appropriate, 4.17
clarity type, 18.23
conclusion, 4.33
consequence, 5.14
controlled, 18.23
craving, 18.24
defered to
Krishna, 12.6
desireless, 18.23
disciplined, 4.32
distressful, 14.16
essential, 3.8
factors,
18.13-15,18
faulty, 18.3
forceful, 18.60
God created?, 5.14
ignorant, 14.16
implication transcended,
5.7
impulsion, 14.9
impulsive, 18.24
inappropriate 4.17
incomprehensible,
4.17
Krishna, 4.14
material nature,
3.33; 13.28,
15.2; 18.41
misconception 18.25
modes, 14.16
mundane energy,
3.27, 28

**Action/activity,**
Nature-produced,
5.14
necessary, 6.1
non-action,
4.18,20
non-defective, 14.16
non-defiling, 5.10
obligatory, 6.1
offering to Krishna,
9.27
parts of, 18.18
performance
required, 16.24
questioned, 4.16
reduced, 4.37
regulation, 3.3
results, 2.51
Sat type, 17.27
seer's, 2.54
spiritual, 4.24
transcending, 9.28
types,
18.9,19,23-25
unmotivated,
18.23
yoga mood, 2.48
acts of sacrifice, charity,
austerities, 17.24
Ādityas, 10.21
**affections,**
crippling, 2.57
yogic type, 14.26
agency, 13.21
**agent,**
factor, 18.14,18
Krishna's 11.33
types, 18.19,26-28
Agni, 11.3
agreeable / disagreeable,
12.17
agriculture, 18.44
air, regulation, 4.30
Airāvata, 10.27
airs, 4.29
all-pervasive Form, 11.20

**Almighty God,**
consequence free,
5.15
Krishna, 6.38;
9.11; 10.3
alone, yogi, 6.10
alphabet, 10.33
alternatives, Arjuna's, 2.6
ambidextrous, 11.33
Ananta, 10.29
anantavijayam, 1.16
ancestors, , 9.25
ancient person, 8.9
ancient spirit, 11.38
angel, 11.22
**angelic kingdom,**
king, 9.20
paradise, 9.21
sovereignty, 2.8
warriors attain, 2.35
**anger,**
absence of, 16.2
cause; 2.62,63; 5.28
cherished, 16.12
eliminated, 4.10
endured, 5.23
hell, 16.21
tendency; 16.4,18
animals, 10.30
antelope skin, 6.11
anxieties, 2.56,57; 12.16
aquatics, 10.29
**Arjuna,**
-Also see Indexed
Names of Arjuna
agent, 11.33
amazed, 11.14
ambidextrous, 11.33
appreciations, 11.1
bowing, 11.14
bowman,1.4; 18.78
conch blown, 1.14
confusion, 18.73
death preferred, 1.45
depression, 2.8
devotion, 9.33

**Arjuna continued,**
disoriented, 11.25
fear-free, 11.49,50
frightened, 11.35
God vision 11.45
hopelessness, 2.1
instructed, 2.37
intimidation, 2.35
Krishna , 10.37
liberated, 11.1
lost?, 18.58
loved, 18.64,65
majestic form 11.3
material nature, 18.59
monkey insignia, 1.20
normalized, 11.51
obeisance, 11.39,40
ordered 11.33,34
overwhelmed, 1.27,46
past birth, 4.5
refuses to fight, 2.9
repulsed, 1.35
request, 1.21,22; 4.42
sense of duty, 2.7
shifty vision, 6.33,34
sickly emotion, 2.2
sinless one, 14.6
sits down, 1.46
stunned, 1.28
submits, 2.7; 18.73
trembles, 1.29, 11.45,48
Universal Form seen, 11.15
work, 4.15
armored warriors, 11.32,34
arms, 11.19, 23
army, destroyed, 11.32,34
arrogance, 16.4,17,18
Aryamā, 10.29
āsana, 6.11-13
**ascetic,**
Krishna related, 7.9
sacrifice, 4.30
temptations, 2.59
yogi superior, 6.46
Asita, 10.13
assertion, false type, 18.52
assertive attitude, 18.17
assurance, 12.8
astral region, 9.20
aśvattha tree, 10.26; 15.1-3
Aśvatthāmā, 1.8
atmosphere, 7.8
**attachment,**
as Cause, 13.22
cause, 2.62; 11.55
conquered, 15.5
discarded, 5.10,11
finished, 4.23
freedom from, 3.9; 12.18
idleness, 2.47
attack, superiors, 2.4
attainment, 6.22, 8.21
**attention,**
drift / restraint, 6.26
Krishna absorbed, 7.1
**attractive objects,**
addictive, 15.9
detachment, 6.4
living space, 13.6
senses interlocked,5.9
audiences, 18.67
austerities, enjoyer, 5.29
**austerity,**
abandoned?, 18.3
asat, 17.28
categories, 17.7-10
faith in, 17.17
godly nature 16.1
impulsive type, 17.18
ineffective, 11.48,53
invented ones, 17.1
Krishna derived, 7.9; 10.5
mistaken type, 17.19
motivation, 4.23
purificatory, 4.10,30; 18.5
rain, 3.14
realistic type, 17.17
religion, 3.14; 4.23
sacrifice, 4.25
tendency, 18.42
terrible type, 17.5
tricky type, 17.18
types, 17.14-17
Universal Form, 11.48
authority, besides Krishna, 9.30; 10.38
avenues of depression, 16.22
axe, 15.3

# B

battle formation, 1.33; 2.31
beasts, 10.30
begetting, 10.28
begging, 2.5
beginning of creation, 7.27
beginningless, Krishna, 10.3
behavior, codes of, 12.20
**beings,**
disintegration, 13.28
independent, 9.4
influenced, 7.27
Krishna produces, 9.7
Krishna's energy sustains, 9.4
origin / ruination, 11.2
production, 9.8
psychological supremacy, 9.5
relation, 4.35
Supreme Lord inhabits, 13.28
types, 16.6
belief in God, 18.42
belief in Krishna, 3.31
belief in others, 7.21
beliefs of wicked people, 16.8,13-15
bellies, 11.16,23
**benefit,**
abandoned, 12.11
detachment from 4.20,22; 17.17
disinterest in, 17.25
luck, 4.22
types, 17.11-23; 18.12
best of gods, 11.31
bewitching energy, 7.14
**Bhagavad Gītā,**
hearing of, 18.67,71
preachers, 18.67
study, 18.70
Bhīma, 1.4,10,15
Bhishma, 1.8,10-12,25;. 2.4; 11.26,34
Bhṛgu, 10.25
Bhṛhat Sama Melody, 10.35
birds, 10.30
**birth,**
certain, 2.27
rebirth, 4.4,5
liberation from, 5.19; 7.19; 14.20
birthless, Krishna, 10.3,12
blockheads, 16.20

**body,**
acquirement / departure from, 2.13; 15.8
assumption of, 2.22
detachment, 14.23
head-neck balance, 6.13
living space, 13.2
maintenance necessary, 3.8
purification usage, 5.11
restriction, 3.7
terminal, 2.18
bondage tendencies, 16.5
boys, 10.6
Brahma Sūtras, 13.5
**Brahmā,**
day / night, 8.17-19; 9.7
Krishna as father, 11.39
Krishna greater, 11.37
Krishna identity, 10.33; 11.39
procreator,3.10
Universal Form 11.15
world of, 8.16
**brahmin,**
compared, 5.18
ordained, 17.23
perceptive, 2.46
praised, 9.33
respected, 17.14
branches of imperishable tree, 15.2
breathing, nature function, 5.8
Bṛhaspati, 10.24
brilliant consciousness, 5.24
brothers, 1.26
brow chakra, 8.10
brute force, 16.18, 17.5
buddy, 11.41,44
business men, 9.32

# C

cakes, 1.41
cannibals, 17.4
cardinal points, 11.25
career categories, 4.13
caste, 4.13; 18.41
categories of elements, 13.6
**cause,**
non-deteriorating, 9.18
destruction, 11.32
elaborated, 13.21
series of, 16.8
Cekitāna, 1.5
celebrity, 3.21
celestial body, 9.19
celestial delights, 9.20
celestial musicians, 11.22
celestial regions, 6.40,41
celestial sea, 10.27
**celibacy,**
austerity17.14
destination, 8.11
yogi's, 6.14
celibate boys, 10.6
ceremonial articles, 4.24
ceremonial rites, 2.43
-see religious ceremony
cessation, 5.25,26
changes of living space, 13.20
chaos, societies', 3.24
chariot, Arjuna's, 1.21
charitable disposition, 18.43
**charity,**
abandoned?, 18.3
categories, 16.1; 17.7-10
ineffective, 11.48,53
Krishna derived, 10.5
purificatory, 18.5
Universal Form, 11.48
yogi bypasses, 8.28
cherish the imperishable, 12.3
choice, Arjuna's, 2.6
chum, 11.44
circular process, 3.16
Citraratha, 10.26
clan, 1.37-42
**clarity,**
captivating, 14.6
disease-free, 14.6
expertise, 14.6
happiness produced by, 14.6,9
illuminating, 14.6
influence, 14.5
lack of, 14.13
**clarity continued,**
predominating, 14.10,11
class, 1.40,41,42
clay, 6.8; 14.24
cleanliness, 16.7; 18.42
cleansers, 10.31
clear-minded people, 17.8
cloud comparison, 6.38
club, 11.17, 46
cold, 2.14; 6.7
colors, 11.5
command, 2.47
commerce, 18.44
common factor, 5.18
comparative view, 6.33
**comparison,**
lamp, 6.19
mind / wind, 6.34
yoga methods, 12.1,2,3
compassion, 1.27; 12.13; 16.2
compensation, 17.21
competence, 12.16
compulsion to act, 3.36, 37
conceit, 16.3
concentrated mental focus, 7.30
concentration, lacking, 2.66
concepts, discipline, 9.15
conclusion, 4.33;10.32; 13.1,2
condemnation, resisted, 12.19; 14.24
conditions, 2.15
conduct, 14.21
confidence, 12.10; 17.3,13
confidential teaching 4.3
**confusion,**
devoid of, 15.5
impulsion, 14.17
production, 14.13
congratulations, 14.24
**consciousness,**
detachment, 14.22
Krishna 10.22
living space, 13.7
purifier, 9.2

**consequence,**
abandonment, 16.2
aftermath, 2.47
Almighty God, 5.15
freedom from
3.31; 9.28
rejection, 18.1,2,4
types, 18.12
contact, happiness, 18.37
contentment,
2.71; 10.5; 12.14
continuation, 10.32
controller, I, 16.14
conviction, 13.7
coping, 2.14
core self, 6.18; 8.12
cosmic destroyers, 10.23
couch, 11.42
cow, 5.18; 10.28; 18.44
cowardice, 2.3; 18.43
**craving,**
abandoned, 2.55
cause, 2.62; 3.37
cherished, 16.12,16
degrading, 16.18,21
eliminated,
4.10; 8.11; 12.17
endured, 5.23
freedom from,
3.30; 6.18; 16.2
impulsion, 14.11
possession of, 17.5
resisted, 2.70
transcended, 2.70,71
created being, 10.39; 16.6
creation, 10.32; 14.2
creative power, 8.3
creator, 9.17
**creature,**
disintegrated, 8.20
evolution, 10.6
Krishna knows, 7.26
Krishna related, 7.9
nourishment, 3.14
origination, 7.6
spirit habitat, 6.29
crippling emotions,
2.48, 57
criticism, 16.2
crowds, 13.11
crown, 11.46
culprit, 4.36
**cultural activity,**
cause of, 3.15
creative power, 8.3
**cultural activity con't,**
exemption, 3.17; 18.49
inferior, 2.49
Krishna 4.13,14; 9.9
mandatory, 4.15
mental / physical, 3.1
perfection related,
3.20
production, 3.14
purification usage,
5.11
questioned, 4.16
religious type, 3.9
rewards abandoned,
5.12
social affairs, 3.4
transcended, 4.41
value, 7.29
yoga method, 6.3
cultured man, 2.2
cumulative intellectual
interest, 6.43
cutting instrument, 4.42
cycles of rebirth, 16.19
cynical, 9.1

# D

dairy farming, 18.44
damage, 18.25
danger of birth/death,
13.9
danger, avoidance, 2.56
Danu, 10.14
dark moon, 8.25
darshan, 11.53
day / night, 8.17-19,24
**death,**
attainments, 2.72
certainty, 2.27
devotee, 12.7
devotion applied,
8.10
duty, 3.35
eyebrow focus, 8.10
Krishna, 4.9; 8.5; 9.19;
10.34; 15.8
liberation,
7.29; 8.25; 14.20
modes influence,
14.14,15
psychology taken 15.8
rebirth, 9.3
repetitive, 8.16
supervisor, 11.39
**death continued,**
texture of existence
recalled, 8.6
deceit, 13.8; 16.4; 17.5
deceiver, 3.6
December, 10.35
decision, 9.30
deeds of Krishna, 4.9
defeat, victory, 2.38
defect universal, 18.48
deity worship, 7.21
deity, outsmarting, 17.12
deliverer, 12.7
**delusion,**
banished, 4.35
cause / production,
2.63
experience, 18.22
overpowering, 16.16
saturated mind, 2.52
demigods, 7.23; 11.52;
16.20
-also see supernatural
rulers
demons, 11.36; 16.20
- also see wicked people
departed spirits,
1.41; 7.26; 9.25
departure of yogis, 8.23
depressed people, 17.10
**depression,**
detachment from,
14.22
predominating,
14.10,12
release from, 16.22
depressive mode,
**desire,**
abandoning, 6.24
contrary ones, 7.20
desire for pay-off,
4.14
eliminated, 5.28
freedom from, 6.18
impulsive type, 2.5
living space, 13.7
motivated action,
5.12
productions, 14.8
resistance, 5.20
restrained, 4.19
satisfaction, 2.70
desireless, 6.10
despair, 18.35
destination, highest, 18.50

destiny, factor, 18.14
destroyers, 11.6
destruction, 7.6
**detachment,**
axe, 15.3
conditions resisted, 6.7
recommended, 3.7,9; 12.19
detection device, 15.7
**determination,**
tendency, 18.43
types, 18.29, 33-35
yoga practice, 6.23
Devadatta, 1.15
Devala, 10.13
devas,
-see supernatural rulers
deviation, 6.37
devilish people, 9.12
**devotee ,**
categorized, 7.16-18; 12.17
dear, 12.20
delivered, 12.7
guarantees, 18.68-70
Krishna attraction 9.28
Krishna enlightens, 10.11
Krishna protects, 9.22
Krishna's favorite, 9.29
Krishna's proximity, 13.19
offerings, 9.26
ruination, 9.31
yogi, 12.14
**devotion,**
dear to Krishna, 12.18
extolled, 12.17
great soul's, 9.14
Krishna, 4.3; 11.55; 18.65
offerings related, 9.26
opportunity, 9.33
required, 12.20; 13.11
supreme type, 18.54,55
unique, 11.54
yogic type, 14.26
devotional practice, 12.8-11
devotional relationship, requirement, 8.22
devotional service, 9.27
devotional worship, 9.29
dharmakṣetre, 1.1
Dhātā, 10.33
Dhṛṣṭadyumna, 1.17
Dhṛṣṭaketu, 1.5
Dhṛtaraṣṭra, 1.1,18,35,45; 2.9; 11.26
Dhṛti, 10.34
diet restraint, 4.30
differences, 18.21
digestive heat, 15.14
dimensions beyond, 4.40
dining, 11.42
direction, 11.25
directive self, 6.7
disc, 11.46
**discernment,**
adjusted, 3.39
constant type, 2.68
maintained, 3.41
senses affected, 2.67
uncontrolled person, 2.66
disciplic succession, 4.34
**discipline,**
accomplishment, 4.32
body, 17.14
concepts, 9.15
continuous, 6.15
mind, 17.16
offering to Krishna, 9.27
speech, 17.15
types, 17.11-13
disciplined behavior, 3.26
disciplined person, 6.36; 9.26
discredit Krishna, 3.32
discrimination, 2.52; 18.42
discus, 11.17
discussion, 10.10
disease, 13.9
disgrace, 2.2
disgusted / tradition, 2.52
disintegration, 13.28
dislikes / likes, 3.34; 4.22
dispassion, 12.18,19; 18.52
dissolution, 14.2
distinction, 6.9
**distress,**
cessation, 2.57,65
happiness, 2.38
remover, 6.17
transcended, 12.15; 14.20
distressed person, 7.16
Diti, 10.30
divine form, 11.52, 54
Divine Supreme Person, 8.8,10
divinity, 2.72
doctors, 11.22
dog, 5.18
doubt, 4.40; 6.39
Draupadī, 1.6,18
Droṇa, 1.7,25;2.4; 11.26,34
Drupada, 1.3,4,18
dry food, 17.9
duality, 2.14; 6.7,32
duration of life, 17.8
Duryodhana, 1.2,12
**duty,**
abandoned?, 18.48
alternatives, 2.31
another's, 3.35
discipline, 6.17
necessary, 3.35; 6.1
neglect, 2.33
perfection, 18.45-48
preferred, 3.19
sin-resistant, 2.38
dying person, 8.5


# E


earth, resonated, 1.19; 7.9; 8.15; 15.13
easy to practice, 9 .2
eatables, 17.7-10
eating, yoga method, 5.8; 6.16,17; 9.27
educated people, 3.39
**education,**
purificatory, 4.10
ineffective, 11.48,53
Krishna, 9.17; 13.18
elements, categories, 13.6
elephant, 5.18; 10.27
**embodied soul,**
-see also Spirit
nine-gate city, 5.13
embryo, 3.38
emotional detachment, 13.10
emotional distress, 2.65

emotional stability, 2.66
emotional weakness, 2.3
emotions,1.19; 2.38,48
**endeavor,**
intention free, 4.19
Krishna, 10.36
righteous type, 2.40
ending, 10.32
enemy killed, 16.14
enemy, passion, 3.37
energizing airs, 4.29
energizing breath, 8.10,12
energy, 7.4-6; 14.13
enjoyable aspects, 1.32
enjoyer, I, 16.14
enjoyment, 2.43,57,58
enlightened parents, 6.42
enlightenment, 14.22
enthusiasm, 14.22
environment of psyche, 13.4
envy-free person, 4.22
equally-disposed, 12.13; 14.25
equanimity, 12.18,19; 14.24,25
era to era, 4.8
essential nature, 17.3
eternal divine person, 10.12
eternal abode, 18.56
eternal life, 9.19; 13.13
eternal peace, 9.31
evacuation, 5.9
even-minded, 12.4; 13.10
everlasting principle, 2.17
evil action forced, 3.36,37
evil-doers, 7.15
evolution, 14.18
example, 3.21
excitement, 2.56,57; 5.20; 12.15; 14.23
exclusive worship, 9.30
exemption, 18.49
exertion, 14.11
exhalation, inhalation, 4.29; 5.27
**existence,**
ceaseless, 2.12
enduring/ non-enduring, 2.16; 4.24
Krishna originates, 10.5,41
Krishna upholds, 7.7
existential arrangement, 6.29
existential conditions, 10.5
existential residence, 9.18
expectations, 16.12
**experience,**
depression obscures, 14.9
explained, 13.13
ignorance, 5.16
illuminating, 4.27
impetus, 18.18
incomparable, 4.38
Krishna gave, 7.2
overshadowed, 7.20
spirit's, 13.22
Supreme Spirit, 13.15
types, 7.2; 18.19-22
experiencer, 13.1,2,23,27
expertise, 18.43
eye movement, 5.9
eyebrows, 5.27
eyes, 11.2,10,16,19


# F


faces, 11.16
facilities of species, 6.32
factors, five, 18.13-15
failure/ success, 2.48; 4.22
**faith,**
experience yielding, 4.39
Krishna awards, 7.21
nature based, 17.3
required, 9.3
undisciplined persons, 6.37
faithfulness, 10.34
faithless person, 4.40; 9.3
fallen yogi, 6.37,41
fame, 10.5,34
familiarity, 11.41
family duties, 1.42
family, fallen yogi, 6.41-43
fantasy, 16.13
father, Krishna, 9.17; 11.43; 14.4
fathers, 1.26,33
faults, 3.13; 4.21; 5.17,25; 6.28; 10.3
fear, 2.56; 4.10; 5.28; 10.5; 12.15; 17.20; 18.35
fearlessness, 10.5; 16.1
features, 14.21
fee, 17.13
feelings, 10.34; 13.7
feet, 11.23
feverish mood, Arjuna's, 3.30
fickleness, absence of, 16.2
fig tree, 10.26
financial assets, 1.33
fire ceremony, necessary, 6.1
fire controller, 11.39
**fire,**
comparison, 18.48
Krishna, 9.16
lust compared, 3.39
universal destruction, 11.25
spirit resists, 2.23
splendor, 15.12
supreme residence 15.6
five factors, 18.13-15
flame, 7.4
flower, Krishna accepts, 9.26
focus on Krishna, 12.2
food, categories, 17.7-10,13
foolish people, 9.11
forbearance, 16.3
forced action, 3.36,37
forgiveness, 11.42
Form of everything, 11.16
Form of Mine, 11.47
formation, 10.32
**forms,**
Krishna inhabits, 6.30
unlimited, 11.5
womb produced, 14.4
fortune, 10.34
**foundation,**
material nature, 9.8
future, 10.34
singular, 13.31
yogi compared, 6.38
four celibate boys, 10.6
four kinds/people, 7.16
four-handed Form, 11.52
fresh air, 4.30
friend, 1.26; 3.21; 9.18; 11.41,44; 12.13
friendship, with Krishna, 4.3
fright, 11.35
fruit, 9.26

fulfillments, 7.22
functional work, 4.15
future productions, 10.34

# G

gain, 3.18
gambling, 10.36
Gāṇḍīva, 1.29
garlands, 11.11
garments, 2.22; 11.11
Garuḍa, 10.30
gas, 7.4
Gāyatrī, 10.35
geniuses, 7.10
gentleness, 16.2, 17.16
ghastly form, 11.49
ghee, Krishna, 9.16
ghosts, 9.25; 17.4
gift, 17.20-22
glorification, resisted, 12.19
glory, 11.41
goal of invisible reality, 12.5
God form, 11.45
God of gods, 11.13
god of romance, 10.28
God Vishnu, 11.24, 30
**God,**
  action free, 5.14
  described, 10.12; 11.11; 18.46
  Krishna, 10.15
  location in body, 8.2
  near / far, 13.16
  pervader, 9.4
goddess of counsel, 10.34
goddess of faithfulness, 10.34
goddess of fame, 10.34
goddess of fortune, 10.34
goddess of patience, 10.34
goddess of recollection, 10.34
goddess of speech, 10.34
godly nature, 16.1-3
gods, 7.22
  --see also supernatural rulers
gold, 6.8, 14.24
good feelings, 1.31
good people, 7.18
governing tendency, 18.43
Govinda, 2.9
grace, 11.47
grandfather Krishna, 9.17
grandfathers, 1.26,33
grandsons, 1.26
grasping, 2.45; 4.21
great person, 3.21
Great Personality, 11.12
**great soul,**
  rare, 7.19
  rebirth exemption, 8.15
  reliance, 9.13
greed, mental obsession, 1.37; 14.11,17; 16.21
grossness, free of, 8.9
grudge, 17.21

# H

habits ,4.12
hairs on end, 18.74
*Hanumān*, 1.20
**happiness,**
  achievement, 2.66
  detachment, 5.23
  distress, 2.38
  endless type, 6.28
  non-fluctuating, 5.21
  production of, 14.6,9
  spiritual type, 5.24
  superior type, 6.27
  types, 18.36-39
  ultimate, 5.2
Hari, 11.9; 18.77
harmony, 6.31
hatred, 16.3
hazy season, 8.25
head posture, 6.13
health, 17.8
**hearing,**
  about soul, 2.29
  austerity, 4.26
  perception, 13.26
  nature function, 5.8
  valid method, 13.26
heat, 2.14; 9.19
**heaven,**
  attainment, 9.20,21
  material nature, 18.40
  open, 2.31
  sickly emotion, 2.2
hell, avenues, 1.43; 16.16,21
hereafter, 4.31; 14.14,15,18
heroes, 1.9
heroism, 18.43
highest living state, 6.15
highest reality, 5.17
highest well-being, 3.11
Himālaya, 10.25
holding, 5.9
home, 13.10
honor / dishonor, 6.7
honored man, 2.34
hope, 2.41; 4.21
hordes of ghost, 17.4
horses, 10.27
hostility, 11.55; 16.20,21
Hṛṣikeśa, 1.15,21,24; 11.36
**human being,**
  Brahman realization, 12.5
  creation of, 3.10
  Krishna affects, 4.11
  material nature, 15.2
  perfection, 7.3
  regard for Krishna, 10.3
  world of, 11.48
  worship gods, 4.12
human body of Krishna, 9.11
Brahmā instructed, 3.10,11,12
hygiene, 12.16
hymns, 10.35
hypocrisy, 16.10

# I

idea of Krishna, 3.31
ideas, overpowering, 16.16
identity-confusion, 3.27
idiot, 15,1018.16
idleness, 2.47
**ignorance,**
  defined, 13.12
  doubt, 4.42
  impulsion, 14.17
  knowledge shrouded, 5.15
  Krishna banishes, 10.11
ignorant person, 4.40
Ikṣvāku, 4.1
illusion, 7.14
immortality, 14.20
impartiality, 5.19; 10.5; 12.16;14.24,25; 18.54
impatience, 12.15

imperishable destination, 8.11
imperishable invisible existence, 12.1,3
impersonal existence, 12.1,3
impetus, 18.18
implication, avoidance, 4.22; 5.3; 9.28
**impulsion,**
activity produced by, 14.6
attachment, 14.6
desire, 14.6
endured, 5.23
influence, 14.5,10,13
mentality adjusted, 2.60
passion, 14.6
impulsiveness, 2.71
impure objectives, 16.10
impurities, 4.30; 9.1
inattentiveness, 14.8,13,17
inconceivable reality, 12.3
independence, 4.20
indestructible factor, 2.17
indetermination, 3.26
indifference, 5.3;6.9,35; 12.16; 13.9
individual existence, 2.12
individualized conditioned beings, 15.7
infamy, 10.5
inferior energy, 7.4,5
influence, 10.12; 17.2
**information,**
God, 13.18
highest, 11.1; 14.1
informed person, 7.16
Krishna's, 7.2; 10.42
liberating, 14.1
secret, 15.20; 18.63,64
Supreme Spirit, 13.12
ultimate, 9.2; 10.1
inhalation, 4.29; 5.27
inherent nature, 18.47
initiate action, 5.8
initiative, 7.4; 13.6,9
innate tendency, 17.2
inner peace, 2.66
inquisitive person, 7.16
insensibility, cause, 14.8
**insight,**
Arjuna bestowed, 11.8
blocked, 3.38,40
Krishna gives, 10.11
protects, 2.40
reaction-resistant, 2.39
reality-piercing, 2.50
steady type, 2.55
view different, 2.41
instruments, 18.14,18
**intellect,**
controlled, 5.28
defective type, 18.16
detached type, 18.49
grasped, 6.25
living space, 13.6
self-focused type, 2.44
spiritual happiness, 6.21
types, 18.29-32
intellectual discipline, 2.49
**intelligence,**
compared, 3.42
grasped, 6.25
Krishna anchored, 8.7
Krishna derived, 10.5
Krishna related, 7.10
mundane, 7.4
passion fostered, 3.40
purification, 5.11
stable, 2.65
intelligent statements, 2.11
**intentions,**
Krishna's, 11.31
restrained, 4.19
wicked ones, 17.6
interaction, 2.68
interim, 2.28
intoxication, 16.10
introspection, 8.11
intuitive perception, 10.35
invisible existence, 8.18,21;.12.1,3,5;
isolation, 6.10; 13.11; 18.52
item of research, 18.18


# J


Jāhnavī, 10.31
Jahnu's daughter, 10.31
Janaka, 3.20
Janārdana, 11.51
japa, 10.25
Jayadrath, 11.34
jinxed, 3.32
joke, 11.42
joy, 5.25
judgment, 6.9


# K


Kāmadhuk, 10.28
Kandarpa, 10.28
Kapila, 10.26
karma yoga, 3.7; 4.2
Karṇa, 1.8; 11.26,34
Kaśi, 1.5,17
Keshava, 2.54; 10.14; 13.1; 18.76;
Keśi, 18.1
Killed/ killer, 2.19
killing, Arjuna repulsed, 1.34; 18.17
kinfolk, Arjuna, 1.31
king, 4.2; 10.27
king's son, 2.31
Kīrti, 10.34
knower of reality, 5.8
**knowledge,**
clarity produces, 14.17
control, 4.33
defined, 13.8-12
derived, 12.12
experience, 9.1
fiery force, 4.19
Krishna produced, 10.5; 15.15
Krishna represented, 10.38
lack of, 16.4
of Krishna, 4.14
**Krishna, Lord,**
-also see ***Indexed Names of Krishna***
A – letter, 10.33
actions of, 4.11
Ādityas, 10.21
Agni, 11.39
Airāvata, 10.27,29
Almighty God, 10.3
ancient person, 11.18
appeasers of, 9.25
approach to, 8.15,16
aquatics, 10.29
Arjuna and, 18.78
Arjuna identity, 10 37
Arjuna loved by, 18.64,65
Arjuna's welfare, 10.1

**Krishna continued,**
armies shown, 1.25
Aryamā, 10.29
ascetics, 7.9
aspiration-free, 3.22
association, 18.55
Aśvattha, 10.26
atmosphere, 7.8
austerity, 7.9
authority, 10.38
basis supreme, 11.37; 14.27
beasts identity, 10.30
beautiful-haired, 1.30
begetting, 10.28
beginningless, 11.19
beings caused by, 9.5
best of gods, 11.31
beyond range, 7.24
birds identity, 10.30
birth transcended, 7.25
birthless, 4.6; 10.12
births, 4.5
body situated, 13.32
Brahmā compared, 10.33; 11.37,39
Bṛhaspati, 10.21
Bṛhgu identity, 10.25
cause of integration, 9.18
cause ultimate, 7.6
celestial sea, 10.27
chanting, 10.25
chariot driver, 1.24
chief of cowherds, 1.32; 2.9
Chitraratha, 10.26
clansman of Vrishnis, 1.40
cleansers, 10.31
commanders, 10.21
conch blown, 1.14
conclusion, 10.32
condition of existence, 8.5
consciousness, identity, 10.22
constant factor, 9.13
continuation, 10.32
contrasting, 11.26
cows identity, 10.28
creations, 10.32
creator, 9.17

**Krishna continued,**
creatures, 7.9
death producer, 9.19
December, 10.35
dependence on, 7.1,29; 11.55
descendant of Madhu, 1.14 ,36
detachment, 9.9
devoted to, 6.14
devotee approaches, 9.28
devotee delivered by, 12.7
devotee guarantee, 9.31
devotee yogi, 12.16
devotion to, 9.14; 13.11; 18.55
devotional worship 9.29
Dhātā, 10.33
digestion, 15.14
disciplines, 10.25
disliked, 16.18
Diti identity, 10.30
divine form, 11.50
divine glory, 10.7
duty-free / duty-bound, 3.22
earth, 7.9; 15.13
easy to reach, 8.14
education, 9.17
elephants, 10.27
endeavor,9.27; 10.36
ending identity, 10.32
endless, 11.16
enjoyer, 5.29
entered, 15.15
equally-disposed, 9.29
eternal life, 9.19
everything, 7.19; 11.40
exclusive worship. 9.30
exemplary, 3.23
existential level, 4.10
existential residence, 9.18
exists in body, 8.4
eyes, 11.2,19
fame, 11.36
father, 9.17
father of world, 11.43

**Krishna continued,**
favorites, 9.29
fig tree identity, 10.26
fire, 9.16
First God, 11.38
focus on, 4.10; 7.30; 8.7; 11.38; 12.8
Form Infinite, 11.16,38
formation, 10.32
foundation, 9.18
four-armed Form, 11.46
fraction, 10.42
friend, 5.29 ; 9.18
gambling, 10.36
garlands, 11.11
garments, 11.11
Garuḍa, 10.30
Gāyatrī, 10.35
geniuses, 7.10
ghastly Form, 11.49
ghee, 9.16
glorified, 9.14; 11.2,9
God of gods, 10.15 ; 11.13
god of romance, 10.28
Govinda, 2.9
grace, 18.56,58
grandfather, 9.17
great souls, 9.13
handsome-haired, 3.1; 11.35
happiness, 14.27
heat producer, 9.19; 11.19
herb, 9.16
higher exisitence, 7.24; 9.11
highest reality, 7.7
Himalaya, 10.25
honored, 11.39
horses identity, 10.27
Hṛṣikeśa, 1.15
human-like Form, 11.49,51
hurls the wicked, 16.19
hymns identity, 10.35
idea, 3.31
impartial, 9.29
important, 12.6
indifference, 9.9
infallible, 11.42

**Krishna continued,**
infinite Lord of gods, 11.37
infinite, 11.11,16
influence, 9.6; 10.12
intelligence, 7.10
items accepted, 9.26
Jāhnavī, 10.32
Jahnu's daughter, 10.32
Janārdana, 11.51
japa identity, 10.25
Kāmadhuk, 10.28
Kandarpa, 10.28
Kapila, 10.26
killer of Madhu, 2.1
king identity, 10.27
king of beasts, 10.30
Knower, 11.38
Knowledge, 10.38
knowledge of, 4.14
known, 7.1
known at death? 8.2
knows Himself, 10.15
Kuvera identity, 10.23
law guardian, 11.18
liberated, 9.9
liberation offered, 18.66
life energy focus, 10.9
life, 7.9
light, 10.21
limitless, 10.19
lion identity, 10.30
logicians, 10.32
longevity, 9.19
Lord of created beings, 10.15
lord of creatures, 4.6
Lord of gods, 11.37
Lord of beings, 7.30
Lord of supernatural rulers and powers, 7.30
Lord of the earth, 1.21
Lord of universe, 10.15
Lord of yoga, 18.75,78
maintainer, 10.15
manifestation, 4.7; 10 40
manliness, 7.9
Marīci, 10.21

**Krishna continued,**
master of religious ceremony, 9.24
master, 9,18
medicinal herb, 9.16
meditation upon, 8.12; 10.8; 12.6
men, 7.9
mental productions, 10.6
Meru identity, 10.23
mind, identity, 10.22
monitors, 10.30
monsters, 10.31
moon, 7.8; 10.21; 15.13
morality, 7.11; 10.38
mother, 9.17
motivator of humans, 1.38
motivator, 1.38; 10.18
mountain, 10.23
mystic discipline, 10.7
mystic master, 7.25; 10.7,17
Nārada, 10.26
nature of, 14.2
non-dependent, 7.12
non-deteriorating cause, 9.18
not fruitive, 4.14
not recognized, 7.26
not visible, 7.25
November, 10.35
obeisance to, 11.37, 39
objective, 9.18
oblation, 9.16
observer, 9.18
ocean, 10.21
odor, 7.9
offering, 9.27
ointments, 11.11
Oṁ, 7.8 ; 9.17
omni vision 9.15
omni-directional, 11.11
one-syllable sound 10.25
opinion, 18.6
opponents, 3.32
opulences, 10.40
origin, 9.18; 10.39
originator, 9.13; 10.8
ornaments, 11.10
Pāṇḍavas, 10.37

**Krishna continued,**
partner, 15.7
Pāvaka, 10.23
penetrates, 11.40
perfected souls, 10.26
perfumes, 11.11
Person of incomparable splendor, 11.43
Person of universal dimensions, 11.46
plants, 15.13
poets identity, 10.37
Power Infinite, 11.40
Prahlāda, 10.30
praised, 11.44
prayers, 10.25
priests identity, 10.21
Primal God, 10.12
Primal Person, 11.31
primeval cause, 7.10
priority, 12.20
procreators, 10.6
punishment, 10.38
purifier, 9..17
rainfall control, 9.19
Rakṣas identity, 10.23
Rāma identity, 10.31
rarely known, 7.3
recalled at death, 8.5
reciprocates, 4.11
recognizing, 5.29
Refuge, 11.38
relation to, 4.35
reliance effective, 9.32
reliance on 4.10; 7.14;18.56
remembered, 8.7
reproduction 10.28
research of, 10.17
reservoir of energies, 9.18
residence, 15.6
resort of world, 11.37
Respected, 11.31
responsibility, 3.24; 10.20
Rig Veda, 9.17
rivers identity, 10.32
romance, 7.11; 10.28
rulers identity, 10.38
rules of social conduct, 14.27

**Krishna continued,**
sacrificial ceremony, 9.16
Sāma Veda, 9.17; 10.22,35
sanctified offering, 9.16
sanctuary ultimate, 11.38
Śaśāṅka, 11.39
sciences, 10.32
sea identity, 10.21,27
sea monsters, 10.31
season identity, 10.35
secrets identity, 10.38
self disciplinary, 10.18
self-declaration, 10.13
self-sufficient, 7.12
senses, identity, 10.22
serpents, 10.28
service to 14.26
shark identity, 10.31
shelter, 9.18; 11.18,43
shielded, 7.25
Shiva identity, 10.23
silence identity, 10.38
Singular Basis, 9.15
Skanda identity, 10.21
slayer of Madhu, 1.34
smiling, 2.10
snakes identity, 10.29
sound, 7.8; 9.16; 10.25
speech about, 10.9
spirits identity, 10.29
spiritual master, 11.43
splendor, 7.10; 10.36,41; 11.19,43
spring identity, 10.35
stars, 10.21
strength, 7.11
subduers, 10.29
sum total, 11.37,40
sun, 10.21
sunlight, 7.8,9
supernatural power, 4.6
supernatural rulers, 10.2,22
supervisor, 9.10
supporter, 9.18
Supreme Being, 9.9
Supreme Form, 11.9
Supreme God, 5.29

**Krishna continued,**
Supreme Master, 7.30; 8.4
Supreme Objective, 6.14
Supreme Person, 10.15; 15.18,19
Supreme Reformer, 10.12
Supreme Refuge, 10.12
supreme residence, 8.21
Supreme Soul, 10.32
sustains, 9.5
swindlers, 10.36
taste, 7.8
thick-haired, 1.24
think about, 10.10
thinking of, 6.14; 18.57,58
thousand-armed, 11.46
thunderbolt, 10.28
thunderstormers, 10.21
time, 10.30,33
titan identity, 10.30
trend-setter, 3.23
troubled in psyche, 17.6
Uccaiḥśrava, 10.27
unaffected, 1.21; 7.13,25
unbiased, 9.29
uncontaminated, 13.32
under-estimated, 7.24
unique, 11.43
universal father, 9.17
Universal Form, 11.7
universal, 10.12
universal influence, 4.11; 10.39
universally available, 6.30
universe reality, 11.13
unrecognized, 7.13; 9.24
Usana identity, 10.37
Vaiśvānara, 15.13
Vajra identity, 10.28
Variety, 9.15
Varuṇa, 10.29; 11.39

**Krishna continued,**
Vāsava Indra, 10.22
Vāsudeva, 10.37
Vāsuki identity, 10.28
Vasus identity, 10.23
Vāyu, 11.39
Vedas, 7.8; 9.17; 10.22; 15.18
Vedic ritual, 9.16
victory, 10.36,38
Vinata identity, 10.30
Vishnu, 10.21; 11.9,24
Vitteśa identity, 10.23
Vṛṣṇis identity, 10.37
Vyāsa identity, 10.37
water, 7.8
weapon, 10.28,31; 11.10
wind identity, 10.31
wise men, 10.38
word, 10.25,33
work of, 11.55; 12.10
worship ,7.28; 9.14,15,20,22,23,29; 12.6; 15.19
Yajur Veda, 9.17
Yakṣas identity, 10.23
Yama, 10.29; 11.39
yoga master, 11.4,9
yoga process, 12.10
yogi attainment, 12.4
yogi dear, 7.17; 12.14
yogi sages, 10.2,25,26,37
yogi sages' cause, 10.6
Kṣamā, 10.34
Kuvera, 10.23
Kuntī, 1.16,27; 2.14,37,60; 3.9,39; 5.22; 8.16; 9.7; 13.2; 14.4
Kuntibhoja, 1.5
Kuru, 1.25; 2.41; 4.31; 6.43
kurukṣetre, 1.1
kuśa grass, 6.11

# L

laborers, Krishna
facilitates, 9.32
lamentation, 2.25; 12.17
lamp, 6.19
language, 16.4
lawlessness, 1.40
laziness, 14.8
leaf, 9.26

left-over food, 17.10
leisure, 6.17
letters, 10.33
levels of reality, 9.15
liberated person,
4.23; 14.2,23-26
**liberation,**
dedication to, 5.28
knowers of, 10.35
many births, 6.45
perpetual type, 5.28
described, 13.24
godly talent, 16.5
status, 14.2
life, Krishna, 7.9
life-duration, 9.21
life-giving codes, 12.20
light of luminaries, 13.18
light, , 7.8; 10.21; 15.12
liking, , 3.34; 4.22; 7.27
lion, , 10.30
liquids, 7.4
listeners, 18.67
lives, sacrificed, 1.33
living beings, 2.28; 9.8
living space,
13.1,2,6,7,20,27,35
location of yogi, 6.11
location, 18.14
logic, 13.5
logicians, 10.32
Lord of all beings, 18.61
Lord of gods, 11.25,37,45
Lord of supernatural
rulers and powers, 8.4
Lord of yoga, 18.75,78
lotus leaf, 5.10; 11.2
lover, 11.44
low opinion, 9.11
luck, warrior's, 2.32
lust, resistance, 2.71
lusty enjoyment, 16.11
lusty urge, 3.39; 16.10
luxuries, 2.5; 9.21

# M

Madhu, 1.14,34; 2.1;
6.33; 8.2
majesty, 18.43
managers, 18.41,44
manifestations, 10.16,19
manifested energies,
4.6; 8.18,19
Maṇipuṣpaka, 1.16
manliness, 7.8
Manu, 4.1
Marīci, 10.21
mass of splendor, 11.17
masses, 2.69
master, Krishna, 8.4; 9.18
master, spirit is, 15.8
masters of philosophical
theory, 6.46
material energy, 4.6; 7.14
material existence,
cessation, 5.25,26
**material nature,**
–also see modes of
material nature
action bound, 3.9
actions, 9.12
as cause, 13.21
beginningless, 13.20
forces, 18.59
foundation, 9.8
imperceptible, 15.3
influence banished,
10.11; 18.19
inquiry, 13.1
Krishna's womb,
14.3,4
Krishna's, 9.7
moods, 13.20
overpowering, 9.8
performer, 14.19
producer, 9.10
productions, 13.27
reliance on, 9.12
restrictive, 7.20
retrogression into, 9.7
spirit transcends,
14.20
sponsors hopes 9.12
submission to, 3.33
supernatural level,
9.13
Supreme Spirit, 13.15
universal, 18.40
Medhā, 10.34
**meditation,**
compared, 12.12
death method, 8.10
deep type, 8.8
energization, 8.10
God as subject, 8.9
on Krishna, 2.61; 9.22;
10.17; 12.8
**meditation continued,**
pleasure-prone
people, 2.44
power-seeking
people, 2.44
scriptural
information, 2.53
steady type, 2.55-56
superficial type, 3.6
valid type, 3.7
meditator, inquiry of, 2.54
**memory,**
Krishna produced,
15.15
indulgences, 2.59
men, 7.8; 10.27
mental approach, 3.1
mental concepts, 16.1
mental dominance, 2.54
mercy, 11.1, 25,31,44,45
merit-based world, 9.20
Meru, 10.23
**mind**
6th . device, 15.7
compared, 3.42
control absolute, 8.14
control difficult,
6.34,35
controlled, 5.28; 6.35
drift / restraint, 6.26
impulsive, 6.34
interiorized, 8.8
Krishna anchored, 8.7
passion fostered, 3.40
purification, 5.11
regulation, 3.3
resistant, 6.34
restricted, 8.12
troublesome, 6.34
unsteady, 6.35
wanderings, 6.26
mindal energy, 7.4
minute factor, 8.9
mirror, 3.38
miserable conditions, 2.56
misery-free place, 2.51
misfortune, 6.40
misplaced self identity,
16.18; 17.5
misty season, 8.25
moderation, 6.16,17
modes of material nature,
14.10,23
modesty, 16.2

money, 16.12,17
monitor, 10.30
monkey insignia, 1.20
month, 10.35
**moods,**
detachment, 14.22
extraction, 2.58
hindrance, 3.34
like / dislike, 3.34
material nature's, 13.20
mood,
motivation, 3.29
phases, 2.45
yogic, 5.2
**moon,**
death, 8.24,25
eye, 11.19
Krishna, 7.8; 10.21
lord, 11.39
mundane, 15.6
sap, 15.13
splendor, 15.12
moral action,
recommended, 3.8
morality,7.11; 10.38; 18.78
mother, 9.17
motivation, 2.47; 6.4
mountain, 10.23
mourning, 2.11
mouth, 11.10,25
mouth of spiritual existence, 4.32
mouth of Universal Form, 11.19
movement, 18.14
multiplicity, 18.21
multitude of beings, 8.19
mundane affinity, 6.15
mundane energy, 3.5; 7.4
mundane influences, 15.2
musical instruments, 1.13
musicians, 11.22
mystic seers, 2.16

# N

Nakula, 1.16
Nārada, 10.13,26
Narāyana Form, 11.46,52
natural resources, 11.22
**Nature,**
Krishna's, 14.2
producer, 5.14
types, 16.3,4
neck posture, 6.13
nectar, 18.37
needy person, 7.16
negligence, 14.9
nervousness, 3.30
night of Brahmā, 8.17-19
nighttime, death, 8.25
nine-gate city, 5.13
no possessions, 6.10
non-acting factor, 4.18
non-attachment, 3.28; 6.4; 15.3
non-existence, 10.5
non-reliance, 3.18
non-violence, 10.5; 13.8; 16.2; 17.14
northern sun passage, 8.24
nose, breath, 5.27
nose-tip gazing, 6.13
nourishment, 3.14
November, 10.35

# O

obeisance, 11.21,35,39,44; 18.65
objective, Krishna, 9.18
oblation, 9.16; 11.19; 17.28
obligatory action, 6.1; 18.7
observer of reality, 14.19
observer, 13.23
ocean, absorption, 2.70
ocean, Krishna
represented, 10.24
odor, Krishna related, 7.9
offering, 3.12; 9.16
ointments, 11.11
old age, 13.9, 14.20
Oṁ, 7.8; 8.13; 9.17; 17.24
Oṁ tat sat, 17.23
one imperishable being, 18.20
oneness, 18.20
openings of body, 8.12
opinion of Krishna, 9.11
**opportunity,**
devotion, 9.33
rejection, 18.1,2
renunciation, 18.49
usage, 5.2
opposite features, 5.3
opulences, 10.40
origin, 9.18; 10.39; 11.2; 14.3
ornaments, 11.10
overheated food, 17.9

# P

pacified mind, 2.65
**pain,**
Krishna derived, 10.5
periodic, 2.14
pleasure related, 5.22
spirit cause, 13.21
pancajanya, 1.15
Pandava, 6.2; 10.37
pandit, 4.19
Pāndu, 1.1,3,14; 4.35; 11.55; 14.22; 16.5
parentage, 9.32
partial insight, 3.29
partner, 15.7
**passion,**
avoidance, 2.56
emotion, 3.37
insight blocked, 3.38
rooted out, 3.43
ruins discernment. 3.41
squelched, 3.41
warehouse, 3.40
past life impetus, 6.43,44
paths, hereafter, 8.26,27
patience, required, 10.5,34; 12.13; 13.8; 18.42
Pauṇḍra, 1.15
Pāvaka, 10.23
pay-off, 4.20
peace, , 5.12; 12.12; 17.16
pearls, 7.6
peer pressure, 2.34,35
penance, 4.28
**people,**
deluded, 5.15
four kinds, 7.16
peppery food, 17.9
**perception,**
clear type, 14.11
dangers, 13.9
hearing method, 13.26
mystic, 13.25; 15.10,11
spiritual, 15.10,11
Supreme Lord, 13.28
perceptive impurities, 14.6
perceptive person, 10.3
perceptive speakers, 5.4
perfected souls, 11.36
**perfection,**
supreme, 8.15
work, 12.10

**performance,**
detachment from, 6.4
recommended, 3.8
types, 18.10
**performer,**
confusion, 3.27
types, 18.19,26-28
perfumes, 11.11; 15.8
permitter, 13.23
Person of universal dimensions, 11.46
Person, knowing everything, 8.9
**personal energies,**
controlled, 3.43
friend / enemy, 6.6
yoga control, 4.1
personal existence, Supreme Soul, 8.3
personal initiative, 13.6,9
personal undertakings, 12.16
personality, 2.12; 13.1,2
Personified Veda, 3.15
philosophers, 6.3,46
physical activity, 6.1
pious merits, 9.21
pious person, 6.40
piously-departed spirits, 10.29
plants, 15.13
**pleasure,**
cause sin, 1.44
family, 1.32
Krishna derived, 10.5
objective, 9.21
pain, 6.7
poetic quotation, 2.42
sensual contact, 5.22
spirit cause, 13.21
terminal 5.22
poets,poetry, 10.35,37
poison, 18.37,38
political affairs, 1.1
political power, 1.31,32; 2.43
population, 7.25
**possessions,**
absent, 6.10
austerity, 4.28
detachment towards, 12.13
freedom from, 2.45
indifference, 2.71
potential, 13.4
power, anger, 3.37
practice, mind control, 6.35
Prahlāda, 10.30
prāṇāyāma, 18.33
pratyāhar, 8.11
prayers, 10.25; 11.14
predominating influences, 14.10
pressure of change, 7.25
pride, 13.8; 15.5; 16,10,17; 18.35
priest, 4.24; 11.22
priestly teachers, 18.41,42
Primal God, 10.12
Primal Person, 11.31; 15.4
primeval unmanifested states, 8.20
priority, 3.2
Procreator Brahmā, - see Brahmā
procreators, 10.6
producer God, 13.17
production, 7.6; 13.27
property control, 4.33
proposal, two-way, 3.2
prosperity, 18.78
prosperous parents, 6.41
prostrations, 11.35
Pṛthā, 1,25,26; 2.3,21,39,42,55,72; 3.16; 4.11; 6.40; 7.1; 8.8,14,19; 9.32; 10.24; 12.7; 18.6
**psyche,**
described, 13.6,7
directive part, 6.7
friend / enemy, 6.6
God inhabits, 18.61
Krishna entered, 15.15
perceiver different, 10.35
spirit powered, 10.34
psychological core, 13.18
psychological environment, 13.19
psychological perfection, 7.3
psychological power, 8.10
psychological results of sacrifice, 4.31
psychological supremacy, 9.5
psychologically pacified, 6.27
pungent food, 17.9
punishment, 10.38
purificatory acts, 18.5
purified parents, 6.41
**purifier,**
consciousness, 9.2
experience, 4.38
Krishna, 9.17
purity of being, 16.1; 17.16
purity, 13.8; 17.14
Purujit, 1.5

# Q,R

questions, 4.34; 5.1
radiance, 8.9; 11.17
rage, 17.5
rain, 3.14; 9.19
Rakṣas, 10.23
Rāma, 10.31
range of Supreme Spirit, 13.14-18
reactionary work, 4.19
realism, 16.7
**Reality,**
indefinable, 12.3
Krishna highest, 7.7
Krishna represented, 10.36
Krishna's womb, 14.3,4
One, 11.7,13
perceiving person, 3.28
reality-piercing vision, 2.57,58
science, 13.12
realized knowledge, 4.37,42
reasoning, 15.15
rebels, 11.22
**rebirth,**
avoidance, 5.17
cessation, 15.4,6
exemption, 4.9; 8.15,16
faithless person, 9.3
formula for, 8.6
freedom from, 2.51
heaven prior, 9.21
planetary effect, 8.25
promised, 2.43
repetitive, 8.16
transcended, 13.24

**rebirth continued,**
wicked peoples', 16.19
yogi's, 6.41
recitation of scripture, 16.1; 17.15
reciters, 2.42,43
recognition of reality, 10.34; 16.2
reference, senses, mind, intelligence, spirit, 3.42
reference, 5.17
reform, 9.31
reformed persons, 9.20
Refuge Supreme, 11.38
regulation,
--see mind regulation,
--see action regulation
**reincarnation,**
devotee, 12.7
formula for, 8.6
Krishna, 7.26
resisted, 5.17
rejection of consequences, 18.1,2,4
rejection of opportunity, 18.1,2
relation, 5.7
relatives, war field, 1.26
reliance on Krishna, 9.32
religion, 9.24
**religious ceremony,**
-see also ritual action
austerity, 4.28
categories, 17.7-10
enjoyer, 5.29
false type, 16.17
invented ones, 17.1
Krishna / master, 9.24
ordinances, 3.9,10; 17.23
prescribed, 17.25
purifies, 4.30
sacrifice, 4.25
types, 17.11-13
unapproved type, 9.23
yogi bypass, 8.28
religious fulfillment, 3.9,10
remembering, objects, 3.6
**renouncer,**
charity, 18.10
consistent type, 5.3
defined, 6.1
**renunciation,**
compared, 12.12
cultural activity, 5.2
defined, 18.11
insufficient, 3.4
mental type, 5.13
social activity?, 5.1
social opportunities, 5.2
to Krishna, 18.57
types, 18.7-9
yoga applied, 6.2
renunciation of opportunities, 5.6
reproduction 10.28
repulsion, 12.15
reputation, 2.34-36; 17.18
research, 18.18
reservoir of energies, 9.18
residence, supreme, 15.6
resident of body, 5.13
resort of the world, 11.37
Respected Person, 11.31
restlessness, 14.11
**restraint,**
bodily limbs, 3.6
questioned, 3.33
tendency, 18.42
**result,**
best one, 3.2
giving up, 18.6
motivation resisted, 2.47
transcended, 6.1
types, 18.12
yogi bypass, 8.28
retardation, 14.5
retarded people, 14.18; 17.4
retrogression, 9.7
revelation, 11.53
reverence, 11.40,44
reversion, 8.18
reward, 17.21
Rig Veda, 9.17
righteous behavior, 9.3
righteous duty, 3.35
--also see duty
righteous lifestyle, 9.21
righteous method, 9.2
righteous practice, 2.40
righteousness, 4.7
**ritual action,**
conditional, 4.12
results rapid, 4.12
Universal Form, 11.48
ritual performers, 6.46
ritual regulation, 4.33
rivers, Krishna represented, 10.31
romance, 7.11; 10.28
rotten food, 17.10
ruination, 11.2
rulers, 10.38
ruling sector, 18.41,43

## S

sacred thread, 17.14
**sacrifice,**
abandoned?, 18.3
purificatory, 18.5
results, 4.31
to Krishna, 18.65
types, 17.11-13
value, 4.30
sacrificial ceremony, 9.16; 11.48,53
sacrificial fire, 3.38
sacrificial ingredients, 4.24
Sādhyā, 11.22
Sahadeva, 1.16
Śaibya, 1.5
saint / wicked person, 9.30
saintly people, 4.8
salty food, 17.9
Sāma Veda, 9.12; 10.22,35
sāṁkhya philosophy, 2.39; 13.25; 18.3,19
sāṁkhya, yoga practice, 5.4,5
sanctification, 3.13
sanctified offering, 9.16
sanctuary, 11.38
sanity, 10.5
Sanjaya, 1.1,2,24; 2.1,9; 18.74,76
sannyāsa, 18.2
Śaśaṅka, 11.39
sat, 17.26,27
satisfaction, 2.70; 4.20; 10.18
Sātyaki, 1.17
science of reality, 13.12
sciences, 10.32
scriptural injunctions, 16.23,24; 17.1

scripture, 2.53
sea, 10.24,27
sea monsters, 10.31
seasons, 10.35
seat of yogi, 6.11,12
seclusion, 13.11
secret, 9.1,2; 10.38
security, 6.15; 16.2; 18.62
seeing what was never seen, 11.45,47
seeing, 5.8
**seer,**
attainment, 5.25,26
common factor, 5.18
destination, 2.51
inquiry of, 2.54
**self,**
concentration on, 6.10
core, 6.18
enemy, 6.5
evaluation, 6.5
fixed on, 6.25
friendship, 6.5
pacified, 6.14
self-composed, 4.41
self-conceited, 16.17
self-content, 2.55
self-control, 5.7; 6.7; 10.5
self-denial, 4.28
self identity, 16.18, 17.5
self-image, 18.16
selfishness, 3.30
self-perception, 6.20
self-purification, 6.12
self-realization, 4.38
self-restraint, 12.11; 13.8; 16.1; 17.16
self-satisfaction, 6.20
self-situated, 3.17
**sensations,**
alternating, 2.14
coping, 2.14
detachment, 5.21
sense control, 2.69
senseless, 3.32
**senses,**
attractive objects, 5.9
compared, 3.42
death baggage, 15.8
Krishna represented, 10.22
like / dislike, 3.34
living space, 13.6
mind affected, 2.67
**senses continued,**
passion fostered, 3.40
purification usage, 5.11
regulating, 3.41
restraint, 2.61
torment ascetic, 2.60
withdrawn, 2.58
sensual activity, withdrawal, 6.25
sensual contacts, 5.27
sensual energy control, 5.28; 6.12; 12.4
sensual energy, restraint, 4.39; 6.24
sensual feelings, retraction, 2.68
sensual objects, 2.62
sensual potency, 13.21
sensual powers, 4.26
sensual pursuits, 4.26
sensual range, 7.24
sensuality, controlled, 2.61; 5.24
sensuality, perpetual, 7.27
separation, from emotion, 6.23
serpents, 10.28; 11.15
service sector, 18.44
serving, 4.34
sexual intermixture, 1.40
sexual restraint, 6.14
sexual urge, 16.8
Shankara, 10.23
shark, 10.31
shelter, 9.18; 18.62
ship, 2.67
Shiva, 10.23
sickness, 17.9
Śikhandī, 1.17
silence, 10.38; 17.16
simpletons, 3.26; 5.4
**sin,**
considered, 1.36,38
God's resistance, 5.15
sinful propensities, 7.28
singers, 10.26
sins terminated, 5.25
situations, 13.22
sixth device, 15.7
Skanda, 10.24
skills destroyed, 1.42
sky resonated, 1.19
sleep regulator, 10.20
sleep, 5.8; 6.16,17; 14.8; 18.35
smelling, 5.8
smoke, 18.48
smoky season, 8.25
Smṛti, 10.34
snakes, 10.29
social circumstance, 6.41
social life, 13.10
social values, 18.34
society, maintenance, 3.25
solids, 7.4
soma drinkers, 9.20
Somadatta, 1.8
son of charioteer, 11.26
son, 1.26,33; 11.44
sorcerers, 17.4
sorrow, 18.35
soul, embodied, adaptations, 2.13
soul, see spirit
soul-situated, 2.45
**sound,**
austerity, 4.26
Krishna related, 7.8; 10.25
Oṁ, 17.24
sour food, 17.9
**space,**
comparison, 9.6; 10.33
mundane, 7.4
pervaded, 11.20
**species,**
as facility, 6.32
comparison, 5.18
ignorant type, 14.15
Krishna inhabits, 6.30; 7.26
rebirth, 14.15
spirit caused, 7.6
spirits inhabit, 15.8
**speech,**
control, 18.51,52
disciplined,17.15
Krishna, 10.34
spinning machine, 18.61
**spirit,**
addicted, 15.9
affected, 15.16
amazing, 2.29
beginningless, 13.20
body energizer, 10.34
cannot be killed, 2.19
cannot kill, 2.19
captivated, 14.5

**spirit continued,**
compared, 3.42
condition-resistant, 2.23
confused, 3.40
considered temporary, 2.26
creature habitat, 6.29
death impossible, 2.20,21
degradation, 16.21
dry-less, 2.23
elevate self, 6.5
eternal, 2.20; 15.7
experience, 13.22
fantastic, 2.29
faultless, 5.19
going to Krishna, 4.9
governor of psyche, 15.9
higher energy, 7.5; 13.23; 15.17
immeasurable, 2.18
imperishable, 2.21
impulsion captivates, 14.6
incombustible, 2.23
indestructible, 2.17
individual, 15.7
Krishna represented, 10.29
Krishna's partner, 15.7
master of body, 15.8
material nature captivates, 14.5
material nature transcended, 14.20
mourning unworthy, 2.30
movements, 15.10
non-actor, 5.13
non-doer, 13.28
non-killable, 2.30
not born, 2.26
not killed, 2.26
origin of species, 7.6
perception, 13.25,28
permanent,2.24
primeval, 2.20
seen / unseen, 15.11
self upliftment, 13.28
sensation cause, 13.21
stable type, 15 16,

**spirit continued,**
stable, 2.24; 15.16
transcendental, 13.33
types, 15.16
unaffected ones, 10.33; 15.16
undetected, 2.28
undisplayed, 2.25
unimaginable, 2.25
universe sustained by 7.5
unknown, 2.29
wet-less, 2.23
wonderful, 2.29
spiritual core self, 6.18
spiritual delight, 5.24
spiritual discernment, 18.37
**spiritual existence,**
known, 7.29
mouth of, 4.32
sacrifice support 4.24,25
spiritual level, 5.10
spiritual master, 4.34; 11.43; 17.24; 18.68,69
spiritual peace, 5.29
spiritual perfection, 3.4
spiritual plane, 5.19,20
**spiritual reality,**
description, 6.44
designation, 17.23
question of, 8.1
unaffected, supreme, 8.3
spiritual religion, 4.31
spiritual self, 2.55
spiritual teacher, 17.14
spiritual world, 8.20,21,24
spirituality, 5.24-26
spiritually content, 3.17
spiritually-pleased, 3.17
splendor, 7.10; 10.36; 18.78
spring, 10.35
Śrī, 10.34
stability, 13.8
stale food, 17.10
standard position, 6.33
standard, two-fold, 3.3
stars, 10.21
states of being, 7.12; 13.31
status of next life, 8.6
stone, 6.8; 14.24

stormers, 11.22
straightforwardness, 13.8; 16.1; 17.14; 18.42
strength, 7.11
string comparison, 7.6
strong-mindedness, 16.3
stubborn, 16.17
student, 4.34
stupified at death, 2.72
subduers, 10.29
Subhadra, 1.6,18
substantial things, 2.16
subtle body, 9.19
success/ failure, indifference, 2.48; 4.22
suffering, 13.9
Sughoṣa, 1.16
sum total, 8.1,4
summer season, 8.24
**sun,**
comparison, 5.16; 10.34
death affected by, 8.25
eye, 11.19
Krishna related, 7.8,9; 10.21
Krishna's splendor, 15.12
mundane, 15.6
thousands, 11.11
super-fantastic form, 18.77
Supermost Personality, 8.1
supernatural destroyers, 11.6
supernatural manifestations, 10.40
**supernatural rulers,**
appeasers of, 7.4,.20,23; 9.23,25
Divine Form not seen, 11.52
human relation, 3.11,12
Krishna represented by, 10.22
Krishna unknown to, 10.2,14
respect, 17.14
source, 10.2
Universal Form 11.6,15,21
supernatural sight, 11.8
supernatural stormers, 11.6
supernatural wondrous manifestations, 10.16,19

supernatural, material nature, 9.13
supernaturally disposed, 11.33,34
**Supersoul,**
beings inhabited by, 13.28
described, 13.14-18,23
disliked, 16.18
transmigration, 18.61
troubled, 17.6
supporter, 9.18
Supreme Being, 9.4-6,9; 18.62
-see also Krishna
supreme destination, 13.28; 16.23
Supreme Form, 11.9,47
supreme goal, 6.45; 9.32
Supreme God, 5.29; 16.18
supreme information, 10.1
Supreme Lord, 13.23,28,32; 16.8
supreme objective, 6.14; 7.18; 8.21
supreme peace, 4.39
supreme perfection, 8.15; 14.1
**Supreme Person,**
action free, 5.14
cause of all causes, 8.22
defined, 15.18
described, 8.9
Krishna, 10.15
reached, 8.8
Supreme Primal State, 8.28
Supreme Reality, 10.12; 11.18; 13.13-18
Supreme Reformer, 10.12
Supreme Refuge, 10.12
Supreme Regulator of religious ceremonies and disciplines, 8.2,4
**Supreme Soul / Spirit,**
association, 15.5
austerity, 3.15
described, 15.17
explained, 11.1
information, 13.12
known, 7.29
Krishna, 10.32
meditate upon, 3.30
**Supreme Soul / Spirit continued**
mundane world producer, 8.3
permitter, 13.23
personal existence, 8.3
Personified Veda, 3.15
question of, 8.1
religious ceremony, 3.15
supporter, 15.17
Supreme Supernatural Person and Power, 8.1
Supreme Supervisor, 8.9
Supreme truth, 5.16,17
supreme yoga, 18.75
supreme destination, 10.35
Supreme, pure world, 14.14
Surendra, 9.20
surrender, 18.62
sustainer, God, 13.17
svarga angelic world, 2.43
swindlers, 10.36
syllable, 10.25
synthesis, 13.27

# T

take note of it, 9.31
talents, 16.3
talking, 5.9
taste, 7.8
tat, 17. 25
**teachers,**
Gītā, 18.68,69
lineage, 4.2
reality-conversant, 4.34
social, 1.26,33
teaching, best, 4.3; 15.20
teeth, 11.23,25
temptation, 2.59
**tendencies,**
elaborated, 18.42-44
eliminated, 6.27
innate, 17.2
overcome, 4.36
texture of existence, 8.6
thief, 3.12
thighs, 11.23
**thinking,**
controlled, 6.10,12
restrained, 5.26
stoppage, 6.20,25
wicked people, 16.13,14
thought controlled, 6.18
thoughts on Krishna, 12.9
threefold influence, 16.21
thunderbolt, 10.28
time, 10.30,33; 11.32
time cycle, 8.17-19
titan, 10.30
tortoise, 2.58
torture, 17.6,19
touching, 5.8
trading, 18.44
**tradition,**
abandoned, 18.66
Arjuna considers, 1.39
destroyers of, 1.43
disgust with, 2.52
trance, 6.22
tranquility, 10.5; 18.42
transcendent person, 14.21
transformation of psyche, 14.2
transmigration, 18.61
tree, 10.26; 15.1-3
trend, 17.3
trickery, 17.18
truth, 9.1
truthfulness, 10.5
truths of existence, 2.16
tyāga, 18.2

# U

Uccaiḥśrava, 10.27
unavoidable circumstance, 2.27
uncles, 1.26
uncontrolled person, 2.66
undisciplined person, 6.36
undivided God, 13.17
unintelligent person, 7.24
universal destruction, 11.25
**Universal Form,**
displayed, 11.3,5-47
Sanjaya, 18.77
supernatural rulers terrified, 11.21
viewers listed, 11.22
universal integration, 9.18
Universal Soul, 13.14-18

**universe,**
Krishna supports, 10.42; 11.38
one reality, 11.7
operations, 9.9
production / destruction, 7.6
rejoices, 11.36
spirit sustained, 7.5
three partitions, 11.43
unmanifested energy, 13.6
unmanifested states, 8.20
unpleasant things, 5.20
Upanishads, 13.5
upper class, 16.15
Uśanā, 10.37
Uttamauja, 1.6

# V

Vaiśvānara, 15.14
vajra, 10.28
Vāk, 10.34
vanity, 18.26
vapor bodies, 11.22
variations, 3.28,29
Variety, 9.15
Varuṇa, 10.29; 11.38
Vāsava, 10.22
vast existence of death, 12.7
Vāsudeva, 7.19; 10.37; 11.50
Vāsuki, 10.28
Vasus, 10.23
Vāyu, 11.39
Veda knower, 8.11; 9.20; 15.1
**Veda,**
Krishna knows / known, 15.15
Krishna related, 7.8; 10.22
offers of 2.45
ordained, 17.23
Personified, 3.15
spoken description, 6.44
surpassed, 6.44
Vedānta, 15.15
worth, 2.46
yogi beyond, 8.28
Vedic education,
Universal Form, 11.48
Vedic hymns recited, 13.5; 15.1; 17.13
Vedic injunction, 9.21; 16.17
Vedic ritual, 9.16
Vedic ceremonies, 11.48
Vedic study, 11.53
Vedic verses, 2.42
vibration, necessary, 3.5
vices, terminated, 5.25
**victory,**
defeat, 2.38
Krishna represented, 10.36,38 ; 18.78
not desired, 1.31
viewers, 2.19
vigor, 16.3
Vikarṇa, 1.8
Vinata, 10.30
violence, 5.10; 18.25
Virāṭa, 1.4,17
virtue, deviation, 9.24
virtuous acts, 6.40
virtuous character, 9.31
virtuous people, 3.13
Vishnu, 10.21
visible world, 8.18,19
vision of reality, 15.10,11
vision of yogi, 2.61
vision, Arjuna given, 11.8
visitation of Krishna, 4.9
visual focus, 5.27
Viśvadeva, 11.22
Vitteśa, 10.23
Vivasvāt, 4.1,4
void, 2.69
vows, ascetics of, 4.28; 7.28; 9.14
Vṛṣṇis, 1.40; 3.36; 10.37
Vyāsa, 10.13,37; 18.75

# W

walking, 5.8
war, 2.33,34
**warriors,**
battle hungry, 1.22
heaven, 2.32
supernaturally disposed, 11.33
**water,**
Krishna accepts, 9.26
Krishna related, 7.8
lotus leaf, 5.10
master of, 11.39
psychic type, 1.41
weapon carriers, Krishna represented, 10.31
weapons, 2.23; 10.28,31; 11.10
weather, 2.14
welfare of all, 12.4
well (water), 2.46
what to do, 16.7
whole multitude, 9.8
wicked persons, 4.8; 16.7
wickedness, 4.7
wife, 13.10
will power, 18.60
**wind,**
Krishna compared, 9.6; 10.31
mind compared, 6.34
regulator, 11.39
ship, 2.67
spirit compared, 15.8
**wise person,**
condition-resistant, 2.15
duty, 3.25
immortality. 2.15
Krishna represented, 10.38
realization, 2.13
womb, Krishna's, 14.3,4
wombs of wicked people, 16.20
women, 1.40; 9.32; 10.34
wonders, 11.6
wood, 4.37
word compound, 10.33
**work,**
discarded, 2.50
material nature, 13.21
tendency, 4.13
working power, 3.30
work-prone people, 14.15
**world,**
action bound, 3.9
God pervades, 9.4
maintenance, 3.20
other, 4.31
production, 8.18,19
spirit pervaded, 2.17
stupefied, 7.13
trembles, 11.20,23
types, 14.14,15
utilized, 4.31
worries, 2.56; 16.10,11
**worship,**
ceremony, 16.1
exclusive, 9.22
God, 18.46

**worship continued,**
Krishna's,
7.16,28; 12.2
procedure, 3.10-12
supernatural rulers',
9.23
types, 17.4,11-13
worshippers of gods, 7.23
worshippers of Krishna,
7.23
worshippers rated, 9.25
worthless person 3.16

# Y

Yadu family man, 11.41
Yajur Veda, 9.17
Yakṣas, 10.23
Yama, 10.29; 11.38
yearning, 3.39; 18.49
**yoga practice,**
application lost, 4.2
application,
5.1; 6.2,28;,16.1
austerity, 4.28
celibacy required,
8.11
concentration, 8.12
controlling force, 4.1
cultural activities,
3.7; 4.41
determination, 18.33
deviation, 6.37
distress-remover, 6.17
exertion, 12.5
expertise, 6.3
harmonized, 10.7
indifference, 2.48
insight applied, 2.39
intellectual discipline,
2.49; 18.57
interiorization, 8.8
Krishna worship, 9.22
Krishna's, 11.47; 12.11
mastery, 2.53; 6.23,36
methods, 6.3
moderation, 6.16
mood, 2.48,50
perfected, 4.38; 6.43
performance skill,
2.50
preliminary, 12.9
proficiency, 5.7,8,12;
6.4,18,29
purpose, 6.12

**yoga practice continued,**
recommended,
7.1;.8.27; 12.9
renunciation, 9.28
required, 13.11
requirements, 12.4
sāṁkhya, 5.4
spiritual plane, 5.21
skill described, 4.18
technique, 4.3,42; 12.2
undistracted, 12.6
**yogi,**
action austerity, 4.27
actions antiseptic,
5.10
Arjuna, 6.46
attainment, 8.23
austerities bypassed,
8.28
baffled, 6.38
births end, 7.19
breath, 4.27
charity, 8.28
death, 8.10,13,24
defined, 6.1
destination, 4.31; 8.28
deviant, 6.37
devotee, 12.14,17
discipline, 6.8; 18.51
distinguished, 7.17
Divine Supreme
Person, 8.10
existential position,
6.15
experience, 6.8
faults ended, 6.28
fond to Krishna 7.17
happiness, 5.21; 6.28
hearing, 4.26
highest type, 6.32
informed type, 7.17
inquiry, 2.54
intention, 6.2
isolation, 6.10
kings, 4.15; 9.33
knowledge, 4.28
Krishna / everything,
7.19
Krishna attracts, 6.47
Krishna contact,
6.30; 8.14
Krishna devoted, 6.47
Krishna
remembrance, 8.13

**yogi continued,**
Krishna seen, 6.30
Krishna worship,
6.47; 12.6
Krishna's
representative, 7.18
Krishna-knowing,
7.30
lamp, 6.19
liberation,
5.26-28; 6.15
meditation, 6.12
memory, 3.6
methods, 12.1,2,3
non-actor, 5.13
past life impetus,
6.43,44
perfection, 6.43
philosophers, 10.37
philosophical / non-
philosophical, 3.3
planetary influence,
8.26
possessions, 4.28
proficiency, 6.4
psychologically
pacified, 6.27
purification, 5.11
release, 7.29
religion, 4.25
religious ceremonies,
8.28
seat, 6.11
sensual austerity, 4.26
sound austerity, 4.26
spiritual plane, 5.6
steadiness, 6.21
supernatural
authority4.25
supreme primal state,
8.28
tendencies, 6.45
two standards, 3.3
valid type, 3.7
Veda austerity, 4.28
Veda bypassed, 8.28
vision of species, 6.29
yoga austerity, 4.28

**yogi sages,**
aśvattha tree, 15.1-3
Krishna praised, 10.13; 11.21
Krishna represented, 10.25,26

**yogi sages, continued**
Krishna unknown, 10.2
seven, 10.6
source, 10.2
Universal Form, 11.15

Yudhāmanyu, 1.6
Yudhiṣṭhira, 1.16
Yuyudhāna, 1.4

# Index to Commentary


## A

abandonment, 454
abhiniveśa, 350
abode of universe, 321
aborigines, 258
absence of anger, 413
abusive language, 419
acquisition, 77
action, 215
action-prone, 106
action-reaction, 80
addiction, 99
Adhakṣena, 270
adhibhūtam, 247, 249
adhidaivam, 247
adhiṣṭhānam, 460
Adhiyajñah, 248, 249
adhyātma yoga, 162
Adhyātman, 247
ādyam puruṣam, 399
agent, attention, 460
Agni devata, 240
Agnidra, 435
ahamkāra, 134, 460
ahbyāsena, 217
alcohol, 469
all pervading reality, 267, 342, 366
aloneness, 134
alphabet, 258
alternate influence, 399
alternatives, 347
analytical switching device, 206
ancestor, 40
anesthetics, 390
angelic women, 363
**anger,**
  absence, 413
  passion, 419
animal rebirth, 388, 446
animal sacrifice, 439
antah karaṇa, 148, 404
antar ātmanā, 223
antar jyotih, 184, 208, 215
antelope skin, 199
anti-material sky, 401
Anu Gītā, 246
archanam, 340
**Arjuna,**
  actions condemned? 389
  agent only, 326
  apology, 332
  convinced, 488
  dear to Krishna, 485
  dilemma, 482
  divine forms seen, 333
  great soul, 488
  Krishna as, 305
  meeting Krishna, 341
  memory inadequate, 138
  mission, 30
  not cynical, 266
  obeisances, 329
  passive means, 67
  reincarnation forgotten, 138
  scorcher of enemy, 47
  siddha? 378
  supernatural vision, 216
  Universal Form, 316
  worshipped, 251
  yogi? 280
army, 42
arrogance, 418
ārya, 47
ascetics, listed, 158
ashram life, 199
Asita Devala, 294, 295
**association,**
  changes required, 427
  higher type, 414
  required, 363
  restricted, 364
aṣṭanga yoga, 148
astral body, 469
asuras, 190, 257
aśvattha tree, 398
ātma, 367
ātma buddhi prasādajam, 471
ātmasamyama, 157
ātma śuddha yoga, 140
ātmavan, 77
ātmavinigrahah, 443
**ātma yoga,**
  jñāna yoga, 140
  spirit perception, 371
  technique, 205
ātmayogat, 333
attachment to Krishna, 249
**attention energy,**
  curbed, 460
  details, 134
  research of, 383
attraction, 362
**austerity,**
  God's representative, 231
  limited, 337
  mistakes in, 412
  motive, 445
**author,**
  blessed, 24
  Nityānānda contact, 20, 64-66
  psychic association, 434
autonomy, 239
avenues of sensuality, 429
Ayodhyā, 141

## B

back log of reactions, 79
Bāli, 140
bankers, 325
Bardo Thodol, 387
beads of golden effulgence, 433
beginningless Supreme Reality, 365
behaviors, 132, 181, 360
being, 420
belief, 229
belief in God, 474
best of gods, 324
bestowals, practice required, 292
**Bhagavad Gītā,**
  alert, 381
  bearers' requirement, 485-486
  study of, 487

**Bhagavān,**
Krishna, 64
Nityānānda, 64
bhajate, 283
**bhakti yoga,**
bhakti + yoga, 364
buddhi yoga compliments, 442
details, 140, 251
highest, 349
modern type, 91
**bhakti,**
defined, 142
purity essential, 142, 290
bhaktim mayi parām, 486
bhaktyā, 279-281,
Bharata, 418
bhāsvatā, 293
bhāva, 250, 251, 252, 289, 482
bhāvasamśuddhi, 443
Bhīmasena, 417
**Bhishma,** 262, 417
karma yoga unknown, 137
treasury of advice, 18
yoga misuse, 48
bhogān, 109
bhoktārama, 188
Bhṛgu, 299
bījam, 305
bird of prey, 429
**body,**
composite, 359
preference, 55
spirit-opposed, 59
sunlight type, 262
brahma mahat, 379
brahma reality, 246
Brahma Sūtras, 350
**brahma yoga,**
blindness required, 12
note-taking, 14
obsession, 419
requirements, 12, 131
stages, 151
**brahma yogi,**
advanced one, 299
teaching discouraged, 468
**Brahmā, Lord,**
human creator, 107
lifespan, 257
mental energy primal, 258
mouth of spiritual existence, 161
Over-soul? 248
position, 299,
primal, 111
purpose of, 13
representative, 329
warning of, 109
worship of, 240
brahmākṣara, 111
brahman spiritual world, 446
brahman, focus, 240
brahmarandra, 465
brahmavādinām, 447
brahmavido, 261
breath, 470
bridge construction, 411
brilliant light, 215
buddhi organ, 91
**buddhi yoga,**
adherents, 340
appraised, 480
available, 388
basic, 278
bhakti yoga, 442
defined, 80
insight cleared, 129
Krishna originator, 203
main hub, 469
mastery, 353
objective, 128, 211
proficiency, 348
recommended, 345
result, 478
summary, 470
budha, 147

# C

casino, 277
caste, flawed, 39
caterpillar , 425
**causal body,**
details, 361
explained, 356
flaws, 362
initiative embedded, 362
celestial body, 277
**celibacy,**
details, 416, 465
privacy, 418
required, 202, 253, 441
subtle body curbed, 363
celibates, 90
center of eyebrows, 202
chakra, 361
Chandikā, 316
chanting, 292
character, 16, 284
charity, 337, 411
Chitti Devī, 174
chivalry, 47
Christ, Jesus, 248
circumscription, 239
citta, 205-207, 400
cittavṛtti, 210, 211
cittih, 174
city father, 275
city, nine gates, 177
civilization, 41
clarifying force, 384, 385
class, 39
club, 361
coconut, 439
color, 359
commodity, 459
communication, after death, 66
compartment, consciousness, 381
compassion, 414
conceit, 419
concepts, discipline, 273
condiments, 438
**confidence,**
appraised, 372
development, 229
immortality? 380
confusion, 133, 387
conscience, 43
consciousness, 381
**consequences,**
avoidance of, 411
complexity of, 79
inconvenient returns, 458
rejection, 451
consideration, 93
constant reality, 342
contentment, 291
convention, 240

**core self,**
attention, 134
finite, 369
location, 199
questioned? 17
correcting others, 48
cow, 231, 438
crane, 104
**craving,**
details, 129
essential force, 452
freedom from, 253
prāṇāyāma cures, 386
root of, 415
created beings, 267
creation, 289
creature, 359
**criminal,**
nature, 38
saintly? 283
critical energy, 14
cucumber, 439
cultural accounts, 452
**cultural activity,**
inferior? 101
material nature feeds on, 398
questioned, 247
waiver, 452, 457
cynicism, 266

# D

daivam, factor, 460
daivīm prakṛtim, 271
Damayanti, 109
**death,**
mental condition, 387
providence, 59
psychological condition, 250
salvation? 403
soul escapes, 50
debates, 365
deceit, 361, 418
defiance, 323
degradation, 39
Deity, 215
Deity Worship, 124, 272, 340
demigods, 144, 240
departed ancestor, 40
depressive energy, 387
**desire,**
causal body, 361
dormant, 148
impulsion, 383
tracing, 98
**destiny,**
clear, 23
elimination of, 415
factor, 460
hazy, 23
joke of, 24
perverse, 24
**detachment,**
application, 351
details, 121
material nature subdued by, 399
required, 59
resistance gained, 406
sensual resistance, 402
social life, 169
detection device, 401
determination, unreliable, 151
devabhogan, 276
devadeva, 314
Devakī, 30, 375
devarṣiṇām, 300
**devas,**
respected, 110
sight of, 109
Devayani, 191
Devotedness, 237
**devotee,**
emphasized, 351
greatest, 486
qualifications, 338
requirements, 272
types, 234-237
**devotion,**
defined, 142
insufficient, 218, 281
insight caused by, 338
purification, 142
purity, 290
supreme type, 480
dhāma paramam, 401
dharma, 192
dharmātma, 284
dharmyāmṛtam, 353
dhīmatām, 221
**Dhṛtaraṣṭra,**
conceited, 23
mother's fault, 12
past life prejudices, 13
stymied, 28
Dhruva, 435
dhruvam, 342,
dhyāna, 254, 371
dhyāna yoga, 479
dhyānayogaparo, 479
dhyāyato, 92
diet, non-violence, 412, 438, 479
digression, 346
dimensional travel, 261
disc, 361
disciple-teacher relation, 165
discipline of concepts, 273
discipline, brahma yoga rules, 34
disciplines of accomplishment, 161
discrimination,
disempowered, 392
disgust, 99
disputations, 365
divine force, 405
Divine Form, 333
divine harassment, 414
divine love, 414
divine mission, Arjuna's, 30
divyam cakṣuh, 312
divyān divi, 276
doṣavat, 453
doubts, 166
dreams, 392
**Droṇa,**
invincible? 417
karma yoga unknown, 137
yoga misuse, 48
drowsy body, 469
duhkhāntam, 471
dulling force, 384, 385
**Durgā,**
divine form, 333
goddess of nature, 24
Kamsa, 109
Over-soul? 248
Universal Form, 316
Yoginis, 416

Duryodhana, 13
Dushana, 141
dust, 130
duty, 127, 476

# E

eating, 292
education, 24, 378
eggs, 438
ekabhaktih, 237
elderly persons, 18
elevation, at death, 250, 251, 252
embryo, 130
**emotion,**
biased, 93
conversion, 81
expansive, 19
family promoted by, 31
fluid of, 51
impregnation, 379
repository, 131
distress separation, 210
end of sorrows, 471
energizer supreme, 367
energizing energy, 470
energy, 63
entrepreneur, 258
environment, 356, 387
eternal tree, 398
**evolution,**
celestial type, 112
creation, 289
species, 428
exemption, details, 113
**experience,**
essential, 164
hunt for, 89
experiential energy, 463
extensive mundane reality, 379
external, 182

# F

factors, 462
**faith,**
effective, 372
explained, 165
highest, 444
insufficient, 218, 308
**family,**
predominant, 144
security, 30
spiritual type, 30-31, 253
utility, 34
fate, mandatory, 64
father, 275
fearfulness, 410
fearlessness, 410
femininity, 230
fickleness, 415
firegod, 130
flavor, 359, 362
**flaws,**
causal form, 362
psychic, 222
flower, 280
fluid of emotions, 51
food, 437
forbearance, 416
formative energies, 411
fortune, 24
four-armed form, 333
freedom from conceit, 417
freedom from hatred, 417
fruit, 280
**frustration,**
energy, 419
heaven, 277
fusion of attention, 383

# G

gambler, 277
garbham, 379
Gautama Rishi, 246
Gāyatrī, 304
generals, 325
gentleness, 415, 442
geography, 172, 261
ghee, 273
ghoṣa, 211
glorification, 272
**God,**
accountable, 119
kingdom, 277
responsibility, 177
Supreme Person, 407
unique, 241
God of gods, 314
Goddess of education, 24
Goddess of fortune, 24
Goddess of nature, 24,
gods, 239
golden effulgence, 433
gopis, 253, 480
Gorakshanatha, Mahāyogi, 90, 201, 254
gorge, 411
Govardhana Hill, 240, 273
governing skill, 137
Govinda, 52
grace of God, 224
grace of providence, 94
grasping tendency, 151
great danger, 72
Greatest of persons, 357
greed, 386
**guarantee,**
details, 345
limited, 281
guardian of law, 317
guilt, sensitivity, 43
**guru,**
claims, 380
substitute, 282
gut feelings, 79

# H

Hanumān, 25, 240
**happiness,**
attachment to, 381
child's pursuit, 36
harassment, 15
Hari, 312
hashish, 438
Haṭha Yoga Pradīpika, 201
haṭha yoga, 68
hearing, 266, 308, 319
**heaven,**
qualifications, 276
value, 70
sex attraction, 392
yogi bypass, 276
hermitage life, 199
horse, wild, 421
**human being,**
body important, 392
influenced, 326
providence restricts, 59
reliant, 111
humility, 449

# I

identifier, 57
identity, 133
Ikṣvāku, 137
images, mental, 194
**imagination**
chamber, 194
orb, 206
theft assistant, 12
immorality, 398
immovable constant reality, 366

immovable existence, 342
immunity, explained, 375
impatience, 361
imperishable existence, 342, 366
imperishable tree, 398
impersonalist, 342
impetus, 462
**impressions,**
  details, 442
  development, 194
  lure of, 411
  theft, 12
imprints, sensual, 92
impulsion, 390
inconceivable, 366
indefinable, 366
independence, 459
indestructible supreme reality, 317
India, 240
indifference, 457
Indra, 240, 299
indriyagrāman, 211
industrialists, 325
infusement, 246
**initiative,**
  attention, 150
  individualized, 359
innate tendency, 432
inner instruments, 404
inquiry, individualized, 355
insecurity, 410
**insight,**
  acquired, 293
  bestowal, 292
  buddhi yoga necessary, 129
  details, 310
  intellect conversion, 176
  revelation, 419
  shrouded, 131
  spiritual form, 223, 226
  spiritual vision, 209, 251, 252
  Supreme Being's, 146
instruments, 460
**intellect,**
  blankness required, 211
  capability, 468
  compliant? 94
  curbed, 479
  ever active, 151
**intellect, continued,**
  jñāna dīpa, 176
  mandatory, 217
  operation, 150
  parts, 206
  permanent, 468
  pulled backwards, 82
  reconverted, 176
  resistance described, 86, 87
  self focus, 75, 76
  senses control, 193
  senses influence, 128
  senses separated, 85
  trained, 115
  transcendental? 209
  transformed, 293
intellectual discipline, 80
intentional determination, 73
introspection, 85
invisible existence, 258, 343, 366
invisible matter, 257
irreligious actions, 243
**isolation,**
  conditions for, 416
  required, 364, 478
  sensual data reduced, 93
īśvarapraṇidhānāni, 252

# J

Janak, 117
Janaloka, 276
japa, 82
Jehovah, 248
Jesus Christ, Lord, 248
jewel, 23
jīva, 463
jñāna dīpa, 176, 179
**jñāna yoga,**
  details, 411, 451
  karma yoga supports, 140
jñānacakṣuṣā, 376, 403, 412
jñānadīpa, 157, 293
jñānī, 290
justice, 119

# K

Kacha, 191
kaivalyam, 134, 151
Kālī, 316
kalyāṇakṛt, 220
kāma, 129
kāmakāmī, 120, 122
kāmarāga, 232
kāmarūpa, 148, 193, 232, 382, 383
Kamsa, 109
kāmyānām, 452
Kapila Rishi, 300
karaṇam, 460
**karma yoga,**
  buddhi yoga, 105
  clarified, 170
  contrasted, 120
  expertise, 147
  inferior? 101
  Krishna established, 137
  limitations, 203
  requirements, 166, 285
  unconscious performance, 77
  yoga unnecessary? 173
**karma yogi,**
  buddhi yoga required, 481
  details, 451
**karma,**
  question, 247
  strand, 23
karmasannyāsa, 170
karmic package, 23
Karṇa, 191
kartā, 460
kevalam, 151
Khara, 141
Krishna Bhakti Religion, 256
Krishna consciousness, 230, 298
**Krishna,**
  Abode of universe, 321
  accountable, 119
  acyuta, 26
  appearance, 139
  best of gods, 324
  Bhagavān, 64
  denied, 278
  Everything, 329
  evolutionary force, 127
  God in Person, 26
  Govinda, 52
  Great Person, 357
  greatest of persons, 357
  indestructible supreme reality, 317

**Krishna, continued,**
interference, 31
Lord of Gods, 321
Mahāpuruṣa, 357
master of yoga, 309, 312
memory, 138
origin, 305
Oversoul, 248
Parameśvaram, 373
perceived, 91
Primeval Being, 107
reality supreme, 317
religion regulator, 249
residence, 401
responsibility ultimate, 278
spiritual existence unavailable, 91
spiritual form, 252
Supreme Lord of world, 373
standard reference, 396
Supreme Being, 331
unaffected, 26
unbiased, 239
unique, 240
unknown, 287
yoga practice, 156
Yogeśvara, 309, 312
yogi supreme, 21, 312
**kriyā yoga,**
buddhi yoga, 99, 149
critical energy, 14
details, 201
jñāna yoga, 140
mystic actions, 413
purpose, 362
stages, 151
Kṛpalvānānda, Swami, 224
Kumbhakaraṇa, 435
kundalini chakra, 134, 151, 159
**kundalini yoga,**
antarjyotih, 184
celibacy, 416, 465
life energy contol, 291
objective, 127
preliminary, 76
purpose, 362
required, 405
touch points, 201
Kurukshetra, 12
kusha grass, 199
ku-yogi, 191

# L

lack of knowledge, 419
lack of pride, 360
lamentation, unnecessary, 64
Land of Buddhas, 387
law, 317
leader, 118
leaf, 280
liability, 164
**liberation,**
conditions, 378, 379
details, 347
impulse primitive, 425
intentional, 420
self achieved, 369
souls threatened, 380
temporary? 370
**life,**
Brahmā's world, 256
God's representative, 231
**life force,**
family promoted by, 31
prāṇāyāma, 76
purification, 127
lifespan, 256
light energy, 359
light of luminaries, 367
lightning, 111
līlā, 139
limited spirits, 401
limits, 239
link, 318
living beings, 239
living space, 356
**location**
factor, 460
mantra, 201, 207
psychological, 387
supernatural type, 318
Lord of gods, 321
lord of the earth, 26
lunatic, 461
lust, 99
luxury resort, 276

# M

madbhaktim parām, 480
Madhvācāya, author, 20, 64-66
Mahabharata, 199, 257, 293, 381
mahāpuruṣa, 357
Maharaloka, 276
mahārṣi, 287, 319
mahātmanah, 488
mahātmānas, 271
mahāyogeśvarah, 312
manager, 258
maneuvers, 18
maṇi, 23
manifestation, 257
Maṇipuṣpaka, 23
manliness, 230
manogatām, 85
mantra, 199
mantra, location, 201, 207
Manu, 137
Markandeya, 258
martyalokam, 277
martyr, 43
martyrdom, 67
mass of splendor, 317
master of yoga, 309
mat samsthām, 203
Matanga Rishi, 141, 142
**material nature,**
contrary, 482
details, 379
potency, 369
tree, 398
material world, 43
matter, 247
**meditation,**
details, 200, 253, 254
mind-set, 105
revelation, 124
stages, 131
membrane, embryo, 130
**memory,**
camera, 12
causal mouth, 442
curbing process, 115
details, 390
impressions produced by, 56
imprint storage, 92
indulgences, 89
intimidating, 94
limited, 30
psychic nexus, 460
recorder, 12
torments yogi, 443
troublesome, 406
unknown initially, 89
mental dominance, 85
mental muscles, 89

mento-emotional energy, 350, 400
merit-based world, 276
merits, 411
milk, 230
**mind,**
6th device, 401
chamber order, 211
components, 213
control rigid, 217
details, 194
device, 401
energy of, 213
rim of, 96
scrapped, 13
self handled by, 21
sensual orbs, 401
struggle with, 212
mirror, 130
modes of material nature, 384, 385
modesty, 415
Mohammed, 248
mokṣa, 187
mokṣakāṅkṣibhih, 447
monkey insignia, 25
moods, 81
**moon,**
stars, 297
transmigration effect, 261
moral restraints, 132
**morality,**
limited, 415
psychological type, 181
subtle body, 360
mother, 21
motivation, 435, 444
mouth of spiritual existence, 161
movements, 460
movie stars, 276
Mr. President, 299
muktasaṅgah, 107
mulādhāra, 202
muni, 97
Murti Form, 124

# N

**naad sound,**
attention to, 28, 85
biography, 22
essential, 211
initial focus, 104
Om sound, 255
Nakula, biography, 22
Nala, 109
nama'stu te devavara, 324
Nanda, 240
Nārada, 293, 294, 295, 299, 300
narcotic, soma? 276
nāsikāgrama, 200
national power, 325
**nature,**
criminal, 38
deity, 24
nectar, poison, 472
need energy, 462
nexus, 460
nine-gate city, 177
nirahankārah, 99
nirmānamohā, 400
niryogakṣena, 77
Nityānānda, 24,64
nityasamnyāsi, 171
nityayuktah, 237
niyama, 132, 360
niyatasya karmaṇo, 455
noise, mental type, 443
non-appropriation, 77
non-violence, 67, 412, 441
nose, 200
notation, 133
note-taking, 14

# O

obeisances, 272
objectivity, 19, 97
obligation, 455
observances, 132, 360
odor, 359
Oṁ tat sat, 446
Oṁ, 255, 304, 447
opium, 438
opportunities, 451, 459
outside focus, inside, 123
over-exertion, 386
overseer, supreme, 270
Over-soul, 247, 248

# P

pacifists, 67
padam avyayam, 400
Pandavas, 25
pandit, 147
Pantañjali, 224
paradise, 70, 277
**Paramātma,**
category, 407
directive self, 197
parameśvaram, 373
Parāśar, 305
Paraśurāma, 191
partners, 401
**passion,**
defective, 384, 385
impulsion, 382
repository, 131
**Patañjali,**
131, 132, 174, 207, 210, 211, 231, 233, 252, 410, 460, 472
God described by, 102
paths of salvation, 140
patience, 361
pepper, 438
perception, 376
perfection right, 227
performer of pious acts, 220, 221
performer, 392
Personality of Godhead, 252
pious act, 389
pitri, 40
pleasure, vices, 41
poison, nectar, 472
political skill, 137
popularity, 386
Prajāpatih, 107, 240
prajñām, 96
praṇava, 255
prāṇāyāma, 133, 159
prasādam, 94, 442
pratyāhār, 148
pravṛttih marga, 439
prayatātmanah, 280
predator, 425
preference, 55
**prejudice,**
memory's, 133
sensual energy's, 133
president, 299, 325
pressures, 39

pride, 360
priest, 74
Primal Creative Cause, 379
Primal Person, 399
Primal Reality, 379
privacy, 418
Procreator Lord, 258
procurements, 362
progeny, 422
propensity, 445
props, 201
pros and cons, 49
**prostitute,**
old age, 277
heavenly world, 276
protection, 38
**providence,**
begrudged? 14
design of, 458
facilitator, 59
independent, 35
indispensible, 417
offerings rejected, 35
unpredictable, 417
upper hand, 37
**proximity,**
elevation through, 145
spirit's, 369
pṛthakceṣṭā, 460
pṛthivīpate, 23
**psyche,**
chaos, 21
component locations, 115
components, 83, 443
details, 350, 376
energy ingested, 419
flaws of, 222
operations, 463
questioned? 356
self control, 196
sorted, 466
study, 389
war within, 15
psychic geography, 261
psychological compartment, 420, 421
psychological environment, 356
psychological organs, 404
psychological strength, 252
psychological weakness, 93
pujārī, 272, 425
puṇyam loka, 276
Purāṇas, 57, 257, 435
pure devotee service, 272
**purification,**
obsession, 419
on-going, 243
required, 142
stages, 132
purifier of consciousness, 266
**purity,**
desired, 353
essential, 291, 417
external type, 441
yogi's priority, 417
puruṣa, 371
Puruṣottama, 247, 407
pūtā, 142

# R

radio frequencies, 359
rāga, 382
rain, 111
**rāja yoga,**
buddhi yoga, 99
jñāna yoga, 140
rājaguhyam, 266
rajarṣis, 136, 287
rājavidyā, 266
rajoguṇa, 129
**Rāma,Śrī**
ideal karma yogi, 140, 141
Over-soul? 248
war of, 25
Rāmāyaṇa, 25, 133, 141, 199, 240
rash undertaking, 386
Rāvaṇa, 25, 141, 435
**reaction,**
arbitrary? 36
back log, 79
psychological, 154
Reality, 304, 317
**rebirth,**
animal to human, 446
circular, 266
consciousness, 388
eliminated? 370
enlightened type, 256
instinct prominent, 250
Krishna's association, 141
rules of, 141
yogi's, 220, 221
recitation of scripture, 411
recognition of reality, 413
recycling, 63
regulative principles, 415
**reincarnation,**
circular, 266
consciousness affects, 388
details, 40, 54-55, 391
rejection, 451
relationships, 253
release, 448
reliance on God, 399
religion, 230, 426
**religious ceremony,**
effectiveness, 110
recommended, 439
regulator, 248, 249
religious leaders, 278
religious principles, 415
**renunciation,**
details, 477
development, 191
psychological, 177, 190
repentance, 422
research, 367
resentments, 14
resort, 276
**responsibility,**
hedge, 40
induced, 362
ultimate type, 278
rest in peace, 469
restlessness, 386
restraint, 126
result-expectant course, 102
**revelation**
achieved, 419
insufficient, 355
methods, 247
requirements, 332, 335
required, 124
varied, 273
righteous duty, 69
righteousness, 139
rights of living beings, 239
root chakra, 202
ruler, 300
rūpam, 252

# S

sacrifice, 439
sacrificial offering, 273
sadhu saṅga, 163

Sahadeva, 23
**salvation,**
details, 448
God promotes, 140
requirements, 346
**samādhi,**
fuss over, 214
required, 254
residual effect, 154
Samkhya, yoga, 172
samnyāsi, 190
samphātaś, 359
samsāra, 266
samsiddhim, 117
samyama, 157, 254
samyamī, 97-99, 120
Sanjaya, 12, 489
sannyāsa, 452
Sanskrit, 276, 426
santah, 110
śāntih, 414
Sarasvatī, 24
Śāśaṅka, 329
sat guru, 94
Sat Puruṣa, 162
Sat, 448
satisfaction, 98, 198
Satyaloka, 276
Satyavati, 305
savior, 424
science, 41
scriptural injunctions, 432
scripture, 411
security, 414
self focus, 113
**self realization,**
course, 408
details, 133
essential, 270
stages, 133,134
self, intellect's stooge? 129
self-conquest, 419
self-evaluation, 388
self-focus, 366
self-restraint, 411, 443
self-situated, 77
sense objects, subtle, 362
sense of identity, factor, 99, 460
sense of ownership, 248
**senses,**
conquest, 194
elongated, 156
grows out, 194
non-cooperative, 82
resistant, 94
restraint, 97
shrinkage, 156
spiritual type, 123
surface of mind, 96
**sensual energy,**
components, 115
directive, 193
dominant, 402
intellect separated, 85
purification, 127
sensuality, 91
**separation,**
core self's, 134
emotional distress, 210
servant, described, 35
service to devotee, 272
sex chakra, 202
sexual function, 422
sexual intercourse, 40, 363
Shabari, 141, 142
shakti, 213
shaktipat, 246
Shakuni, 323
Shankaracharya, Śrīpad, 379
ship, 96
Shiva, 248, 333, 416, 449
Shuka, 480
Shukracharya, 191
siddha saṅghāh, 327
siddha, 378
siddhaloka, 276
silence, 305, 443
Sītā, 25
sixth detection device, 401
smell sense, 231
smoke, 129
smṛti, 53
snake, 104
social values, 415
soma drinkers, 276
soul-situated, 77
sound, 359, 478
**species,**
body type, 55
explained, 214
power supply, 180
speech, 442, 479
speed, subtle, 133
**spirit self,**
bewildered, 401
categories, 214
commodity? 459
congregates, 433
deathless, 60
degradation, 373, 429
down-sourced? 62
exhausted? 62
finite, 369
grades, 214
influenced, 401
insecurity of, 410
liberation, 369
material nature fusion, 268
minute, 463
numerous, 367
observer, 96
psyche directs, 194
senses dominate, 402
senses non-cooperation, 82
spiritual light, 215
susceptible, 407
transformation, 380
wonderful, 65
spiritual eye, 157
spiritual form, 252, 333
spiritual vision, 28
**spiritual master,**
disciple, 165
substitutes for, 282, 416, 417
spiritual perceptions, 223, 226
spiritual security, 414
spiritual senses, 123
spiritual vision, 91, 215, 251, 252,
śraddhayā parayā, 444
śrīmatām, 221
static electricity, 111
stooge, 129
straightforwardness, 412, 441
stress, 214
strong-mindedness, 417
student-teacher relation, 165
study of psyche, 132, 365

**subtle body,**
alterations, 62
anatomy, 156
bed-rock, 360
components, 227
curbed, 363
deathless? 60
enjoyment facilities, 402
explained, 356
influences upon, 381
objectivity lacking, 392
resistant, 336
rest of, 469
transmigration, 261
**subtle organs,**
organized, 291
speed of, 133
subtle perception, 357
success, 79
śucīnām, 221
sudurācāro, 284
Sughoṣa, 22
Sugriva, 140
sum total gross reality, 247
**sun,**
God's representative, 231
influential, 143
sungod, 136
transmigration effect, 261
Supermost Personality, 247
supernatural formations, 312
supernatural plane, 247, 310, 324
supernatural rulers, 110
supernatural world, 313
Supersoul, 297
**Supreme Being,**
immunity, 375
limitations, 178
non-involved, 178
non-relational, 178
powers, 269
providence observer, 38
responsibilities, 119
service to, 477
singled out, 139
Supreme Divine Person, 253
Supreme Lord of world, 373
Supreme overseer, 270
Supreme Person, 407
supreme secret, 486
Supreme Soul, 247
--- see also Supreme Being
Supreme Spirit, 180
--- see also Supreme Being
Supreme Supernatural Person / Power, 247
**supreme will,**
buffered? 79
pious acts, 389
pressures, 322
surasaṅghā, 319
Surendra, 276
surface, 359
surrender, 125, 281
suśumnā nāḍi, 127
suśumnā, 253
sūtram, 161, 228, 379
sva, 248
svabhāva, 432, 482
svacakṣuṣā, 311
svādhiṣṭhānam 202
Svarga world, 47, 70, 277
synthesis, 372

# T

tamo dvāraih, 429
Tapoloka, 276
taste, child's, 230
tattvavit, 122
teacher, substitutes for, 416, 417
technical insight, 73
techniques, 112, 113
tejah, 333
temple worship, 272
temptations, 88
**tendency,**
impressions produce, 56
rebirth, 258
texture of consciousness, 250
theft, imprints, 92
theft,
senses, 12
universal, 459
theism, 474
thinking/thought
details, 148
location, 207
thousand-armed Person, 333
Tibetan Book of the Dead, 387
Tibetan yoga, 387
**time,**
drama of, 43
respected, 302, 303
ruinous, 25
tortoise, 87
transcendental form, 294
**transmigration,**
attachments, 249, 250
causeless? 60
details, 40, 54-55
discussed, 112
land of Buddhas, 387
lower species, 214
prejudices, 13
providence controls, 37
psychology intact, 402
subtle body, 261
transposition, 63
tree, 398
trends, 118
tyāgis, 480

# U

Uddhava, 480
ultimate source, 366, 367
unconsciousness, 390
unimaginable form, 252
**Universal Form,**
attractive, 323
cooperation required, 475
details, 311
entrusting to Him, 125
functional basis, 120
insufficient, 355
male beings, 316
mass of splendor, 317
pious acts, 389
power of, 313
threatening, 320, 321
viewers, 320
unmanifest selves, 241
Upanishads, 57, 133, 240, 246
up-grade existence, 378
upside-down tree, 398
ūrdhva reta, 418
utility of time, 34

# V


vaiśvānara, 405
vāk mayam tapa, 442
Vālmīki, 133, 141, 199
vanasprastha, 117
vanity, 419
Varuṇa, 240, 329
Vasiṣṭha, 435
Vasudeva, 304, 375
Vāsudeva, 304
Vāyu, 240, 329
Vedanta, 406
Vedic gods, 240
Vedic ritual, 273
Vedic study, 337
vegetation, 63, 388
vexation, 419
vigor, 416
**violence,**
  explained, 361
  God's, 361
  supernatural? 361
vipaścitah, 91
Vishnu, 248, 312
vision of reality, 403
vision, 109, 209, 215
visualization organ, 22, 206
Viśvāmitra, 435
Viśvamūrte, 333
vitamin, 412
Vivasvat, 136, 137
vows, insufficient, 272
vows, listed, 158
Vṛndāvan, 273
vṛtti, 76, 207
vulture, 429
Vyāsa, 293, 294, 295, 305


# W


waiver, 452, 457
war, 15
wasp, 425
water, 230, 280
weapons, 17
White Yajur Veda, 432
wicked person, 283
**will power,**
  neutralized, 90
  sensuality defeats, 91
wind, 96, 267
womb, 179
women, 363
worship, 292, 411
worship of Krishna, 276, 290
worship of others, 239


# Y


Yahweh, 248
yajña, defined, 159
Yajñavalka, 246, 432
yama, 132, 360
Yatra, 207
yearning, 12
**yoga practice,**
  application, 167
  bhakti highest, 349
  complete, 136
  details, 254
  discovery, 155
  distress remover, 204
  individual, 201
  learning required, 406
  license, 190
  mentioned frequently, 281
  misuse, 48
  moderation, 204
  motive, 435
  props, 201
  psyche purification, 138
  rebirth recall, 138
  resting, 204
  Samkhya contrasted, 172
  stages, 191
  superfluous? 371
  Tibetan, 387
  types, 102
  uncertainties, 213
yoga siddha body, 262
yogabalena, 252
yogabhraṣṭah, 220, 221
yogadhāraṇām, 254
yogamāya, 174
yogāruḍhah, 192
yogasamsiddha, 164
yogeśvara, 309
yogi kings, 136
**yogi**
  bypassing heaven, 276
  chit akasha penetration, 139
  death reviewed, 263
  devotee type, 343, 344
  dispensable, 28
  dried out, 210
  duty, 417
  endeavor required, 224, 362
  fallen type, 220, 221
  flawed practice, 210
  grace of God, 224
  heavenly life, 392
  humility required, 449
  indifference, 457
  Krishna devoted, 203
  mind entry by others, 21
  motivation, 190, 191
  struggle, 93
  parents, 221
  problem internal, 461
  providence sensitive, 35
  return to society, 176
  revelation, 336
  satisfaction, 198
  son of Shiva, 416, 418
  transmigration, 263
  types, 136
  unsuccessful type, 219
yogini, 416, 418
Yudhiṣṭhira, , 22, 42
yukta, defined, 90

## LIST OF TEACHERS

**Gaudiya Vaishnava teacher:**
*Śrīla* Bhaktivedanta Swami Prabhupada
***Haṭha* yoga teacher:**
Swami Vishnudevananda
**Kundalini yoga teacher:**
*Mahāyogī Śrī* Harbhajan Singh
**Celibacy yoga teachers:**
Swami Shivananda,
*Śrīla* Yogiraj Yogeshwarananda
**Purity-of-the-psyche yoga teacher:**
*Śrīla* Yogiraj Yogeshwarananda
***Kriyā* yoga teachers:**
*Śrīla Bābāji Mahāśaya*,
Siddha Swami Muktananda
**Brahma yoga teacher:**
Siddha Swami *Nityānānda*

# About the Author

*Michael Beloved (Yogi Madhvāchārya) took his current body in 1951 in Guyana. In 1965, while living in Trinidad, he instinctively began doing yoga postures and trying to make sense of the supernatural side of life.*

*Later on, in 1970, in the Philippines, he approached a Martial Arts Master named Mr. Arthur Beverford, explaining to the teacher that he was seeking a yoga instructor. Mr. Beverford identified himself as an advanced disciple of Rishi Singh Gherwal, an astanga yoga master.*

*Mr. Beverford taught the traditional Aṣṭanga Yoga with stress on postures, attentive breathing and brow chakra centering meditation. In 1972, Madhvāchārya entered the Denver Colorado Ashram of Kundalini Yoga Master Śrī Harbhajan Singh. There he took instruction in Bhastrika Prāṇāyāma and its application to yoga postures. He was supervised mostly by Yogi Bhajan's disciple named Prem Kaur.*

*In 1979 Madhvāchārya formally entered the disciplic succession of the Brahmā-Madhava Gaudiya Sampradaya through Swami Kirtanananda, who was a prominent sannyāsi disciple of the Great Vaishnava Authority Śrī Swami Bhaktivedanta Prabhupada, the exponent of devotion to Sri Krishna.*

*After carefully studying and practicing the devotional process introduced by Śrī Swami Bhaktivedanta Prabhupada, Madhvāchārya was inspired to do a translation of the Bhagavad Gītā, which is published with commentary, under the title of Bhagavad Gītā Explained. The same translation without commentary is published as Bhagavad Gītā English. And the same with Sanskrit text and word-for-word meanings, is published as Bhagavad Gītā Revealed. He published a second commentary for Kriyā yogins, under the title of Kriyā Yoga Bhagavad Gītā.*

*This publication, his third commentary, is for brahma yogins. It was dictated to him by Mahāsiddha Swami Nityānānda, who no longer uses a gross body and whose contact he experienced through clairvoyance and clairaudience. Regarding those who carefully study the Gītā and those who hear it with confidence, Śrī Krishna said this:*

> ***I would be loved by the devotee who by sacrifice of his knowledge, will study this sacred conversation of ours. This is My opinion. (18.70)***
>
> ***Even the person who hears with confidence, without ridiculing is freed. He should attain the happy worlds where persons of pious actions reside. (18.71)***

*Śrī Gopāl Krishna*

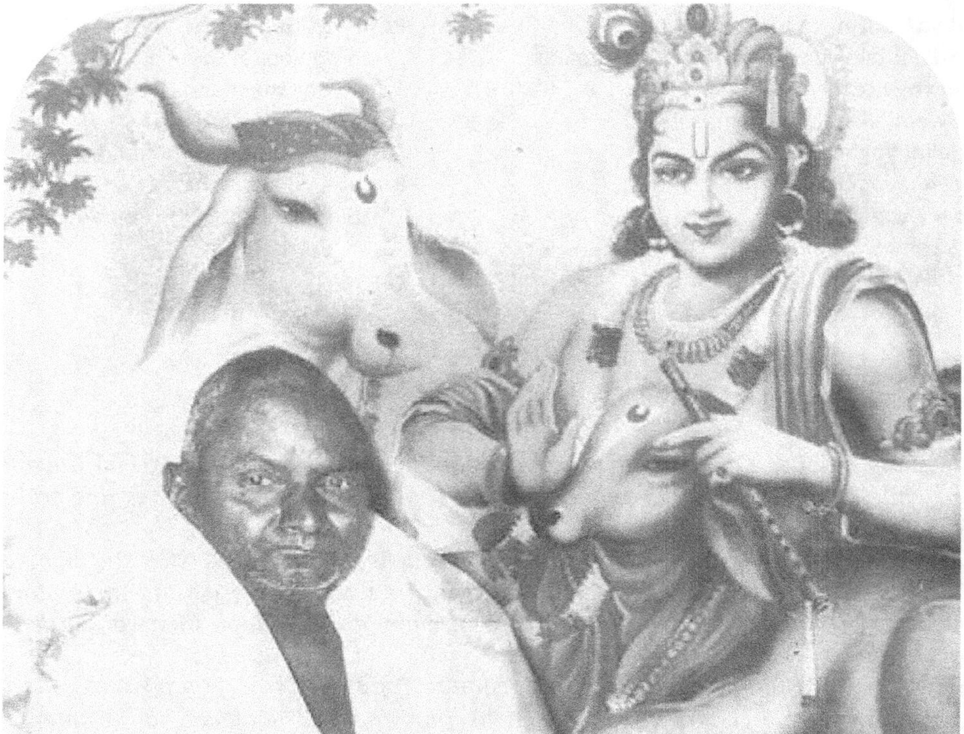

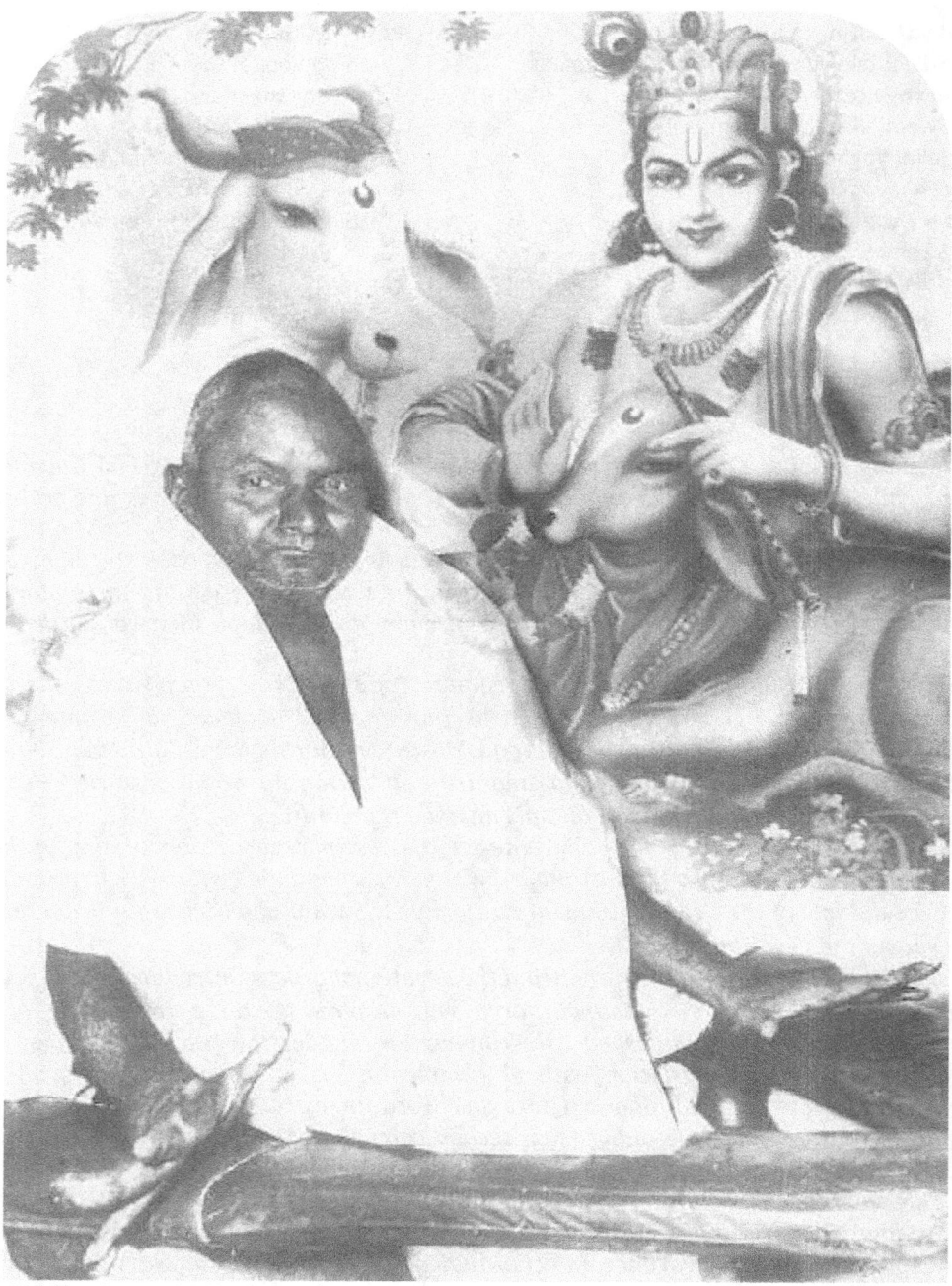

*Siddha Swami Nityānānda*

# Publications

## English Series

Bhagavad Gita English

Anu Gita English

Markandeya Samasya English

Yoga Sutras English

Uddhava Gita English

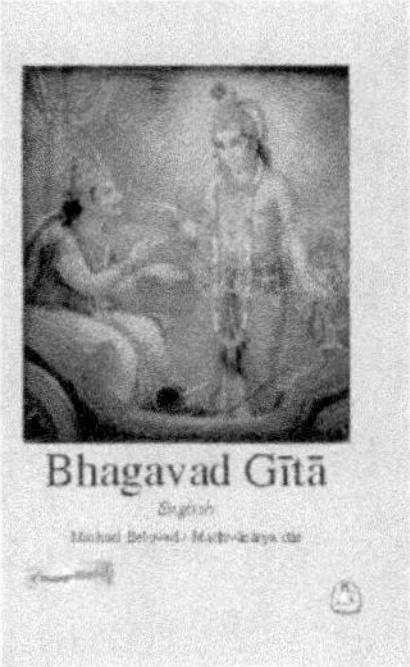


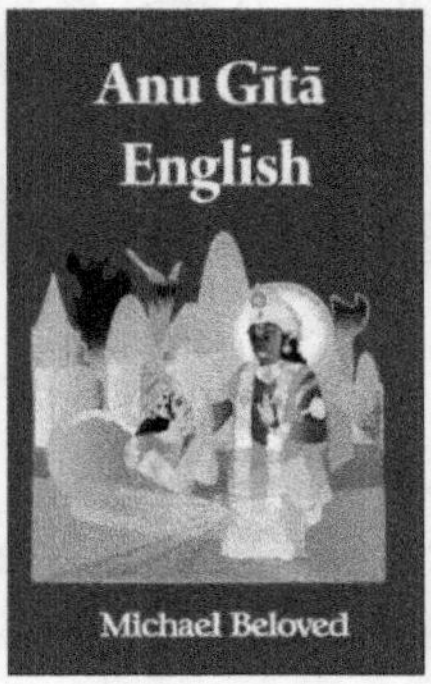


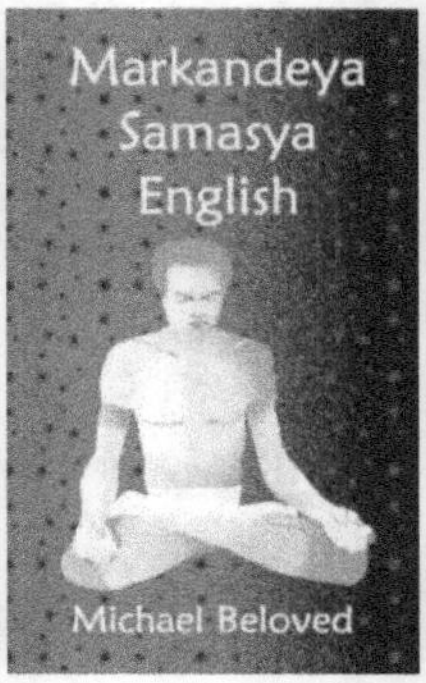


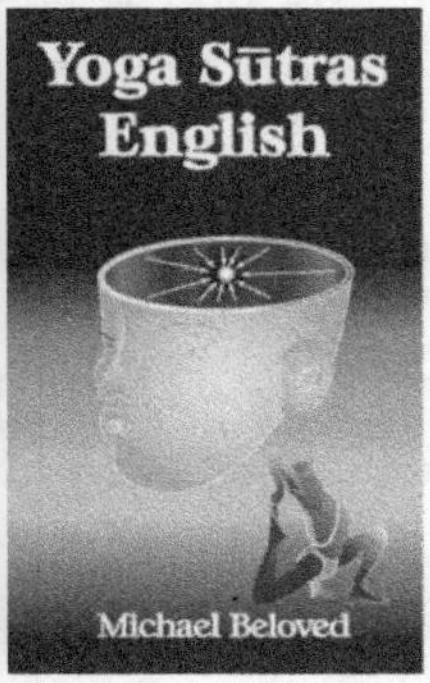


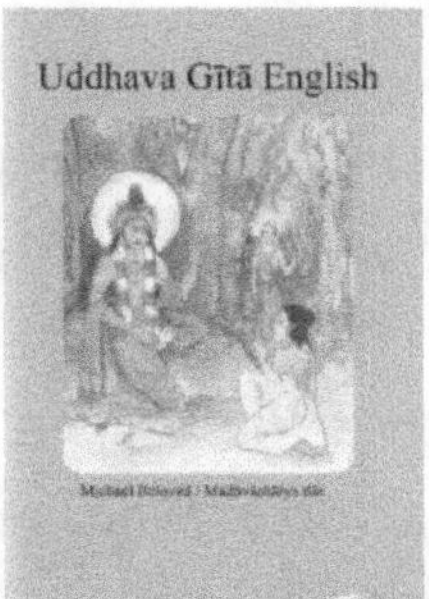


These are in 21st Century English, very precise and exacting. Many Sanskrit words which were considered untranslatable into a Western language are rendered in precise, expressive and modern English, due to the English language becoming the world's universal means of concept conveyance.

Three of these books are instructions from Krishna. **In Bhagavad Gita English** and **Anu Gita English**, the instructions were for Arjuna. In the **Uddhava Gita English,** it was for Uddhava. Bhagavad Gita and Anu Gita are extracted from the Mahabharata. Uddhava Gita was extracted from the 11th Canto of the Srimad Bhagavatam (Bhagavata Purana). One of these books, the **Markandeya Samasya English** is about Krishna, as described by Yogi Markandeya, who survived the cosmic collapse and reached a divine child in whose transcendental body, the collapsed world was existing. Another of these books, the **Yoga Sutras English,** is the detailed syllabus about yoga practice.

My suggestion is that you read **Bhagavad Gita English**, the **Anu Gita English, the Markandeya Samasya English,** the **Yoga Sutras English** and lastly the **Uddhava Gita English**, which is much more complicated and detailed.

For each of these books we have at least one commentary, which is published separately. Thus your particular interest can be researched further in the commentaries.

The smallest of these commentaries and perhaps the simplest is the one for the Anu Gita. We published its commentary as the Anu Gita Explained. The Bhagavad Gita explanations were published in three distinct targeted commentaries. The first is Bhagavad Gita Explained, which sheds lights on how people in the time of Krishna and Arjuna regarded the information and applied it. Bhagavad Gita is an exposition of the application of yoga practice to cultural activities, which is known in the Sanskrit language as karma yoga.

Interestingly, Bhagavad Gita was spoken on a battlefield just before one of the greatest battles in the ancient world. A warrior, Arjuna, lost his wits and had no idea that he could apply his training in yoga to political dealings. Krishna, his charioteer, lectured on the spur of the moment to give Arjuna the skill of using yoga proficiency in cultural dealings including how to deal with corrupt officials on a battlefield.

The second commentary is the Kriya Yoga Bhagavad Gita. This clears the air about Krishna's information on the science of kriya yoga, showing that its techniques are clearly described free of charge to anyone who takes the time to read Bhagavad Gita. Kriya yoga concerns the battlefield which is the psyche of the living being. The internal war and the mental and emotional forces which are hostile to self-realization are dealt with in the kriya yoga practice.

The third commentary is the Brahma Yoga Bhagavad Gita. This shows what Krishna had to say outright and what he hinted about which concerns the brahma yoga practice, a mystic process for those who mastered kriya yoga.

There is one commentary for the **Markandeya Samasya English**. The title of that publication is Krishna Cosmic Body.

There are two commentaries to the Yoga Sutras. One is the Yoga Sutras of Patanjali and the other is the Meditation Expertise. These give detailed explanations of the process of Yoga.

For the Uddhava Gita, we published the Uddhava Gita Explained. This is a large book and requires concentration and study for integration of the information. Of the books which deal with transcendental topics, my opinion is that the discourse between Krishna and Uddhava has the complete information about the realities in existence. This book is the one which removes massive existential ignorance.

## Meditation Series

Meditation Pictorial

Meditation Expertise

Core-Self Discovery

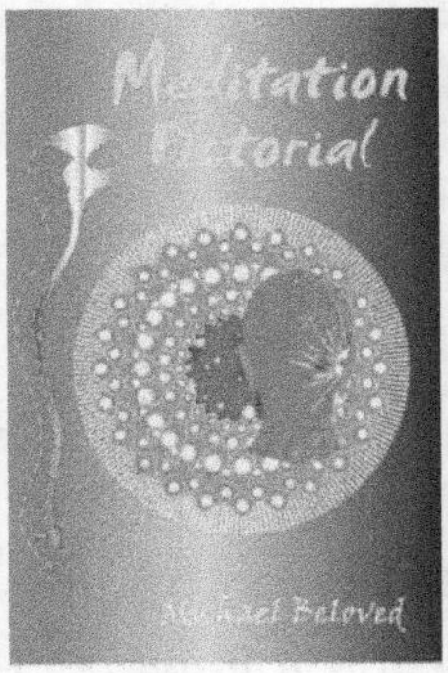

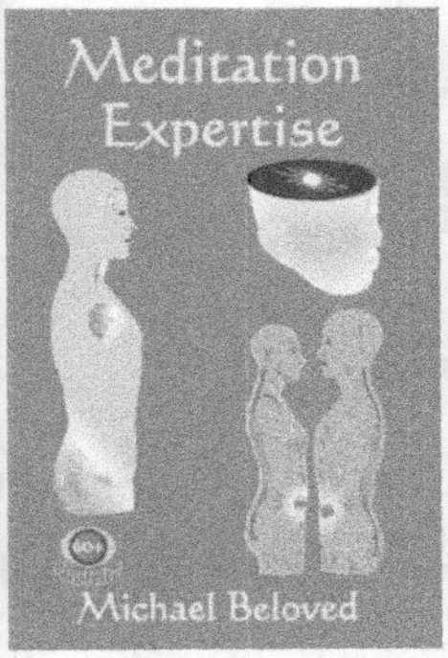

The specialty of these books is the mind diagrams which profusely illustrate what is written. This shows exactly what one has to do mentally to develop and then sustain a meditation practice.

In the **Meditation Pictorial**, one is shown how to develop psychic insight, a feature without which meditation is imagination and visualization, without any mystic experience per se.

In the **Meditation Experti**se, one is shown how to corral one's practice to bring it in line with the classic syllabus of yoga which Patanjali lays out as the ashtanga yoga eight-staged practice.

In **Core-Self Discovery**, one is taken though the course of pratyahar sensual energy withdrawal which is the 5th stage of yoga in the Patanjali ashtanga eight-process complete system of yoga practice. These events lead to the discovery of a core-self which is surrounded by psychic organs in the head of the subtle body. This product has a DVD component for teachers and self-teaching students.

These books are profusely illustrated with mind diagrams showing the components of psychic consciousness and the inner design of the subtle body.

## Explained Series

Bhagavad Gita Explained

Uddhava Gita Explained

Anu Gita Explained

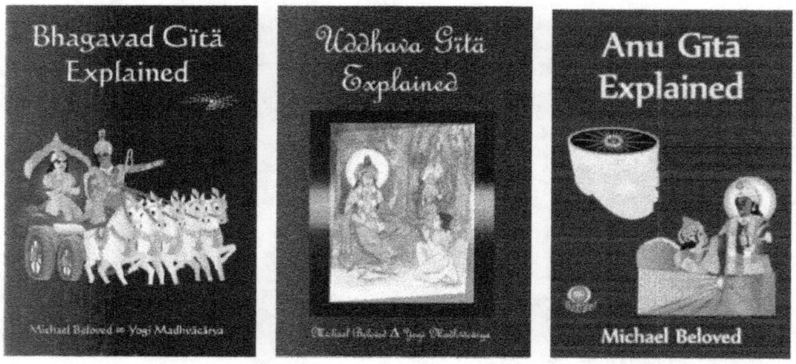


The specialty of these books is that they are free of missionary intentions, cult tactics and philosophical distortion. Instead of using these books to add credence to a philosophy, meditation process, belief or plea for followers, I spread the information out so that a reader can look through this literature and freely take or leave anything as desired.

When Krishna stressed himself as God, I stated that. When Krishna laid no claims for supremacy, I showed that. The reader is left to form an independent opinion about the validity of the information and the credibility of Krishna.

There is a difference in the discourse with Arjuna in the Bhagavad Gita and the one with Uddhava in the Uddhava Gita. In fact these two books may appear to contradict each other. In the Bhagavad Gita, Krishna pressured Arjuna to complete social duties. In the Uddhava Gita, Krishna insisted that Uddhava should abandon the same.

The Anu Gita is not as popular as the Bhagavad Gita but it is the conclusion of that text. Anu means what is to follow, what proceeds. In this discourse, an anxious Arjuna request that Krishna should repeat the Bhagavad Gita and again show His supernatural and divine forms.

However Krishna refuses to do so and chastises Arjuna for being a disappointment in forgetting what was revealed. Krishna then cites a celestial yogi, a near-perfected being, who explained the process of transmigration in vivid detail.

## Commentaries

Yoga Sutras of Patanjali

Meditation Expertise

Krishna Cosmic Body

Anu Gita Explained

Bhagavad Gita Explained

Kriya Yoga Bhagavad Gita

Brahma Yoga Bhagavad Gita

Uddhava Gita Explained

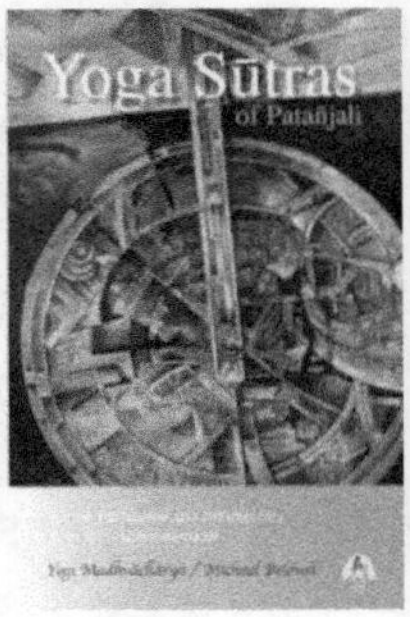

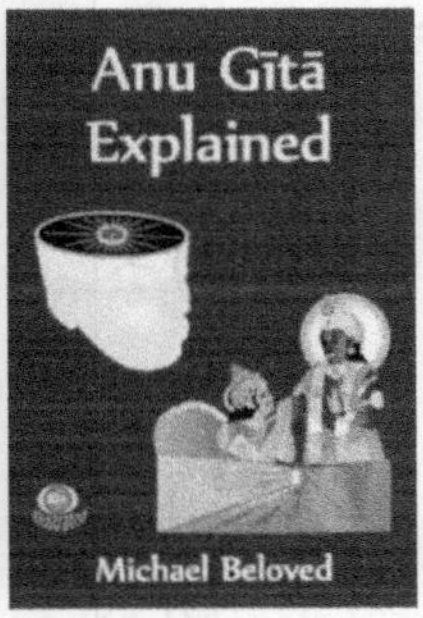

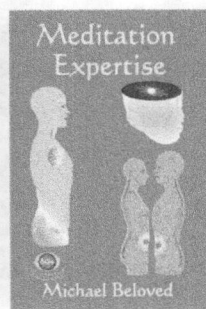

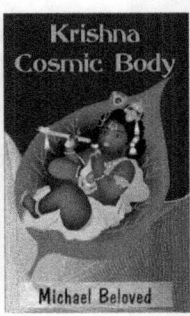

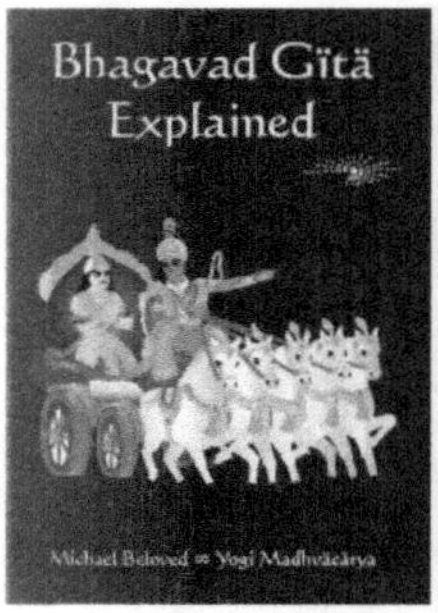


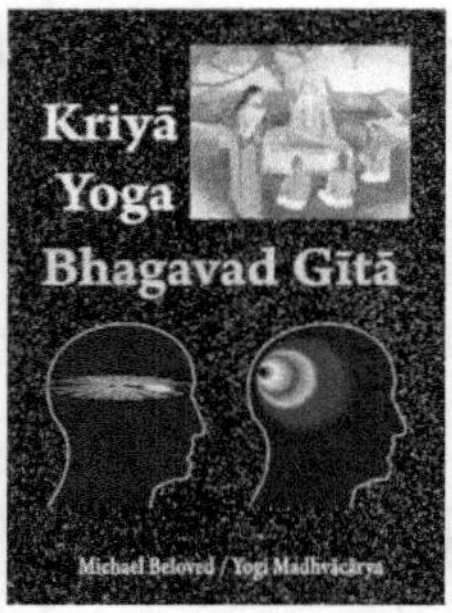


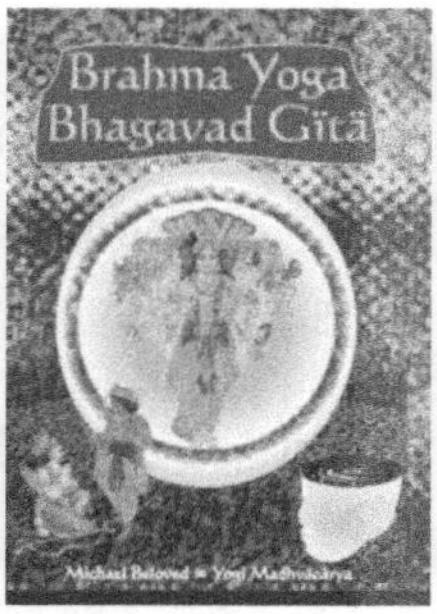


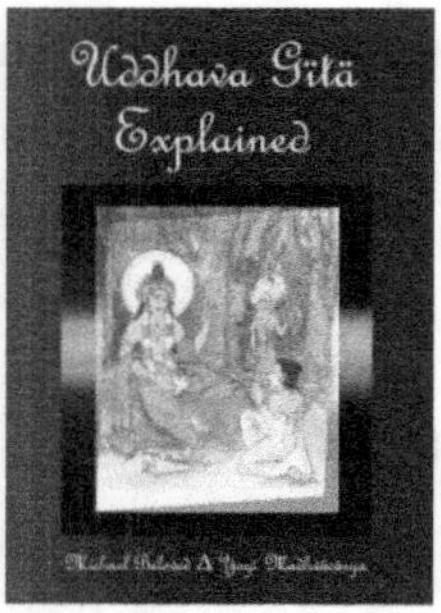


**Yoga Sutras of Patanjali** is the globally acclaimed text book of yoga. This has detailed expositions of yoga techniques. Many kriya techniques are vividly described in the commentary.

**Meditation Expertise** is an analysis and application of the Yoga Sutras. This book is loaded with illustrations and has detailed explanations of secretive advanced meditation techniques which are called kriyas in the Sanskrit language.

**Krishna Cosmic Body** is a narrative commentary on the Markandeya Samasya portion of the Aranyaka Parva of the Mahabharata. This is the detailed description of the dissolution of the world, as experienced by the great yogin Markandeya who transcended the cosmic deity, Brahma, and reached Brahma's source who is the divine infant, Krishna.

**Anu Gita Explained** is a detailed explanation of how we endure many material bodies in the course of transmigrating through various life-forms. This is a discourse between Krishna and Arjuna. Arjuna requested of Krishna a display of the Universal Form and a repeat narration of the Bhagavad Gita but Krishna declined and explained what a siddha perfected being told the Yadu family about the sequence of existences one endures and the systematic flow of those lives at the convenience of material nature.

**Bhagavad Gita Explained** shows what was said in the Gita without religious overtones and sectarian biases.

**Kriya Yoga Bhagavad Gita** shows the instructions for those who are doing kriya yoga.

**Brahma Yoga Bhagavad Gita** shows the instructions for those who are doing brahma yoga.

**Uddhava Gita Explained** shows the instructions to Uddhava which are more advanced than the ones given to Arjuna.

Bhagavad Gita is an instruction for applying the expertise of yoga in the cultural field. This is why the process taught to Arjuna is called karma yoga which means karma + yoga or cultural activities done with a yogic demeanor.

Uddhava Gita is an instruction for apply the expertise of yoga to attaining spiritual status. This is why it is explains jnana yoga and bhakti yoga in detail. Jnana yoga is using mystic skill for knowing the spiritual part of existence. Bhakti yoga is for developing affectionate relationships with divine beings.

Karma yoga is for negotiating the social concerns in the material world and therefore it is inferior to bhakti yoga which concerns negotiating the social concerns in the spiritual world.

This world has a social environment and the spiritual world has one too.

Right now Uddhava Gita is the most advanced informative spiritual book on the planet. There is nothing anywhere which is superior to it or which goes into so much detail as it. It verified that historically Krishna is the most advanced human being to ever have left literary instructions on this planet. Even Patanjali Yoga Sutras which I translated and gave an application for in my book, **Meditation Expertise**, does not go as far as the Uddhava Gita.

Some of the information of these two books is identical but while the Yoga Sutras are concerned with the personal spiritual emancipation (kaivalyam) of the individual spirits, the Uddhava Gita explains that and also explains the situations in the spiritual universes.

Bhagavad Gita is from the Mahabharata which is the history of the Pandavas. Arjuna, the student of the Gita, is one of the Pandavas brothers. He was in a social hassle and did not know how to apply yoga expertise to solve it. Krishna gave him a crash-course on the battlefield about that.

Uddhava Gita is from the Srimad Bhagavatam (Bhagavata Purana), which is a history of the incarnations of Krishna. Uddhava was a relative of Krishna. He was concerned about the situation of the deaths of many of his relatives but Krishna diverted Uddhava's attention to the practice of yoga for the purpose of successfully migrating to the spiritual environment.

# Specialty

These books are based on the author's experiences in meditation, yoga practice and participation in spiritual groups:

Spiritual Master

sex you!

Sleep **Paralysis**

Astral Projection

Masturbation Psychic Details

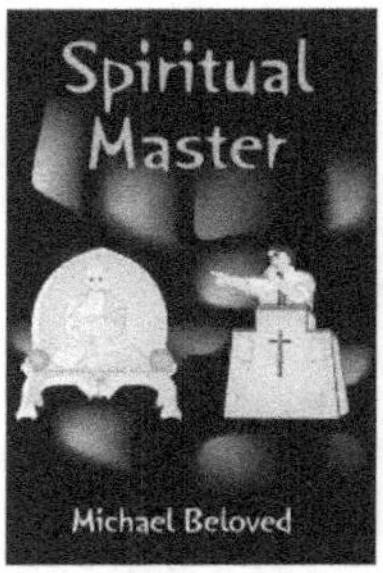

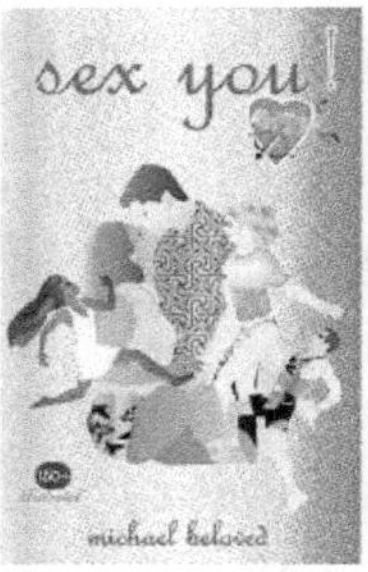

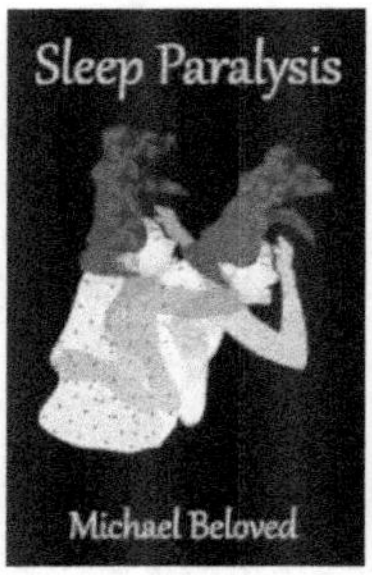

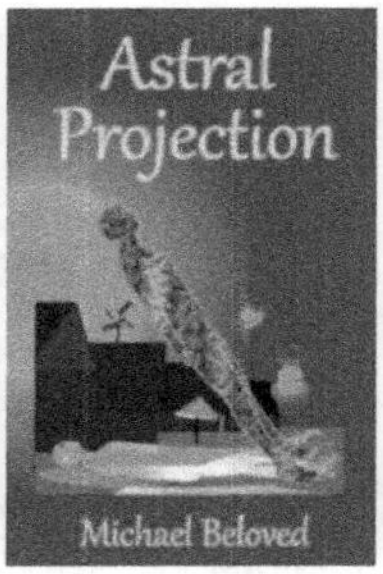

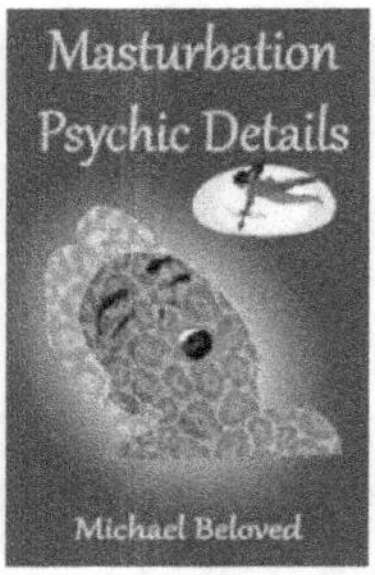


In **Spiritual Master**, Michael draws from experience with gurus or with their senior students. His contact with astral gurus is rated. He walks you through the avenue of gurus showing what you should do and what you should not do, so as to gain proficiency in whatever area of spirituality the guru has proficiency.

**sex you!** is a masterpiece about the adventures of an individual spirit's passage through the parents' psyches. The conversion of a departed soul into a sexual urge is described. The transit from the afterlife to residency in the emotions of the parents is detailed. This is about sex and you; learn about how much of you comprises the romantic energy of your would-be parents!

**Sleep Paralysis** clears misconceptions so that one can see what sleep paralysis is and what frightening astral experience occurs while the paralysis is being experienced. This disempowerment has great value in giving you confidence that you can and do exist even if you are unable to operate the physical body. The implication is that one can exist apart from and will survive the loss of the material body.

**Astral Projection** details experiences Michael had even in childhood, where he assumed incorrectly that everyone was astrally conversant. He discusses the life force psychic mechanism which operates the sleep-wake cycle of the physical form, and which budgets energy into the separated astral form which determines if the individual will have dream recall or no objective awareness during the projections. Astral travel happens on every occasion when the physical body sleeps. What is missing in awareness is the observer status while the astral body is separated.

**Masturbation Psychic Details** is a surprise presentation which relates what happens on the psychic plane during a masturbation event. This does not tackle moral issues or even addictions but shows the involvement of memory and the sure but hidden subconscious mind which operates many features of the psyche irrespective of the desire or approval of the self-conscious personality.

# Online Resources

**Visit The Website And Forum**

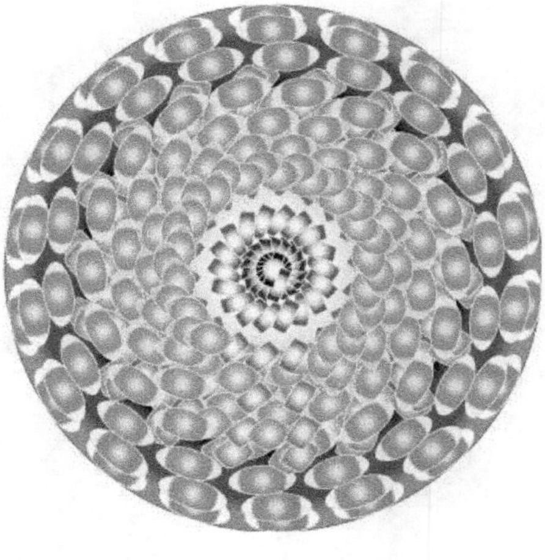


| | |
|---|---|
| ***Email:*** | michaelbelovedbooks@gmail.com<br>axisnexus@gmail.com |
| ***Website*** | michaelbeloved.com |
| ***Forum:*** | inselfyoga.com |

www.ingramcontent.com/pod-product-compliance
Lightning Source LLC
Chambersburg PA
CBHW082141230426
43672CB00016B/2928
*9780979391651*